Gynecologic and Obstetric Pathology

HIGH-YIELD PATHOLOGY

Christopher P. Crum, MD
Professor of Pathology, Harvard Medical School
Vice Chair and Director, Women's and Perinatal
   Pathology
Department of Pathology
Brigham and Women's Hospital
Boston, Massachusetts

Anna R. Laury, MD
Department of Pathology & Laboratory Medicine
Cedars-Sinai Medical Center
Los Angeles, California

Michelle S. Hirsch, MD, PhD
Associate Professor of Pathology
Brigham and Women's Hospital
Department of Pathology
Division of Women's and Perinatal Pathology
Boston, Massachusetts

Charles Matthew Quick, MD
Assistant Professor of Pathology
Director of Gynecologic Pathology
University of Arkansas for Medical Sciences
Little Rock, Arkansas

William A. Peters III, MD
Clinical Professor of Obstetrics & Gynecology,
   University of Washington
Swedish Medical Center
Seattle, Washington

SAUNDERS

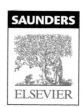

ELSEVIER

ELSEVIER

1600 John F. Kennedy Blvd.
Ste 1800
Philadelphia, PA 19103-2899

GYNECOLOGIC AND OBSTETRIC PATHOLOGY:
HIGH-YIELD PATHOLOGY

ISBN: 978-1-4377-1422-7

International Standard Book Number: 978-1-4377-1422-7

Content Strategist: William R. Schmitt
Senior Content Development Specialist: Jennifer Ehlers
Publishing Services Manager: Catherine Jackson
Design Direction: Paula Catalano

Printed in China.

Last digit is the print number: 9   8   7   6   5   4   3   2   1

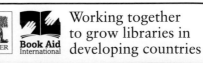

CONTRIBUTORS

Odise Cenaj, MD, PhD
Resident in Pathology
Department of Pathology
Brigham and Women's Hospital
Boston, Massachusetts

Brooke E. Howitt, MD
Instructor in Pathology
Department of Pathology
Brigham and Women's Hospital
Boston, Massachusetts

Emily E.K. Meserve, MD, MPH
Fellow in Women's and Perinatal Pathology
Department of Pathology
Brigham and Women's Hospital
Boston, Massachusetts

Jelena Mirkovic, MD, PhD
Fellow in Women's and Perinatal Pathology
Department of Pathology
Brigham and Women's Hospital
Boston, Massachusetts

Bradley J. Quade, MD, PhD
Associate Professor of Pathology
Department of Pathology
Division of Women's and Perinatal Pathology
Brigham and Women's Hospital
Boston, Massachusetts

Kathleen Sirois, BA
Pathology Specialist
Women's and Perinatal Pathology
Brigham and Women's Hospital
Boston, Massachusetts

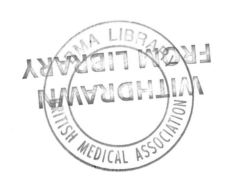

PREFACE

Consultations, whether intradepartmental or extradepartmental, are a vital component of patient care and are designed to come as close as possible to the theoretical ideal of an error-free practice. This book is intended to touch on both routine and potentially problematic areas of diagnosis; hence, the "pitfalls" designation for many of the chapters and the appendix, which summarizes many of the problems we have encountered in our experience. No summary can possibly cover all of the potential traps awaiting the practitioner, but the following guidelines (the seven Cs are offered based on our own experience) are intended to reduce errors in interpretation. They are as follows:

1. When examining a case as consultants, are we paying attention to the submitter's *concerns*? This is an aspect that can be quite variable and requires careful review of the submitted records. In particular, the letter from the person requesting the consultation must be read carefully to ascertain not only the history but also the reasons for the consultation request. In many cases the reason for the consultation may not be clearly stated but implied in the preliminary diagnosis. It is imperative that the concerns of the submitter be ascertained.

2. Is the suspected entity *cryptic* as in rare or unusual? In most cases the entity under review or the question being asked is a common one. Is this an endometrial intraepithelial neoplasia/atypical hyperplasia or a benign proliferation? Is it differentiated VIN or lichen simplex chronicus; atypical leiomyoma or STUMP? Such cases *usually* do not have a hidden pitfall. For others, the process or the question is not readily apparent, that is, the features on the slide do not conjure up an instant differential.

3. Are we getting *consultation* from other colleagues or experts, including nongynecologic pathologists? Every pathologist knows that discussion with other pathologists is particularly helpful with unusual, or rarely encountered, problematic lesions. When obtaining consultation, the pathologist must consider three things. First, they obviously must make sure that the pathologists are experienced; second, they must make sure that the pathologists are fully attentive to the case; and third they must make certain that the opinion of their consultant(s) is reasonable. Ultimately, the pathologist seeking consultation must formulate the diagnosis, and this goes for not just the original pathologist but also the "expert" who is being asked to review the case. The value of additional consultation from the literature cannot be overestimated, notwithstanding the limitations in illustration. A "perfect match" between the slide and an image in the literature should be viewed with caution!

4. Are we about to *contradict* the diagnosis of the submitter? Pathologists are by nature independent in their assessments, a natural and necessary aspect of maintaining objectivity. That being said, the submitting pathologist has often gone to considerable effort to understand and describe the difficulties of a particular case. In a nonreferral routine practice, problematic cases are less common and thus receive careful scrutiny. The consultant is well advised to carefully consider the impressions of the submitter and be certain when he or she contradicts their diagnosis. In our experience the submitter is correct in the large proportion of cases.

5. Are we exercising *caution* in our interpretation? One of the biggest threats to a correct diagnosis is overconfidence and a "snap diagnosis" because it short-circuits the slower but more orderly process of weighing the differential diagnoses, obtaining confirmatory opinions, and making the soundest judgment possible.

6. Is a *creative* diagnosis being considered, that is, one that is not in the books? Most of the diagnoses rendered pertain to common questions as discussed earlier. When a consultant encounters something that is particularly unusual, there may be the temptation to apply a diagnosis that is nonstandard. The risk is that the consultant is missing an unusual presentation of something more common. Creative diagnoses should always be made with care, especially if the diagnosis implies a specific line of therapy.

7. Have we reviewed the mundane but critical clerical component? Always verify that the slides sent belong to the patient whom they should represent. Similarly, always make sure that the abnormality belongs to the patient by excluding laboratory contaminants (floaters).

Much of the above information is intuitive to most pathologists, but it is intended to reinforce the great value of taking an organized approach to pathologic diagnosis, whether one is the initial reviewer or consultant. This book will address as many of the potential problems as possible. There will certainly be more, and we welcome input from the readers as we hope to include them in a subsequent edition.

Christopher P. Crum, MD

CONTENTS

SECTION I.   LOWER ANOGENITAL TRACT

A. Inflammatory Disorders

Eczematous Dermatitis, 3

Lichen Simplex Chronicus and Prurigo Nodularis, 5

Psoriasis, 7

Seborrheic Dermatitis, 9

Lichen Sclerosus Including Early Lichen Sclerosus, 11

Lichen Planus, 14

Zoon's Vulvitis, 16

Bullous Pemphigoid, 18

Pemphigus Vulgaris, 20

Hailey-Hailey Disease, 22

Darier's Disease, 24

Epidermolytic Hyperkeratosis, 26

Hidradenitis Suppurativa, 28

Crohn's Disease of the Vulva, 30

Vulvodynia, 32

B. Vulvar Infections

Vulvovaginal Candidiasis, 34

Bacterial Vaginosis, 36

Molluscum Contagiosum, 38

Acute Herpes Simplex Virus Infection, 40

Chronic Erosive Herpes Simplex **PITFALL**, 42

Syphilis **PITFALL**, 44

Chancroid, 46

Granuloma Inguinale, 48

Schistosomiasis, 50

Bacillary Angiomatosis, 52

Necrotizing Fasciitis, 54

Varicella Zoster, 55

C. Vulvar Adnexal Lesions

Bartholin's Duct Cyst, 57

Mucous Cyst of the Vagina, 59

Ectopic Breast Tissue, 61

Fibroadenoma, 63

Hidradenoma **PITFALL**, 65

Syringoma, 68

Hyperplasia of Bartholin's Gland, 70

Bartholin's Adenoma, 72

Adenoid Cystic Carcinoma, 74

Bartholin's Gland Carcinoma, 76

D. Vulvar Epithelial Neoplasia

Condyloma, 79

Verruciform Xanthoma, 82

Warty Dyskeratoma, 84

Fibroepithelial Stromal Polyp, 86

Seborrheic Keratosis, 88

Pseudobowenoid Papulosis **PITFALL**, 90

Flat Condyloma (VIN1), 92

Classic (Usual) Vulvar Intraepithelial Neoplasia, 94

Classic Vulvar Intraepithelial Neoplasia with Lichen Simplex Chronicus **PITFALL**, 98

Classic Vulvar Intraepithelial Neoplasia (Bowenoid Dysplasia), 100

Pagetoid Vulvar Intraepithelial Neoplasia **PITFALL**, 102

Vulvar Intraepithelial Neoplasia with Columnar Differentiation **PITFALL**, 104

Epidermodysplasia Verruciformis–Like Atypia **PITFALL**, 106

Polynucleated Atypia of the Vulva, 108

Differentiated Vulvar Intraepithelial Neoplasia, 110

Verruciform Lichen Simplex Chronicus, 114

Vulvar Acanthosis with Altered Differentiation (Atypical Verruciform Hyperplasia), 116

Early Invasive Squamous Cell Carcinoma, 118

Vulvar Squamous Carcinoma: Basaloid and Warty Patterns, 122

Vulvar Squamous Carcinoma: Keratinizing Pattern, 124

Verrucous Squamous Cell Carcinoma, 128

High-Grade Squamous Intraepithelial Lesion (Vulvar Intraepithelial Neoplasia III) with Confluent Papillary Growth, 131

Giant Condyloma of the External Genitalia **PITFALL**, 134

Pseudoepitheliomatous Hyperplasia **PITFALL**, 137

Keratoacanthoma **PITFALL**, 139

Basal Cell Carcinoma, 141

Adenosquamous Carcinoma, 144

Paget's Disease of the Vulva, 146

Merkel Cell Carcinoma, 149

Cloacogenic Neoplasia, 151

Metastatic Carcinoma of the Vulva, 153

E. Pigmented Lesions

Lentigo, 155

Genital-Type Nevus, 157

Dysplastic Nevus, 159

Melanoma, 161

F. Soft Tissue Vulvar Neoplasia

Angiomyofibroblastoma, 163

Aggressive Angiomyxoma **PITFALL**, 165

Superficial Angiomyxoma, 166

Cellular Angiofibroma, 168

Dermatofibroma (Fibrous Histiocytoma), 170

Dermatofibrosarcoma Protuberans, 172

Low-Grade Fibromyxoid Sarcoma, 174

Lipoma, 176

Liposarcoma, 177

Synovial Sarcoma of the Vulva **PITFALL**, 179

Rhabdomyoma, 181

Angiokeratoma, 183

Granular Cell Tumor, 185

Prepubertal Vulvar Fibroma, 187

G. Anus

Anal Condyloma, 190

Anal Intraepithelial Neoplasia II and III, 193

Anal Carcinoma, 195

Anal Paget's Disease, 197

H. Vagina

Prolapsed Fallopian Tube, 200

Granulation Tissue, 202

Vaginal Adenosis, 204

Polypoid Endometriosis, 206

Vaginal Papillomatosis (Residual Hymenal Ring) **PITFALL**, 208

Low-Grade Vaginal Intraepithelial Lesion (Vaginal Intraepithelial Neoplasia I and Condyloma), 210

High-Grade Vaginal Intraepithelial Lesion (Vaginal Intraepithelial Neoplasia II-III), 212

High-Grade Vaginal Intraepithelial Neoplasia III, 215

Radiation-Induced Atrophy, 217

Papillary Squamous Carcinoma, 219

Clear-Cell Adenocarcinoma, 221

Metastatic Adenocarcinoma, 223

Melanoma **PITFALL**, 226

Spindle Cell Epithelioma **PITFALL**, 228

Embryonal Rhabdomyosarcoma, 230

SECTION II. CERVIX

A. Squamous Lesions

Exophytic Low-Grade Squamous Intraepithelial Lesion, 235

Low-Grade Squamous Intraepithelial Lesion (Flat Condyloma/Cervical Intraepithelial Neoplasia I), 237

High-Grade Squamous Intraepithelial Lesion (Cervical Intraepithelial Neoplasia II and III), 240

Low-Grade Squamous Intraepithelial Lesion (Giant Condyloma) **PITFALL**, 243

Low-Grade Squamous Intraepithelial Lesion (Immature Condyloma), 245

Mixed-Pattern Squamous Intraepithelial Lesion (Low- and High-Grade Squamous Intraepithelial Lesions), 247

Atrophy Including Squamous Intraepithelial Lesion in Atrophy, 249

Minor p16-Positive Metaplastic Atypias, 252

Squamous Intraepithelial Lesion, Not Amenable to Precise Grading (QSIL), 255

Superficially Invasive Squamous Cell Carcinoma, 259

Conventional Squamous Cell Carcinoma, 262

Pseudocrypt Involvement by Squamous Cell Carcinoma, 266

Lymphoepithelial-Like Squamous Carcinoma, 268

B. Glandular Lesions

Superficial (Early) Adenocarcinoma In Situ, 270

Conventional Adenocarcinoma In Situ, 273

Stratified Adenocarcinoma In Situ, 276

Intestinal Variant of Adenocarcinoma In Situ, 278
> *Brooke E. Howitt*

Cervical Endometriosis, 280

Pregnancy-Related Changes in the Cervix, 282

Reactive Atypias in the Endocervix, 284

Radiation Atypias, 286

Villoglandular Adenocarcinoma of the Cervix, 288

Superficially Invasive Endocervical Adenocarcinoma, 290

Extensive Adenocarcinoma In Situ vs Invasion, 292

Infiltrative Endocervical Adenocarcinoma, 295

Clear-Cell Carcinoma of the Cervix, 298

Atypical Lobular Endocervical Glandular Hyperplasia and Invasive (Minimal Deviation) Adenocarcinoma of the Cervix with Gastric Differentiation, 300

"Serous" Carcinoma of the Cervix, 302

Signet-Ring Cell Carcinoma of the Cervix, 305

Adenoid Basal Carcinoma, 308

Mesonephric Remnants, 310

Mesonephric Carcinoma, 312

Prostatic Metaplasia of the Cervix, 315

Endocervical Glandular Hyperplasia, 317

Metastatic Serous Carcinoma to the Cervix, 319

Metastatic Endometrioid Carcinoma to the Cervix, 321

Atypical Endocervical Polyp, 324
> *Brooke E. Howitt*

Adenomyoma of the Cervix, 326

Microglandular Hyperplasia of the Cervix, 328

Adenosarcoma of the Cervix, 331
> *Brooke E. Howitt*

C. Miscellaneous Lesions

Cervical Schwannoma, 333

Glial Polyp of the Cervix, 335

SECTION III. UTERUS

A. Benign Endometrium

Dysfunctional Uterine Bleeding (Early or Mid-Cycle Breakdown), 339

Breakdown Mimicking Neoplasia, 341

Anovulatory Endometrium with Persistent Follicle, 343

Benign Endometrial Hyperplasia, 345

Telescoping Artifacts Mimicking Neoplasia, 347

Mixed-Pattern Endometrium, 349

Adenomyomatous Polyp, 351

Chronic Endometritis, 353

Pseudoactinomycotic Radiate Granules, 355

Pyometra, 357

Tubercular Endometritis, 359

Submucosal Leiomyoma, 361

Exfoliation Artifact, 364

Perforation, 366

Ablation Artifact, 368

B. Endometrial Glandular Neoplasia and Its Mimics

Endometrial Intraepithelial Neoplasia (Atypical Hyperplasia), 370

Atypical Polypoid Adenomyoma, 374

Endometrial Involvement by Endocervical Glandular Neoplasia, 376

Degenerative Repair, 378

Proliferative Repair, 380

Mucinous Metaplasia of the Endometrium, 382

Squamous and Morular Metaplasia, 384

Ichthyosis Uteri, 387

Squamous Carcinoma of the Endometrium, 389

Tubal and Eosinophilic (Oxyphilic) Metaplasia, 391

Microglandular Endometrial Adenocarcinoma in Curettings, 393

Endometrioid Adenocarcinoma, 396

Lower Uterine Segment Adenocarcinoma, 400

Lynch Syndrome Screening, 403
  Brooke E. Howitt

Myoinvasion in Endometrial Adenocarcinoma, 406

Intraperitoneal Keratin Granuloma, 410

Endometrial Histiocytes and Foamy Stromal Macrophages, 412

Serous Cancer Precursors, 414

Serous Endometrial Intraepithelial Carcinoma, 417

Ischemic Atypias of the Endometrium, 419

Reactive Atypia in the Endometrium, 421

Uterine Serous Carcinoma, 423

Mixed-Pattern Adenocarcinoma, 426

p53-Positive Endometrioid Adenocarcinoma, 428

Neuroendocrine Differentiation in Endometrial Carcinoma, 430

Undifferentiated Carcinoma of the Endometrium, 432

Clear-Cell Carcinoma, 434

Endometrioid or Clear-Cell Carcinoma? 437

Carcinosarcoma, 440

Adenocarcinoma with Spindle Cell Features, 445

Wilms' Tumor of the Endometrium, 447

C. Mesenchymal Lesions of the Uterus

Endometrial Stromal Nodule, 449

Stromomyoma, 451

Endometrial Stromatosis, 453

Low-Grade Endometrial Stromal Sarcoma, 455

Uterine Tumor Resembling Sex Cord Stromal Tumor, 459

High-Grade Endometrial Stromal Sarcoma, 461

Undifferentiated Uterine Sarcoma, 464

Adenosarcoma of the Endometrium, 466
  Brooke E. Howitt

Atypical Endometrial Polyp, 469
  Brooke E. Howitt

Adenomatoid Tumor, 472

Lipoleiomyoma, 475

Cellular Leiomyoma, 477

Hydropic Leiomyoma, 479

Mitotically Active Leiomyoma, 481

Atypical Leiomyoma (Leiomyoma with Bizarre Nuclei), 483

Leiomyomatosis, 485

Intravenous Leiomyoma, 487
  Bradley J. Quade

Intravenous Leiomyomatosis, 489
  Bradley J. Quade

Morcellation-Related Dissemination of Smooth Muscle Neoplasia, 491
  Bradley J. Quade

Disseminated Peritoneal Leiomyomatosis, 493
  Bradley J. Quade

Pathology Following Uterine Artery Embolization, 495
  Bradley J. Quade

Hereditary Leiomyomatosis and Renal Cell Carcinoma Syndrome **PITFALL**, 497

Leiomyosarcoma, 499

Myxoid Leiomyosarcoma, 501

Epithelioid Leiomyosarcoma, 503

PEComa, 505

Reproductive Tract Lymphoma, 507
Emily E.K. Meserve

SECTION IV. FALLOPIAN TUBE

A. Benign, Inflammatory/Reactive

Adrenal Rest, 511

Pseudoxanthomatous Salpingiosis, 513

Xanthogranulomatous Salpingitis, 515

Follicular Salpingitis, 517

Salpingitis Isthmica Nodosum, 519

Granulomatous Salpingitis, 520

Torsion of the Tube and Ovary, 522

Tubal Arias-Stella Effect **PITFALL**, 524

B. Neoplastic and Preneoplastic

Adenofibroma, 527

Benign Epithelial Hyperplasia (Secretory Cell Outgrowths), 529

p53 Signatures, 532

Low-Grade Serous Tubal Intraepithelial Neoplasia (Serous Tubal Intraepithelial Lesion), 535

Papillary Hyperplasia, 539

High-Grade Serous Tubal Intraepithelial Neoplasia (Serous Tubal Intraepithelial Carcinoma), 541

The Risk Reducing Salpingo-Oophorectomy, 545

Salpingoliths, 547

Adenocarcinoma of the Fallopian Tube, 549

Endosalpingeal Implants from Remote Tumors, 552

Female Adnexal Tumor of Wolffian Origin, 554

SECTION V. OVARY

A. Benign

Tangentially Sectioned Ovarian Follicle **PITFALL**, 559

The Ovary in Pregnancy, 561

Solitary Luteinized Follicle Cyst, 564

Polycystic Ovarian Syndrome, 566
Emily E.K. Meserve

Cortical Stromal Hyperplasia and Hyperthecosis, 569

Endometrioma with Mucinous Metaplasia, 571

Endometrioma with Atypia, 573

Decidualized Endometrioma **PITFALL**, 575

Serous Cystadenomas and Cystadenofibromas, 577

Cortical Inclusion Cysts, 580

Endosalpingiosis, 582

Malakoplakia, 584

B. Epithelial Neoplasia

High-Grade Serous Carcinoma, Classic Type, 586
Brooke E. Howitt

High-Grade Serous Carcinoma with "SET" Patterns, 588
Brooke E. Howitt

Low-Grade Endometrioid Adenocarcinoma with Squamotransitional or Spindle Features, 590

Carcinosarcoma, 592

Adenosarcoma of the Ovary, 594

Serous Borderline Tumor (SBT), 597

Serous Borderline Tumor with Complex Architecture, 600

Low-Grade Invasive Serous Carcinoma of the Ovary, 602

Invasive Implants of Low-Grade Serous Tumor, 605

Mucinous Carcinoma, 607

Mucinous Tumors with Mural Nodules, 610

Mucinous Borderline Tumor, 613

Mucinous Borderline Tumor with Intraepithelial Carcinoma, 615

Low-Grade Endometrioid Adenocarcinoma, 617

Endometrioid Adenofibroma, 620

Proliferative (Borderline) Endometrioid Adenofibroma, 622

Müllerian Mucinous and Seromucinous Tumors of the Ovary, 625

Benign Brenner Tumor, 629

Malignant Brenner Tumor, 631

Clear-Cell Carcinoma, 633

Ovarian Adenocarcinoma with Yolk Sac Differentiation **PITFALL**, 636

Brooke E. Howitt

Borderline Clear-Cell Adenofibroma, 638

Metastatic Carcinoma to the Ovary, 640

Pseudomyxoma Peritonei, 644

C. Germ Cell Tumors

Mature Cystic Teratoma: Normal Neural Differentiation, 646

Fetiform Teratoma, 648

Odise Cenaj and Jelena Mirkovic

Struma Ovarii, 650

Malignant Struma, 653

Strumal Carcinoid, 656

Metastatic Carcinoid, 659

Malignancy Arising in Teratomas, 662

Dysgerminoma, 664

Yolk Sac Tumor, 667

Embryonal Carcinoma, 670

Immature Teratoma, 672

Mixed Germ Cell Tumor, 675

D. Sex Cord Stromal Tumors

Thecoma-Fibroma, 677

Fibroma with Minor Sex Cord Elements, 680

Sclerosing Peritonitis, 682

Granulosa Cell Tumor, 684

Granulosa Cell Tumor Variants **PITFALL**, 687

Juvenile Granulosa Cell Tumor **PITFALL**, 690

Sertoli-Leydig Cell Tumor, 693

Retiform Sertoli-Leydig Cell Tumor **PITFALL**, 696

Leydig Cell (Hilar) Tumor, 698

Stromal Luteoma, 701

Pregnancy Luteoma, 703

Sclerosing Stromal Tumor, 705

Small Cell Carcinoma of Hypercalcemic Type, 707

Small Cell Carcinoma of Pulmonary (Neuroendocrine) Type, 709

Sex Cord Tumor with Annular Tubules, 711

E. Miscellaneous Tumors

Solitary Fibrous Tumor, 713

Gastrointestinal Stromal Tumor, 715

Primitive Neuroectodermal Tumor, 717

Desmoplastic Small Round Cell Tumor, 719

Benign Cystic Mesothelioma, 721

Papillary Mesothelioma, 723

Papillary Mesothelial Hyperplasia, 725

Malignant Mesothelioma, 727

SECTION VI. GESTATIONAL

A. Early Gestation

Gestational Sac, 731

Fresh Implantation Site **PITFALL**, 733

Implantation Site Nodule, 735

Spontaneous Abortion, 737

Ectopic Pregnancy, 739

B. Trophoblastic Neoplasia

Complete Hydatidiform Mole **PITFALL**, 741

Invasive Hydatidiform Mole, 745

Partial Hydatidiform Mole, 748

Mesenchymal Dysplasia **PITFALL**, 750

Choriocarcinoma, 752

Intraplacental Choriocarcinoma **PITFALL**, 754

Placental Site Trophoblastic Tumor **PITFALL**, 757

Molar Implantation Site, 759

Epithelioid Trophoblastic Tumor, 761

Chorangioma, 764

C. Second and Third Trimester Placenta

Knots in the Umbilical Cord, 766

Single Umbilical Artery (SUA), 768

Hypercoiled and Hypocoiled Umbilical Cord, 769
Kathleen Sirois

Variations on Cord Insertion (Marginal, Membranous, Furcate), 770
Kathleen Sirois

Circummarginate and Circumvallate Placentas, 772
Kathleen Sirois

Fetal Vascular Thrombosis **PITFALL**, 774

Amniotic Bands, 776

Maternal Floor Infarct/Massive Perivillous Fibrin Deposition, 778

Chorioamnionitis, 780

Gestational *Candida* Infection, 783

Listeria Placentitis **PITFALL**, 785

Chronic Villitis, 787

Chronic Histiocytic Intervillositis, 789

Congenital Syphilis, 791

Lysosomal Storage Disorder, 793

Inflammatory Abruption, 795

Hypertensive Bleeding (Ball-in-Socket) Infarct, 798

Congenital Parvovirus Infection, 800

Fetal Leukemia, 802

Placenta Creta, 804

Placenta Previa, 807

Toxoplasmosis, 808

Toxemia, 810

Placental Infarction, 812

Meconium Staining, 814

Distal Villous Pathology, 816

Fetal to Maternal Hemorrhage, 818

Appendix: Common Pitfalls in Diagnostic Gynecologic and Obstetric Pathology, 821

Lower Anogenital Tract

ECZEMATOUS DERMATITIS

DEFINITION—A constellation of inflammatory conditions caused by a reaction to exogenous or endogenous factors. Including, but not limited to, exogenous dermatitis, irritant contact dermatitis, allergic contact dermatitis, atopic dermatitis, and nummular dermatitis.

CLINICAL FEATURES

EPIDEMIOLOGY

- Seen in all demographic groups.

PRESENTATION

- Clinically, the disorders follow a progression starting with erythema, pruritus, and discomfort, followed by vesicle and bulla formation.
- A superficial yellow crust can form after vesicle rupture.

PROGNOSIS AND TREATMENT

- Prognosis—excellent, responds well to treatment.
- Treatment—avoidance of irritants, hygiene, and steroid ointments.

PATHOLOGY

HISTOLOGY

- Epidermal spongiosis is the defining feature.
- Three phases can be seen histologically: acute, subacute, and chronic.

- In the acute phase a mixed inflammatory infiltrate can be seen in the epidermis and papillary dermis. Spongiosis can progress to vesicle and bulla formation. Necrotic keratinocytes can be seen.
- The subacute phase is marked by acanthosis (frequently psoriasiform) and variable hyperkeratosis and hypergranulosis.
- In the chronic phase the degree of spongiosis decreases; however, the acanthosis, hyperkeratosis, and hypergranulosis become more pronounced.
- Not uncommonly, these lesions can progress to resemble lichen simplex chronicus.

IMMUNOPATHOLOGY (INCLUDING IMMUNOHISTOCHEMISTRY)

- Noncontributory.

MAIN DIFFERENTIAL DIAGNOSIS

- Fungal infection.

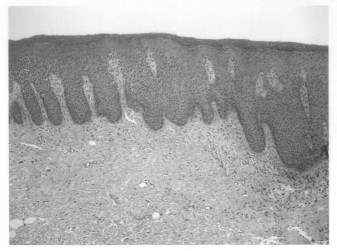

FIGURE 1

Eczematous dermatitis. Acanthosis, hypergranulosis, and hyperkeratosis are present. Note the superficial inflammatory infiltrate in the right aspect of the photo.

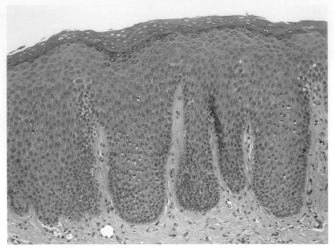

FIGURE 2

Eczematous dermatitis. Acanthosis, hypergranulosis, and spongiosis are present.

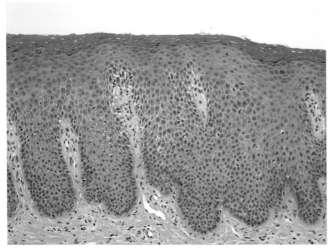

FIGURE 3

Eczematous dermatitis. Marked spongiosis is present in the central aspect, as well as parakeratosis and hyperkeratosis, which are associated with mechanical irritation.

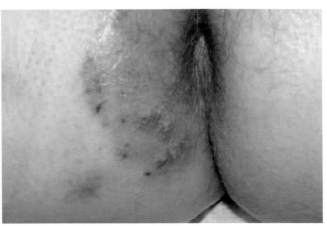

FIGURE 4

Eczematous dermatitis presenting as a pruritic reddened scaly rash in the perianal area. *(Photo courtesy Hope Haefner, MD.)*

LICHEN SIMPLEX CHRONICUS AND PRURIGO NODULARIS

DEFINITION—A cutaneous reaction related to scratching, often superimposed on other dermatoses.

CLINICAL FEATURES

EPIDEMIOLOGY

- Lichen simplex chronicus (LSC) is not a distinctive disease but a clinical and pathologic response to repeated physical trauma such as rubbing or scratching.
- Often superimposed on eczematous dermatitis.
- Also seen in patients who habitually scratch.
- In the absence of other pathology, it is termed neurodermatitis.
- More commonly seen at perimenopause and postmenopause, but can present at any age.
- Associations have been made with both classic and differentiated vulvar intraepithelial neoplasia (VIN) and certain human leukocyte antigen (HLA) haplotypes.

PRESENTATION

- Chronic pruritus, often accentuated at night.
- LSC presents as thickened skin that has erythema and scaling that is plaquelike, often with overlying excoriation.
- Physiologic skin markings are exaggerated, and visual excoriations are present (Fig. 4). Hyperpigmentation may also be seen.
- Associations have been made with VIN and certain HLA haplotypes.

PROGNOSIS AND TREATMENT

- Prognosis is good with attention to alleviating the symptoms (topical steroids) and interrupting the itch–scratch cycle.
- Recognition and treatment of the underlying cause when present (fungal infection, tinea cruris, chronic eczematous dermatitis, and psoriasis).

PATHOLOGY

HISTOLOGY

- The epidermis shows hyperkeratosis and hypergranulosis.
- Superimposed excoriation and scale crust may be present with vigorous scratching.
- Typically, the rete ridges are elongated.
- Sparse mononuclear infiltrates in the dermis and neutrophils in the epidermis in some cases.

IMMUNOHISTOCHEMISTRY

- Usually noncontributory. In cases with superimposed lichen sclerosus or epithelial atypia, stains for p16ink4 (which will be positive—strong linear staining) and p53 (strong continuous staining of basal cells) may help to rule out a human papillomavirus (HPV)–associated classic VIN or differentiated VIN, respectively.

MAIN DIFFERENTIAL DIAGNOSIS (OR UNDERLYING CONDITIONS)

- Eczematous dermatitis—prominent spongiosis will be seen.
- Yeast infections—clusters of neutrophils in the keratin layer, excluded with fungal stains.
- Psoriasis—uniform "test-tube" rete and microabscesses in the apical keratin layer.
- Classic or differentiated VIN—atypia will be present in the basal one-third of the epithelium.

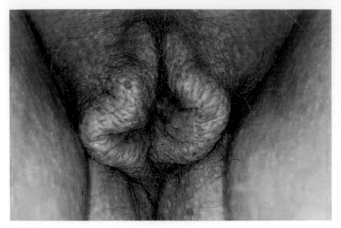

FIGURE 1

LSC. Note the marked symmetrical epithelial thickening due to chronic scratching. *(Photo courtesy Hope Haefner, MD.)*

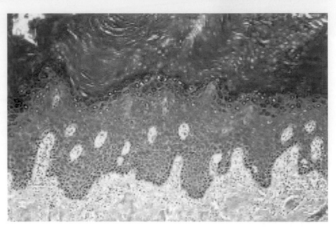

FIGURE 2

LSC. There are prominent acanthosis, hypergranulosis, and hyperkeratosis with a mild dermal mononuclear infiltrate.

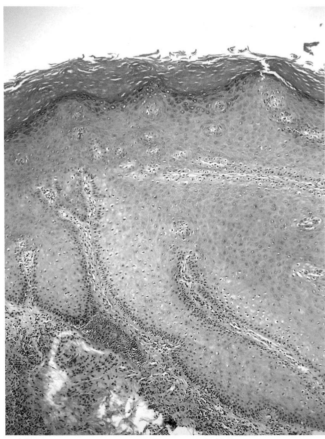

FIGURE 3

LSC. This field shows mild verruciform change.

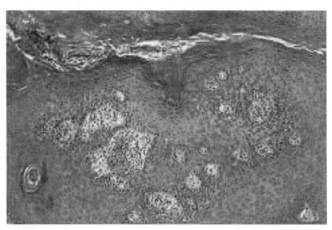

FIGURE 4

Candida infection with superimposed LSC. When suspected, the sections should be evaluated with fungal stains to exclude this treatable cause.

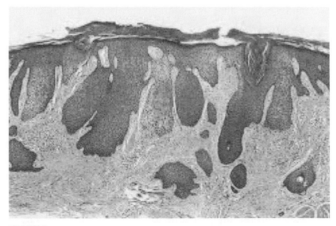

FIGURE 5

LSC. There is prominent epithelial hyperplasia. This pattern overlaps with that of prurigo nodularis, a chronic highly pruritic condition of multiple etiologies characterized by multiple cutaneous nodules and also associated with a severe itch–scratch cycle.

PSORIASIS

DEFINITION—A chronic, hyperproliferative, papulosquamous disorder with a relapsing course.

CLINICAL FEATURES

EPIDEMIOLOGY

- Affects 1% to 2% of Caucasians.
- Onset is usually in the late 20s.
- A genetic component is likely, as first-degree relatives are also often affected.
- At least one third of the female patients have vulvar involvement, although isolated vulvar involvement is uncommon.

PRESENTATION

- In general, classical (plaque-type) psoriasis is characterized by symmetrically distributed erythematous plaques covered with a silver scale.
- These plaques can be reflected, which results in pinpoint bleeding (Auspitz sign).
- Plaque-type psoriasis is the most common form of psoriasis to affect the vulva, but the lesions are shiny because they lack the silvery scale.
- Guttate psoriasis occurs in young patients, including children, and arises after infection with β-hemolytic streptococcus.
- Guttate psoriasis presents as crops of small subcentimeter erythematous papules without a scale.
- Guttate psoriasis may herald the onset of plaque-type disease.
- Pustular psoriasis displays plaques and superimposed pustules, and is also notable for its prominent systemic symptoms (i.e., fever).
- The development of psoriatic lesions is associated with the Koebner's phenomenon, when the lesions arise at the site of prior trauma.

PROGNOSIS AND TREATMENT

- Prognosis—variable, as this is a chronic disease with a protracted clinical course.
- Debilitating psoriatic arthritis may develop after years of skin disease.
- Treatment—topical or systemic steroids, topical antiproliferative agents, methotrexate, cyclosporine, and other immunomodulatory drugs.

PATHOLOGY

HISTOLOGY

- Epidermal acanthosis with regular elongation and fusion of the rete ridges, also known as psoriasiform hyperplasia, is characteristic.
- Psoriasiform hyperplasia has a "test-tube" appearance due to the regularity of the elongated rete, which can also have rounded club shape.
- Loss of the granular cell layer and confluent parakeratosis, which often contains a neutrophilic infiltrate with intraepidermal pustules, is common.
- Microabscesses or pustules formed in the corneal layer are named Munro's microabscesses.
- When the spinous layer is spongiotic and contains collections of neutrophils, they are termed spongiform pustules of Kogoj.
- The spongiform pustules of Kogoj are more often seen in the pustular variant, as are confluent Munro's microabscesses, which can form macropustules.
- The lesions of guttate psoriasis have more subtle, irregular psoriasiform hyperplasia, and often maintain the granular cell layer.
- The superficial dermal papillae contain ectatic tortuous vessels, and this is often associated with thinning of the overlying epidermis. These areas of the epidermis are very susceptible to trauma and likely account for the Auspitz sign seen clinically.
- The very early changes of psoriasis include superficial vascular plexus dilation accompanied by a mild lymphocytic perivascular and dermal infiltrate.

- Established lesions show marked acanthosis and parakeratosis, with increased epidermal mitotic activity.

IMMUNOPATHOLOGY (INCLUDING IMMUNOHISTOCHEMISTRY)

- Noncontributory.

MAIN DIFFERENTIAL DIAGNOSIS

- Fungal infection.
- Chronic eczematous dermatitis.
- Psoriasiform drug eruption.
- Lichen simplex chronicus.

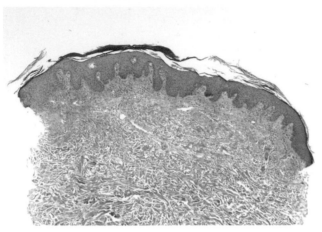

FIGURE 1

Vulvar psoriasis. Acanthosis with regular elongated rete ridges. The rete has round bulbous tips. A mild dermal lymphocytic infiltrate is present.

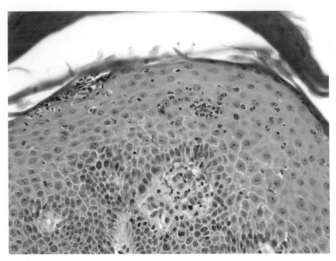

FIGURE 3

Vulvar psoriasis. Munro's microabscesses, which consist of collections of neutrophils within the corneal layer, are present. Spongiosis is prominent.

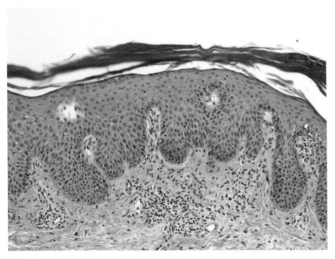

FIGURE 2

Vulvar psoriasis. Confluent parakeratosis with a collection of neutrophils present on the surface. Collections of neutrophils are seen in the superficial epidermis. The bulbous rete is fused.

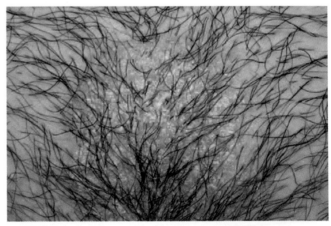

FIGURE 4

Vulvar psoriasis. This close-up view illustrates a typical plaque composed of confluent reddish bumps with a silvery scale. *(Photo courtesy Hope Haefner, MD.)*

SEBORRHEIC DERMATITIS

DEFINITION—A chronic, recurrent dermatitis occurring in areas where sebum is produced marked by red plaques with a yellow scale.

CLINICAL FEATURES

EPIDEMIOLOGY

- Common.
- Affects all demographic groups.
- Immunosuppressed patients and patients with some chronic conditions (including congestive heart failure and Parkinson's disease) have more severe disease and may develop generalized seborrheic dermatitis.
- The disease characteristically flares in winter and spring, with the resolution of symptoms during the summer months.

PRESENTATION

- A red plaque with a greasy yellow scale is noted on the vulva or perineum of adults.
- The surface is frequently "shiny" in genital lesions.
- Patients may report intermittent burning or itching of the area.

PROGNOSIS AND TREATMENT

- Prognosis—excellent, readily responds to treatment.
- Treatment—medicated shampoo and steroid lotions or creams.

PATHOLOGY

HISTOLOGY

- Variable spongiosis with an underlying dermal lymphocytic infiltrate.
- The epithelium may display psoriasiform acanthosis and parakeratosis.
- Clusters of neutrophils are present, particularly around the follicular ostia.

IMMUNOPATHOLOGY (INCLUDING IMMUNOHISTOCHEMISTRY)

- Noncontributory.

MAIN DIFFERENTIAL DIAGNOSIS

- Fungal infection (candidiasis).
- Eczematous dermatitis.
- Psoriasis.

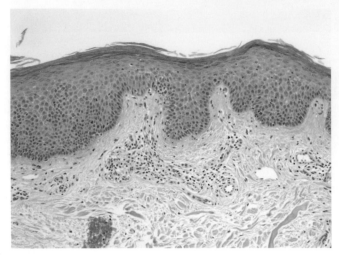

FIGURE 1

Seborrheic dermatitis. Acanthosis with mild hyperparakeratosis and a patchy dermal lymphocytic infiltrate.

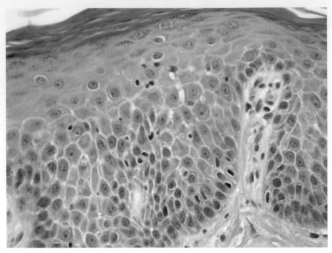

FIGURE 2

Seborrheic dermatitis. Spongiosis and a mild superficial dermal lymphocytic infiltrate.

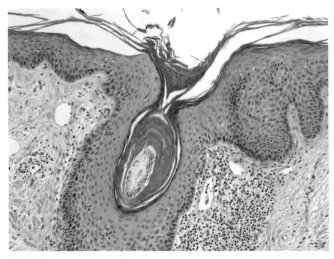

FIGURE 3

Seborrheic dermatitis. Follicular keratosis and perifollicular inflammation, including neutrophils.

LICHEN SCLEROSUS INCLUDING EARLY LICHEN SCLEROSUS

DEFINITION—A chronic inflammatory dermatosis of unknown etiology that commonly affects the vulva.

CLINICAL FEATURES

EPIDEMIOLOGY

- More commonly seen in perimenopausal and postmenopausal patients; however, can be seen at any age.
- Associations have been made with vulvar intraepithelial neoplasia (VIN) and certain human leukocyte antigen (HLA) haplotypes.

PRESENTATION

- Frequently asymptomatic, but can present with pruritus, burning, and pain.
- Clinically, the lesion appears as a symmetrical white patch that has been compared with parchment or cigarette paper.
- Progressive disease can lead to distortion of the normal architecture with progressive stenosis of the introitus and anus.
- Involvement may be seen in areas of previous trauma (Koebner's phenomenon).

PROGNOSIS AND TREATMENT

- Prognosis—a small, but definite, risk of squamous cell carcinoma (~5%) has been associated with lichen sclerosus (LS).

PATHOLOGY

HISTOLOGY

- Early lesions show vacuolar interface changes with scattered lymphocytes and necrotic keratinocytes.
- The lymphocytic infiltrate may be denser and "band-like" in early lesions.
- Dermal edema or hyalinization involving the superficial reticular dermis or papillary dermis may be present in lesions of any age.
- In well-established lesions, the amount of dermal inflammation can decrease, and there is frequent thinning of the epidermis with loss of rete ridges.
- Changes seen in lichen simplex chronicus (LSC) (hyperkeratosis, hypergranulosis) can be seen in traumatized LS.

IMMUNOPATHOLOGY (INCLUDING IMMUNOHISTOCHEMISTRY)

- Noncontributory.

MAIN DIFFERENTIAL DIAGNOSIS

- Lichen planus (especially early LS lesions).
- Vitiligo (clinically).
- Radiation-related changes.

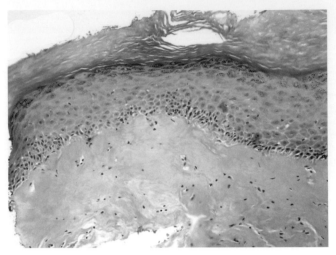

FIGURE 1

LS. Vacuolar changes in the basal layer, as well as loss of the rete ridges and hyalinization of the dermis, are seen.

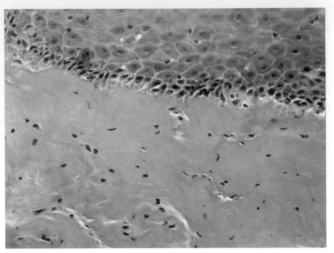

FIGURE 2

LS. High magnification accentuates the vacuolar changes in the basal cells.

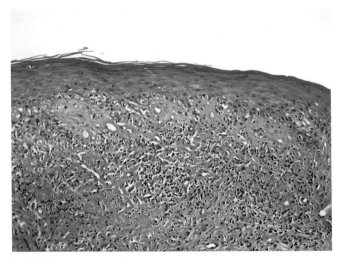

FIGURE 3

Early LS. There is thinning of the epidermis and early basal cell dropout at the interface. The stromal hyalinization change is less conspicuous, and the inflammatory infiltrate is still at the interface.

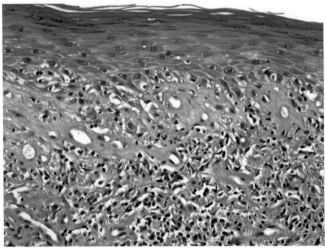

FIGURE 4

Early LS. Higher magnification showing the vacuolar basal cell changes and early subepithelial sclerosis.

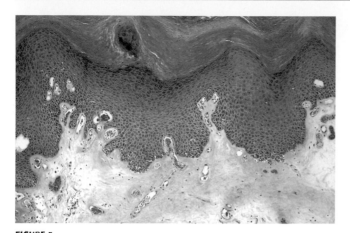

FIGURE 5

LS with superimposed LSC. Note the marked epidermal thickening. This lesion is considered at greater risk for subsequent squamous cell carcinoma.

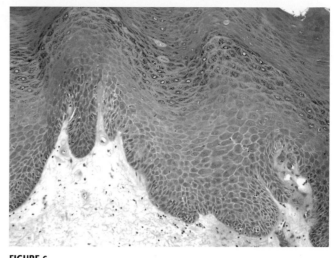

FIGURE 6

LS with superimposed LSC. There is prominent hyperkeratosis and mild spongiosis.

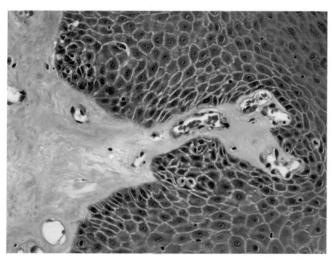

FIGURE 7

LS with superimposed LSC. There is focal basal cell dropout at the interface.

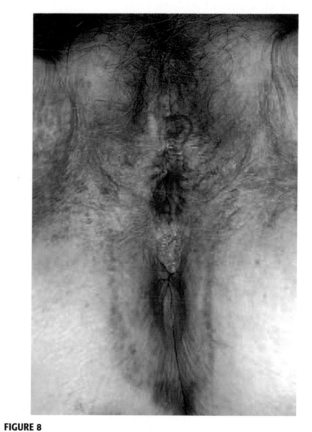

FIGURE 8

LS. Note the atrophy of the labium minus in this clinical picture. *(Photo courtesy Hope Haefner, MD.)*

LICHEN PLANUS

DEFINITION—An uncommon idiopathic mucocutaneous inflammatory dermatosis with a prototypical lichenoid tissue reaction pattern, and a wide range of clinical presentations.

CLINICAL FEATURES

EPIDEMIOLOGY

- Women at ages of 30 to 60 years.

PRESENTATION

- Papular lichen planus (LP) is characterized by small, intensely pruritic, polygonal violaceous papules.
- Chronic erosive LP (the most common vulvar variant) presents with dyspareunia and clinically appears as a desquamative, ulcerating lesion that can extend into the vagina.
- Vulvar involvement is much less common than cutaneous or oral disease, but a significant number of patients with vulvar disease may also have oral lesions.

PROGNOSIS AND TREATMENT

- Topical steroids and emotional support.
- Papular lesions typically resolve within 2 years, often leaving behind pigmentation.
- Chronic erosive LP is not therapy responsive and may persist for years; it is occasionally associated with squamous cell carcinoma.

PATHOLOGY

HISTOLOGY

- Bandlike lymphocytic infiltrate with interface change (lichenoid reaction pattern), parakeratosis, keratinocyte necrosis in the lower layers of the epidermis, and characteristic loss of the basal layer (squamatization).

- The rete pegs may become pronounced ("saw-tooth" pattern); however, this feature is not always prominent in vulvar lesions; the wedge-shaped hyperkeratosis seen in the cutaneous lesions is not seen in the vulvar lesions.
- The dermal infiltrate is composed predominantly of lymphocytes, with a few macrophages, some of which contain melanin (melanophages).
- Erosive lesions show central ulceration with nonspecific chronic inflammation; the classic features of LP are present at the periphery of the lesion.

IMMUNOPATHOLOGY (INCLUDING IMMUNOHISTOCHEMISTRY)

- Direct immunofluorescence of erosive LP shows only fibrin deposition at the dermal–epidermal junction (no immunoglobulin).

MAIN DIFFERENTIAL DIAGNOSIS

- Early lichen sclerosus (papular LP).
- Bullous disorders (erosive LP).
- Zoon's vulvitis.
- Candida.
- Lichenoid drug eruption.

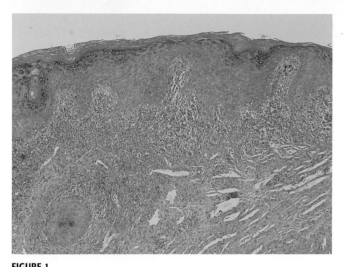

FIGURE 1

LP. A bandlike lymphocyte-predominant lichenoid infiltrate fills the dermis.

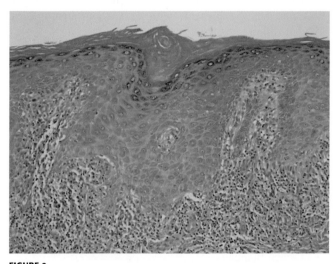

FIGURE 2

LP. The basal layer is not apparent. There is a jagged contour to the epithelial base due to pronounced rete ridges.

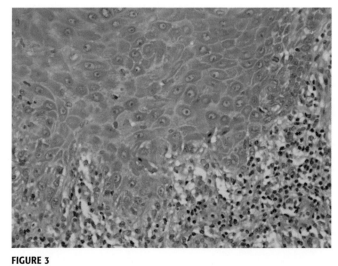

FIGURE 3

LP. Dying keratinocytes (Civatte bodies) can be seen in the bottom layers of the epithelium.

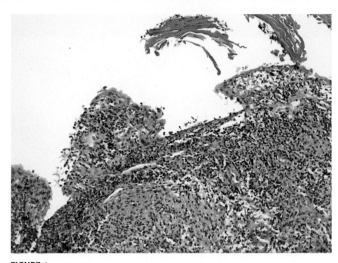

FIGURE 4

LP. Vulvar LP with superficial erosion and a thick, bandlike lymphocytic infiltrate.

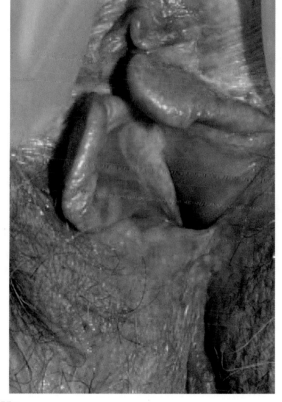

FIGURE 5

LP of the vulva with a white lacelike pattern and erythema. (*Photo courtesy Hope Haefner, MD.*)

ZOON'S VULVITIS

DEFINITION—Plasma cell–mediated vulvitis of unknown etiology.

CLINICAL FEATURES

EPIDEMIOLOGY

- A rare condition.
- Has also been reported in men, as balanitis chronica circumscripta plasmacellularis.
- Age range is from 25 to 70 years, with middle-aged women most commonly being affected.

PRESENTATION

- A well-defined, shiny red to brown macule.
- Lesions are usually solitary.
- Some cases are asymptomatic; however, itching, burning, and soreness may occur.

PROGNOSIS AND TREATMENT

- Prognosis is favorable.
- Not associated with the development of carcinoma in women, although carcinoma may occur in association with plasma cell balanitis in uncircumscribed male patients.
- The treatment consists of steroids: topical, intravaginal, or intralesional injections.

PATHOLOGY

HISTOLOGY

- A lichenoid infiltrate consisting predominantly of plasma cells within the lamina propria; longstanding lesions have the greatest numbers of plasma cells.

- Lymphocytes, mast cells, and eosinophils are also noted.
- Interface change is absent.
- Spongiosis of the epidermis is frequently present.
- Increased vascularity with extravasation of red blood cells may be present, with or without hemosiderin deposition.
- Epidermal atrophy with loss of the granular cell layer and surface keratin occurs.
- Dermal fibrosis is also seen in the longstanding lesions.

IMMUNOPATHOLOGY (INCLUDING IMMUNOHISTOCHEMISTRY)

- Noncontributory.

MAIN DIFFERENTIAL DIAGNOSIS

- Syphilis.
- Lichen planus.

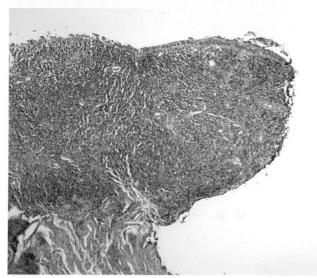

FIGURE 1

Zoon's vulvitis. A dense lichenoid infiltrate is present in the dermis.

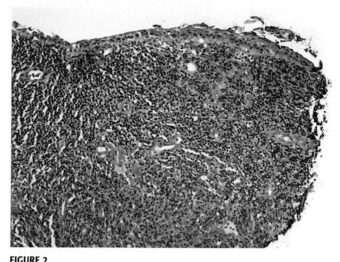

FIGURE 2

Zoon's vulvitis. The overlying epidermis is markedly atrophic. Surface keratinization and the granular cell layer are absent.

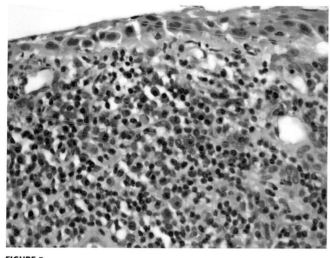

FIGURE 3

Zoon's vulvitis. The infiltrate is composed predominantly of plasma cells. Rare eosinophils are present. Epidermal spongiosis is evident.

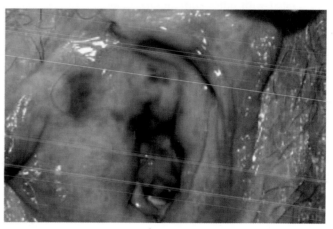

FIGURE 4

Zoon's vulvitis in the introitus. *(Photo courtesy Hope Haefner, MD.)*

BULLOUS PEMPHIGOID

DEFINITION—An autoimmune blistering disorder that is the most common cause of subepidermal blisters. Caused by antibodies to a 230 kD plakin (BPAg1) and a 180 kD glycoprotein (BPAg2).

CLINICAL FEATURES

EPIDEMIOLOGY

- Primarily seen in older patients and is commonly associated with other autoimmune disorders (lupus, diabetes, primary biliary cirrhosis, ulcerative colitis, and alopecia areata).

PRESENTATION

- Tense vesicles (due to subepidermal nature of the blister) that do not expand with pressure (Nikolsky's sign).
- Vesicles are most frequently seen on the lower abdomen, flexural surfaces of the arms and legs, and the groin.
- The disease can extend to involve mucosal surfaces.
- Onset might be heralded by erythema and urticaria.

PROGNOSIS AND TREATMENT

- Prognosis—chronic disease with periods of remission; however, may become refractory to treatment.
- Steroids are the most common form of first-line treatment.
- Severe cases may require immunomodulatory drugs, plasmapheresis, or intravenous immunoglobulin (IvIg).
- Separation of the labia and vaginal dilation may be used to prevent adhesions.

PATHOLOGY

HISTOLOGY

- Unilocular, subepidermal bullae.
- Numerous eosinophils and neutrophils, admixed with serum and fibrin, are seen within the blister.
- Re-epithelialization may be confused as intraepidermal blister formation.

IMMUNOPATHOLOGY (INCLUDING IMMUNOHISTOCHEMISTRY)

- Immunofluorescence—linear IgG and C3 deposition along the basement membrane.

MAIN DIFFERENTIAL DIAGNOSIS

- Cicatricial pemphigoid.
- Pemphigus vulgaris.
- Lichen planus.

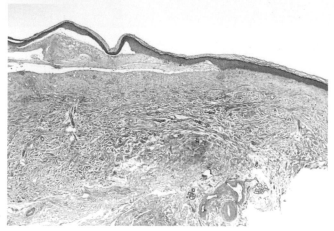

FIGURE 1

Bullous pemphigoid. Low-power view of a single, unilocular vesicle in bullous pemphigoid.

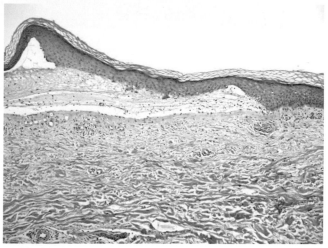

FIGURE 2

Bullous pemphigoid. Note the separation of the epidermis from the underlying dermis (subepithelial split).

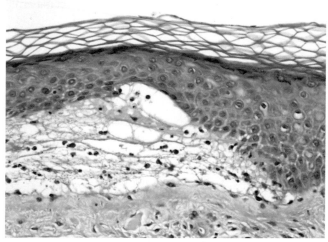

FIGURE 3

Bullous pemphigoid. Eosinophils along with fibrin and rare neutrophils can be seen in the vesicle.

PEMPHIGUS VULGARIS

DEFINITION—An acquired autoimmune (anti–desmoglein 3 antibodies) blistering disorder that is marked by flaccid bullae and mucosal erosions.

CLINICAL FEATURES

EPIDEMIOLOGY

- Incidence is rare and the disease may affect all age groups.

PRESENTATION

- Mucosal-based erosions, which can be painful, can be seen involving the mucosa of the mouth, nose, and anogenital region.
- Nikolsky's sign, which is extension of the border of the blister with pressure, is commonly present.
- The blisters are fragile and flaccid.
- Vulvar involvement can lead to scarring.

PROGNOSIS AND TREATMENT

- Prognosis—favorable, the disease responds to treatment in most cases.
- Treatment—topical and\or oral steroids. Methotrexate may be used in severe cases.

PATHOLOGY

HISTOLOGY

- Acanthosis with suprabasal blister formation.
- Basal cells may be intact and resemble a "row of tombstones."

- Blister formation overlying vascular papillae may create a "pseudopapillary" pattern.

IMMUNOPATHOLOGY (INCLUDING IMMUNOHISTOCHEMISTRY)

- Immunofluorescence is positive for IgG and C3 in the intercellular regions of the epidermis "fish net pattern."

MAIN DIFFERENTIAL DIAGNOSIS

- Bullous pemphigoid.
- Cicatricial pemphigoid.
- Hailey-Hailey disease.
- Darier's disease.
- Warty dyskeratoma.
- Acantholysis of the vulvocrural area.

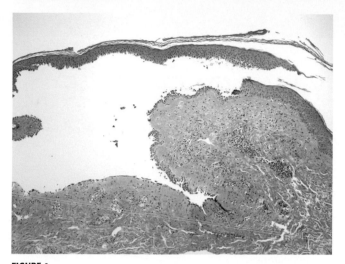

FIGURE 1

Pemphigus vulgaris. Intraepithelial (suprabasal) blister formation.

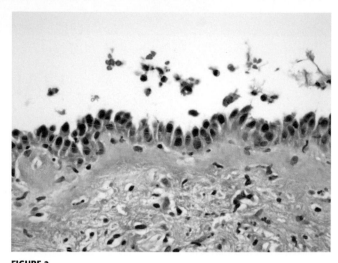

FIGURE 2

Pemphigus vulgaris. Intact basal cells showing a "row of tombstones" formation.

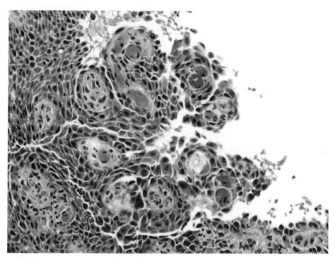

FIGURE 3

Pemphigus vulgaris. Clefting overlying vascular papillae creating a pseudopapillary growth pattern.

HAILEY-HAILEY DISEASE

DEFINITION—An autosomal dominant, acantholytic dermatosis with a predilection for moist body creases.

CLINICAL FEATURES

EPIDEMIOLOGY

- It is a rare autosomal dominant disease.

PRESENTATION

- Pruritic erosions involving or extending to the vulva that extend centrifugally.
- Over time, a foul-smelling crust can form and depigmentation can occur.
- Scarring is rare.

PROGNOSIS AND TREATMENT

- Currently there is no cure for Hailey-Hailey disease.
- Avoidance of triggers (sunburn, sweat, friction), topical steroid, and antibiotics.
- Topical tacrolimus, systemic steroids, and antibiotics may be used in severe cases.

PATHOLOGY

HISTOLOGY

- Early cases show suprabasal lacunae with evolution into vesicles and bullae that are intraepidermal and have an orderly appearance, referred to as a "brick wall appearance."
- Dyskeratotic cells may be present.
- Variable amounts of acanthosis and hyperkeratosis may be seen.

IMMUNOPATHOLOGY (INCLUDING IMMUNOHISTOCHEMISTRY)

- Immunofluorescence is negative.

MAIN DIFFERENTIAL DIAGNOSIS

- Pemphigus vulgaris.
- Bullous pemphigoid.
- Cicatricial pemphigoid.
- Darier's disease.
- Acantholytic vulvar intraepithelial neoplasia.

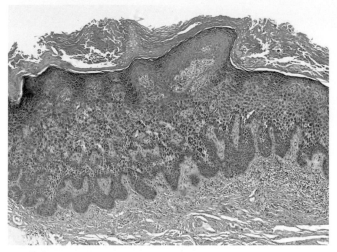

FIGURE 1

Hailey-Hailey disease. Acantholysis of the keratinocytes can be appreciated at low power (brick wall appearance). Several lacunae are present. Note the associated acanthosis, hyperkeratosis, and superficial dermal inflammatory infiltrate.

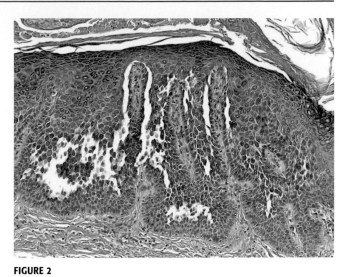

FIGURE 2

Hailey-Hailey disease. Prominent acantholysis forming small clefts.

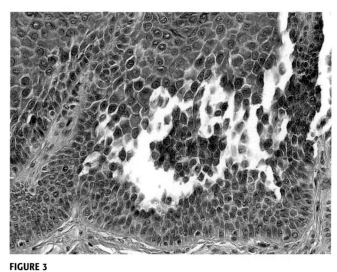

FIGURE 3

Hailey-Hailey disease. Acantholysis with detached cells filling the clefts.

DARIER'S DISEASE

DEFINITION—Autosomal dominant genodermatosis marked by numerous hyperkeratotic papules that usually involve the trunk.

CLINICAL FEATURES

EPIDEMIOLOGY

- Patients present around puberty; however, they can present later in life.
- Men are more severely affected; however, the incidence is equal in men and women.

PRESENTATION

- Pruritic and warty lesions associated with a foul odor are present.
- Secondary irritation by scratching, as well as superinfection by bacteria or fungi, may occur.
- Patients may suffer from thin, brittle nails.

PROGNOSIS AND TREATMENT

- Currently there is no cure, and long-term remission is rare.
- Avoidance of triggers (sunlight, maceration), sunscreen, and oral retinoids.
- Topical steroids and moisturizers with urea or lactic acid may be used to help with symptoms.

PATHOLOGY

HISTOLOGY

- Acanthosis with parakeratosis (frequently seen in columns) and acantholysis.
- The acantholysis is usually suprabasal and forms small lacunae.
- Overlying epidermis may display hyperkeratosis.
- Dyskeratotic cells (corps ronds and grains of Darier) may be seen in the stratum spinosum and stratum corneum, respectively.

IMMUNOPATHOLOGY (INCLUDING IMMUNOHISTOCHEMISTRY)

- Immunofluorescence is negative.

MAIN DIFFERENTIAL DIAGNOSIS

- Hailey-Hailey disease.
- Warty dyskeratoma.
- Acantholysis of the vulvocrural area.
- Pseudobowenoid papulosis (dyskeratotic cells).

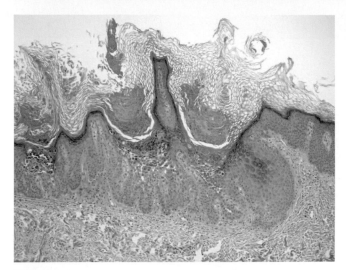

FIGURE 1

Darier's disease. Columnlike acanthosis and parakeratosis. Note the marked hyperkeratosis.

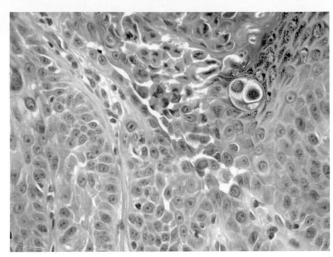

FIGURE 2

Darier's disease. Dyskeratotic cells, identified by their eosinophilic cytoplasm. Suprabasal acantholysis is pronounced.

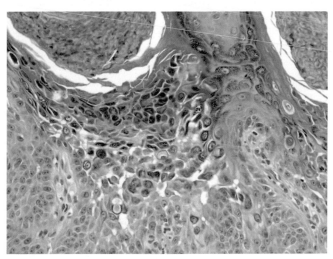

FIGURE 3

Darier's disease. Acantholysis of the superficial keratinocytes.

EPIDERMOLYTIC HYPERKERATOSIS

DEFINITION—Hyperkeratosis marked by discrete, flesh- to white-colored papules to plaques. This entity overlaps with what is called acantholytic dyskeratosis (a term under which other dyskeratoses might fall). In this section we discuss a process that is encountered sporadically.

CLINICAL FEATURES

EPIDEMIOLOGY

- Epidermolytic hyperkeratosis is an uncommon condition with no demographic predilections.

PRESENTATION

- Single to multiple (can become confluent) flesh- to white-colored papules that may be associated with erythema and pruritus. It can also be encountered as an incidental finding when examining vulvar skin for other disorders.

PROGNOSIS AND TREATMENT

- Prognosis—chronic disease with variable response to treatment. When encountered as an incidental finding, no therapy is required.
- Treatment—topical steroids (rarely effective), electrocautery, and surgical excision, as needed.

PATHOLOGY

HISTOLOGY

- Marked compact hyperkeratosis.
- Acantholysis with separation of intracellular bridges between keratinocytes.

- Scattered dyskeratotic cells may be noted by their brightly eosinophilic cytoplasm (corps ronds and grains of Darier).

IMMUNOPATHOLOGY (INCLUDING IMMUNOHISTOCHEMISTRY)

- Immunofluorescence is negative.

MAIN DIFFERENTIAL DIAGNOSIS

- Darier's disease—a familial disorder, corps ronds usually more conspicuous, and parakeratosis common.
- Hailey-Hailey disease—familial, bullae formation, and disordered keratinocytes forming a "dilapidated brick wall."
- Viral vulvar warts (or VIN1)—prominent keratohyalin granules as seen in acantholytic dyskeratosis would not be expected, and some superficial cell atypia would be more likely.
- Other verruciform acanthoses (e.g., lichen simplex chronicus, verruciform xanthoma) will not demonstrate the prominent combination of acantholysis and keratohyalin granule formation with grains of Darier.

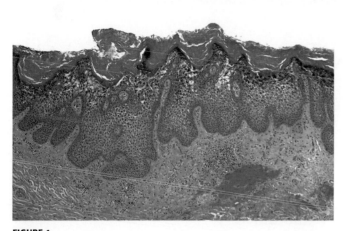

FIGURE 1

Epidermolytic hyperkeratosis. There is thickening of the epidermis (acanthosis) with compact hyperkeratosis and prominent keratohyalin granules.

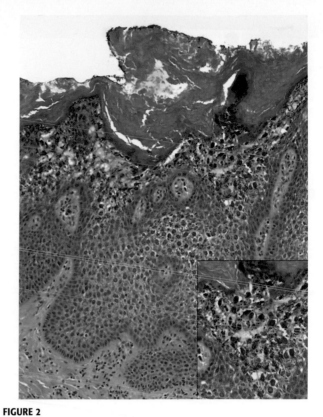

FIGURE 2

Epidermolytic hyperkeratosis. The superficial epidermis shows acantholysis with prominent spaces and vacuoles located between keratinocytes, noted by their intensely eosinophilic cytoplasm (inset).

HIDRADENITIS SUPPURATIVA

DEFINITION—A suppurative inflammatory process that can be associated with fistula tract or abscess formation.

CLINICAL FEATURES

EPIDEMIOLOGY

- Most commonly seen in young women.
- The most common sites of involvement are the axilla and groin.

PRESENTATION

- Presents with a solitary painful papule.
- Over time, ulceration, abscess, or fistula formation may occur.
- Bacterial superinfection may occur.
- Scarring may occur in severe, chronic cases.

PROGNOSIS AND TREATMENT

- Variable prognosis; severe disease can be chronic and debilitating.
- Antibiotics, topical antiseptics, and compresses are common first-line treatments.
- Severe disease may require systemic corticosteroids and immunomodulatory drugs, in addition to surgery.

PATHOLOGY

HISTOLOGY

- Abscess or sinus tracts with abundant necroinflammatory debris.
- A partial squamous lining may be present.
- Fibrosis and granuloma formation may occur.
- Pseudoepitheliomatous hyperplasia may be present and mistaken for squamous cell carcinoma.

IMMUNOPATHOLOGY (INCLUDING IMMUNOHISTOCHEMISTRY)

- Noncontributory.

MAIN DIFFERENTIAL DIAGNOSIS

- Other causes of abscess formation.
- Vulvar Crohn's disease.
- Fox-Fordyce disease.
- Lymphogranuloma venereum.

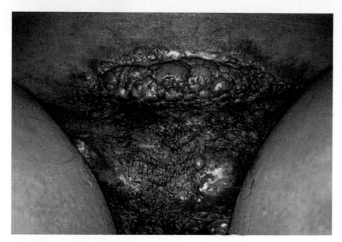

FIGURE 1

Severe case of hidradenitis suppurativa.

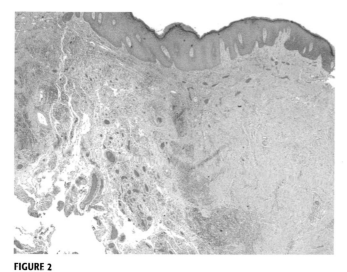

FIGURE 2

Hidradenitis suppurativa. Abscess and granulation tissue formation can be seen on the left side of the photo. Note the presence of acanthosis and hyperkeratosis in the overlying epithelium.

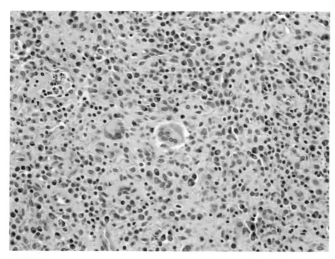

FIGURE 3

Hidradenitis suppurativa. A mixed inflammatory cell infiltrate with occasional foreign body giant cells.

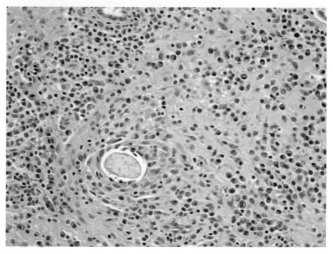

FIGURE 4

Hidradenitis suppurativa. Fragments of foreign material may be present. In this case hair from an adjacent ruptured follicle is seen, surrounded by inflammation.

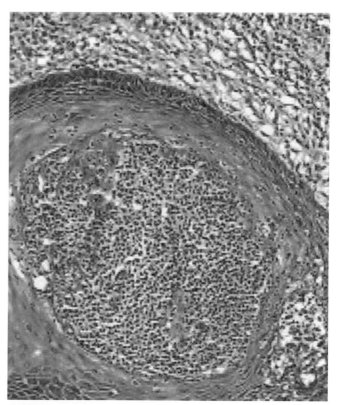

FIGURE 5

High-power view of a sinus with abscess formation.

CROHN'S DISEASE OF THE VULVA

DEFINITION—A granulomatous, inflammatory bowel disease that may spread to involve other sites such as skin and mucosa.

CLINICAL FEATURES

EPIDEMIOLOGY

- Seen in patients with Crohn's disease.
- Crohn's disease has no gender predilection and usually manifests in the second to third decade of life.
- Vulvar involvement may be contiguous (i.e., fistula formation) or may be isolated (metastatic Crohn's disease) with lower gastrointestinal symptoms.

PRESENTATION

- Edema, drainage, ulceration, and occasionally mass-forming lesions.

PROGNOSIS AND TREATMENT

- Crohn's disease is a progressive disease with tremendous associated morbidity. Immunosuppressants, 5-aminosalicylic acid (5-ASA), and topical steroids are used for treatment.
- Antibiotics may be added for difficult-to-treat cases.
- Surgical excision is an option.

PATHOLOGY

HISTOLOGY

- Nonspecific; consisting of a mixed inflammatory infiltrate composed of histiocytes, giant cells, and plasma cells.
- Superficial ulceration and occasional fistula formation may be present.
- Occasionally, granuloma formation is present.

IMMUNOPATHOLOGY (INCLUDING IMMUNOHISTOCHEMISTRY)

- Noncontributory.

MAIN DIFFERENTIAL DIAGNOSIS

- Herpes virus infection (ulcerative lesions).
- Widespread tuberculosis.
- Inflammation secondary to an irritant (foreign body).

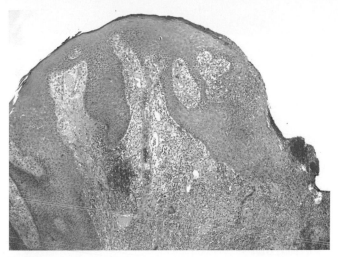

FIGURE 1

Crohn's disease of the vulva. Low-power magnification shows acanthosis and an increased inflammatory infiltrate in the lamina propria. Giant cells can be seen even at scanning magnification.

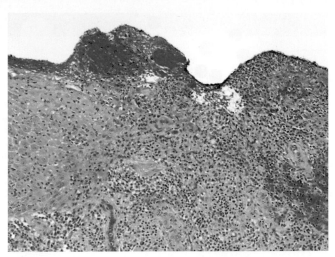

FIGURE 2

Crohn's disease of the vulva. Ulceration or fistula formation may be present.

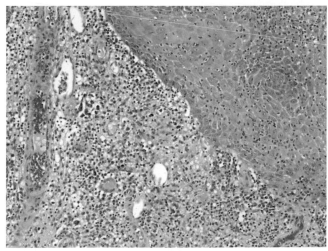

FIGURE 3

Crohn's disease of the vulva. An intense, mixed inflammatory infiltrate is present within the lamina propria. A single giant cell is present.

VULVODYNIA

DEFINITION—The sensation of pain localized to the vulvar vestibule.

CLINICAL FEATURES

EPIDEMIOLOGY

- Once thought to be a relatively rare condition, it is now known to affect millions of women.

PRESENTATION

- Localized vulvodynia has no clinically identifiable features other than the patient's report of pain.
- Occasional erythema is described; however, the diagnosis of vulvodynia cannot be made in the presence of grossly abnormal vulvar structures.

PROGNOSIS AND TREATMENT

- Due to unknown etiology in the vast majority of cases, prognosis and treatment vary greatly from patient to patient.
- Treatments have ranged from avoidance of irritation, topical treatment, injection of anesthetics, and even surgery.

PATHOLOGY

HISTOLOGY

- The histologic findings are entirely nonspecific.
- If a biopsy of the sample is performed, the results may be normal.
- A mixed inflammatory infiltrate composed of T-lymphocytes, monocytes, and plasma cells has been identified in some resection specimens.
- Occasionally, nonspecific findings such as glandular inflammation, squamous metaplasia, hyperkeratosis, and parakeratosis are identified.

IMMUNOPATHOLOGY (INCLUDING IMMUNOHISTOCHEMISTRY)

- Noncontributory.

MAIN DIFFERENTIAL DIAGNOSIS

- Varies greatly depending on the clinical scenario.

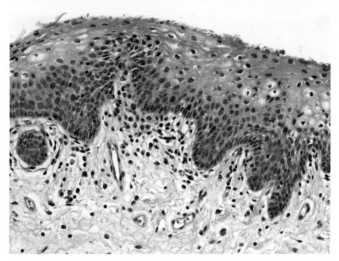

FIGURE 1

Squamous mucosa with mild nonspecific change. There is mild parakeratosis and a mild chronic inflammatory infiltrate in the upper dermis composed of lymphocytes and plasma cells.

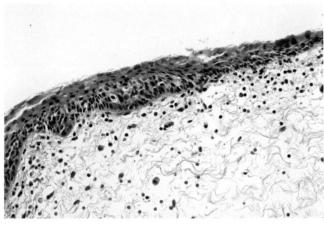

FIGURE 2

Squamous mucosa with mild dermal edema and a mild dermal infiltrate composed of lymphocytes and plasma cells. Mild parakeratosis is also present.

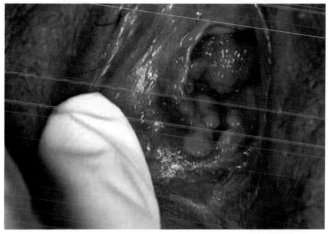

FIGURE 3

Photo of localized vulvodynia showing introital mucosa edema. *(Courtesy Hope Haefner, MD.)*

VULVOVAGINAL CANDIDIASIS

DEFINITION—A fungal infection caused by any member of the Candida species of fungi.

CLINICAL FEATURES

EPIDEMIOLOGY

- Very common, affecting up to 75% of females starting after menarche and increasing in incidence with peaks in the third or fourth decades.
- Predisposing factors include diabetes; immunocompromised state; and steroid, antibiotic, and oral contraceptive use.

PRESENTATION

- Intense vulvar pruritus, dysuria, edema, erythema, and a white vaginal discharge with a curd-like appearance.

PROGNOSIS AND TREATMENT

- Favorable.
- Treatment with topical (or systemic in severe cases) antifungal medications typically leads to resolution.

PATHOLOGY

HISTOLOGY

- Acanthosis, parakeratosis, psoriasiform epidermal hyperplasia, and neutrophilic infiltration of the epithelium are typically seen.

- Microabscess formation within the epidermis may be noted.
- Variable amounts of spongiosis may be present.

IMMUNOPATHOLOGY (INCLUDING IMMUNOHISTOCHEMISTRY)

- Silver stains or periodic acid–Schiff (PAS) stain (with diastase) may aid in identifying fungal forms.

MAIN DIFFERENTIAL DIAGNOSIS (FUNGAL STAINS SHOULD BE PERFORMED IF CLINICALLY APPROPRIATE)

- Eczematous dermatitis
- Lichen simplex chronicus
- Intertrigo
- Psoriasis
- Atypical verruciform acanthosis—fungal infection should always be excluded with any unresolved verruciform acanthosis in which there is a low index of suspicion for malignancy.

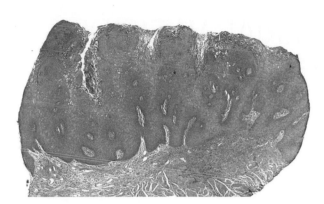

FIGURE 1

Vulvar candidiasis. Marked acanthosis may be seen at low power.

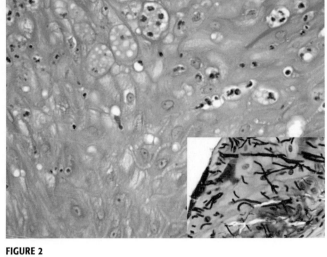

FIGURE 2

Vulvar candidiasis. A neutrophilic infiltrate, with occasional microabscess formation, is typically present. Note the presence of spongiosis in this example. PAS stain highlights organisms *(inset)*.

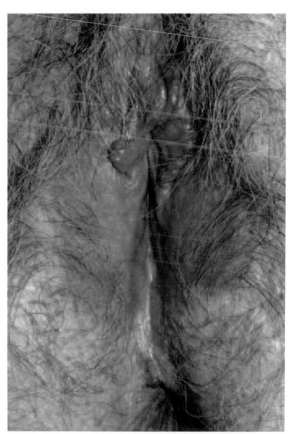

FIGURE 3

Erythema of the labia minora and majora with satellitosis from candidiasis. *(Courtesy Hope Haefner, MD.)*

BACTERIAL VAGINOSIS

DEFINITION—Infection marked by a shift in the vaginal flora. Caused by a decrease in the normal lactobacilli and an increase in numerous other organisms (*Gardnerella vaginalis*, *Mobiluncus*, *Mycoplasma hominis*, *Prevotella*, *Porphyromonas*, *Bacteroides*, and *Peptostreptococcus*).

CLINICAL FEATURES

EPIDEMIOLOGY

- Most commonly present in young, sexually active women; however, it can be seen across a wide age group.

PRESENTATION

- Patients present with a strong, "fishy" odor and increased vaginal discharge.
- This odor may be worse during menses or after intercourse.
- Itching and irritation may be present.

PROGNOSIS AND TREATMENT

- Treatment with antibiotics (metronidazole and clindamycin) yields excellent results.

PATHOLOGY

HISTOLOGY

- Pap smears show characteristic "clue cells" with decreased to absent numbers of lactobacilli and white blood cells.

- Clue cells are squamous epithelial cells with adherent bacteria that create a "fuzzy" border as opposed to the usually crisp epithelial contour.

IMMUNOPATHOLOGY (INCLUDING IMMUNOHISTOCHEMISTRY)

- Noncontributory.

MAIN DIFFERENTIAL DIAGNOSIS

- Candidiasis (clinical).
- Cervicitis (clinical).
- Chlamydia (clinical).
- Gonorrhea (clinical).
- Herpes (clinical).
- Trichomonas (clinical).
- Desquamative inflammatory vaginitis (clinical).

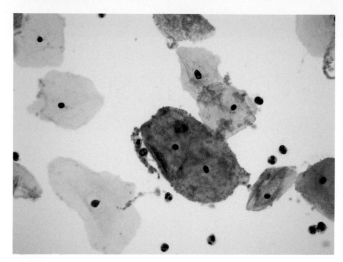

FIGURE 1

Bacterial vaginosis. A clue cell with its characteristic hazy blue color and fuzzy border.

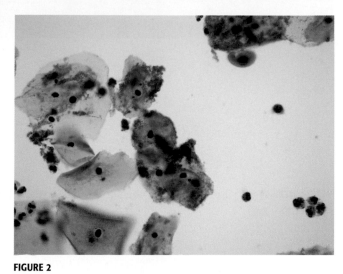

FIGURE 2

Bacterial vaginosis. Multiple clue cells. Note the fragments of bacteria in the left side of the picture as well as the scattered neutrophils.

MOLLUSCUM CONTAGIOSUM

DEFINITION—A viral infection of the skin (often sexually transmitted when involving the genital area) caused by a DNA poxvirus.

CLINICAL FEATURES

EPIDEMIOLOGY

- Genital infection most commonly occurs in young, sexually active individuals.
- In this population it is commonly transmitted by sexual or fomite contact.
- Cases in children are generally not sexually transmitted.

PRESENTATION

- Dome-shaped, flesh-colored papules typically appear a few weeks after contraction.
- Scattered lesions will have a central umbilication with an underlying material with a cheesy consistency.
- The lesions are not painful.

PROGNOSIS AND TREATMENT

- A self-limited disease that can be treated by curettage, cryotherapy, or topical agents if desired.

PATHOLOGY

HISTOLOGY

- Lesions are typically cup shaped and show epithelial hyperplasia.

- The peripheral basal cells mature toward the center of the lesion and shed keratinous debris into the central cavity.
- Molluscum bodies (diagnostic viral inclusions) are eosinophilic to cyanophilic, and as the cells mature, the inclusion displaces the cytoplasm and marginates the nucleus.

IMMUNOPATHOLOGY (INCLUDING IMMUNOHISTOCHEMISTRY)

- In situ hybridization is available.

MAIN DIFFERENTIAL DIAGNOSIS

- Acrochordon.
- Epidermal inclusion cyst.
- Dermatitis herpetiformis.
- Keratoacanthoma.
- Neurofibroma.
- Condyloma.
- Pyogenic granuloma.
- Herpes infection.
- Basal cell carcinoma.

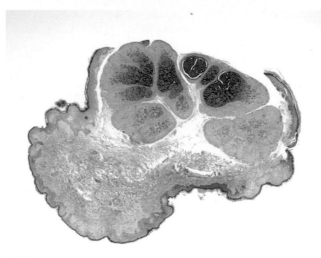

FIGURE 1

Molluscum contagiosum. A cup-shaped lesion with large nests of hyperplastic epithelium.

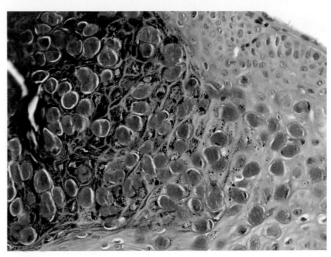

FIGURE 2

Molluscum contagiosum. Orientation of the basal layer of the infected keratinocytes toward the center of the lesion.

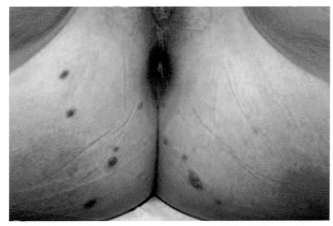

FIGURE 3

Clinical presentation of molluscum, with discrete, dome-shaped, pink-colored papules.

ACUTE HERPES SIMPLEX VIRUS INFECTION

DEFINITION—An ulcerative sexually transmitted disease (STD) caused by the herpes simplex virus (HSV) (double-stranded DNA).

CLINICAL FEATURES

EPIDEMIOLOGY

- The most common ulcerative disease of the genital tract in developed countries. A prevalence of upward of 20 million cases has been reported in the United States. Chronic erosive HSV infection can be seen in human immunodeficiency virus (HIV)–positive patients and is an AIDS-defining illness if lesions last more than 1 month.

PRESENTATION

- Within 3 to 14 days of exposure the infected area becomes red and swollen with numerous vesicles. These vesicles rupture, and open erosions form, which commonly last for 2 weeks. These outbreaks typically heal without scarring.

PROGNOSIS AND TREATMENT

- HSV infection leads to a chronic course with multiple periods of relapse and remission of clinical disease. Antivirals (acyclovir) are useful in controlling outbreaks; however, there is no cure. HSV infection can cause significant morbidity and mortality in immunocompromised patients and fetuses.

PATHOLOGY

HISTOLOGY

- The biopsy specimen shows epithelial necrosis and an eosinophilic aggregate of affected epithelial cells. The interface of the ulcer and necrotic ulcer bed may display characteristic nuclear inclusions marked by multinucleation with basophilic, "glassy" nuclei. The base of the ulcer may show a dermal inflammatory infiltrate (predominantly neutrophilic).

IMMUNOPATHOLOGY (INCLUDING IMMUNOHISTOCHEMISTRY)

- Immunohistochemical stains for HSV I and II are available and stain infected cells.

MAIN DIFFERENTIAL DIAGNOSIS

- Herpes zoster and cytomegalovirus (CMV) can be excluded by immunohistochemistry.
- Aphthous and other ulcers are excluded by the absence of inclusions or HSV antigens. Epithelial necrosis is particularly characteristic of HSV versus nonviral ulceration.

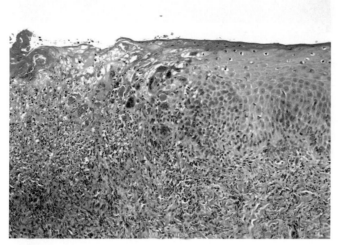

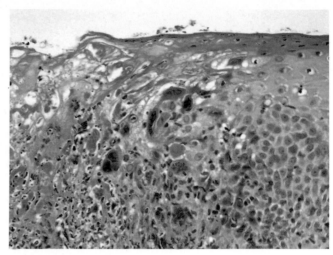

FIGURE 1

Herpes simplex infection of the vulva. Note the frank epithelial necrosis at the left. The herpetic inclusions stand out at the junction of the nonulcerated epithelium and the ulcer.

FIGURE 2

Herpes simplex infection. At higher magnification, mononucleated and multinucleated cells contain densely eosinophilic inclusions with opaque chromatin encased in amphophilic cytoplasm.

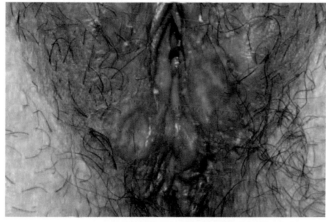

FIGURE 3

Herpetic ulcers with yellow-white bases. *(Photo courtesy Hope Haefner, MD.)*

CHRONIC EROSIVE HERPES SIMPLEX

DEFINITION—A chronic herpes simplex virus (HSV) infection lasting more than 1 month.

CLINICAL FEATURES

EPIDEMIOLOGY

- This is the most common ulcerative disease of the genital tract in developed countries. A prevalence of upward of 20 million cases has been reported in the United States. Chronic erosive HSV infection can be seen in HIV-positive patients and is an AIDS-defining illness if the lesions last more than 1 month.

PRESENTATION

- The lesions present as both ulcers and hypertrophic proliferations of epithelium.

PROGNOSIS AND TREATMENT

- Because these chronic infections may be resistant to thymidine kinase–dependent antiretroviral drugs, they require additional measures such as drugs targeting viral-dependent DNA polymerases. These drugs (e.g., foscarnet, cidofovir) can generate a dramatic improvement in susceptible infections.
- The risk of disseminated HSV is low with chronic herpes infections, even in immunosuppressed individuals.

PATHOLOGY

HISTOLOGY

- Whereas conventional herpes typically has epithelial necrosis with inclusions at the junction of the epithelium and ulcer, chronic herpes presents with epithelial hyperplasia and a striking subepithelial infiltrate, often over a broad area in the anogenital region.
- Inclusions can often be found at the epithelial–stromal junction.

IMMUNOPATHOLOGY (INCLUDING IMMUNOHISTOCHEMISTRY)

- Immunohistochemical stains for HSV 1 and 2 are available and stain infected cells.

MAIN DIFFERENTIAL DIAGNOSIS

- Syphilis, Behcet's disease, and aphthous ulcers will not contain viral inclusions among other exclusions. Herpes zoster and cytomegalovirus (CMV) can be excluded by immunostains.

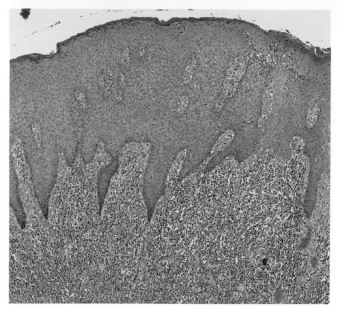

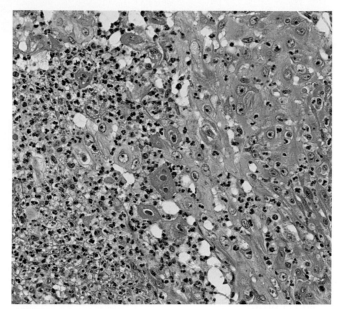

FIGURE 1

Chronic erosive HSV. There is epithelial acanthosis, and an ulcer is not seen in this field. Note the intense inflammatory infiltrate.

FIGURE 2

Chronic erosive HSV. Numerous inclusions are present at the epithelial–stromal interface.

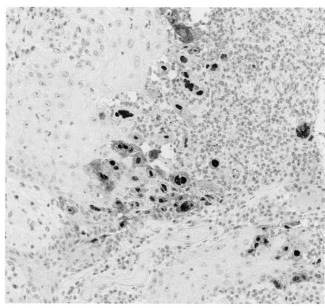

FIGURE 3

Chronic erosive HSV. An immunostain for HSV 1 highlights the inclusions.

SYPHILIS

DEFINITION—A sexually transmitted disease caused by the spirochete *Treponema pallidum*.

CLINICAL FEATURES

EPIDEMIOLOGY

- Primary syphilis typically occurs in young, sexually active adults.
- Secondary and tertiary disease is much less common due to the effectiveness of antibiotic treatment of the primary infection.
- Secondary syphilis develops in weeks to months in untreated individuals.
- Tertiary syphilis will occur in one third of untreated individuals.

PRESENTATION

- Primary syphilis presents with the characteristic chancre at the exposure site; "kissing" chancres can be seen in the vulva.
- The chancre is a sharply circumscribed macule or papule with central ulceration and is often indurated and edematous.
- Superinfection is common with vulvar lesions.
- Chancres are painless, except when traumatized or superinfected, and usually resolve in 2 weeks or less.
- Adenopathy may or may not be present; vulvar disease may cause unilateral inguinal adenopathy.
- Secondary syphilis evolves in weeks to months, and it may present with systemic symptoms including fever and malaise.
- If secondary maculopapular lesions are present, the distribution is more diffuse and often symmetrical.
- Condyloma lata are the vulvar manifestation of secondary syphilis and can easily be confused with traditional condyloma.

PROGNOSIS AND TREATMENT

- Excellent.
- Primary chancres shed large numbers of organisms, and the disease is highly infectious at this stage.

- *T. pallidum* is highly susceptible to high doses of penicillin.

PATHOLOGY

HISTOLOGY

- Primary syphilis is characterized by a dense dermal infiltrate composed of plasma cells, lymphocytes, histiocytes, and neutrophils.
- Plasma cells may be scarce in early lesions but increase in number as the lesion progresses.
- Plasma cells often congregate around small vessels, causing endothelial swelling and prominence.
- Epidermal hyperplasia is present, and pseudoepitheliomatous hyperplasia may develop, particularly at the edges of lesions.
- The classic lesions of secondary syphilis are also characterized by extensive dermal infiltration by histiocytes and plasma cells, with overlying psoriasiform epidermal hyperplasia (often marked in advanced cases) and a plasmacytic perivascular infiltrate with endothelial swelling and injury.
- The histologic patterns of secondary syphilis are highly variable; neutrophils generally diminish as do the numbers of organisms that can be seen on special stains.
- Late secondary lesions are often granulomatous.
- Condyloma lata are nonulcerated and composed of markedly hypertrophic and hyperkeratotic epidermis.
- Plasma cell "vasculitis" with endothelial injury is often seen with condyloma lata.
- The lesions of tertiary syphilis are granulomatous, with admixed plasma cells.
- The "gumma" of tertiary syphilis is centrally necrotic with a rim of inflammation composed of plasma cells, histiocytes, and lymphocytes.
- Eosinophilic "ghost cells" may be seen in the necroinflammatory debris.

IMMUNOPATHOLOGY (INCLUDING IMMUNOHISTOCHEMISTRY)

- Warthin-Starry and Steiner silver stains may be used to demonstrate organisms.
- Darkfield microscopy of secretions may be helpful in early infections when serologic testing is not particularly sensitive.

- Zoon's vulvitis.
- Chancroid.

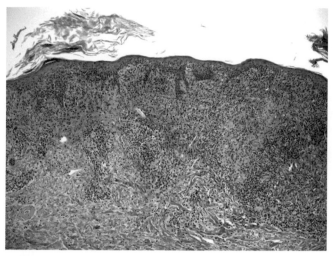

FIGURE 1

Syphilis. Low power of a primary lesion showing a dense superficial and deep lichenoid dermal infiltrate composed of mixed chronic inflammation.

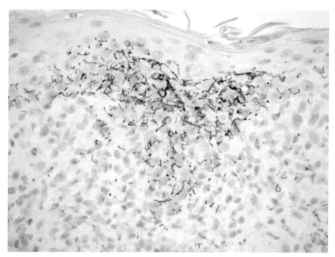

FIGURE 3

Syphilis. Warthin-Starry stain showing spirochetal organisms in the superficial dermis. Organisms can also be identified in the deep dermis (not shown).

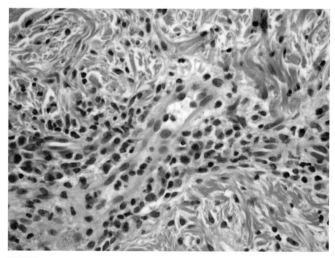

FIGURE 2

Syphilis. Perivascular inflammation composed predominantly of plasma cells. The endothelial cells are plump.

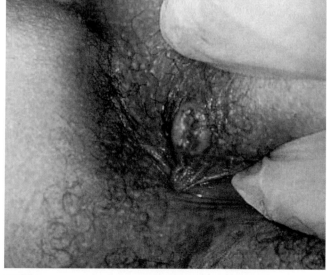

FIGURE 4

Syphilitic chancre in the perianal region. *(From Fiumara NJ: Primary and secondary syphilis. In Rein M, editor: Atlas of Infectious Diseases, Vol. V: Sexually Transmitted Diseases, Philadelphia, 1996, Churchill Livingstone, p 9.7, Fig. 9.19.)*

CHANCROID

DEFINITION—Infection secondary to infection with *Haemophilus ducreyi* marked by painful ulcers and adenopathy.

CLINICAL FEATURES

EPIDEMIOLOGY

- Most common in tropical and subtropical developing countries.
- It is more common in males than females and is commonly seen in the setting of human immunodeficiency virus (HIV) infection.
- Chancroid is a risk factor for heterosexual transmission of HIV.

PRESENTATION

- Papules and pustules develop 3 to 10 days after infection, which later ulcerate as a result of mechanical irritation.
- The ulcerative lesions are painful, with a ragged border and surrounding erythema.
- Smaller ulcers may coalesce into large lesions.
- Adenopathy develops 1 to 2 weeks after the ulcers appear, and if left untreated, the adenopathy may develop into "buboes" with draining sinus tracts.

PROGNOSIS AND TREATMENT

- Favorable.
- Antibiotic treatment causes rapid resolution of the lesions.

PATHOLOGY

HISTOLOGY

- Lesions display a "zonal" distribution.
- The uppermost portion consists of a neutrophilic infiltrate with admixed blood and fibrin, underneath which lies a layer of granulation tissue.
- The base of the lesion consists of a dense band of plasma cells, lymphocytes, and histiocytes.

IMMUNOPATHOLOGY (INCLUDING IMMUNOHISTOCHEMISTRY)

- Noncontributory.

MAIN DIFFERENTIAL DIAGNOSIS

- Herpes.
- Syphilis.

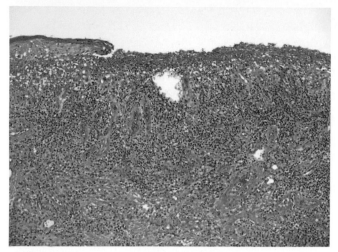

FIGURE 1

Chancroid. The uppermost portion of a chancroid ulcer can be seen here with its accompanying superficial layer of blood and fibrin and underlying granulation tissue.

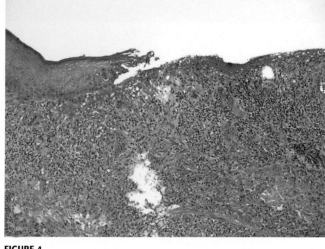

FIGURE 4

Chancroid. In this figure all three layers may be appreciated: the uppermost layer of blood and fibrin, the underlying granulation tissue, and the deep lymphoplasmacytic infiltrate.

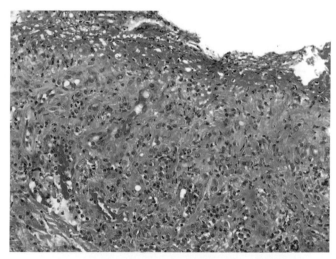

FIGURE 2

Chancroid. Fibrin and granulation tissue in an ulcer bed.

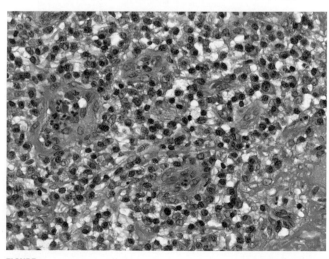

FIGURE 3

Chancroid. Deep to the ulcer a bandlike infiltrate of lymphocytes and plasma cells should be present.

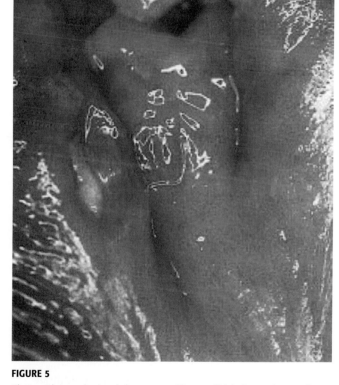

FIGURE 5

Chancroid. Irregular introital mucosa with superficial ulcers. *(From Allen R: Chancroid. In Rein M, editor: Atlas of Infectious Diseases, Vol V: Sexually Transmitted Diseases, Philadelphia, 1996, Churchill Livingstone, p 16.7, Figure 16.18.)*

GRANULOMA INGUINALE

DEFINITION—A sexually transmitted disease, marked by ulceration, caused by the intercellular, gram-negative rod *Klebsiella granulomatis*.

CLINICAL FEATURES

EPIDEMIOLOGY

- Endemic in tropical and subtropical areas in sexually active adults.
- Sporadic outbreaks do occur in Western countries.

PRESENTATION

- Erythematous papules or small nodular lesions that are painless.
- Lesions expand to form "beefy-red" ulcers that are friable and bleed easily.
- Scarring and hypertrophic forms have been noted.

PROGNOSIS AND TREATMENT

- Excellent; however, long treatment with antibiotics may be required for refractory ulcers.

PATHOLOGY

HISTOLOGY

- Marked, mixed, nonspecific inflammatory infiltrate.
- Donovan bodies (vacuoles in histiocytes containing the organism) may be present.
- Acanthosis, ulceration, and pseudoepitheliomatous hyperplasia of the epidermis may be noted.

IMMUNOPATHOLOGY (INCLUDING IMMUNOHISTOCHEMISTRY)

- Noncontributory.

MAIN DIFFERENTIAL DIAGNOSIS

- Lymphogranuloma venereum.
- Syphilis.
- Chancroid.
- Herpes simplex virus (HSV) infection.
- Candidiasis.
- Amebiasis (genital).

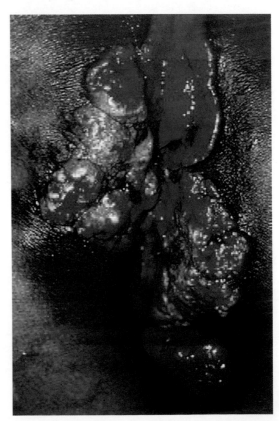

FIGURE 1

Granuloma inguinale, presenting as a combination of hypertrophic mucosa with submucosal edema and focal ulceration. *(From Hart G: Donovanosis: Granuloma inguinale. In Rein M, editor: Atlas of Infectious Diseases, Vol. V: Sexually Transmitted Diseases, Philadelphia, 1996, Churchill Livingstone, p 17.8, Figure 17.21.)*

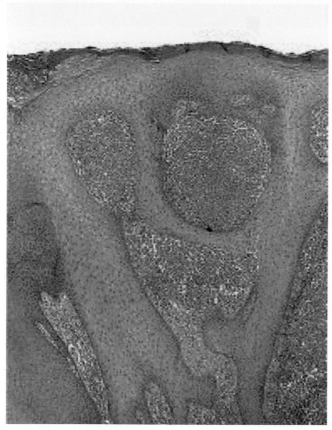

FIGURE 2

Granuloma inguinale. Low-power view of inflammation in granuloma inguinale exhibits both pseudoepitheliomatous hyperplasia and intense submucosal inflammation, corresponding to the clinical presentation (see Figure 1) *(From Crum CP, Nucci MR, Lee KR, editors: Diagnostic Gynecologic and Obstetric Pathology, ed 2, Philadelphia, 2011, Elsevier, Figure 4-20A.)*

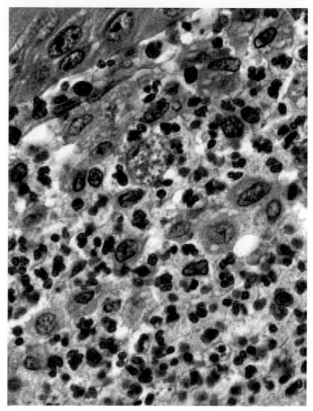

FIGURE 3

Granuloma inguinale. Donovan bodies are discrete cytoplasmic vacuoles containing organisms (center) seen here on hematoxylin and eosin staining. *(From Crum CP, Nucci MR, Lee KR, editors: Diagnostic Gynecologic and Obstetric Pathology, ed 2, Philadelphia, 2011, Elsevier, Figure 4-20B.)*

SCHISTOSOMIASIS

DEFINITION—Infection by trematodes that belong to the superfamily schistosomatidae (*Schistosoma haematobium*, *Schistosoma japonicum*, and *Schistosoma mansoni*).

CLINICAL FEATURES

EPIDEMIOLOGY

- Endemic in Egypt and the Middle East.
- Genital lesions occur in approximately 5% of patients infected by the trematode.
- Vulvar manifestations are more commonly seen in younger women.
- Infection may be acquired by freshwater swimming in endemic areas.

PRESENTATION

- Swelling and ulceration may or may not be painful, but pruritus is common.
- Skin often has a nodular or eroded surface.
- Clitoromegaly may be seen.
- Papules or warts might be described in patients from nonendemic areas, with patients reporting the presence of an "itchy wart."
- Chronic infection leads to tumorlike masses associated with ulceration and pain.
- Labia majora involvement is most common as the trematodes have easier access to veins in this site.

PROGNOSIS AND TREATMENT

- Favorable.
- Antihelminthic drug treatment cures the infection.
- Skin manifestations resolve a few weeks after initiation of treatment.

PATHOLOGY

HISTOLOGY

- Immature schistosome eggs with intensely basophilic internal structures.
- An intense granulomatous, eosinophilic, and acute inflammatory reaction is usually associated with the eggs.
- Epithelioid histiocytes and noncaseating granulomas may form.

IMMUNOPATHOLOGY (INCLUDING IMMUNOHISTOCHEMISTRY)

- Periodic acid–Schiff (PAS) staining identifies the chitin within the egg structure.

MAIN DIFFERENTIAL DIAGNOSIS

- Nematode infection, including trichuriasis.
- Carcinoma—may be confused clinically.
- Condyloma—may be confused clinically.

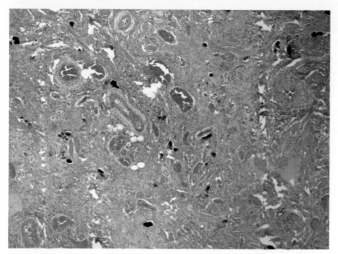

FIGURE 1

Schistosomiasis. At low power a large number of densely basophilic structures can be seen embedded within the vascular soft tissue of the labia majora.

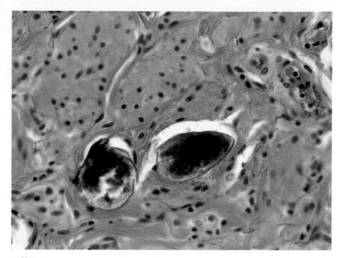

FIGURE 2

Schistosomiasis. Two calcified schistosoma ova.

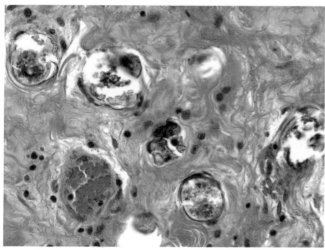

FIGURE 3

Schistosomiasis. Multiple calcified schistosoma ova.

BACILLARY ANGIOMATOSIS

DEFINITION—An opportunistic infection that commonly occurs in the backdrop of human immunodeficiency virus (HIV)/AIDS infection caused by the organisms *Bartonella henselae* or *Bartonella quintana*.

CLINICAL FEATURES

EPIDEMIOLOGY

- This is a rare, opportunistic disease seen in immuno-compromised individuals.

PRESENTATION

- Small red papules that increase in size.
- Larger lesions can ulcerate.
- Deeper, subcutaneous lesions may develop that tend to be lighter (flesh to pink in color).

PROGNOSIS AND TREATMENT

- Favorable; antibiotic therapy (erythromycin) will typically lead to resolution within a week, with longer courses of therapy required for advanced mucosal disease.

PATHOLOGY

HISTOLOGY

- In immunocompetent people a necrotizing granulomatous disease develops within the draining lymph nodes.
- In immunocompromised people a distinct vascular proliferation occurs that is composed of capillaries with "histiocytoid" endothelial cells, which have been noted to protrude into the vessel lumen.
- Scattered endothelial cells, neutrophils, and karyorrhectic debris are noted within edematous stroma.
- Collections of organisms, which may appear as a hazy purple area surrounding vessels, may be seen (best on Warthin-Starry staining).

IMMUNOPATHOLOGY (INCLUDING IMMUNOHISTOCHEMISTRY)

- Silver stains (Warthin-Starry) may help to identify organisms.

MAIN DIFFERENTIAL DIAGNOSIS

- Kaposi's sarcoma.
- Angiosarcoma.
- Ulcerated pyogenic granuloma.

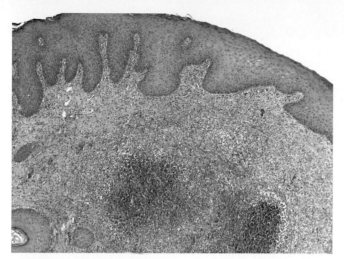

FIGURE 1

Bacillary angiomatosis. At low power a nodular infiltrate of inflammatory cells and vessels is often present.

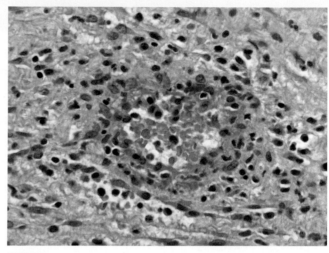

FIGURE 2

Bacillary angiomatosis. Vessels display "histiocytoid" endothelial cells that slough into the lumen. A mixed inflammatory infiltrate is present.

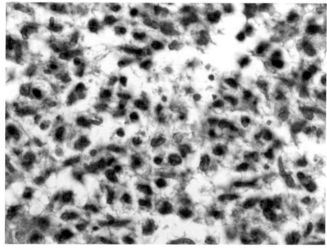

FIGURE 3

Bacillary angiomatosis. An edematous area with a mixed inflammatory infiltrate and a hazy purple background that is composed of clumps and clusters of organisms.

NECROTIZING FASCIITIS

DEFINITION—An aggressive infection of the subcutis and fascia.

CLINICAL FEATURES

EPIDEMIOLOGY

- Commonly seen in the setting of diabetes.
- Predisposing factors include obesity, hypertension, immune compromise, and history of previous trauma.

PRESENTATION

- Localized erythema and pain that rapidly expands.
- The infected skin will break down and ulcerate and slough.
- Sepsis may occur late in the course of the disease.

PROGNOSIS AND TREATMENT

- Unfavorable; rates of mortality range from 0% to 75% in the literature.
- Aggressive surgical debridement and systemic antibiotics are required.

PATHOLOGY

HISTOLOGY

- Nonspecific; however, the inflammatory exudate may be sparse to abscess forming.
- When present, abscesses are noted along the fascia and dissecting into fat lobules.
- Sheets of bacteria may be noted in the subcutaneous tissue.
- Skeletal muscle necrosis, as well as vessels with fibrin thrombi, may be noted.

IMMUNOPATHOLOGY (INCLUDING IMMUNOHISTOCHEMISTRY)

- Gram stains may be useful in identifying organisms.

MAIN DIFFERENTIAL DIAGNOSIS

- Superficial cellulitis (early).
- Pyoderma gangrenosum.

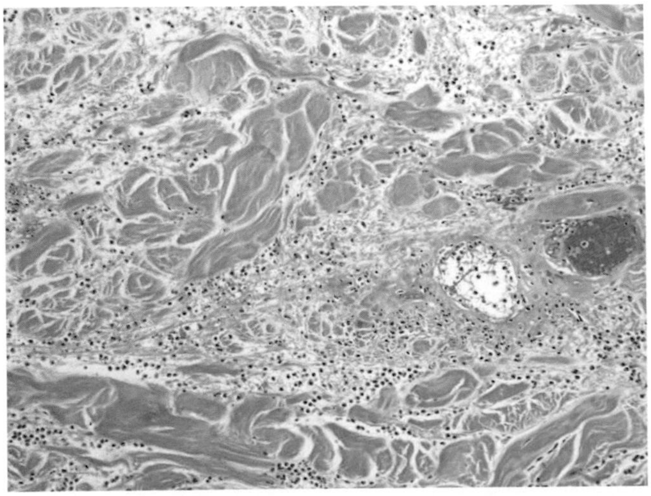

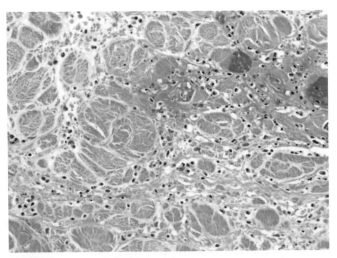

FIGURE 1

Necrotizing fasciitis. Inflammatory cells are present in and around bundles of muscle.

FIGURE 2

Necrotizing fasciitis. A scattered, mixed, inflammatory cell infiltrate with a central area of coagulative necrosis.

VARICELLA ZOSTER

DEFINITION—Infection by the neurotropic varicella-zoster virus (VZV), an alpha-herpesvirus.

CLINICAL FEATURES

EPIDEMIOLOGY

- Primary VZV infection, commonly known as chickenpox, occurs predominantly in children.
- Recurrences occur later in life.
- Severe, recurrent infections can be seen in the setting of immunodeficiency.
- Herpes zoster (shingles) is the secondary manifestation of VZV infection.

PRESENTATION

- In primary disease a vesiculobullous rash occurs 10 to 21 days after exposure.
- Skin lesions progress from macules to papules and finally to vesicles which rupture, dry, and crust over.
- Lesions are present at a variety of stages in the acutely affected patient.
- Secondary disease is heralded by a prodrome or pain and paresthesias; itching, burning, or tingling, usually in a dermatomal distribution.
- The prodrome is followed by an acute vesiculobullous eruption.
- Fever and headache may or may not be present in secondary reactivation.
- Patients may present with chronic vulvar pain or clitorodynia.

PROGNOSIS AND TREATMENT

- Primary infection is nearly always self-limited in immunocompetent patients.
- Primary infection in immunocompromised patients may be fatal, and high-dose acyclovir is required.
- High-dose acyclovir is also required in any patient with disseminated or visceral zoster, which can (rarely) occur even in immunocompetent patients.
- Secondary VZV reactivation can result in postherpetic neuralgia, and chronic pain may persist for months or years.

PATHOLOGY

HISTOLOGY

- The histologic appearance of VZV is identical to the changes seen in herpes simplex virus (HSV) infection.
- Early lesions are characterized by bullous formation, with acantholysis of keratinocytes.
- Epithelial necrosis with extensive debris in the ulcer bed is seen in later stages.
- Viral inclusion may be seen at the interface of the ulcer and normal epithelium or within the acantholytic cells in bullae.
- The viral inclusions are histologically identical to those seen in HSV infection; they are seen as large glassy pink-red nuclear inclusions.

IMMUNOPATHOLOGY (INCLUDING IMMUNOHISTOCHEMISTRY)

- Immunohistochemistry for VZV is positive.
- Immunohistochemistry for HSV is negative.

MAIN DIFFERENTIAL DIAGNOSIS

- HSV infection—this can be distinguished best by immunohistochemistry.

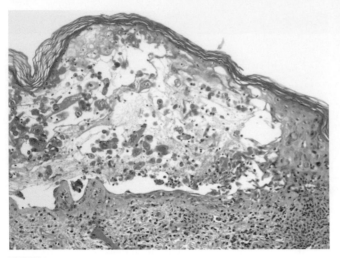

FIGURE 1

Varicella zoster. Bulla formation with epidermal necrosis and necrotic debris.

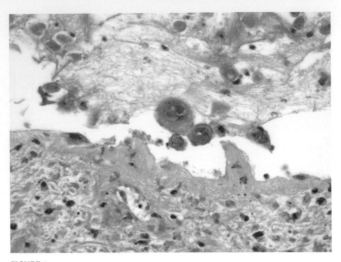

FIGURE 2

Varicella zoster. Glassy nuclear viral inclusions.

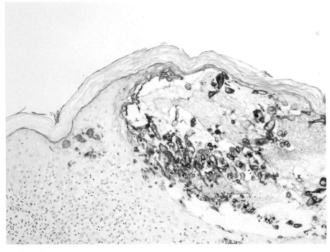

FIGURE 3

Varicella zoster. Immunohistochemical stain for VZV.

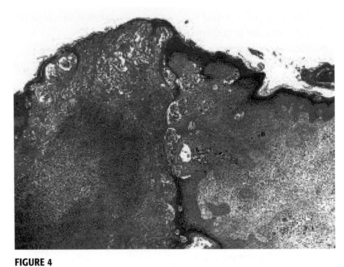

FIGURE 4

Varicella zoster. At low power there is pronounced submucosal edema and epithelial hyperplasia. Ulceration is inconspicuous.

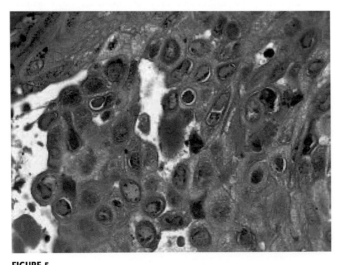

FIGURE 5

Inclusions are conspicuous at higher power, similar in appearance to herpes simplex.

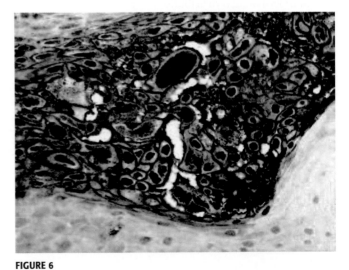

FIGURE 6

Immunohistochemical staining for zoster will discriminate this from herpes simplex.

BARTHOLIN'S DUCT CYST

DEFINITION—Cyst formation follows occlusion of Bartholin's duct, which drains Bartholin's glands.

CLINICAL FEATURES

EPIDEMIOLOGY

- Common lesions that happen in all age groups.

PRESENTATION

- May present as mass lesions with or without tenderness based on accompanying inflammation (or abscess formation).
- Cysts are located in the posterior introitus around the orifices of the ducts that drain Bartholin's glands

PROGNOSIS AND TREATMENT

- Excellent.
- The majority of the lesions can be treated by catheter insertion and marsupialization, the latter of which is not recommended in abscesses.
- Antibiotics may be utilized for accompanying cellulitis.

PATHOLOGY

HISTOLOGY

- Variable-sized cysts lined by squamous-, mucinous-, or transitional-type epithelium in varying proportions.
- An adjacent Bartholin's gland may be present.

IMMUNOPATHOLOGY (INCLUDING IMMUNOHISTOCHEMISTRY)

- Noncontributory.

MAIN DIFFERENTIAL DIAGNOSIS

- Skene's duct cyst—periurethral location.
- Epidermal inclusion cyst—subepithelial, no accompanying Bartholin's gland.
- Mucous cyst—usually vaginal in location.
- Benign adnexal tumors—hidradenoma and syringoma, may be confused clinically.
- Soft-tissue tumors—may be confused clinically.
- Bartholin's adenoma/carcinoma—may be confused clinically.

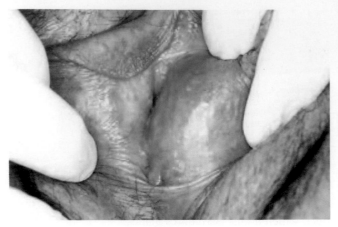

FIGURE 1

Clinical appearance of Bartholin's duct cyst. *(From Marzano DA, Haefner HK: The barthol gland cyst: past, present and future, J Low Genit Tract Dis 8(3):195-204, 2004.)*

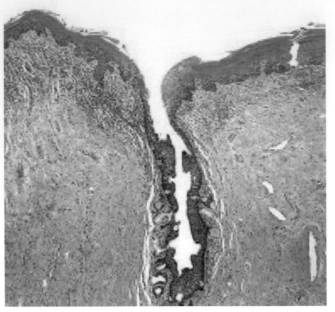

FIGURE 2

Bartholin's duct cyst. Low-power microphotography illustrating the transitional epithelium.

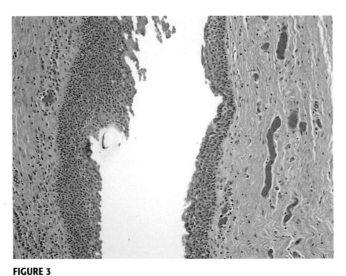

FIGURE 3

Higher magnification of a prominent cyst with transitional epithelium.

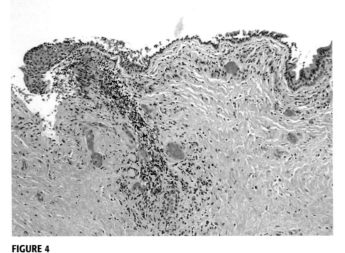

FIGURE 4

Bartholin's duct cyst. In this image there is attenuation of the epithelium and some underlying inflammation.

MUCOUS CYST OF THE VAGINA

DEFINITION—Vaginal cyst of müllerian origin.

CLINICAL FEATURES

EPIDEMIOLOGY

- Relatively uncommon.
- Derived from müllerian remnants.
- Wide age range with a median in the fourth decade.

PRESENTATION

- Lateral and posterior wall.
- Patient may notice a swelling and experience dyspareunia and stress incontinence.

PROGNOSIS AND TREATMENT

- Excision is curative.

PATHOLOGY

HISTOLOGY

- Variable size lined by müllerian (endocervical-type) mucinous epithelium.
- Squamous metaplasia is common.

IMMUNOPATHOLOGY (INCLUDING IMMUNOHISTOCHEMISTRY)

- Noncontributory.

MAIN DIFFERENTIAL DIAGNOSIS

- Skene's duct cyst—periurethral location.
- Epidermal inclusion cyst—squamous epithelium that may be confused with squamous metaplasia, but keratinaceous debris is more typical.
- Benign adnexal tumors—hidradenoma and syringoma may be confused clinically but are more typically situated in the vulva.
- Gartner's duct cyst—cuboidal lining and no mucin.

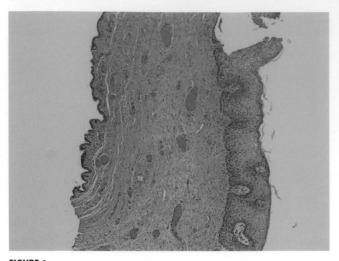

FIGURE 1

Mucous cyst lined by a low columnar mucin-producing epithelium. Surface squamous mucosa is on the right.

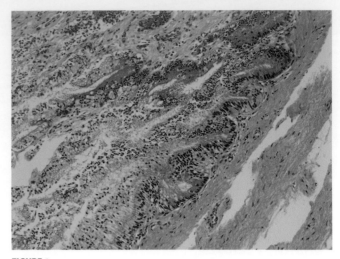

FIGURE 2

Mucous cyst. Abundant mucin-producing epithelium.

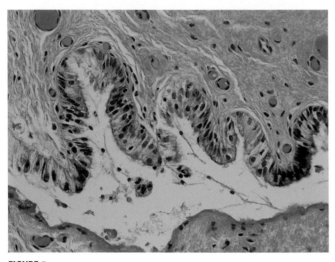

FIGURE 3

Mucous cyst. Note the resemblance to endocervical epithelium.

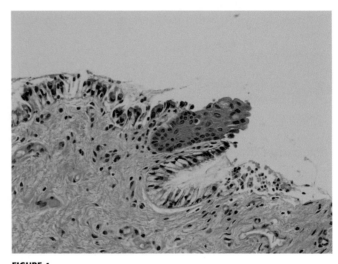

FIGURE 4

Mucinous cyst with focal squamous differentiation.

ECTOPIC BREAST TISSUE

DEFINITION—Adnexal tissue with mammary differentiation in the vulvar region.

CLINICAL FEATURES

EPIDEMIOLOGY

- Rare.
- The most popular theory is that it reflects a rudiment of caudal mammary buds (in the "milk line") that did not completely regress during development.
- Other theories include mammary-like anogenital glands that concentrate in the labial sulcus and give rise to "ectopic breast tissue."

PRESENTATION

- Typically presents as a smooth well-circumscribed mass resembling a Bartholin's duct cyst or hidradenoma. May be seen during pregnancy.

PROGNOSIS AND TREATMENT

- Excision is curative.

PATHOLOGY

HISTOLOGY

- Appearance is that of normal breast tissue.
- Glandular epithelium including ducts and lobules.

IMMUNOPATHOLOGY (INCLUDING IMMUNOHISTOCHEMISTRY)

- Usually noncontributory; but in less discrete cases, p63 immunostaining will highlight basal–reserve cells confirming a benign process.

MAIN DIFFERENTIAL DIAGNOSIS

- No diagnostic problems are expected on histology. However, the lesion may clinically be confused with adnexal cysts or benign tumors.
- Fibroadenomas and other neoplasms can arise in the breast tissue (see fibroadenoma).

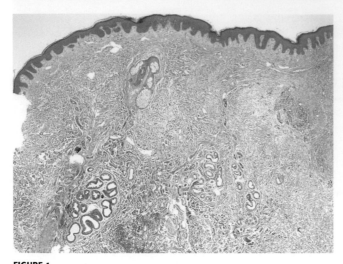

FIGURE 1

Ectopic breast tissue. Mammary differentiation is seen with small ducts and acini, including a focus with apocrine metaplasia *(lower left)*.

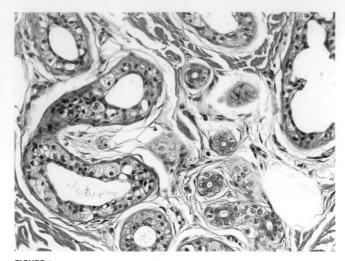

FIGURE 2

Ectopic breast tissue. Higher magnification depicts ductal structures.

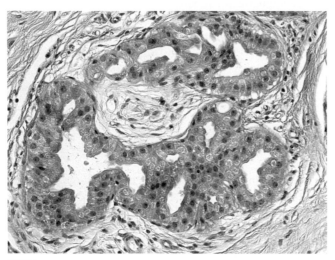

FIGURE 3

Ectopic breast tissue. Apocrine differentiation.

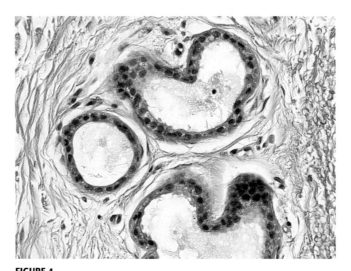

FIGURE 4

Small ectatic ducts in ectopic breast tissue.

FIBROADENOMA

DEFINITION—Tumor of mammary phenotype arising in ectopic breast tissue.

CLINICAL FEATURES

EPIDEMIOLOGY

- Rare.
- The most popular theory is that this tumor arises in a rudiment of mammary tissue (in the "milk line") that did not completely regress during development.

PRESENTATION

- Young patients typically.
- Typically presents as a smooth well-circumscribed mass resembling an adnexal duct cyst or hidradenoma. May be seen during pregnancy.

PROGNOSIS AND TREATMENT

- Excision is curative.

PATHOLOGY

HISTOLOGY

- May be associated with recognizable normal breast tissue.

- Glandular epithelium including ducts and lobules within a characteristic benign appearing fibromatous stroma.
- Some glandular proliferation may be seen.
- Some fibroadenomas may appear complex, raising the possibility of a phyllodes tumor. However, stroma cells are usually not atypical.

IMMUNOPATHOLOGY (INCLUDING IMMUNOHISTOCHEMISTRY)

- Usually noncontributory; but in less discrete cases, p63 immunostaining will highlight basal–reserve cells confirming a benign process.

MAIN DIFFERENTIAL DIAGNOSIS

- Hidradenoma—this may exhibit similar differentiation but exhibits the characteristic acinar/papillary architecture without the more typical concentric fibrous component of a fibroadenoma.

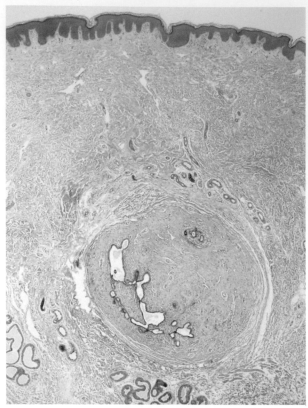

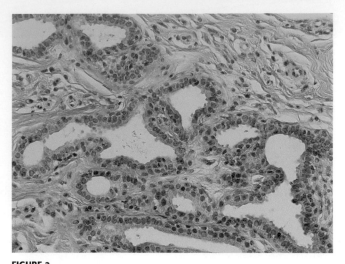

FIGURE 2

Ectopic breast tissue with fibroadenoma. There is some mild increase in glandular proliferation.

FIGURE 1

Ectopic breast tissue with fibroadenoma. Note the central fibrous nodule with mild glandular hyperplasia.

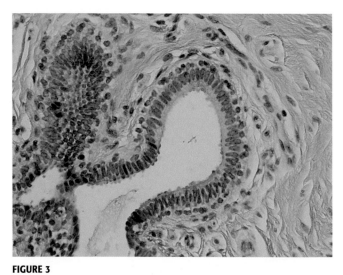

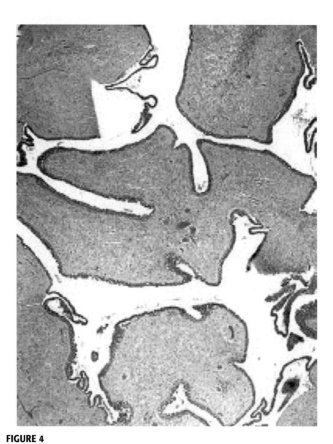

FIGURE 3

Ectopic breast tissue with fibroadenoma. Note the benign cytologic features.

FIGURE 4

Mildly complex fibroadenoma. Note the somewhat phyllodiform appearance. There is no stromal atypia.

HIDRADENOMA

PITFALL

DEFINITION—An unusual benign adnexal tumor that exhibits both apocrine and eccrine differentiation and occurs almost exclusively in the vulva.

CLINICAL FEATURES

EPIDEMIOLOGY

- Uncommon.
- Nearly always seen in postpubertal, but premenopausal, adult women.
- More frequent in Caucasians.

PRESENTATION

- A small- to medium-sized (<2 cm), discrete, painless nodule located in the sulcus between the labium minus and majus.

PROGNOSIS AND TREATMENT

- Excision is curative.

PATHOLOGY

HISTOLOGY

- Most are well-circumscribed papillary-to-cribriform proliferation of glandular epithelium.

- The characteristic two-layer epithelium has a strikingly uniform appearance.
- The surface epithelial cells exhibit distinctive "decapitation secretion."
- Myoepithelial cells and fibrovascular cores are evident.
- Overlying acanthosis is occasionally prominent.
- Beware occasional cases that are not discrete and may be intermixed with fibrosis, mimicking malignancy.
- Some will exhibit prominent apocrine differentiation.

IMMUNOPATHOLOGY (INCLUDING IMMUNOHISTOCHEMISTRY)

- Usually noncontributory; but in less discrete cases, p63 immunostaining will highlight basal–reserve cells confirming a benign process.

MAIN DIFFERENTIAL DIAGNOSIS

- Adenocarcinoma (such as metastatic endometrioid) when gland proliferation is prominent.
- Infiltrating adenocarcinoma when fibrosis with gland entrapment occurs (exclude with staining for p63).
- Mesenchymal neoplasms (clinical).

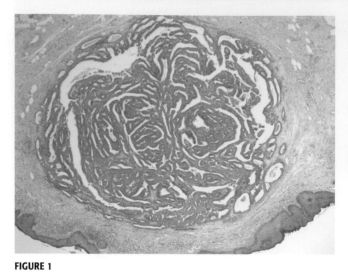

FIGURE 1

Hidradenoma papilliferum (HP). A well-circumscribed nodule of glandular epithelium.

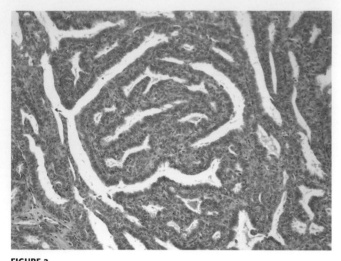

FIGURE 2

HP. Higher magnification depicts regularly arranged but variable lumens.

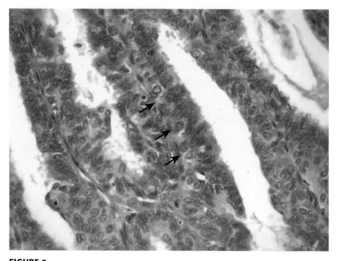

FIGURE 3

HP. Uniform cells arranged focally into conspicuous two cell layers *(arrows)*.

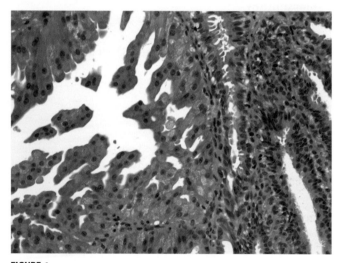

FIGURE 4

Apocrine differentiation in HP.

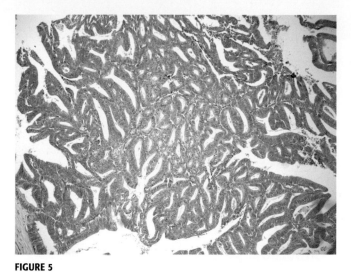

FIGURE 5

Metastatic endometrioid carcinoma for comparison.

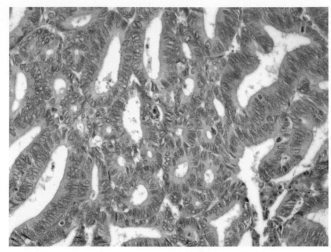

FIGURE 6

At higher magnification, metastatic carcinoma with a single neoplastic cell type devoid of two cell layers.

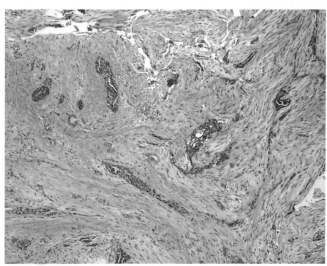

FIGURE 7

Sclerotic HP mimicking an infiltrative carcinoma.

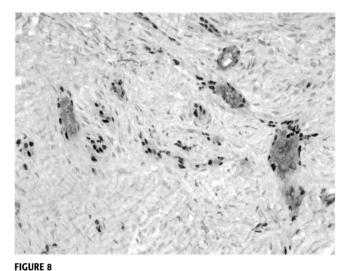

FIGURE 8

p63 immunostaining of field in Figure 7 highlights reserve cell layer, confirming a benign HP and excluding invasive carcinoma.

SYRINGOMA

DEFINITION—A benign adnexal tumor with eccrine differentiation.

CLINICAL FEATURES

EPIDEMIOLOGY

- Higher incidence in women and Asians.
- More frequently identified in trisomy 21 patients.

PRESENTATION

- Small (<4 mm) flesh-colored papules with a symmetrical distribution.
- Most commonly found on the lower eyelid but can also affect the vulva.
- Often appear around puberty.
- Can be pruritic, which is exacerbated by pregnancy and warm weather.

PROGNOSIS AND TREATMENT

- Excellent.
- For symptomatic lesions, laser ablation has been used.

PATHOLOGY

HISTOLOGY

- Intersecting epithelial strands and ducts forming comma-shaped structures (tadpoles) set within an eosinophilic fibrous stroma.
- The ductlike structures are characterized by two cell layers.
- The nuclei are bland, and mitoses are infrequent.

IMMUNOPATHOLOGY (INCLUDING IMMUNOHISTOCHEMISTRY)

- Not needed, although p63 highlights the basal epithelial layer.

MAIN DIFFERENTIAL DIAGNOSIS

- Fox-Fordyce disease.

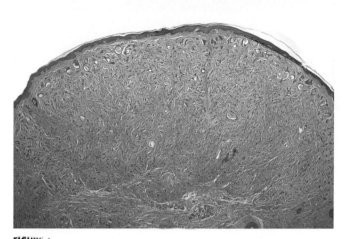

FIGURE 1

Syringoma, seen here at low magnification as a well-circumscribed lesion.

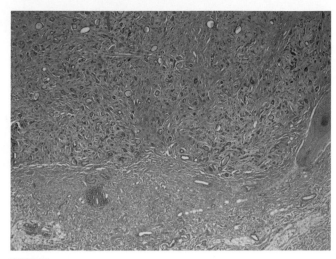

FIGURE 2

Syringoma. The lesion–stromal interface is uniformly demarcated.

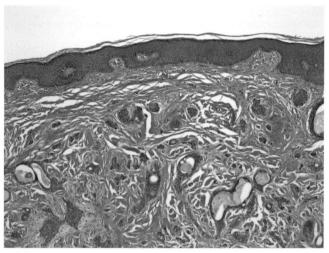

FIGURE 3

Syringoma. Note the angulated comma-shaped epithelial structures.

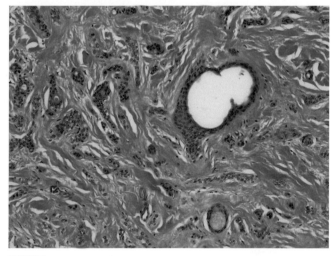

FIGURE 4

Syringoma. Some ectatic ductal structures are admixed with the others.

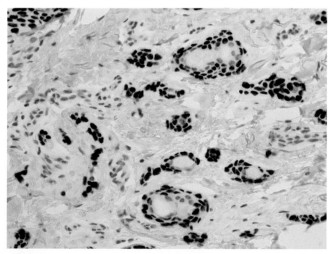

FIGURE 5

Syringoma. A p63 immunostain highlights the basal cells in a two-cell-layered epithelium.

HYPERPLASIA OF BARTHOLIN'S GLAND

DEFINITION—An increase in the number of Bartholin's glands with preservation of normal architecture.

CLINICAL FEATURES

EPIDEMIOLOGY

- Seen in a wide age range.
- Hyperplasia of Bartholin's glands generally occurs at a younger age than adenoma.

PRESENTATION

- May present as a mass-forming lesion.

PROGNOSIS AND TREATMENT

- Excellent prognosis.
- Cured by excision.

PATHOLOGY

HISTOLOGY

- A general increase in the number of Bartholin's glands.
- Ductal and acinar architecture are preserved.

- Coexisting inflammation and squamous metaplasia may also be present.

IMMUNOPATHOLOGY (INCLUDING IMMUNOHISTOCHEMISTRY)

- Noncontributory.

MAIN DIFFERENTIAL DIAGNOSIS

- Bartholin's duct cyst or abscess—may be confused clinically.
- Bartholin's gland adenoma—loss of gland to duct orientation.

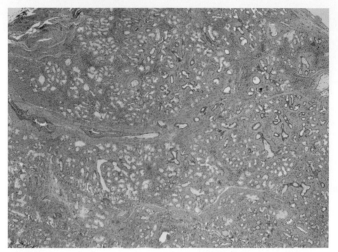

FIGURE 1

Bartholin's gland hyperplasia. Increased numbers of mucinous Bartholin's glands can be seen. There is a preservation of the normal lobular architecture.

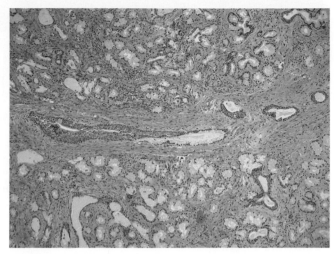

FIGURE 2

Bartholin's gland hyperplasia. At higher power, emphasizing the preservation of the ducts (centrally).

BARTHOLIN'S ADENOMA

DEFINITION—An increase in the number of Bartholin's glands with a generalized loss of architecture.

CLINICAL FEATURES

EPIDEMIOLOGY

- Occurs across a wide age range; however, adenomas generally occur at an older age.
- Very rare.

PRESENTATION

- May present as a mass-forming lesion, mimicking a Bartholin's gland cyst.
- May also present with pain.

PROGNOSIS AND TREATMENT

- Favorable prognosis.
- The majority of lesions are cured by excision.
- Rare cases have been associated with a concomitant malignancy (adenocarcinoma).

PATHOLOGY

HISTOLOGY

- Increased numbers of Bartholin's glands with a loss of the normal architecture (i.e., haphazard growth pattern).

- As in hyperplasia, squamous metaplasia and inflammation may be present.

IMMUNOPATHOLOGY (INCLUDING IMMUNOHISTOCHEMISTRY)

- Noncontributory.

MAIN DIFFERENTIAL DIAGNOSIS

- Bartholin's duct cyst or abscess—may be confused clinically. Gland structures will be seen in the wall of the cyst.
- Bartholin's gland hyperplasia—duct structures are preserved.
- Malignancy (clinically).

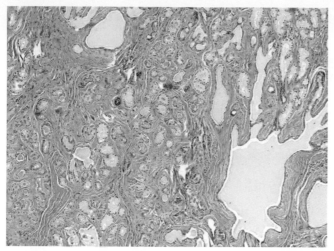

FIGURE 1

Bartholin's gland adenoma. Medium-magnification view of numerous, haphazardly arranged glands comprising a Bartholin's adenoma.

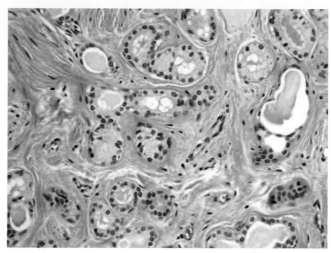

FIGURE 2

Bartholin's gland adenoma. Disorganized glands with abundant eosinophilic cytoplasm and innocuous, regular nuclei.

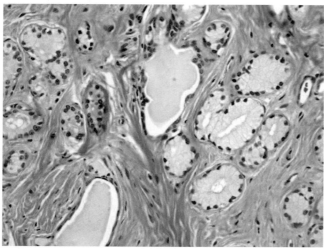

FIGURE 3

Bartholin's gland adenoma. Occasional glands may show cystic dilatation and irregular contours.

ADENOID CYSTIC CARCINOMA

DEFINITION—A slow-growing/indolent malignancy derived from the Bartholin's gland with a tendency for late metastasis.

CLINICAL FEATURES

EPIDEMIOLOGY

- Very rare.
- Accounts for less than 1% of vulvar malignancies.
- Wide age range, with an average age in the fourth decade.

PRESENTATION

- Mass-forming lesion in the area of the Bartholin's gland.
- Slow growing, may be present for months or years.

PROGNOSIS AND TREATMENT

- Treatment includes wide local excision.
- Slow growth, frequent recurrence, and a tendency toward late distant metastases to lymph nodes and lung.
- Reported 5-year survival is 70%.

PATHOLOGY

HISTOLOGY

- At low power the tumor fills and expands the background Bartholin's gland ducts and is composed of small, bland cells arranged in two patterns.
- The first pattern is a cribriform or microcystic pattern in which nests of cells form small pseudoduct-like spaces with thin, delicate septae.
- The second pattern is characterized by nests, cords, or reticular arrangements of small blue cells set in an eosinophilic hyaline matrix.

IMMUNOPATHOLOGY (INCLUDING IMMUNOHISTOCHEMISTRY)

- Luminal secretions are periodic acid–Schiff (PAS) positive.

MAIN DIFFERENTIAL DIAGNOSIS

- Hidradenoma (will exhibit two cell layers with p63+ basal cells).
- Adenoid variant of basal cell carcinoma (located superficial rather than deep).
- Myoepithelioma (benign mixed tumor).
- Poorly differentiated basaloid carcinomas—usually seen in the vagina and cervix.
- Adnexal or apocrine carcinoma—superficial, exhibits marked atypia.

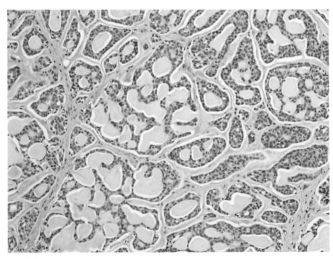

FIGURE 1

Adenoid cystic carcinoma. Adenoid cystic carcinoma showing a predominantly cribriform architecture, marked by large nests of monomorphic tumor cells with pseudoglandular spaces.

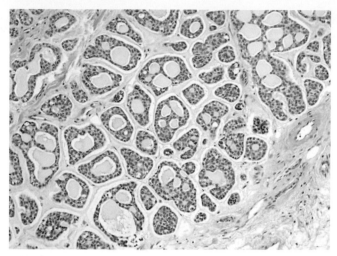

FIGURE 2

Adenoid cystic carcinoma. Small nests of cells without pseudoglandular spaces may be appreciated in the lower half of this photomicrograph.

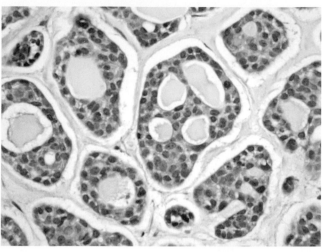

FIGURE 3

Adenoid cystic carcinoma. High-power detail of nests of tumor cells with monomorphic cells with bland nuclei. Note the hazy, amphophilic luminal secretions that will stain positive with PAS.

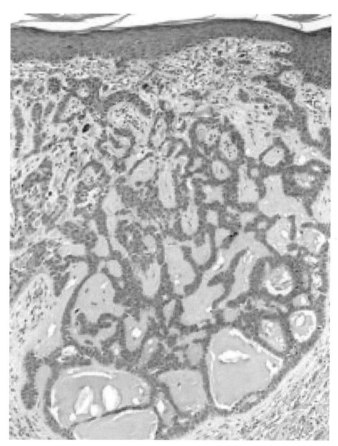

FIGURE 4

Basal cell carcinoma, adenoid variant. This is superficially situated.

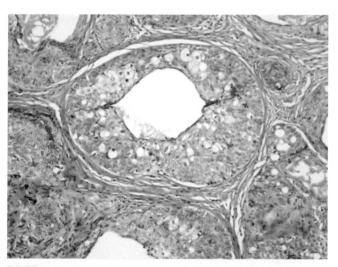

FIGURE 5

Adenocarcinoma with apocrine features. Note the high-grade nuclei.

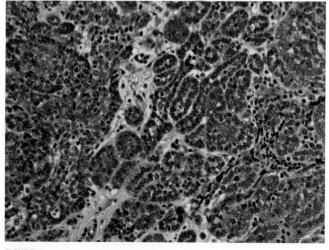

FIGURE 6

Basaloid carcinoma. This tumor consists of a primitive-appearing population of simple glands. It is typically seen in the apex of the vagina or cervix.

BARTHOLIN'S GLAND CARCINOMA

DEFINITION—A malignancy arising in the Bartholin's glands or ducts.

CLINICAL FEATURES

EPIDEMIOLOGY

- Very rare.
- Incidence of approximately one per million.
- Approximately 75% are squamous carcinomas, and the remainder include adenoid cystic carcinoma; adenocarcinoma, not otherwise specified (NOS); epithelial–myoepithelial carcinoma; and neuroendocrine carcinoma.

PRESENTATION

- Typically present as a mass that may be slow growing.

PROGNOSIS AND TREATMENT

- Excision and node dissection, similar to other forms of vulvar carcinoma.
- Prognosis is dependent on stage and tumor type, with neuroendocrine carcinomas having a poor prognosis and most patients dying within 2 years.

PATHOLOGY

HISTOLOGY

- At low power the tumor fills and expands the background Bartholin's gland ducts and is composed of small, bland cells arranged in two patterns.

- The first pattern is a cribriform, or microcystic, pattern in which nests of cells form small pseudoduct-like spaces with thin, delicate septae.
- The second pattern is characterized by nests, cords, or reticular arrangements of small blue cells set in an eosinophilic hyaline matrix.

IMMUNOPATHOLOGY (INCLUDING IMMUNOHISTOCHEMISTRY)

- Luminal secretions are periodic acid–Schiff (PAS) positive.

MAIN DIFFERENTIAL DIAGNOSIS

- Hidradenoma (will exhibit two cell layers with p63+ basal cells).
- Adenoid variant of basal cell carcinoma (located superficial rather than deep).
- Myoepithelioma (benign mixed tumor).
- Poorly differentiated basaloid carcinomas—usually seen in the vagina and cervix.
- Adnexal or apocrine carcinomas—superficial, exhibit marked atypia.

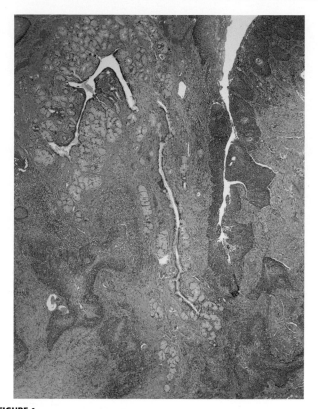

FIGURE 1

Adenoid cystic carcinoma. Adenoid cystic carcinoma showing a predominantly cribriform arrangement, marked by large nests of monomorphic tumor cells with pseudoglandular spaces.

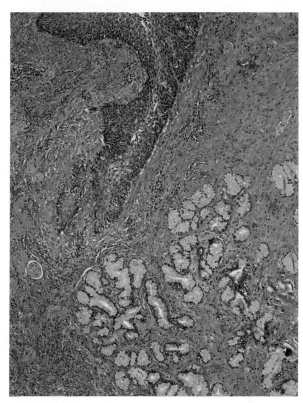

FIGURE 2

Adenoid cystic carcinoma. Small nests of cells without pseudoglandular spaces may be appreciated in the lower half of this photomicrograph.

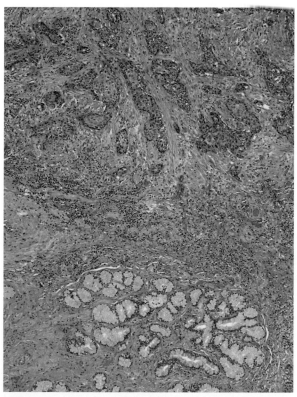

FIGURE 3

Adenoid cystic carcinoma. High-power detail of nests of tumor cells with monomorphic cells with bland nuclei. Note the hazy, amphophilic luminal secretions that will stain positive with PAS.

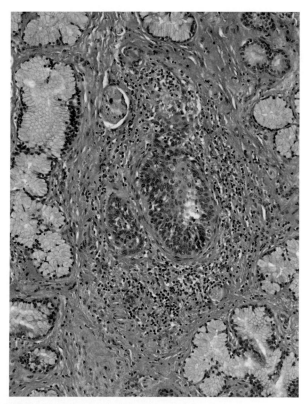

FIGURE 4

Basal cell carcinoma, adenoid variant. This is superficially situated.

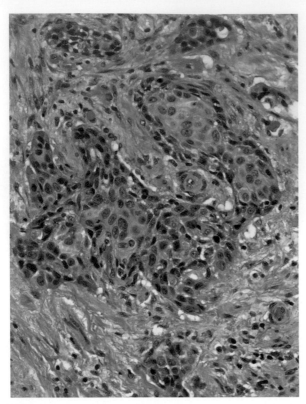

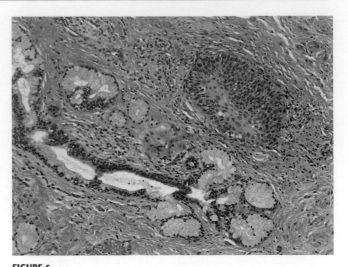

FIGURE 6

Basaloid carcinoma. This tumor consists of a primitive-appearing population of simple glands. It is typically seen in the apex of the vagina or cervix.

FIGURE 5

Adenocarcinoma with apocrine features. Note the high-grade nuclei.

CONDYLOMA

DEFINITION—Benign squamous tumors caused by infection of human papillomavirus (HPV). In this chapter condyloma includes two verruciform variants: classic condyloma and fibroepithelial papilloma. A third, seborrheic, keratosis-like condyloma will be discussed separately.

CLINICAL FEATURES

EPIDEMIOLOGY

- Very common sexually transmitted tumors that are most commonly (~80%) caused by infection of HPV 6 or 11.
- Approximately one million women are affected each year. Disease is most common in young, sexually active women.

PRESENTATION

- Presentation may range from small macules or papules to large lesions that affect the entire vulva.
- Smaller lesions may coalesce.

PROGNOSIS AND TREATMENT

- Excellent; the majority of lesions in patients regress in 6 weeks or less.
- Lesions that progress may be treated with fluorouracil (5-FU), Aldara, cryotherapy, or carbon dioxide laser.

PATHOLOGY

HISTOLOGY

- Classic lesions consist of papillary, "spirelike" proliferations of stratified squamous epithelium supported by fibrovascular stroma.
- Typically acanthosis, parakeratosis, hyperkeratosis, and superficial koilocytosis are present.
- Many lesions, however, will have little to no cytopathic (koilocytic) changes, often termed fibroepithelial papillomas.
- Many "condylomas" will closely resemble seborrheic keratoses seen on skin.

- The combination of papillomatosis and acanthosis is strongly suggestive of the diagnosis of a condyloma.

IMMUNOPATHOLOGY (INCLUDING IMMUNOHISTOCHEMISTRY)

- Ki-67 will show increased proliferative activity in the upper epidermal layers, but it may be subtle.
- Staining with p16 is patchy (as opposed to strong, diffuse staining in high-grade lesions associated with high-risk HPVs).
- In situ hybridization for HPV (low risk) will show nuclear reactivity.

MAIN DIFFERENTIAL DIAGNOSIS

- Fibroepithelial papilloma and seborrheic keratoses are managed (at least in premenopausal women) as variants of condyloma.
- Pseudobowenoid papulosis—an unusual variant of HPV infection (presumably low risk) that manifests with many apoptotic cells.
- Fibroepithelial stromal polyp—lacks the verruciform acanthosis of condyloma.
- Verruciform lichen simplex chronicus—lacks the characteristic cytopathic effect seen in condyloma.
- Vulvar acanthosis with altered differentiation—surface epithelial pallor instead of cytopathic effect.
- Verrucous carcinoma—an important differential when faced with large lesions. Beware the diagnosis of verrucous carcinoma in a young woman.
- Verruciform squamous cell carcinoma—marked atypia is the rule.
- Keratoacanthoma—a cup-shaped acanthosis.
- Classic vulvar intraepithelial neoplasia (VIN)—prominent atypia in at least the basal two thirds of the epithelium.
- Papillary squamous cell carcinoma—high proliferative index and atypia.

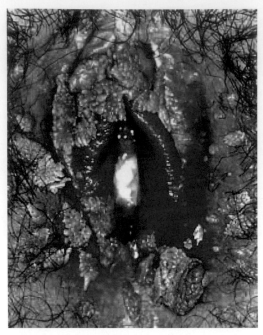

FIGURE 1

Condyloma acuminatum. Multiple small white lesions at the introitus. *(Courtesy Alex Ferenczy.)*

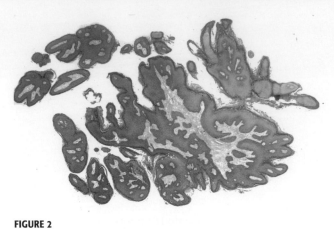

FIGURE 2

Low-power scanning image details the acanthosis and papillomatosis of multiple condylomata.

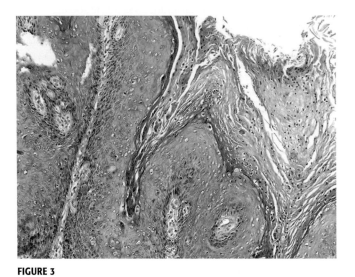

FIGURE 3

Condyloma acuminatum. Prominent "spirelike" projections are present, along with marked acanthosis, hyperkeratosis, and hypergranulosis. Note the lack of conspicuous parabasal nuclear atypia.

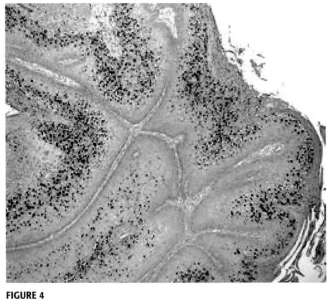

FIGURE 4

Condyloma acuminatum depicting strong nuclear staining for low-risk (corresponding to HPV 6) HPV nucleic acids. *(Courtesy Lisa Jensen-Long, Ventana Medical Systems.)*

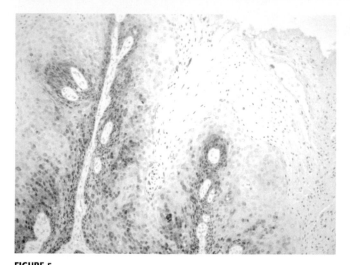

FIGURE 5

Condyloma acuminatum with immunostaining for p16. Note the patchy basal positivity.

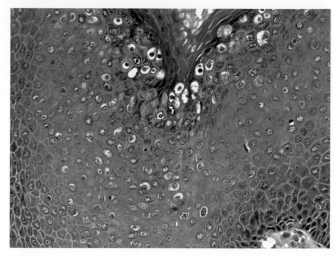

FIGURE 6

This condyloma contains less striking koilocytotic atypia. The acanthosis and papillomatosis are the key features in the diagnosis, since atypia will vary.

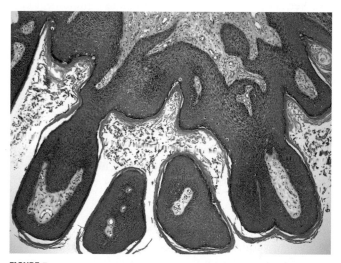

FIGURE 7

Nonkoilocytotic variant of condyloma (fibroepithelial papilloma).

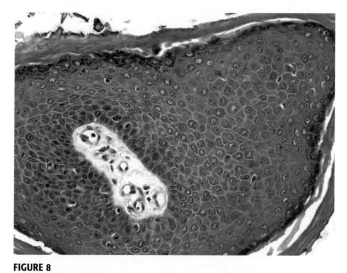

FIGURE 8

At higher magnification, fibroepithelial papilloma displays no atypia. Nonetheless, in this setting it is synonymous with condyloma.

VERRUCIFORM XANTHOMA

DEFINITION—Verruciform xanthoma is a solitary benign verrucous lesion of the vulva that contains foamy histiocytes in the lamina propria.

CLINICAL FEATURES

- Middle-aged women.
- Solitary wartlike growth on the genital area.
- No relationship to human papillomavirus (HPV).

PATHOLOGY

HISTOLOGY

- Uniform repetitive verruciform architecture.
- Superficial dyskeratosis with variable acute inflammatory changes, resembling but not quite the same as parakeratosis.
- The hallmark is numerous foamy histiocytes in the stroma of the papillae.
- Absence of koilocytosis or surface atypia.

IMMUNOHISTOCHEMISTRY

- Not applicable.

DIFFERENTIAL DIAGNOSIS AND PITFALLS

- Condyloma acuminatum, including seborrheic keratosis variants. This entity will manifest with surface atypia.
- Verruciform lichen simplex chronicus—prominent keratohyalin granules and absence of xanthoma cells.
- Candida infection due to the focal surface inflammatory exudate, foam cell absent.
- Psoriasis due to the small plaques of dyskeratotic epithelial cells, foam cell absent.
- Granular cell myoblastoma. This lesion may be associated with epithelial hyperplasia, but the granular cells can easily be distinguished from foamy histiocytes.
- Verrucous carcinoma and its precursor verruciform acanthosis are usually more irregular in growth and lack the foamy histiocytes.

CLINICAL MANAGEMENT/OUTCOME

- Verruciform xanthoma is a benign condition that is not infectious and in rare cases will recur following removal.

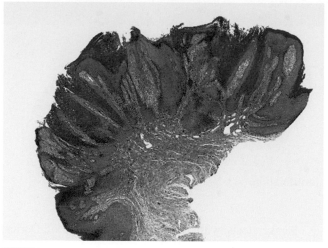

FIGURE 1

Verruciform xanthoma at low magnification. Note the regularity of the verrucous architecture and eosinophilic layers of pseudoparakeratosis (dyskeratosis) on the surface.

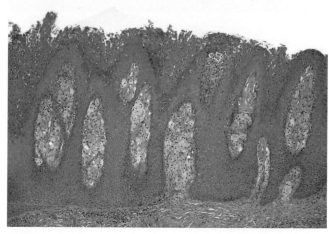

FIGURE 2

At medium magnification the dense layer of surface dyskeratosis is visible, resembling that seen in psoriasis.

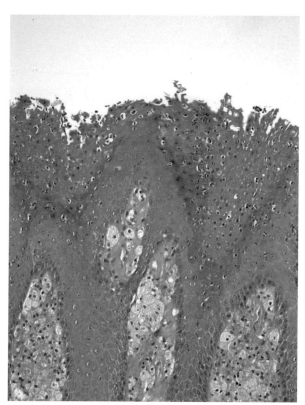

FIGURE 3

At higher magnification the foamy histiocytes in the dermis can be seen.

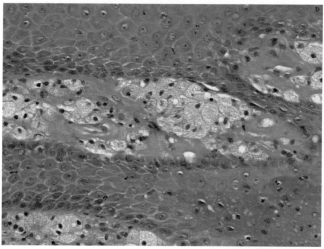

FIGURE 4

High magnification of the foamy histiocytes.

WARTY DYSKERATOMA

DEFINITION—A solitary acanthotic and dyskeratotic epidermal proliferation.

CLINICAL FEATURES

EPIDEMIOLOGY

- Rare disease, most often seen in the head and neck regions.
- Very rarely involves the vulva.
- Not an inherited condition (as opposed to Darier's disease).

PRESENTATION

- Solitary keratotic papule or nodule.
- May be umbilicated.

PROGNOSIS AND TREATMENT

- Prognosis is excellent as these are benign lesions.
- Excision is adequate treatment.

PATHOLOGY

HISTOLOGY

- Acanthotic and hyperkeratotic plaques.
- Dyskeratosis is frequently present, presenting as corps ronds.

- Parakeratosis with retained nuclei (grains of Darier) may be present as well.
- Acantholysis can occasionally lend a prominent pseudopapillary architecture.
- Warty dyskeratoma frequently has a more pronounced papillary architecture than Darier's disease.

IMMUNOPATHOLOGY (INCLUDING IMMUNOHISTOCHEMISTRY)

- Immunofluorescence is negative.

MAIN DIFFERENTIAL DIAGNOSIS

- Darier's disease—multiple lesions, familial.
- Acantholytic hyperkeratosis—does not have the prominent grains of Darier.
- Verruciform vulvar intraepithelial neoplasia (VIN)—exhibits marked atypia.
- Viral warts (condyloma)—lack the prominent grains of Darier and acantholysis.

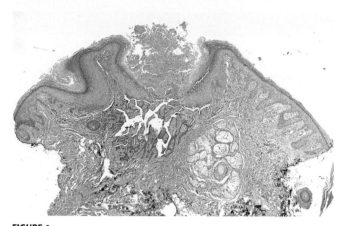

FIGURE 1

Low magnification of a warty dyskeratoma. Note the cup-shaped lesion with dense hyperkeratosis.

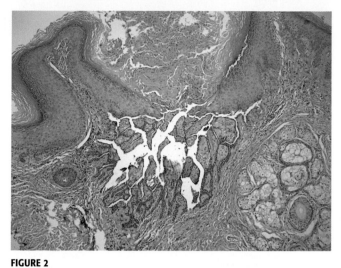

FIGURE 2

Higher magnification reveals the striking acantholysis, revealing the bare dermal papillae in a pseudopapillary conformation.

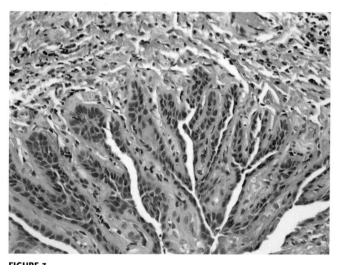

FIGURE 3

Higher magnification of the pseudopapillary appearance at the interface of the acantholysis.

FIBROEPITHELIAL STROMAL POLYP

DEFINITION—Benign polypoid vulvovaginal lesions of young- to middle-aged women with a striking array of histologic appearances, often associated with pregnancy.

CLINICAL FEATURES

EPIDEMIOLOGY

- Young- to middle-aged women.
- Multiple lesions are associated with pregnancy.
- Very rare before menarche.

PRESENTATION

- Pedunculated, polypoid, or occasionally fronded lesion(s) of the vulva, vagina, or (occasionally) the cervix.
- Size varies considerably from small (<1 cm) to very large (>10 cm).

PROGNOSIS AND TREATMENT

- Excellent.
- Complete excision is advised as lesions may recur if incompletely excised.

PATHOLOGY

HISTOLOGY

- Bland overlying squamous epithelium.
- Central fibrovascular core, with thick-walled medium-sized vessels.

- Stellate multinucleate stromal cells that are particularly prominent at the stromal–epithelial interface and a margin that blends imperceptibly with surrounding soft tissue.
- Particularly during pregnancy, the stroma may be more cellular, with strikingly pleomorphic stromal cells and atypical mitotic figures (pseudosarcoma botryoides).

IMMUNOPATHOLOGY (INCLUDING IMMUNOHISTOCHEMISTRY)

- Desmin positive; estrogen and progestin receptors are variable.

MAIN DIFFERENTIAL DIAGNOSIS

- Aggressive angiomyxoma—these are deeper lesions with a zone of normal tissue separating the mucosa, plus a distinct vascular pattern.
- Condyloma—there should be acanthosis and variable verruciform epithelial growth.

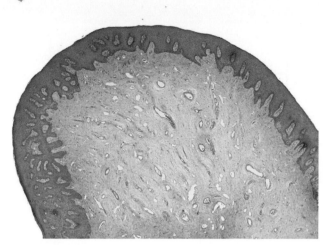

FIGURE 1

Fibroepithelial stromal polyp. A polypoid projection with an unremarkable, albeit acanthotic, squamous lining. The stroma is relatively hypocellular, and there are numerous small- to medium-sized vessels present.

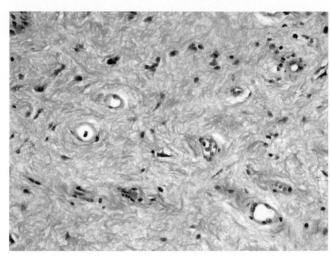

FIGURE 2

Fibroepithelial stromal polyp. Paucicellular stroma with small, bland, stromal cells. Numerous small vessels are present.

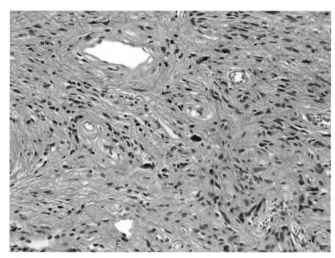

FIGURE 3

Fibroepithelial stromal polyp. Occasional polyps may be more hypercellular or contain atypical stromal cells. These are not signs of malignancy.

SEBORRHEIC KERATOSIS

DEFINITION—A benign, warty proliferation of keratinocytes that is frequently pigmented and often associated with low-risk human papillomavirus (HPV) (types 6 and 11).

CLINICAL FEATURES

EPIDEMIOLOGY

- Can be seen in all age groups.
- A large percentage are associated with HPV types 6 and 11, implying a variant of condyloma (or low-grade squamous intraepithelial lesion). Presumably a subset of HPV-negative lesions also exists.

PRESENTATION

- Maculopapular lesions that appear "stuck on."
- Seborrheic keratosis (SK) may be skin colored or hyperpigmented.
- Usually asymptomatic, although some patients report pruritus or irritation.
- Lesions range in size from several millimeters to several centimeters.

PROGNOSIS AND TREATMENT

- Excellent prognosis.
- Conservative excision is curative but not required.

PATHOLOGY

HISTOLOGY

- A benign epidermal proliferation characterized by acanthosis with hyperkeratosis and pseudohorn cysts, which are invaginations of the epithelial surface.
- The lesions appear raised and are thickened compared with the adjacent normal epithelium.
- The base is flat and exhibits the so-called string sign; one can imagine holding a piece of string taut along the base.

- There is a variable amount of melanin pigment; in hyperpigmented examples most of the pigment has been taken up by the lesional keratinocytes.
- A range of epithelial architectural patterns have been identified in SK, including clonal, reticular, hyperkeratotic, and verrucous. These variants are important only to recognize the variety of appearances possible in SK.
- Reactive epithelial changes are common in traumatized lesions and can include reactive cytologic atypia, dyskeratosis, spongiosis, and increased mitoses.

Diagnostic terms: In younger individuals where the lesion presents as a presumed condyloma the diagnosis of "condyloma with features of SK" is appropriate. For SKs presenting with minimal acanthosis or wartlike features, a diagnosis of unqualified "SK" is appropriate.

IMMUNOPATHOLOGY (INCLUDING IMMUNOHISTOCHEMISTRY)

- p16 immunostains will be patchy or negative, in keeping with low-risk HPV.
- KI67 (MIB1) stains will usually highlight cells in the upper epithelial layers similar to other variants of condyloma.

MAIN DIFFERENTIAL DIAGNOSIS

- Condyloma—typically contains koilocytotic atypia but overlaps etiologically with SK.
- Nevus (epidermal)—linear in distribution and can be seen in young patients.
- Vulvar intraepithelial neoplasia, low grade (VIN I) or "bowenoid dysplasias"—some bland-appearing HPV 16 infections of the vulva may overlap with SK. Typically staining for p16 will be strongly positive in such lesions in contrast to SK.

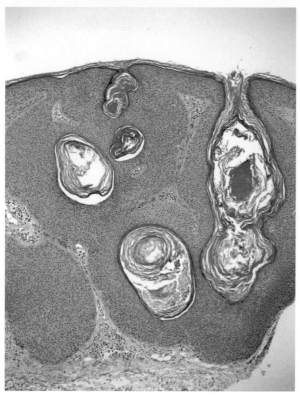

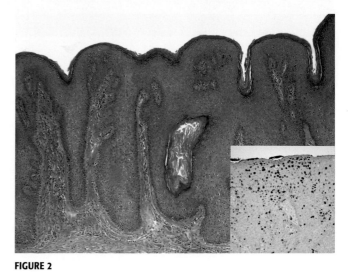

FIGURE 2

Seborrheic keratosis. Slightly more subtle variant but discrete acanthosis. MIB1 immunostaining *(inset)* depicts numerous positive nuclei in the upper epithelial layers.

FIGURE 1

Seborrheic keratosis. Prominent acanthosis with pseudohorn cysts.

PSEUDOBOWENOID PAPULOSIS

PITFALL

DEFINITION—An unusual variant of condyloma that is marked by a striking increase in apoptosis in the upper epithelial layers.

CLINICAL FEATURES

EPIDEMIOLOGY

- Occurs in the same demographic groups as typical condyloma; however, disease is secondary to more uncommon variants of human papillomavirus (HPV) such as types 13 and 32.

PRESENTATION

- Small to large macular or papular lesions.

PROGNOSIS AND TREATMENT

- Favorable, similar outcome as seen in traditional condyloma acuminata.

PATHOLOGY

HISTOLOGY

- The upper epithelial layers display a striking increase in apoptotic cells.

- These cells are in different stages of degeneration, ranging from chromatin dispersal (which may appear similar to a mitotic figure [i.e., pseudomitoses]) to small hypereosinophilic (degenerated) keratinocytes.
- Koilocytic atypia is usually not seen.

Diagnostic terminology: Low-grade squamous intraepithelial lesion (condyloma/VINI).

IMMUNOPATHOLOGY (INCLUDING IMMUNOHISTOCHEMISTRY)

- Ki-67 may be increased in the upper epidermis.
- Staining for p16 is patchy.

MAIN DIFFERENTIAL DIAGNOSIS

- Fibroepithelial papilloma or condyloma—these lesions do not contain apoptosis.
- Seborrheic keratosis—may resemble pseudobowenoid papulosis but lacks apoptosis and pseudomitoses.
- Classic vulvar intraepithelial neoplasia (VIN)—overlaps histologically because of the apoptosis, but the remainder of the keratinocytes will display atypia, unlike pseudobowenoid papulosis.

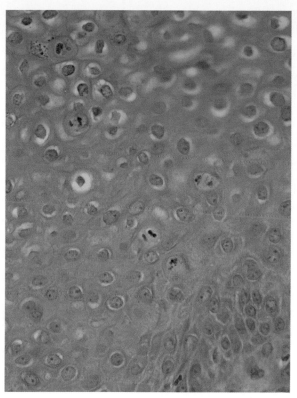

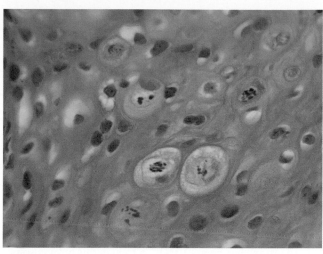

FIGURE 2

Pseudobowenoid papulosis. Apoptotic bodies in different stages of degradation, some of which resemble mitotic figures. The centrally clumped chromatin is surrounded in some by a collapsing cell membrane with another space between the membrane and the interface with the adjacent cells. This creates a targetlike appearance.

FIGURE 1

Pseudobowenoid papulosis. Note the presence of some koilocytes interspersed with pseudomitoses. The remainder of the epithelial cells show minimal atypia.

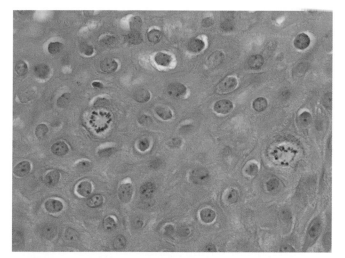

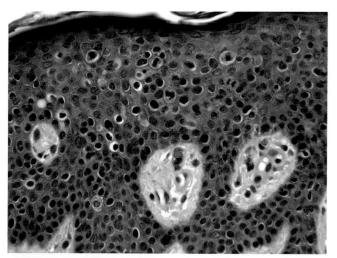

FIGURE 3

Pseudobowenoid papulosis. A few apoptotic cells with uniformly circumferentially dispersed chromatin.

FIGURE 4

This variant of VIN contains a mild to moderate degree of diffuse nuclear atypia with some apoptotic cells in the upper layers and may be confused with the pseudobowenoid papulosis variant of condyloma.

FLAT CONDYLOMA (VIN1)

DEFINITION—Flat condyloma is defined as a macular variant of condyloma that falls within the category of low-grade squamous intraepithelial lesion (LSIL) and displays an identical distribution of atypia as its exophytic counterpart. In contrast to exophytic condylomas, these flat lesions are more likely to be associated with high-risk human papillomavirus (HPV) types, although the majority do not contain HPV 16 and the regression rate is presumably high. Another term for these lesions has been "VIN1," although this term is somewhat problematic. Currently they are under the category of LSILs of the vulva, similar to exophytic condylomas and their variants.

CLINICAL FEATURES

- Reproductive age, sexually active women.
- Small papular or raised vulvar lesions, similar to condyloma.
- Acetowhite.

PATHOLOGY

HISTOLOGY

- Discrete acanthosis.
- Variable cytopathic effect (koilocytosis).
- Mild to moderate hypercellularity in the lower epithelial cell layers.
- In some instances cytopathic effect is minimal, and the lesion resembles a macular seborrheic keratosis.

IMMUNOHISTOCHEMISTRY/MOLECULAR FINDINGS

- Ki-67 expression is moderate, and staining in the upper epithelial layers is present due to expression of viral genes in superficial (koilocytotic) cell nuclei.
- p16ink4 expression is variable and not helpful diagnostically.
- A wide range of HPVs, with HPV 16 present in less than 15%.

DIFFERENTIAL DIAGNOSIS AND PITFALLS

- Koilocytotic (warty) vulvar intraepithelial neoplasia II (VIN II) will have greater atypia in the lower epithelial layers.

CLINICAL MANAGEMENT/OUTCOME

- Most flat condylomas are managed conservatively by observation or with topical (Aldara) therapy.

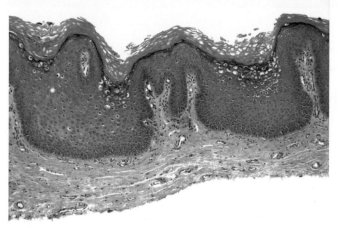

FIGURE 1

Flat condyloma (LSIL) with koilocytotic atypia. Note the basal hypercellularity without appreciable atypia.

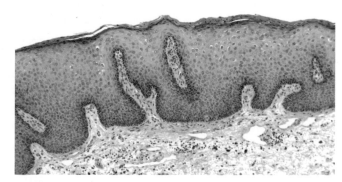

FIGURE 2

A flat condyloma (LSIL) with no evidence of koilocytotic atypia. There is prominent hypercellularity, as well as parakeratosis, present within the basal aspect.

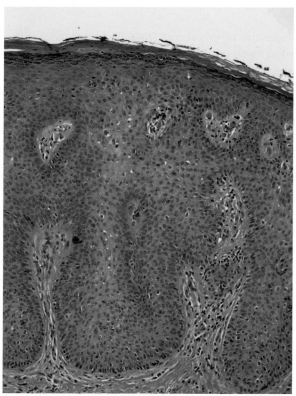

FIGURE 3

A flat lesion resembling seborrheic keratosis, also within the category of LSIL.

CLASSIC (USUAL) VULVAR INTRAEPITHELIAL NEOPLASIA

DEFINITION—Classic (usual) high-grade squamous intraepithelial lesions of the vulva are defined as full-thickness or near full-thickness atypias associated with high-risk or carcinogenic human papillomavirus (HPV) infections, principally HPV 16.

CLINICAL FEATURES

- A wide age range, from second to eighth decade, predominating in the fourth and fifth decades.
- From papular to verrucous in presentation, pigmented or nonpigmented.
- Increased frequency in immunosuppressed women.
- Acetowhite in the mucosal surfaces.

CLINICAL MANAGEMENT/OUTCOME

- Outcome is strongly associated with age, with the risk of both progression and coexistence of invasion (20%) associated with postmenopause.
- Spontaneous regression is associated with pigmented lesions, younger age, and pregnancy.
- Smoking and immunosuppression both are associated with persistence and resistance to therapy.
- Local excision is preferred, followed by laser or in small lesions topical imiquimod (Aldara).

PATHOLOGY

HISTOLOGY

- Increased cellularity with hyperchromasia and a high cell density.
- Anisokaryosis, polychromasia, and coarse chromatin, usually involving at least the lower two thirds of the epithelial thickness.

- Variable maturation ranging from minimal (basaloid) to conspicuous with pseudokoilocytosis (warty).
- Abnormal mitoses (multipolar, irregular, dispersed).
- Pigmentation (variable).

Diagnostic terminology: High-grade squamous intraepithelial lesion (vulvar intraepithelial neoplasia [VIN] II and III).

IMMUNOHISTOCHEMISTRY

- Ki-67 expression is usually near full thickness due to loss of cell cycle control throughout the epithelium but may be less pronounced in some cases.
- p16ink4 expression is usually diffuse and linear in the immature component and typically both cytoplasmic and nuclear.
- p53 staining is negative or patchy (nuclear).

DIFFERENTIAL DIAGNOSIS AND PITFALLS

- Seborrheic keratosis—minimal nuclear atypia, negative for p16.
- Pseudobowenoid papulosis—apoptotic cells (pseudomitoses) may mimic mitotic activity, but basal layers exhibit minimal atypia, negative for p16.
- Multinucleate atypia—polynucleation, which is uncommon in classic VIN; low proliferative index; negative for p16.

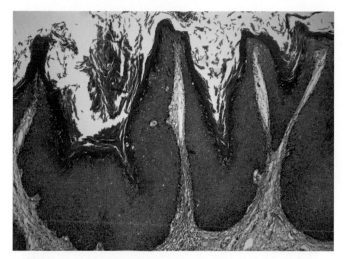

FIGURE 1
Classic VIN. This case exhibits a verruciform or warty pattern.

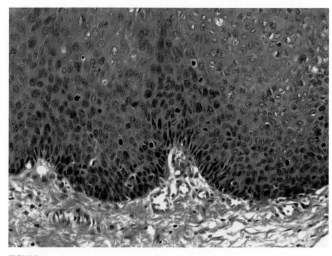

FIGURE 2
Classic VIN. At higher magnification the immature cells show marked atypia.

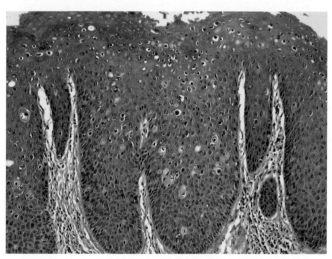

FIGURE 3
Classic VIN. This is a slightly less mature variant of classic VIN.

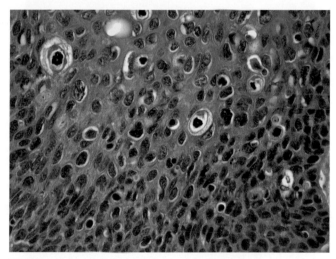

FIGURE 4
Classic VIN. Note the prominent apoptosis and individual cell keratinization.

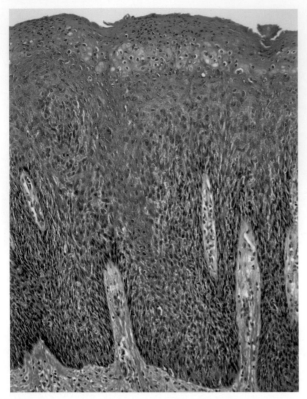

FIGURE 5
Classic VIN. This variant is rather homogeneous in appearance.

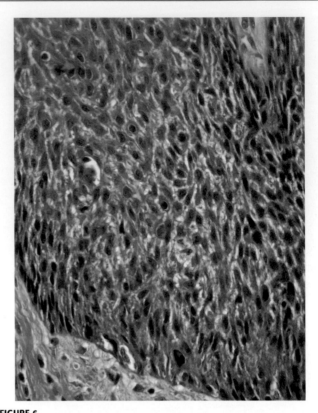

FIGURE 6
Classic VIN. At high power the cells are uniform but in this case uniformly abnormal.

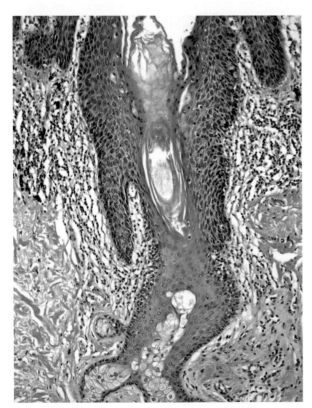

FIGURE 7
Classic VIN. An example of adnexal involvement.

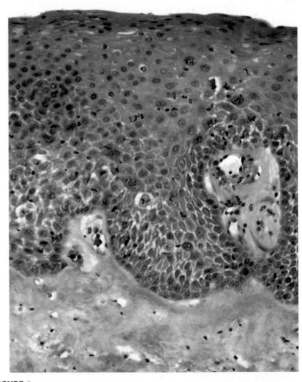

FIGURE 8
Classic VIN. This HPV 16–positive example was associated with lichen sclerosus.

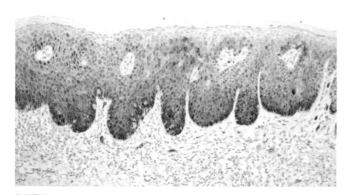

FIGURE 9
Classic VIN. Immunohistochemical staining for p16 shows both nuclear and cytoplasmic positivity in the immature component.

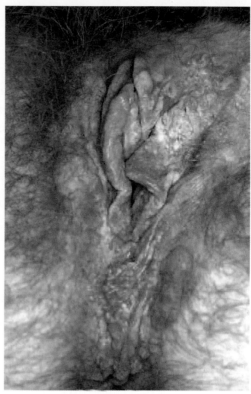

FIGURE 10
Classic VIN presenting as raised, thickened mucosa with hyperkeratosis.

CLASSIC VULVAR INTRAEPITHELIAL NEOPLASIA WITH LICHEN SIMPLEX CHRONICUS

PITFALL

DEFINITION—Human papillomavirus (HPV)-associated squamous intraepithelial lesion (SIL) with superimposed changes of lichen simplex chronicus (LSC).

CLINICAL FEATURES

EPIDEMIOLOGY

- Affects a fraction of the patients with classic vulvar intraepithelial neoplasia (VIN).

PRESENTATION

- Similar to that of classic VIN.
- The plaques, papules, and scaly skin changes seen in LSC are invariably present.

PROGNOSIS AND TREATMENT

- Similar to that of classic VIN.

PATHOLOGY

HISTOLOGY

- Acanthosis with parakeratosis and prominent keratohyalin granules may initially present some confusion because it will be associated with reduced atypia in the upper epithelial layers.
- Variable amounts of chronic inflammatory cells are present within the dermis.

- Squamous cell atypia is mild to moderate and typically more basal in location, mimicking the findings seen in differentiated VIN. In some cases the degree of atypia may be quite subtle.
- Areas with histology more typical of classic VIN are variably present.

DIAGNOSTIC TERMINOLOGY: High-grade squamous intraepithelial lesion (HSIL) (or low-grade squamous intraepithelial lesion [LSIL]) with superimposed LSC. If uncertain as to lesion grade, simply classify as SIL with superimposed LSC and comment that the lesion is of intermediate grade (VIN I–VIN II).

IMMUNOPATHOLOGY (INCLUDING IMMUNOHISTOCHEMISTRY)

- p16 will stain cells diffusely within the basal compartment, with maturing cells in the upper epidermal layers showing a lack of staining.
- Ki-67 demonstrates increased labeling but will be more prominent in the basal epithelial layers.
- p53 immunostains will be weak and patchy.

MAIN DIFFERENTIAL DIAGNOSIS

- LSC—prominent basal atypia is not seen.
- Differentiated VIN—can be more difficult. Immunostaining for p16 (strong) and p53 (weak) may be helpful.

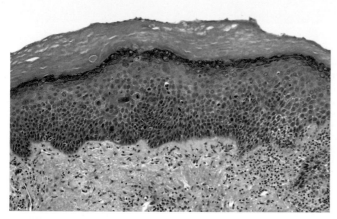

FIGURE 1

Classic VIN with superimposed LSC. Conspicuous hyperkeratosis and hypergranulosis are often present. Expansion of the basal layer and prominent atypia are similar to classic VIN in this case, which would be easily distinguished from differentiated VIN or LSC alone. Note the dermal inflammatory infiltrate.

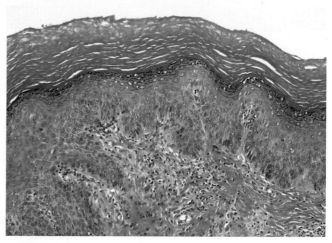

FIGURE 2

A more subtle example of classic VIN with superimposed LSC. Note how much more subtle the atypia is in this case. There is prominent hypergranulosis.

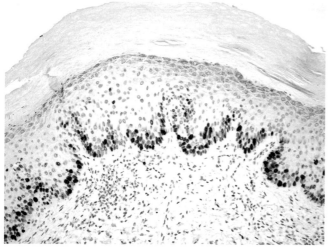

FIGURE 3

MIB-1 immunostain of the case in Figure 2. Note the confinement of the positive cells to the basal portion of the epithelium, similar to LSC.

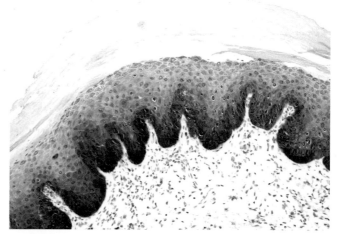

FIGURE 4

Immunostaining for p16 of the above case (in Figure 2) shows intense nuclear and cytoplasmic positivity in the lower half of the epithelium, in keeping with a variant of classic VIN.

CLASSIC VULVAR INTRAEPITHELIAL NEOPLASIA (BOWENOID DYSPLASIA)

DEFINITION—Classic or "usual-type" vulvar intraepithelial neoplasia (VIN) with full-thickness atypia similar to that seen in bowenoid papulosis but with milder atypia.

CLINICAL FEATURES

EPIDEMIOLOGY

- Consists of a fraction of the patients with classic VIN.
- May be seen in younger women.

PRESENTATION

- Similar to that of classic VIN.

PROGNOSIS AND TREATMENT

- Similar to that of classic VIN. Might temporize on management if lesions are small.

PATHOLOGY

HISTOLOGY

- This variant of classic VIN is problematic by virtue of its milder atypia. It overlaps with bowenoid papulosis (i.e., classic VIN).
- Atypia is full thickness but mild.
- An expanded population of basaloid keratinocytes.

Terminology: Squamous intraepithelial lesion, intermediate grade (VIN I-VIN II).

IMMUNOPATHOLOGY (INCLUDING IMMUNOHISTOCHEMISTRY)

- P16 staining should be diffuse.
- Ki-67 demonstrates increased labeling, including cells in the upper epidermis.

MAIN DIFFERENTIAL DIAGNOSIS

- Seborrheic keratosis—p16 stains will be patchy.
- Pseudobowenoid papulosis—similar population of immature keratinocytes. Should be distinguished by the p16 stain.
- Seborrheic keratosis-like condyloma—similar cell population but less atypia; p16 patchy or negative.

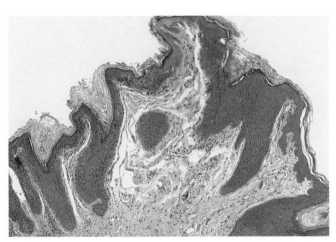

FIGURE 1

Bowenoid dysplasia. Low-power view showing full-thickness loss of maturation but the degree of atypia is mild. Must be distinguished from seborrheic keratosis or pseudobowenoid papulosis.

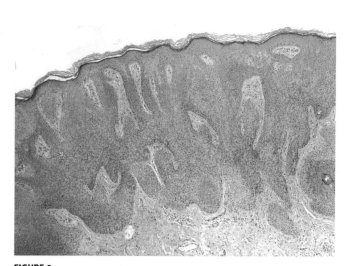

FIGURE 2

Bowenoid dysplasia associated with HPV 16. Another case with acanthosis and monotonous population of immature keratinocytes.

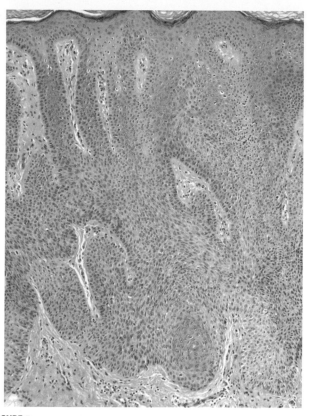

FIGURE 3

Bowenoid dysplasia associated with HPV 16. Note the resemblance to seborrheic keratosis.

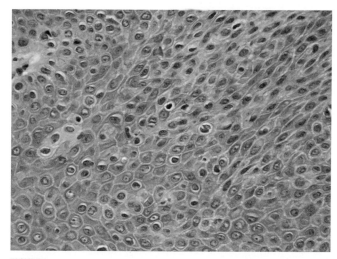

FIGURE 4

Bowenoid dysplasia. At high magnification there is modest variation in nuclear size.

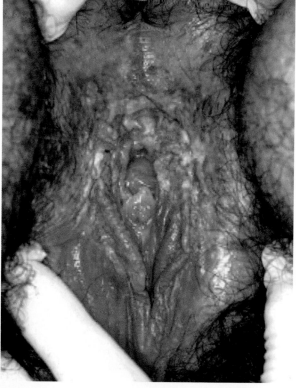

FIGURE 5

Pigmented bowenoid VIN in a reproductive-age woman.

PAGETOID VULVAR INTRAEPITHELIAL NEOPLASIA

PITFALL

DEFINITION—An unusual variant of vulvar intraepithelial neoplasia (VIN) in which the more poorly differentiated cells invade the overlying mature squamous epithelium.

CLINICAL FEATURES

EPIDEMIOLOGY

- Rare, affects a small fraction of the patients with classic VIN.

PRESENTATION

- Similar to that of classic VIN.

PROGNOSIS AND TREATMENT

- Similar to that of classic VIN.

PATHOLOGY

HISTOLOGY

- The less-differentiated cells invade the overlying, mature, squamous epithelium.

- The migrating cells may be seen as single cells or clusters admixed with the mature keratinocytes.
- The distribution of the affected cells mimics that of Paget's disease.

IMMUNOPATHOLOGY (INCLUDING IMMUNOHISTOCHEMISTRY)

- p16 stains the abnormal immature cells in both the basal and upper epidermal layers.
- Ki-67 demonstrates increased labeling, including cells in the upper epidermis.

MAIN DIFFERENTIAL DIAGNOSIS

- Paget's disease (histologically).

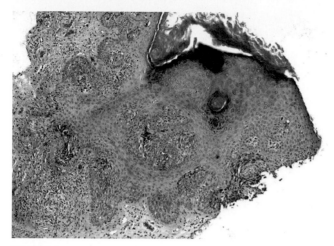

FIGURE 1

Pagetoid VIN. This biopsy specimen depicts discontinuous nests of basophilic cells in the lower epithelium.

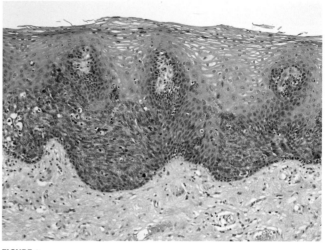

FIGURE 2

Pagetoid VIN. Another pagetoid VIN showing the discontinuous nests of neoplastic squamous cells at higher magnification.

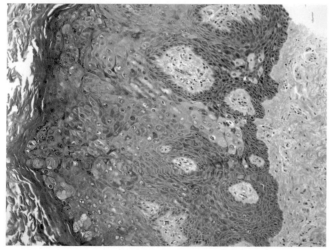

FIGURE 3

A third case of pagetoid VIN showing dyskeratosis in the neoplastic cells.

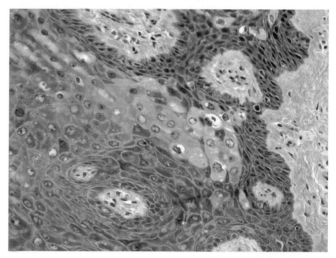

FIGURE 4

Dyskeratotic pagetoid squamous cells at higher magnification.

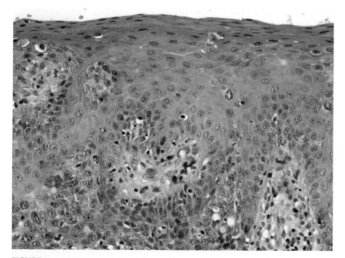

FIGURE 5

Small clusters of neoplastic squamous cells situated higher in the epidermis.

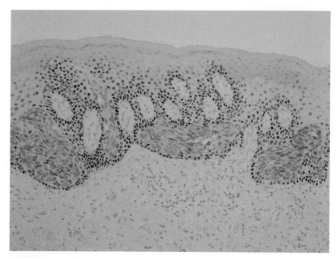

FIGURE 6

This stain for p63 highlights both the normal basal squamous cells and the neoplastic nests, distinguishing them from columnar-derived cells of conventional Paget's disease. The lighter-staining pagetoid squamous cells contrast sharply with the normal basal keratinocytes.

VULVAR INTRAEPITHELIAL NEOPLASIA WITH COLUMNAR DIFFERENTIATION

PITFALL

DEFINITION—A rare variant of vulvar intraepithelial neoplasia (VIN) with lesional columnar (i.e., mucinous) cells.

CLINICAL FEATURES

EPIDEMIOLOGY

- Rare, affects a small fraction of the patients with classic VIN.

PRESENTATION

- Similar to that of classic VIN.

PROGNOSIS AND TREATMENT

- Similar to that of classic VIN.

PATHOLOGY

HISTOLOGY

- Atypical mucinous columnar epithelial cells admixed with typical squamous cells.

- The columnar cells may show only mild pleomorphism.
- May cause diagnostic confusion with Paget's disease or extension from a urothelial carcinoma.

IMMUNOPATHOLOGY (INCLUDING IMMUNOHISTOCHEMISTRY)

- p16 stains the immature cells in both the basal and upper epidermal layers.
- Ki-67 demonstrates increased labeling, including cells in the upper epidermis.
- Mucicarmine highlights mucin-containing cells in difficult cases.

MAIN DIFFERENTIAL DIAGNOSIS

- Paget's disease (histologically).
- Urothelial carcinoma (histologically).

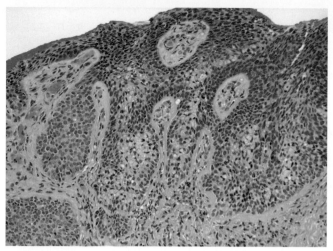

FIGURE 1

Classic VIN with columnar differentiation. Classic, high-grade, basaloid VIN with admixed mucin-containing cells.

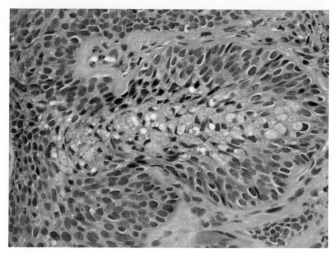

FIGURE 2

Classic VIN with columnar differentiation. Immature, dysplastic squamous cells with admixed mucinous cells. Note the pale blue cytoplasm.

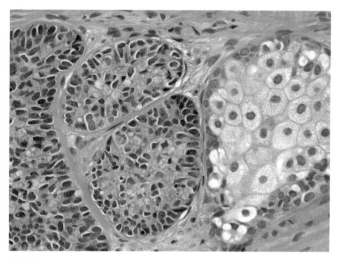

FIGURE 3

Classic VIN with columnar differentiation. In this example the mucinous cells are the predominant component. Increased mitotic figures are present.

EPIDERMODYSPLASIA VERRUCIFORMIS–LIKE ATYPIA

PITFALL

DEFINITION—A variant of epithelial atypia associated with gamma papillomaviruses, classically associated with epidermodysplasia verruciformis (EDV) but now appreciated in immunosuppressed (including human immunodeficiency virus [HIV]–infected) patients and involves the vulva.

CLINICAL FEATURES

- A wide age range.
  - Multiple plaque or papular to verrucous in presentation, pigmented or nonpigmented.
  - May resemble condyloma, seborrheic keratosis, or psoriasis.
- Increased frequency in HIV-infected or immunosuppressed women.
- Can be seen on any cutaneous or mucosal site.

CLINICAL MANAGEMENT/OUTCOME

- Conservative local excision or topical Aldara is the rule.
- Treatment of the underlying immune suppression although it may or may not ameliorate the disorder.
- Risk of progression to malignancy is low.

PATHOLOGY

HISTOLOGY

- Enlarged keratinocytes in the upper epidermis with gray-blue cytoplasm.
  - Enlarged, round nuclei with pale chromatin, and one or multiple nucleoli.
- Basal atypia variable.

IMMUNOHISTOCHEMISTRY

- Ki-67 expression is usually near full thickness due to loss of cell cycle control throughout the epithelium but may be less pronounced in some cases.
- p16ink4 expression may vary. Diffuse staining is not the rule.
- p53 staining is negative or patchy (nuclear).

DIFFERENTIAL DIAGNOSIS AND PITFALLS

- Seborrheic keratosis—minimal nuclear atypia, negative for p16.
- Pseudobowenoid papulosis—apoptotic cells (pseudomitoses) may mimic mitotic activity, but basal layers exhibit minimal atypia, negative for p16.
- Multinucleate atypia—polynucleation, which is uncommon in classic vulvar intraepithelial neoplasia (VIN); low proliferative index; negative for p16.

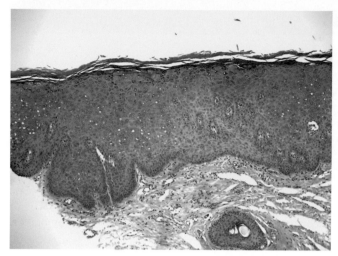

FIGURE 1

EDV-like atypia in an immunosuppressed patient. There is mild hyperkeratosis, and the acanthotic epithelium is punctuated by basophilic clusters of maturing keratinocytes.

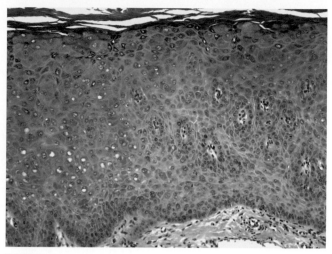

FIGURE 2

EDV-like atypia. At higher magnification of Figure 1, note the clustered groups with basophilia. Note the lower third of the epithelium exhibits minimal crowding or atypia in this field.

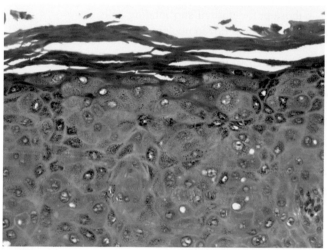

FIGURE 3

Higher magnification of the surface cell layers. The cytoplasm is punctuated by fine keratohyalin granules.

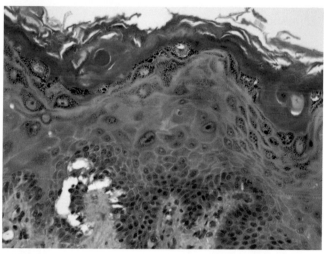

FIGURE 4

In this field there is focal nuclear enlargement, suspended in the middle of the epithelium with prominent nucleoli.

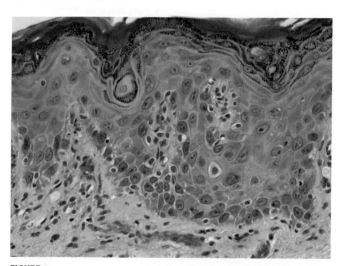

FIGURE 5

This field more closely resembles a classic VIN except for the prominent nucleoli.

POLYNUCLEATED ATYPIA OF THE VULVA

DEFINITION—A reactive epithelial process seen in skin or vulva characterized by a cytoskeletal defect with accumulation of nuclei in individual cells (multinucleation).

CLINICAL FEATURES

EPIDEMIOLOGY

- No particular demographic other than an association with nonspecific, chronic, irritative, or inflammatory changes in the vulva. Similar changes can be seen in cutaneous dermatoses.

PRESENTATION

- Flesh-colored mucocutaneous papules. Lesions may be pruritic or painful in keeping with the underlying condition.

PROGNOSIS AND TREATMENT

- A benign condition likely superimposed on a dermatosis. Management of the dermatological condition will suffice. The impact of this entity lies in its potential misdiagnosis as a condyloma or vulvar intraepithelial neoplasia (VIN).

PATHOLOGY

HISTOLOGY

- Mild acanthosis, normal maturation, and no appreciable nuclear enlargement.

- Keratinocytes in the lower to middle epithelium exhibit multiple nuclei.
- The nuclei are normochromatic and identical in size to those in the normal surrounding cells.
- As many as a dozen nuclei may be seen in a single cell.

Diagnostic Terminology: Benign squamous mucosa with reactive epithelial changes.

IMMUNOHISTOCHEMISTRY

- Not necessary, but Mib-1 and p16ink4 stains will be negative (normal distribution). These cells are human papillomavirus (HPV) negative.

MAIN DIFFERENTIAL DIAGNOSIS

- Condyloma—these have superficial nuclear atypia, and there is nuclear enlargement.
- VIN II and III—these lesions may have multinucleation but like condyloma the nuclei are abnormal, as is the rest of the epithelium.
- Viral (herpetic) changes—characteristic viral cytopathic effect with inclusions.

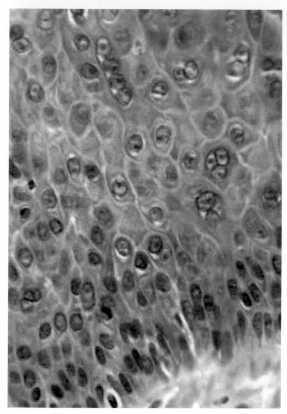

FIGURE 1

Multinucleated atypia of the vulva (MAV). Note the presence of keratinocytes in the lower and middle epithelial layers with two or more nuclei. Note also the lack of chromatin abnormalities and similarities in size to the adjacent normal mononuclear cells.

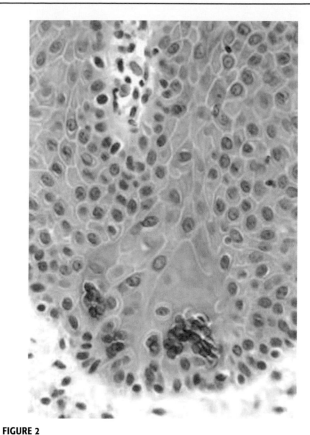

FIGURE 2

MAV. One basal-oriented cell in particular contains numerous nuclei.

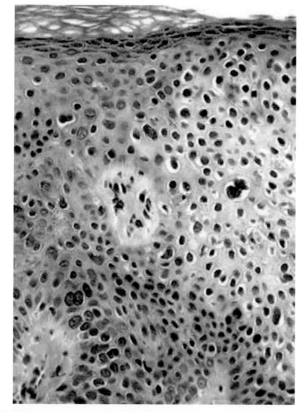

FIGURE 3

VIN with multinucleation. This should be easily distinguished from MAV by the additional nuclear abnormalities.

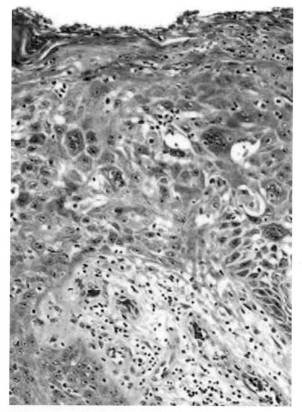

FIGURE 4

Herpetic infections of the vulva can also manifest with multinucleation but are distinguished by the characteristic presentation (usually with inflammation and ulceration) and viral inclusions.

DIFFERENTIATED VULVAR INTRAEPITHELIAL NEOPLASIA

DEFINITION—Vulvar intraepithelial neoplasia (VIN) that likely is secondary to a series of host gene alterations that are discrete from those involved in classic VIN.

CLINICAL FEATURES

EPIDEMIOLOGY

- Occurs in postmenopausal women but can be seen earlier.
- Associated with less than 5% of all diagnosed cases of VIN.
- Typically associated with chronic vulvar inflammatory disease (lichen sclerosus or lichen simplex chronicus).

PRESENTATION

- Typically presents with symptoms and signs associated with lichen sclerosus and lichen simplex chronicus.
- Lesions tend to be less conspicuous clinically.

PROGNOSIS AND TREATMENT

- Most differentiated VINs (DVINs) are found in association with keratinizing squamous cell carcinomas. Outcome of isolated cases is uncertain, but they are approached as cancer precursors.
- Conservative excision of lesions and biopsy of new and/ or suspicious lesions in patients with DVIN are recommended.
- Most are not typically managed with topical therapy due to the severity of the underlying vulvar inflammatory process.

PATHOLOGY

HISTOLOGY

- Best appreciated as variable and sometimes subtle forms of atypia, and there is no sharp cutoff between lichen simplex chronicus and DVIN.

- Basal atypia is the rule and is characterized by variable hyperchromasia, nuclear enlargement, and nucleoli.
- Foci of accentuated keratinization.
- Foci of prominent spongiosis or acantholysis often present.
- Occasional variants demonstrate expansion of the basal cell layer and may mimic classic VIN.

IMMUNOPATHOLOGY (INCLUDING IMMUNOHISTOCHEMISTRY)

- p53 staining is often, if not invariably, diffuse and moderate to marked in degree. Depending on the degree of basal cell expansion, involved cell layers will be from one to several and occasionally near full thickness.
- Ki-67 may also be focally increased in the basal layers but will parallel the degree of immaturity and is not a reliable marker.
- p16 staining is typically negative or patchy, distinguishing DVIN from classic VIN.

MAIN DIFFERENTIAL DIAGNOSIS

- Psoriasis—similar architecture but lacks the basal atypia.
- Spongiotic dermatitis—basal cells will display minimal atypia.
- Candida vulvitis—may mimic a hypertropic DVIN but lacks atypia.
- Lichen sclerosus and lichen simplex chronicus—can be distinguished by degree of atypia. p53 immunostaining might help in making the distinction.

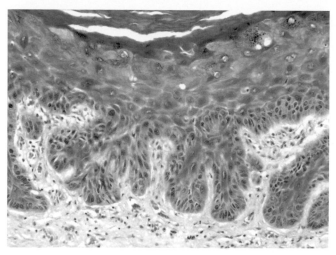

FIGURE 1

DVIN. Striking basal atypia consisting of hyperchromasia and irregular nuclear contours is seen in the first two to three cell layers.

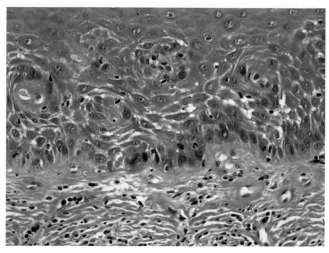

FIGURE 2

DVIN. This DVIN exhibits a more subtle but definite basal atypia.

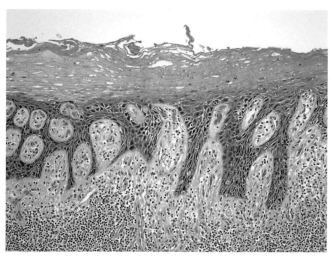

FIGURE 3

DVIN. This example has an expanded basal layer with conspicuous atypia.

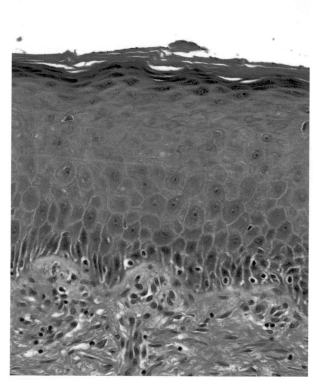

FIGURE 4

Nonneoplastic squamous mucosa for comparison.

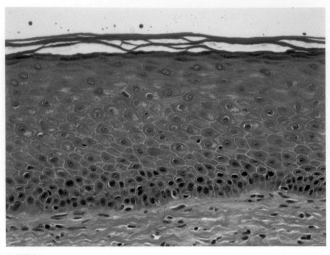

FIGURE 5

First of a series of biopsy specimens from the same patient. This is below the threshold for DVIN.

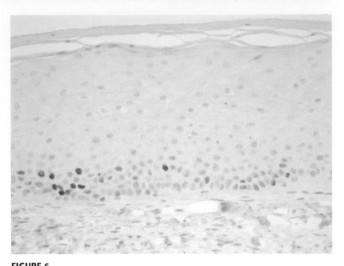

FIGURE 6

Immunostaining of Figure 5 for p53 shows sporadic staining.

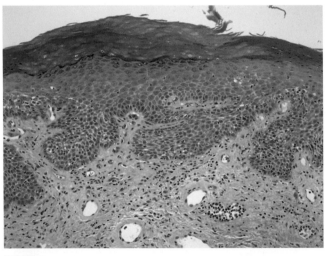

FIGURE 7

An adjacent field shows slightly higher accentuation of the basal layer.

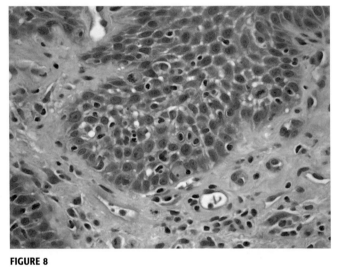

FIGURE 8

At higher magnification the basal cells display subtle enlargement with prominent nucleoli.

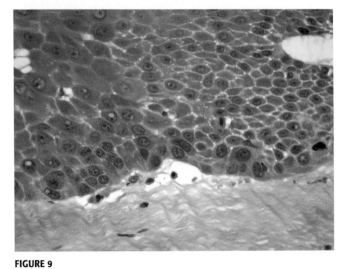

FIGURE 9

An adjacent field displays even greater basal atypia. Note the abnormal keratinization in the upper left of the panel.

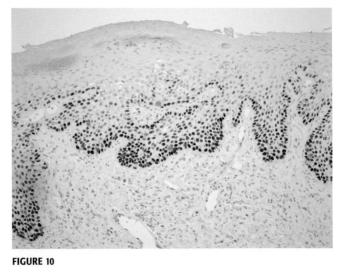

FIGURE 10

A p53 stain of this area (in Figures 7 to 9) shows strong multilayered p53 staining.

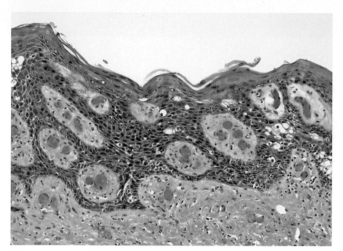

FIGURE 11

Prominent basal cell expansion in a DVIN mimics classic VIN.

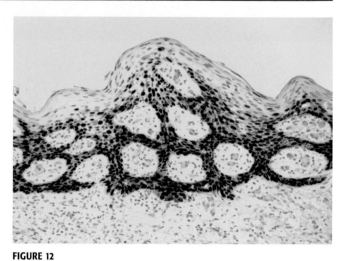

FIGURE 12

A p53 stain is strong in all layers. In essence, the distribution of p53 parallels the degree of basal cell expansion. The latter appears to increase as a function of lesion severity.

VERRUCIFORM LICHEN SIMPLEX CHRONICUS

DEFINITION—A clinical and pathologic response to continued physical trauma comprised of markedly thickened skin with verruciform changes along with erythema and plaquelike scaling.

CLINICAL FEATURES

EPIDEMIOLOGY

- Seen in all demographic groups; however, has been associated with vulvar cancer and verrucous carcinoma.

PRESENTATION

- Patients typically present with a history of irritation/pruritus. Clinically the skin is markedly thickened with surrounding erythema and overlying plaquelike scale. Excoriation is frequently present. Normal physiologic skin markings may be exaggerated.

PROGNOSIS AND TREATMENT

- Prognosis—can be associated with vulvar carcinoma, and regular follow-up (especially in older patients) is warranted.
- Treatment—breaking of the irritant/trauma cycle with or without topical steroids. Patient education and behavioral modification. Close clinical follow-up.

PATHOLOGY

HISTOLOGY

- Acanthosis with hyperkeratosis and hypergranulosis is present in varying degrees. A variable mononuclear cell infiltrate is present in the superficial dermis.
- Verruciform features may mimic other verruciform lesions.

IMMUNOPATHOLOGY (INCLUDING IMMUNOHISTOCHEMISTRY)

- Usually noncontributory, although p53 immunostains should be negative with heterogeneous staining in the lower epithelial layers.

MAIN DIFFERENTIAL DIAGNOSIS

- Verrucous carcinoma—there is less hypergranulosis, with superficial epithelial pallor and bulbous downgrowth (blunt invasion).
- Fungal infection (tinea cruris)—may overlap with verruciform lichen simplex chronicus (LSC). Fungal stains should be considered in the appropriate clinical context.
- Differentiated vulvar intraepithelial neoplasia (VIN)—verruciform variants exist and overlap with verruciform LSC. p53 immunostaining may help (but not always) make this distinction.

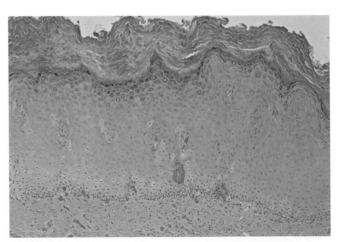

FIGURE 1

Verruciform LSC. There is mild verruciform architecture with hypergranulosis. No atypia is seen.

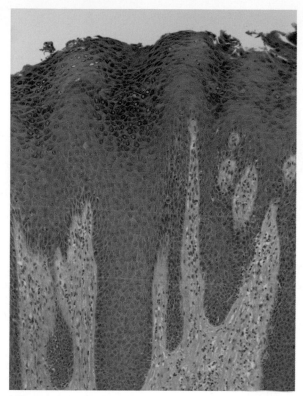

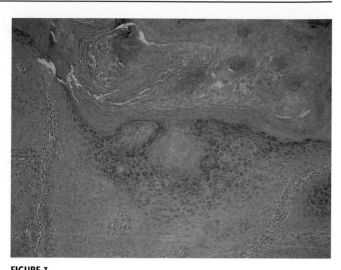

FIGURE 3

Verruciform LSC. Note the thickening of the epithelium with some verruciform architecture and slight papillomatosis.

FIGURE 2

Verruciform LSC. There is mild elongation of the rete.

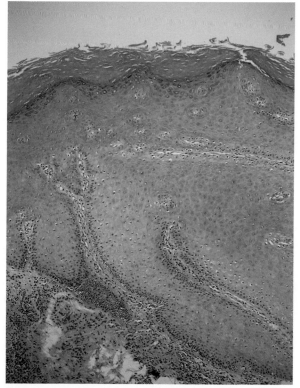

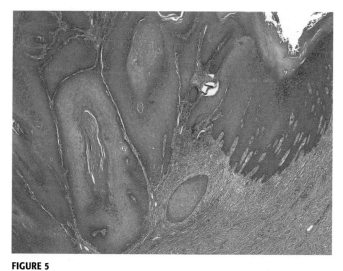

FIGURE 5

Verruciform LSC *(right)* merging with a verrucous carcinoma *(left)*.

FIGURE 4

Verruciform LSC. Again note the absence of basal atypia.

VULVAR ACANTHOSIS WITH ALTERED DIFFERENTIATION (ATYPICAL VERRUCIFORM HYPERPLASIA)

DEFINITION—Vulvar acanthosis with altered differentiation (VAAD) is defined as vulvar acanthosis with variable verruciform architecture that lacks the nuclear atypia characteristic of vulvar intraepithelial neoplasia (VIN) but exhibits abnormalities in keratinocyte differentiation. It is classed as a risk factor for squamous carcinoma. For the purposes of this discussion, we will address this entity and potential mimics.

CLINICAL FEATURES

EPIDEMIOLOGY

- Menopausal and postmenopausal women.
- Associated with lichen sclerosus, lichen simplex chronicus (LSC), and verruciform LSC.

PRESENTATION

- Patchy verruciform or exophytic growth on the vulva.

PROGNOSIS AND TREATMENT

- VAAD may be associated with verrucous carcinoma or well-differentiated squamous carcinoma.
- Conservative removal and follow-up, with attention to any new lesions.

PATHOLOGY

HISTOLOGY

- Acanthosis.
- Variable verruciform architecture.
- Layers of parakeratosis.
- Epithelial cytoplasmic pallor near the surface.
- Limited downward elongation of the rete pegs.
- Virtually no interface atypia.

Terminology: Either epithelial hyperplasia or acanthosis with altered differentiation, with the proviso that this is not considered a precancer (no nuclear atypia) but merits follow up with biopsy of any new or suspicious lesions.

IMMUNOHISTOCHEMISTRY

- Ki-67, p16, and p53 staining will be unremarkable.

DIFFERENTIAL DIAGNOSIS AND PITFALLS

- Differentiated VIN will exhibit *interface atypia*.
- Verrucous carcinoma will demonstrate similar features but will exhibit *blunt invasion*.
- Classic VIN will exhibit conspicuous and usually near full-thickness atypia (excepting classic VIN with superimposed LSC).
- Verruciform LSC will contain prominent keratohyalin granules and does not contain prominent parakeratosis and epithelial pallor.
- Pseudoepitheliomatous hyperplasia lacks either nuclear or cytoplasmic atypia.
- Inverted keratosis—a regular pattern of pearl-like formation without atypical cytoplasmic differentiation (squamous eddies).
- Verruciform xanthoma—foamy macrophages in the lamina propria, pseudoparakeratosis.

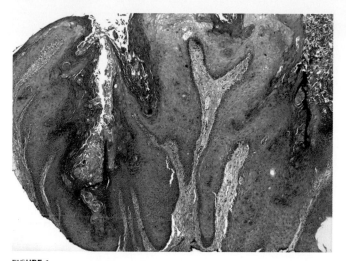

FIGURE 1

VAAD. This low-power image illustrates acanthosis with verruciform architecture.

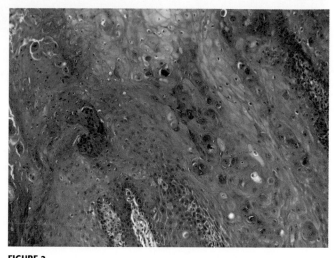

FIGURE 2

Higher magnification of VAAD. Note the prominent dyskeratosis and lack of atypia.

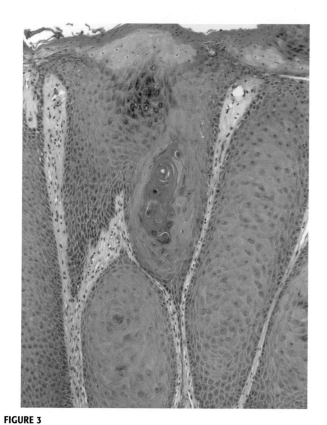

FIGURE 3

VAAD showing some abnormalities in superficial cytoplasmic differentiation with epithelial cell pallor and parakeratosis. This is not specific for this entity because similar changes can be seen in reactive epithelia.

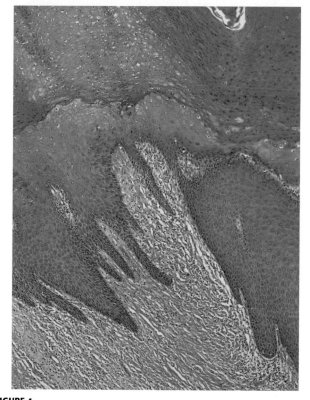

FIGURE 4

VAAD. Note the surface epithelial pallor and parakeratosis.

EARLY INVASIVE SQUAMOUS CELL CARCINOMA

DEFINITION—Invasion less than 2 cm in diameter and to a depth of less than 1 mm below the highest epithelial–stromal interface.

EPIDEMIOLOGY

- A wide age range, from second to eighth decade, predominating in the fifth and sixth decades.
- Patients typically present with vulvar intraepithelial neoplasia (VIN). Approximately 20% of VINs in older women harbor areas of early invasion.

CLINICAL MANAGEMENT/OUTCOME

- Risk of metastases is essentially zero for lesions that fulfill the criteria for "microinvasion."
- Wide local excision is preferred. Regional lymph node sampling may be done if there is regional lymph node enlargement or other clinical concerns, such as multiple foci of invasion or uncertainty regarding lymphovascular invasion (LVI).
- Lesions invading greater than 1 mm or with LVI have an appreciable (5% to 10%) risk of lymph node metastases.

PATHOLOGY

HISTOLOGY

Patterns of early invasion include

- Confluent growth with an irregular epithelial–stromal interface.

- Discrete tongues of neoplastic epithelium with desmoplasia.
- Irregular intersecting nests with variable size and conformation, as seen with basaloid growth.
- Bulbous pushing invasion. This can be difficult to distinguish from noninvasive adnexal involvement.

Diagnostic Terminology: Superficially invasive squamous cell carcinoma, well, moderate, or poorly differentiated. The lesion measures (numeric value) mm in length and invades to a depth of (numeric value) mm beneath the highest epithelial–stromal interface. LVI is present/absent. The invasive focus is (numeric value) mm from the deep margin, and a minimum of (numeric value) mm from the lateral (radial) margins.

IMMUNOHISTOCHEMISTRY

- Usually noncontributory.

DIFFERENTIAL DIAGNOSIS AND PITFALLS

- Appendage involvement by VIN.
- Pseudoepitheliomatous hyperplasia (in VIN).
- Tangential sectioning.
- Traumatic displacement of neoplastic epithelium in stroma.
- Basal cell carcinoma.

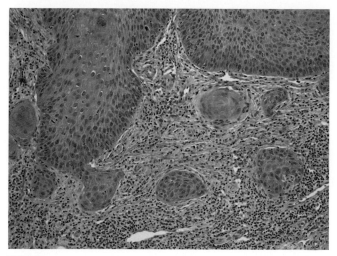

FIGURE 1

Superficially invasive squamous cell carcinoma. Note the small nests beneath the epithelial–stromal interface with a subtle loss of epithelial polarity. One nest is budding from the overlying epithelium.

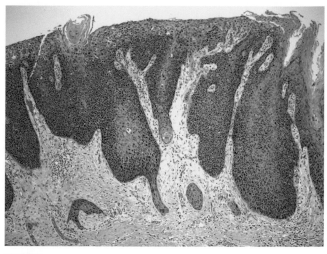

FIGURE 2

Superficially invasive squamous cell carcinoma. These invasive nests are more conspicuous by their irregular shapes, prominent maturation, and desmoplasia.

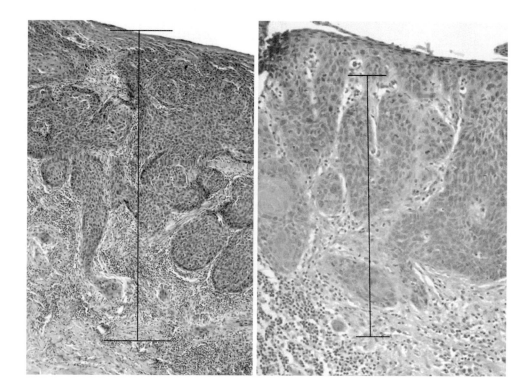

FIGURE 3

Superficially invasive squamous cell carcinoma. Depth is measured, if possible, from the highest adjacent epithelial–stromal interface. If this is not possible a measurement of thickness is sufficient.

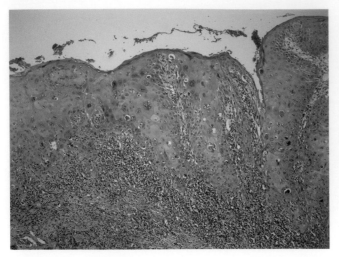

FIGURE 4

Superficially invasive squamous cell carcinoma. This neoplastic epithelium is more difficult to assess because of the inflammation. However, note the obvious loss of epithelial polarity at the base.

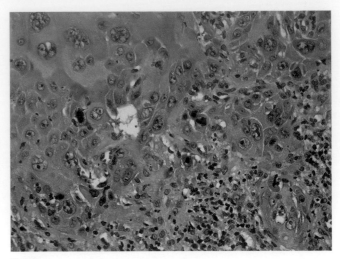

FIGURE 5

Superficially invasive squamous cell carcinoma. The obvious loss of epithelial polarity at the base in Figure 4 is seen at higher power here.

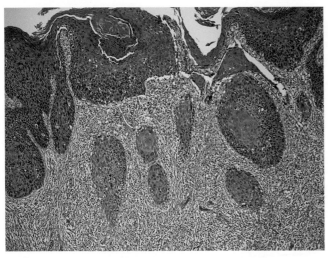

FIGURE 6

Mimic of early invasion. Marked inflammation is present but the nests exhibit a uniform contour.

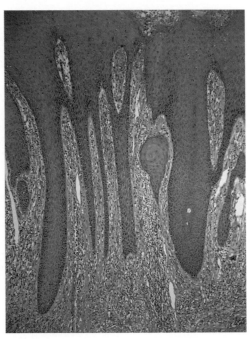

FIGURE 7

Mimic of early invasion. Small foci of dysmaturation within epithelial hyperplasia.

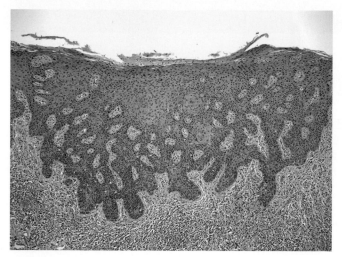

FIGURE 8

Mimic of early invasion. Tangential sectioning of VIN. Note the uniform network of interconnecting basal epithelium.

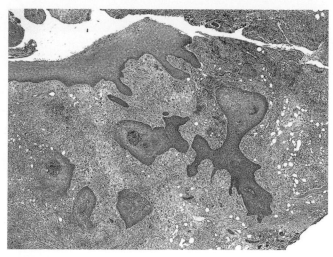

FIGURE 9

Mimic of early invasion. Pseudoepitheliomatous hyperplasia in an inclusion cyst.

VULVAR SQUAMOUS CARCINOMA: BASALOID AND WARTY PATTERNS

DEFINITION—Invasive epithelial neoplasm composed of keratinocytes involving the vulva. Comprise tumors associated with classic vulvar intraepithelial neoplasia (VIN).

CLINICAL FEATURES

EPIDEMIOLOGY

- Typically affects women in their sixth decade but can be seen in women under 40 who are immunocompromised.
- Strong association with human papillomavirus (HPV), particularly HPV 16.
- Usually found associated with classic VIN.
- Some patients present with no history of vulvar neoplasia.
- Strong association with smoking.
- Association with other lesions in the lower genital tract (cervix, vagina).
- Risk increases with increasing age.

PRESENTATION

- May be seen in the clinical context of classic VIN symptoms (pruritus, pain, or bleeding).
- Will often complicate VIN in women aged over 50.

PROGNOSIS AND TREATMENT

- Guarded, patients with localized, resectable disease have a variable recurrence rate.
- Patients with documented nodal spread at the time of first treatment have a recurrence rate of 30% to 70% if they do not receive adjuvant radiation therapy.
- Recurrence in the groin carries a mortality of about 90% even if the groin was not treated at the time of initial diagnosis.
- Localized recurrence may be treated with re-excision or radiation.
- Surgical resection with lymph node dissection is the most common treatment approach.
- There is increasing interest in sentinel lymph node excision to decrease morbidity.

- Tumors that are papillary without stromal penetration have an excellent prognosis.

PATHOLOGY

HISTOLOGY

INVASION CRITERIA
- Differentiating invasive disease from high-grade VIN may be difficult, especially in cases with extensive inflammation.
- Classic features of invasion include irregular epithelial profiles in the stroma, desmoplasia, loss of cellular polarity, and vascular space invasion.
- In addition, the following patterns are strongly suggestive of invasion (and warrant further sampling if invasion is not found):
  1. Cohesive "intraepithelial-like" invasive patterns (associated with classic VIN).
  2. Linear pavementlike clusters of poorly differentiated epithelium with a discrete epithelial–stromal interface but excessive architectural complexity.
  3. Well-differentiated, infiltrative-appearing patterns with high nuclear grade.
  4. Well-differentiated cohesive clusters with a moderate to high nuclear grade.

DIFFERENTIATION PATTERNS
- Well to poorly differentiated cohesive growth patterns (warty or basaloid) with well-circumscribed nests of tumor cells. These nests frequently have smooth, undulating borders and resemble intraepithelial neoplasia (intraepithelial like).
- Papillary carcinomas with striking similarity to papillary squamous cell carcinomas in the cervix. These show exophytic, filiform papillae that are lined by a well-polarized squamous epithelium. These may be difficult to distinguish from high-grade squamous intraepithelial

lesions (HSIL) (VIN2 and VIN3) and may display a sharply defined epithelial–stromal interface.

IMMUNOPATHOLOGY (INCLUDING IMMUNOHISTOCHEMISTRY)

- p16 staining may be helpful in discriminating HPV-associated carcinomas from those that are HPV negative. However, special stains are not routinely used.

MAIN DIFFERENTIAL DIAGNOSIS

- Tangential sectioning of VIN—the nests are regular in contour with preserved polarity.

- Adnexal involvement—similar to tangential sectioning.
- Pseudoepitheliomatous hyperplasia—fine threadlike strands interconnect nests of benign-appearing epithelium. However, similar changes can occur in VIN.
- Artifactual displacement of tumor by trauma/iatrogenic—look for other evidence of trauma, markedly dilated vessels suggesting anesthetic injection, disaggregated fragments of tumor rather than more rounded smooth-bordered tumor conforming to the vessel wall.
- Keratoacanthoma—always a difficult distinction and one that should be made with caution.

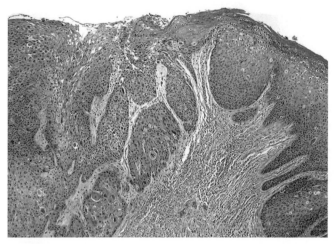

FIGURE 1

Vulvar squamous cell carcinoma. An HSIL on the right merges with an invasive carcinoma at the left.

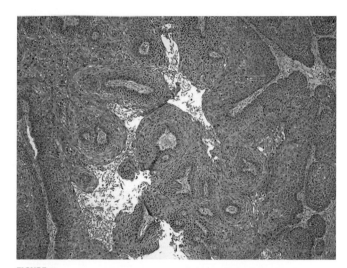

FIGURE 3

Vulvar squamous cell carcinoma. Irregular ill-defined papillary architecture with abnormal parakeratosis lends a warty appearance to this tumor.

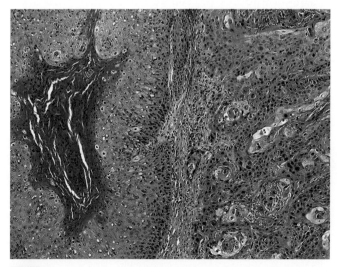

FIGURE 2

Vulvar squamous cell carcinoma. Irregular nests of invasive carcinoma at the right beneath an intraepithelial lesion (VIN, left).

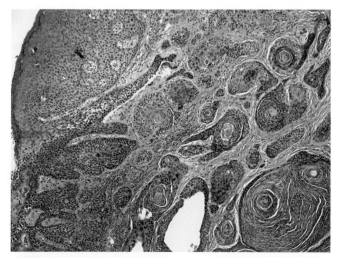

FIGURE 4

Vulvar squamous cell carcinoma. An HSIL (upper left) overlays poorly differentiated infiltrating (basaloid) squamous carcinoma. Note the similarity of the invasive component to the HSIL (intraepithelial like).

VULVAR SQUAMOUS CARCINOMA: KERATINIZING PATTERN

DEFINITION—Invasive epithelial neoplasm composed of keratinocytes involving the vulva. Human papillomavirus (HPV) negative.

CLINICAL FEATURES

EPIDEMIOLOGY

- Typically affects women in their seventh and eighth decades and is usually found associated with inflammatory dermatosis (differentiated vulvar intraepithelial neoplasia [VIN]).
- Some patients present with no history of vulvar neoplasia.
- Not associated with HPV and not associated with squamous neoplasms of the cervix.

PRESENTATION

- Typically emerges in the background of vulvar inflammatory disease.
- Often not preceded by a diagnosis of differentiated VIN.
- May develop rapidly as a nodule.

PROGNOSIS AND TREATMENT

- Guarded, patients with localized, resectable disease have a variable recurrence rate.
- Patients with documented nodal spread or recurrence in the groin have a mortality of 85% to 100%.
- Localized recurrence may be treated with re-excision or radiation.
- Surgical resection with or without lymph node dissection is the most common treatment approach.
- There is increasing interest in sentinel lymph node excision to decrease morbidity.

PATHOLOGY

HISTOLOGY

- Tumors that demonstrate maturation and keratinization toward the epithelial surface (or in the center of invasive nests of tumor).
- Mild to moderate nuclear atypia is usually present in the basal layers as these tumors are often associated with differentiated VIN or inflammatory dermatoses.
- Invasive nests of tumor may range from large, blunt, cohesive cell nests with conspicuous keratinization to small, angular nests of malignant cells.
- Single, invasive, eosinophilic cells may be noted as well.

Diagnostic terminology: Well/moderately/poorly differentiated keratinizing squamous cell carcinoma.

IMMUNOPATHOLOGY (INCLUDING IMMUNOHISTOCHEMISTRY)

- p16 staining will be negative or patchy, therefore is not helpful.
- p53 staining will typically be strong in the immature epithelial layers.
- Lesions will be HPV negative by in situ hybridization or other HPV detection techniques.

MAIN DIFFERENTIAL DIAGNOSIS

- Tangential sectioning of differentiated VIN: This can be highly subjective.

- Pseudoepitheliomatous hyperplasia (PEH): Differentiation from keratinizing cancer can be difficult. Important is the lack of atypia with PEH.
- Inverted keratosis: Lack of atypia at the epithelial stromal interface.

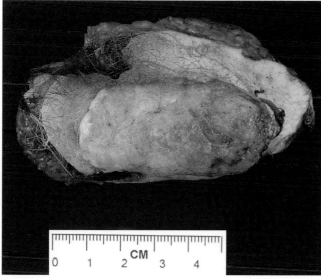

FIGURE 1

Keratinizing vulvar squamous cell carcinoma. A discrete plaquelike tumor on this wide excision.

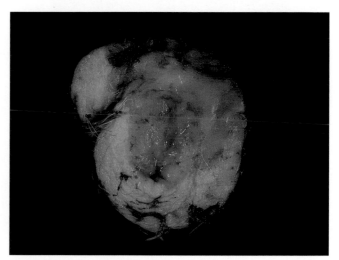

FIGURE 3

Keratinizing vulvar squamous cell carcinoma. This tumor presents as a flat shallow ulcer without exophytic growth.

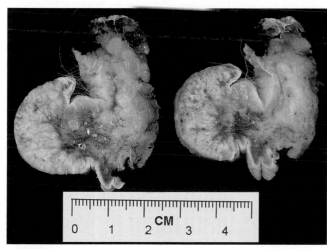

FIGURE 2

Keratinizing vulvar squamous cell carcinoma. Sectioning of the tumor in Figure 1 shows a raised warty or exophytic appearance.

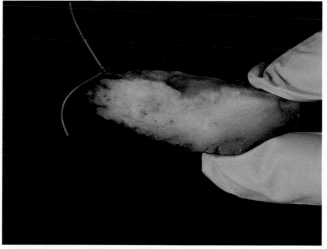

FIGURE 4

Keratinizing vulvar squamous cell carcinoma. Sectioning of the tumor in Figure 3 shows the shallow ulcer with vertical growth into the stroma. This can appear to happen rather quickly in some cases.

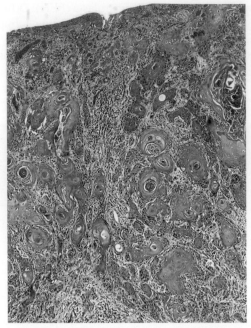

FIGURE 5

Keratinizing vulvar squamous cell carcinoma. Confluent, disorganized tumor nests of variable sizes penetrate the stroma, with focal keratinization.

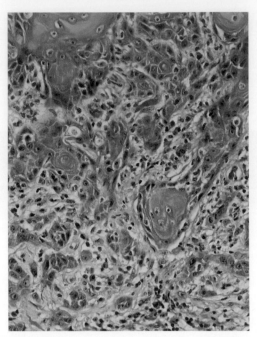

FIGURE 6

Keratinizing vulvar squamous cell carcinoma. Tumor stromal interfaces with conspicuous atypia.

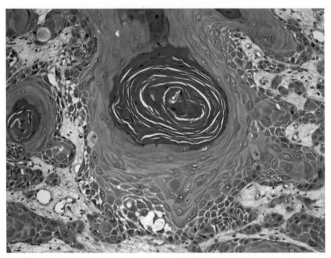

FIGURE 7

Keratinizing vulvar squamous cell carcinoma. Note the sharp transition from basal atypia to a blander mature keratinizing epitheium.

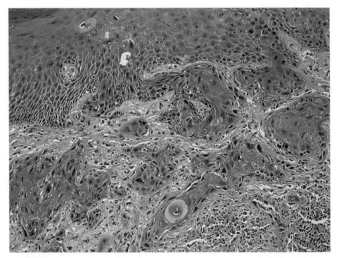

FIGURE 8

Keratinizing vulvar squamous cell carcinoma. The prominent nuclear atypia distinguishes this from pseudoepitheliomatous hyperplasia or tangentially sectioned reactive epithelial changes.

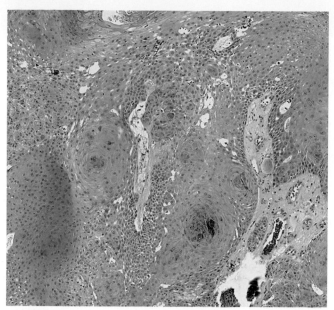

FIGURE 9

Inverted keratosis. This will present an appearance of disorganized keratinizing epithelium. However, note the lack of atypia.

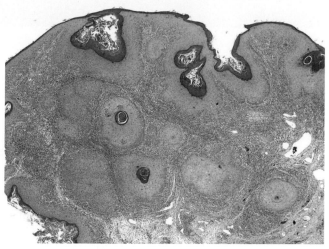

FIGURE 10

PEH with a dense lymphoplasmacytic infiltrate. This may mimic keratinizing carcinoma but raises the possibility of syphilis, which must be excluded.

VERRUCOUS SQUAMOUS CELL CARCINOMA

DEFINITION—Invasive epithelial neoplasm composed of keratinocytes involving the vulva. Exhibits a distinct histology and invasive pattern that is nonmetastasizing.

CLINICAL FEATURES

EPIDEMIOLOGY

- Typically affects women in their seventh and eighth decades and is usually found associated with inflammatory dermatosis. May be associated with atypical verruciform hyperplasia.
- Human papillomavirus (HPV) negative and not linked to other gynecologic (cervical) squamous lesions.

PRESENTATION

- Usually elderly, long-standing inflammatory dermatosis, such as lichen simplex chronicus (LSC) or lichen sclerosus et atrophicus (LSA) may be present with an associated mass lesion.

PROGNOSIS AND TREATMENT

- Good prognosis if resectable and not associated with conventional carcinoma.
- Localized recurrence may be treated with re-excision; radiation to be avoided.
- Surgical resection with or without lymph node dissection is the most common treatment approach.

PATHOLOGY

HISTOLOGY

CARDINAL HISTOLOGIC FEATURES
- Large verruciform mass.
- The absence of atypia in the superficial layers and at the stromal interface.
- Bulbous, blunt pattern of invasion.
- Some inflammation or necrosis common.
- The large lesions must be extensively sampled to rule out concurrent conventional squamous cell carcinoma.

Diagnostic terminology: Extremely well-differentiated squamous carcinoma (verrucous carcinoma [VC]) (with measurements and margins). Comment: This form of squamous carcinoma is not typically associated with lymph node metastases. However, clinical correlation is advised.

IMMUNOPATHOLOGY (INCLUDING IMMUNOHISTOCHEMISTRY)

- p16 staining will be patchy or negative at the stromal interface.
- Ki-67 labeling is not increased, confined to the basal layers.
- p53 immunostaining should be weak and sporadic.
- HPV negative.

MAIN DIFFERENTIAL DIAGNOSIS

- Large (giant) condylomas. These can be seen at all ages including older women. Key features are an exophytic growth pattern without appreciable extension into the underlying stroma and normal keratinocyte maturation relative to VC.
- Deceptively bland keratinizing squamous carcinomas. These will differ from VC by the more irregular interface. Look closely for interface atypia.
- Keratoacanthoma.

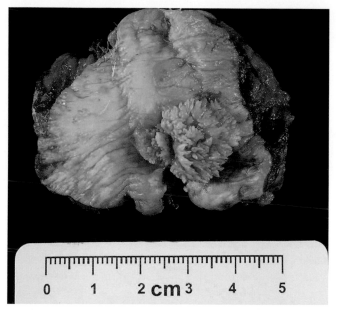

FIGURE 1

VC. Gross photo of a fungating discrete mass on the vulva.

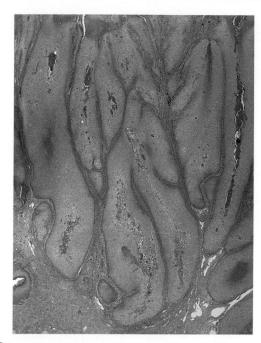

FIGURE 2

Low magnification depicts the bulbous growth pattern.

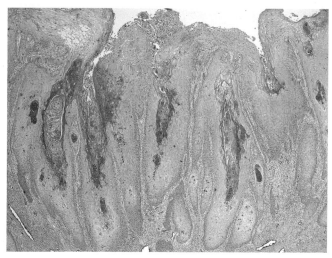

FIGURE 3

This low-power image of a VC illustrates a more narrow growth pattern.

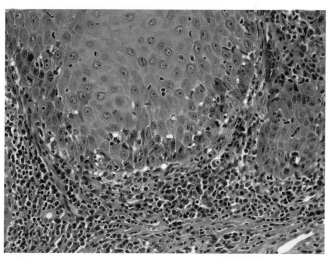

FIGURE 4

At high magnification the basal cells are uniform, albeit with prominent nucleoli.

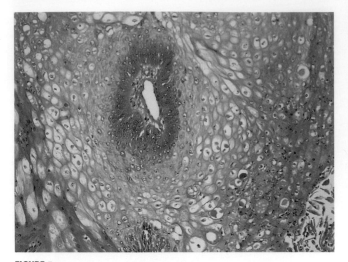

FIGURE 5

The absence of superficial atypia characterizes VC.

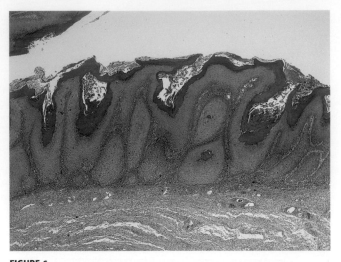

FIGURE 6

An earlier noninvasive component of a VC, adjacent to the main tumor mass.

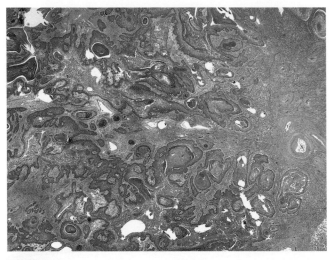

FIGURE 7

Low magnification of a well-differentiated conventional squamous carcinoma.

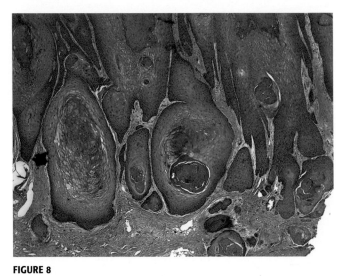

FIGURE 8

This low-power view of a well-differentiated vulvar squamous carcinoma resembles VC but depicts more irregular, angulated invasive epithelium.

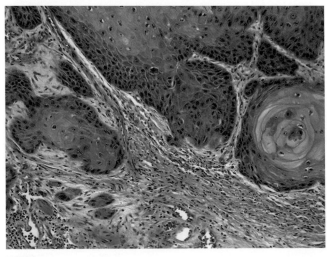

FIGURE 9

A different field of the case in Figure 8 confirms interface atypia and invasion by small groups of cells.

HIGH-GRADE SQUAMOUS INTRAEPITHELIAL LESION (VULVAR INTRAEPITHELIAL NEOPLASIA III) WITH CONFLUENT PAPILLARY GROWTH

DEFINITION—A papillary exophytic squamous lesion similar in morphology to vulvar intraepithelial neoplasia (VIN) III but with risk of underlying invasion.

CLINICAL FEATURES

EPIDEMIOLOGY

- Identical to that of a classic or usual high-grade VIN. May be associated with an invasive carcinoma. Human papillomavirus (HPV) positive, usually HPV 16. Predominating in the fifth and sixth decades of age.

PRESENTATION

- Raised, verruciform- or condyloma-like lesions, may be erythematous and hyperkeratotic.

PROGNOSIS AND TREATMENT

- Managed by excision and lymph node dissection if invasion is present or strongly suspected. If not, wide excision alone will suffice. Risk of lymph node involvement is minimal if there is no invasion.

PATHOLOGY

HISTOLOGY

- High-grade histology, in keeping with a VIN III. Confluent or complex intraepithelial growth pattern with "reduplication" and exophytic features. Confluent growth pattern resembles a carcinoma but may not breach the basal lamina.

IMMUNOHISTOCHEMISTRY

- Not necessary if the histology is characteristic of a high-grade lesion, but MIb-1 and p16ink4 stains will be positive (diffuse distribution). These cells are usually HPV positive (high-risk types mostly HPV 16).

MAIN DIFFERENTIAL DIAGNOSIS

- Condyloma—these might be confused with carcinoma if markedly inflamed or very large.
- Unclassified papillary neoplasms with moderate atypia—this entity is not well defined but falls between condyloma and a papillary carcinoma.
- Verruciform VIN II and III—the epithelial architecture is preserved, and "reduplication" is not seen.
- Verrucous carcinoma—these are very well differentiated.

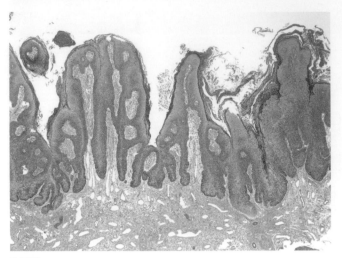

FIGURE 1

Papillary high-grade squamous intraepithelial lesion (HSIL). This is a typical HSIL of the vulva. There is no confluence of papillary growth.

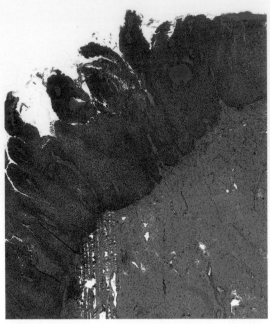

FIGURE 2

Papillary HSIL. There is focal confluence of papillae but the degree is still within the range accepted for an HSIL.

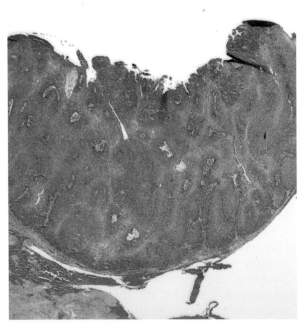

FIGURE 3

HSIL with confluent papillary growth. This is analogous to papillary carcinoma; however, there is no stromal invasion.

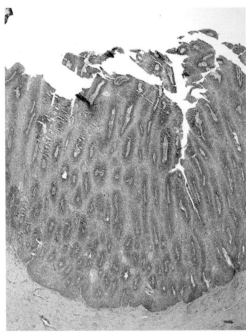

FIGURE 4

HSIL with confluent papillary growth. This is analogous to papillary carcinoma; however, there is no stromal invasion.

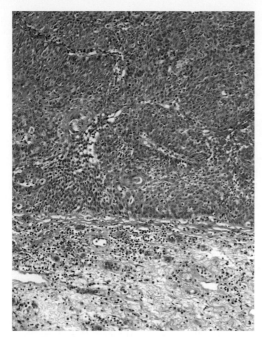

FIGURE 5

Uniform epithelial–stromal interface in a papillary HSIL with complex growth.

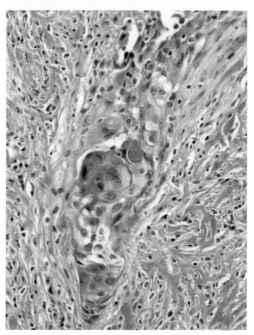

FIGURE 6

A focus of invasion confirms malignancy.

GIANT CONDYLOMA OF THE EXTERNAL GENITALIA

DEFINITION—A papillosquamous lesion of significant size, histologically indistinguishable from generic condyloma.

CLINICAL FEATURES

EPIDEMIOLOGY

- A rare entity that most commonly affects young men.
- Seen more commonly in immunosuppressed patients (human immunodeficiency virus [HIV] positive).
- Can also be seen in older women and may be human papillomavirus (HPV) negative.

PRESENTATION

- Large, diffuse, papillary lesions resembling typical condyloma, with a much more extensive distribution.

PROGNOSIS AND TREATMENT

- Topical and surgical treatments are available; however, the disease has a high local recurrence rate, especially in immunocompromised individuals.
- In elderly patients close follow-up is advised to exclude progression to a more aggressive entity (such as verrucous carcinoma or keratinizing squamous carcinoma).

PATHOLOGY

HISTOLOGY

- Papillary squamous hyperplasia.
- Koilocytosis is variable and may be absent in older women.

- These lesions are differentiated from verrucous carcinoma in that they have uniform cell maturation and lack of fingerlike projections into the underlying stroma.
- Inflammation may be present.

Diagnostic terminology: Extensive (giant) condyloma.

IMMUNOPATHOLOGY (INCLUDING IMMUNOHISTOCHEMISTRY)

- Mib-1 and p16 staining are patchy and not dramatically increased.
- p53 staining will be weak or patchy.
- HPV testing should reveal HPV 6 or 11 in many cases, but some will score negative, suggesting an alternative pathogenesis.

MAIN DIFFERENTIAL DIAGNOSIS

- Condyloma—smaller, has more conspicuous koilocytosis or keratohyalin granules.
- Verrucous carcinoma—bulbous downward growth, epithelial pallor.

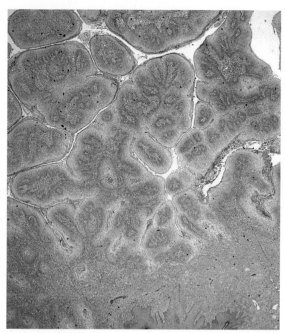

FIGURE 1

Giant condyloma. A large lesion with broad verrucopapillary projections.

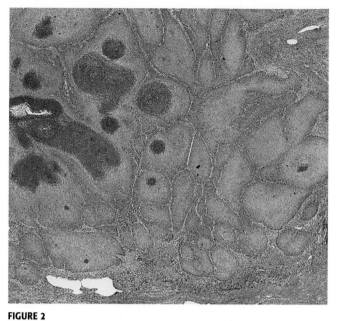

FIGURE 2

Verrucous carcinoma for comparison. Note the numerous rounded epithelial nests penetrating the underlying stroma.

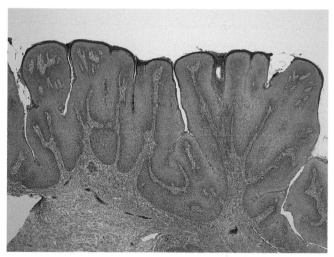

FIGURE 3

Giant condyloma. A less dramatic verrucous growth in this area.

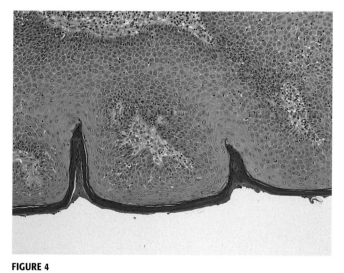

FIGURE 4

Giant condyloma. Superficial growth with uniform maturation. However, note the lack of koilocytotic atypia.

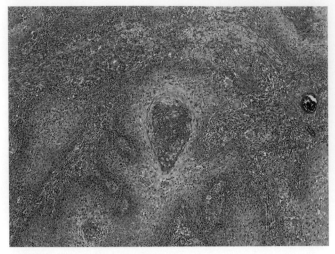

FIGURE 5

Giant condyloma. Note the inflammation at the epithelial stromal interface.

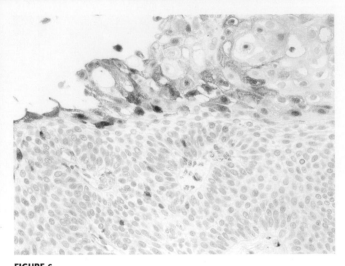

FIGURE 6

Giant condyloma. p16 staining is weak or patchy.

PSEUDOEPITHELIOMATOUS HYPERPLASIA

PITFALL

DEFINITION—A reactive condition marked by acanthosis and irregular epithelial architecture.

CLINICAL FEATURES

EPIDEMIOLOGY

- Noncontributory.

PRESENTATION

- Thickening of the skin, coexisting conditions are usually present (occasionally, granular cell tumor)

PROGNOSIS AND TREATMENT

- Noncontributory.

PATHOLOGY

HISTOLOGY

- Acanthosis with an irregular dermal/epidermal junction.

- Traditionally there is a lack of atypia, and the dermal component consists of thin, irregular squamous projections that frequently have pointed tips.
- Underlying conditions such as a granular cell tumor or inflammatory process should be sought out.

IMMUNOPATHOLOGY (INCLUDING IMMUNOHISTOCHEMISTRY)

- Noncontributory although staining for both p16 and p53 should be negative if there is no coexisting vulvar intraepithelial neoplasia (VIN).

MAIN DIFFERENTIAL DIAGNOSIS

- Squamous cell carcinoma with or without invasion.
- A syphilitic lesion can also present this way (look for abundant plasma cells and do appropriate tests if concerned).
- Rarely, associated with an underlying granular cell tumor.

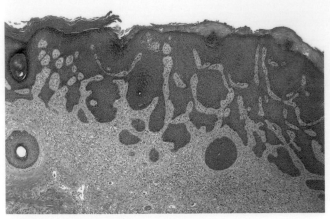

FIGURE 1

Pseudoepitheliomatous hyperplasia (PEH). There are numerous subsurface epithelial nests, connected by thin septae. There may be an element of tangential sectioning in this case.

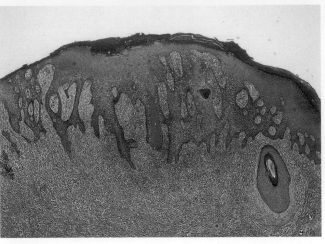

FIGURE 2

PEH. Marked acanthosis with irregular, pointed epithelial projections into the stroma. Abnormal keratinization may be present and is not a sign of malignancy.

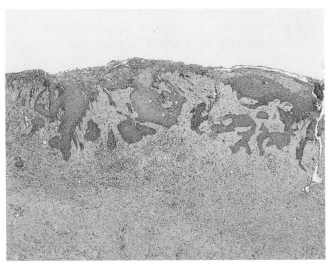

FIGURE 3

PEH. This is a more challenging case and might elicit some controversy as to whether this is PEH or invasive carcinoma. This patient was irradiated for a prior squamous carcinoma. Note the oddly angulated subsurface nests and the *absence* of atypia, loss of polarity, and desmoplasia.

KERATOACANTHOMA

DEFINITION—A neoplastic proliferation of keratinocytes arising in follicular epithelium.

CLINICAL FEATURES

EPIDEMIOLOGY

- Typically occurs in the middle aged to elderly.
- Suspected causes include ultraviolet light, immunosuppression, genetic alterations, chemical exposure, viruses, and trauma.

PRESENTATION

- Papular masses with central umbilication and keratin accumulation form rapidly.

PROGNOSIS AND TREATMENT

- The prognosis is good.
- Most cases left untreated will spontaneously regress; however, rare cases of metastasis have been noted.
- Surgery is curative in the vast majority of cases.

PATHOLOGY

HISTOLOGY

- A discrete, inverted, cup-shaped lesion with central keratin accumulation.
- In general the basal keratinocytes lack atypia when compared with traditional squamous cell carcinoma.

IMMUNOPATHOLOGY (INCLUDING IMMUNOHISTOCHEMISTRY)

- Noncontributory.

MAIN DIFFERENTIAL DIAGNOSIS

- Traditional squamous cell carcinoma—conspicuous atypia is the norm but not invariable.
- Pustular folliculitis.

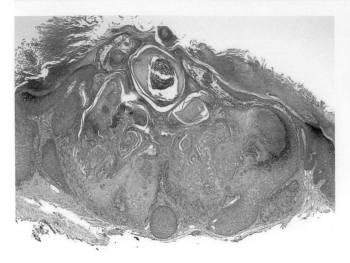

FIGURE 1

Keratoacanthoma. Low-power examination reveals a cup-shaped lesion with pushing borders and central keratinization.

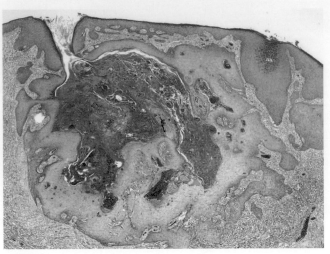

FIGURE 2

Keratoacanthoma. Prominent keratinization may be seen in the center of the lesion. Note the irregular epithelial stromal interface.

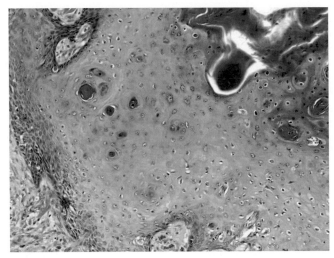

FIGURE 3

Keratoacanthoma. The squamous cells lack conspicuous atypia.

BASAL CELL CARCINOMA

DEFINITION—An uncommon, nonmetastasizing (usually!) but locally destructive carcinoma of basal keratinocytes with characteristic peripheral nuclear palisading.

CLINICAL FEATURES

EPIDEMIOLOGY

- Rare.
- Not human papillomavirus (HPV) associated.
- Elderly women in their 70s and 80s.

PRESENTATION

- Typically a raised, sometimes ulcerated, discoid vulvar lesion.
- Occasionally presents as a polypoid mass.

PROGNOSIS AND TREATMENT

- Wide local excision is appropriate.
- These carcinomas are nonmetastasizing but have a propensity for destructive local recurrence.
- Rare reports of nodal metastases exist.
- May be a candidate for Mohs' surgery.

PATHOLOGY

HISTOLOGY

- Vulvar tumors have the same histologic features as lesions at other sites.

- These carcinomas are characterized by a monotonous, cohesive population of small blue cells with a high nuclear-to-cytoplasmic ratio.
- Cells may be arranged in rounded or elongated nests with peripheral nuclear palisading (classic pattern), or as infiltrative cords and strands set in a myxoid matrix with a reticular architecture (adenoid pattern).
- Nests often show characteristic clefting between tumor cells and surrounding stroma.
- The tumor cells lack significant nuclear atypia, and mitotic figures are rare.

IMMUNOPATHOLOGY (INCLUDING IMMUNOHISTOCHEMISTRY)

- Noncontributory.

MAIN DIFFERENTIAL DIAGNOSIS

- Basaloid squamous cell carcinoma— higher nuclear grade, irregular growth pattern, associated vulvar intraepithelial neoplasia (VIN).
- Pagetoid VIN—discrete foci of neoplastic epithelium but intraepithelial and does not extend into stroma.
- Differentiated VIN with parabasal expansion—nesting is less discrete.
- Adenoid cystic carcinoma—mimicked by adenoid variant of basal cell carcinoma (BCC).
- Syringoma—bland-appearing nests may suggest BCC at low power.

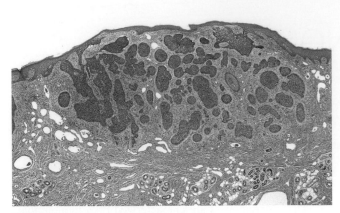

FIGURE 1

BCC. At low power, nests of darkly staining cells are emanating from abnormal basal cells at the epithelial–stromal interface, forming a nodular mass.

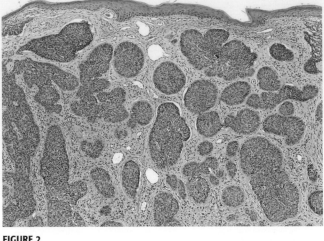

FIGURE 2

At higher magnification, the discrete nests are regularly arranged with minimal stromal reaction.

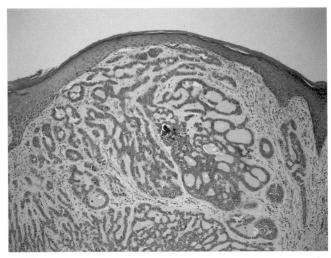

FIGURE 3

BCC with an adenoid pattern with delicate anastomosing strands of neoplastic epithelium. Note the pigment in the center.

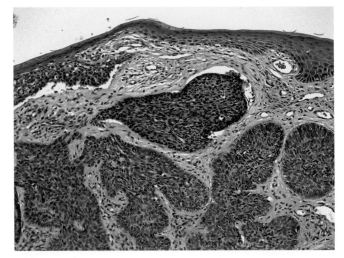

FIGURE 4

BCC. BCC with discrete nests of neoplastic basal cells and minimal stromal reaction in the dermis.

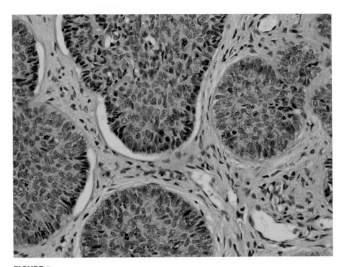

FIGURE 5

BCC at higher power, showing uniformly polarized neoplastic cells and apoptosis.

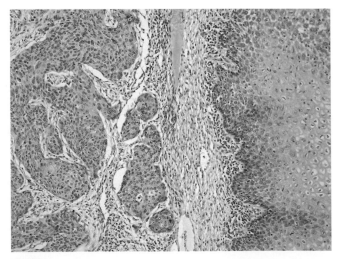

FIGURE 6

Basaloid squamous carcinoma (HPV positive), for comparison, shows an irregular growth pattern and cellular heterogeneity.

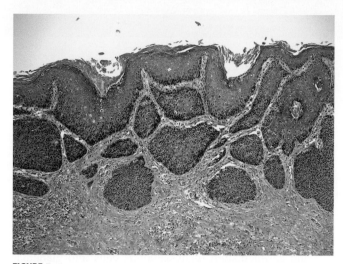

FIGURE 7

Classic VIN, with appendage involvement, for comparison.

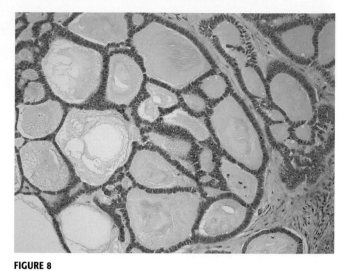

FIGURE 8

High magnification of adenoid BCC of the vulva. Contrast with adenoid cystic carcinoma (see page 74).

ADENOSQUAMOUS CARCINOMA

DEFINITION—An aggressive variant of squamous cell carcinoma with conspicuous glandular differentiation.

CLINICAL FEATURES

EPIDEMIOLOGY

- Uncommon.
- Mean age at diagnosis is 65 to 70 years.
- Associated with chronic vulvar inflammatory disease.
- Human papillomavirus (HPV) link is unclear but likely when coexisting with basaloid carcinomas.

PRESENTATION

- Vulvar mass involving the labium majus and occasionally the minus; may also arise in the Bartholin's duct or gland.
- The majority of patients present with late-stage disease.

PROGNOSIS AND TREATMENT

- A few reports suggest that outcomes are worse than for conventional squamous cell carcinoma.
- The extent of surgical excision depends heavily on disease extent; small lesions (< 2 cm in diameter and 1 mm thickness) may be treated with wide excision and 1 cm margins.
- For larger lesions, partial radical vulvectomy and ipsilateral groin lymphadenectomy or sentinel node sampling is required.
- For nonsurgical (late-stage) disease, combination chemoradiation is the standard of care.

PATHOLOGY

HISTOLOGY

- This tumor is characterized by a blend of squamous and glandular differentiation.

- The squamous component typically exhibits acanthosis and desquamation of dyskeratotic cells into glandular spaces.
- The glandular component is admixed with the squamous and composed of medium-sized to small acinar glandular spaces.
- The glands are lined by one- to two-cell layer of low columnar to cuboidal cells.
- In most cases the tumor is deeply invasive and involves adjacent perineal structures or the vagina.
- In metastatic lesions the dual squamous and glandular differentiation pattern is retained.

IMMUNOPATHOLOGY (INCLUDING IMMUNOHISTOCHEMISTRY)

- p16ink4 immunostaining, when diffuse and strong, would favor if not guarantee an HPV etiology.

MAIN DIFFERENTIAL DIAGNOSIS

- Conventional invasive squamous cell carcinoma with acantholysis.
- Invasive Paget's disease.
- Amelanotic melanoma.
- Sweat gland carcinoma.

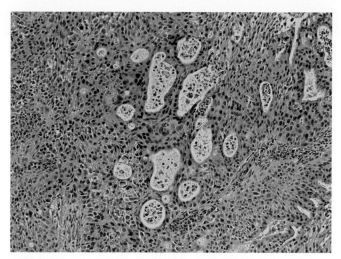

FIGURE 1

Adenosquamous carcinoma. Squamous carcinoma showing acantholysis and desquamation into luminal-like spaces.

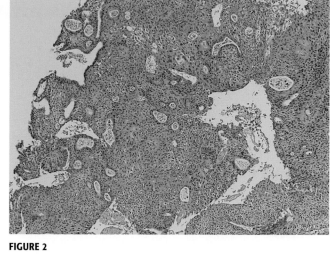

FIGURE 2

Adenosquamous carcinoma. Alternating areas of squamous and glandular differentiation. The glands are frequently lined by low cuboidal epithelium.

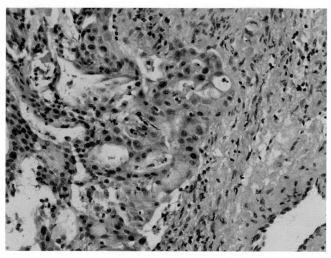

FIGURE 3

Adenosquamous carcinoma. High-power detail of area of adenocarcinoma within an adenosquamous carcinoma. Note the cribriforming glandular spaces lined by low cuboidal to columnar epithelium.

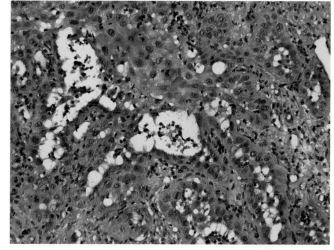

FIGURE 4

Adenosquamous carcinoma. Both carcinoma and adenocarcinoma can be seen here, with the areas of squamous carcinoma denoted by their deeply eosinophilic cytoplasm (keratinization).

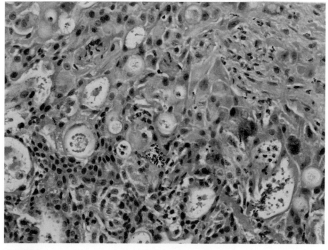

FIGURE 5

Adenosquamous carcinoma. Marked nuclear pleomorphism.

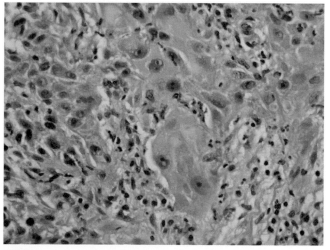

FIGURE 6

Adenosquamous carcinoma. Large keratinizing squamous cells.

PAGET'S DISEASE OF THE VULVA

DEFINITION—Infiltration of the squamous epithelium by mucin-producing neoplastic cells.

CLINICAL FEATURES

EPIDEMIOLOGY

- Uncommon; represents only 1% to 2% of vulvar malignancies.
- The average age at presentation is 65 years; the majority of patients are over 50 years.

PRESENTATION

- Vulvar pruritus is the most common symptom.
- Ill-defined, erythematous plaques on the labium (majus or minus), perineum, or anus.
- Involved skin may exhibit eczematous changes or ulceration.

PROGNOSIS AND TREATMENT

- Radical excision is the treatment of choice and often requires reconstruction.
- Close follow-up is necessary; disease recurs in up to 50% of patients, even with negative margins.
- If stromal invasion is present, recurrence and metastases to distant sites and lymph nodes may occur.
- An associated internal malignancy (e.g., colorectal carcinoma) has been reported in up to 25% of cases.

PATHOLOGY

HISTOLOGY

- Nests and single cells percolate through the epidermis, frequently extending into adnexal structures.

- The neoplastic cells are large, often with abundant pale blue cytoplasm, large vesicular nuclei, and small conspicuous nucleoli.
- Rarely Paget cells may form glands within the epidermis.
- A basal keratinocyte is often present between the Paget's cells and the basement membrane.
- Stromal invasion by Paget's cells may be difficult to distinguish from adnexal involvement.
- The associated squamous epithelium may show benign changes including acanthosis, hyperkeratosis, or papillomatous hyperplasia.

IMMUNOPATHOLOGY (INCLUDING IMMUNOHISTOCHEMISTRY)

- Positive for CK7 and mucin.
- Negative for CK5/6 (positive in squamous epithelium), CK20, S100, and p63.

MAIN DIFFERENTIAL DIAGNOSIS

- Melanoma.
- Urothelial carcinoma (via direct extension).
- Pagetoid vulvar intraepithelial neoplasia.
- Candidal infection (clinically).

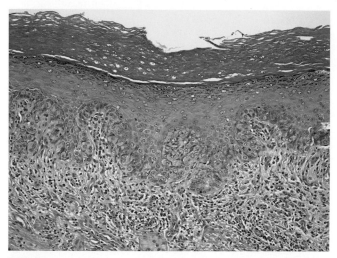

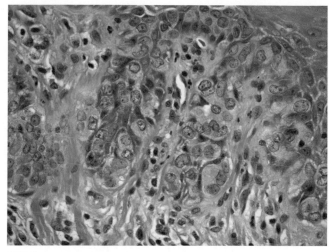

FIGURE 1

Paget's disease. Basal involvement by large cells with abundant hazy blue cytoplasm.

FIGURE 2

Paget's disease. Large cells with abundant blue cytoplasm, large nuclei, and pinpoint nucleoli.

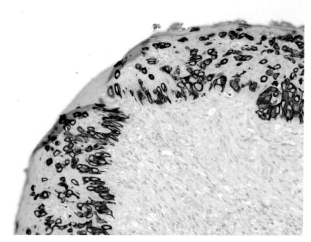

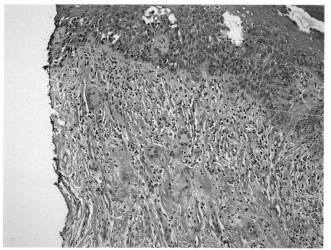

FIGURE 3

Paget's disease. Immunohistochemical staining with CK7, highlighting the neoplastic cells.

FIGURE 4

Paget's disease. Nests of Paget's disease cells within the dermis.

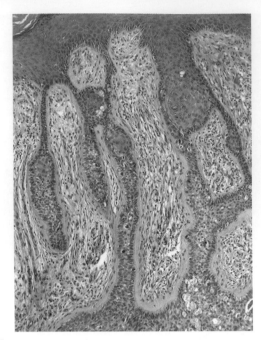

FIGURE 5

Paget's disease. Pseudoepitheliomatous hyperplasia associated with Paget's disease.

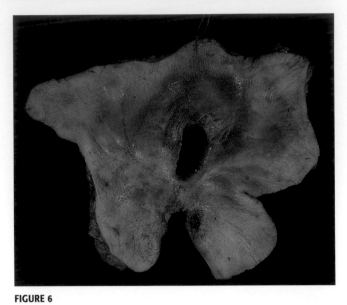

FIGURE 6

Paget's disease. Gross specimen displaying Paget's disease. Note the ill-defined, erythematous plaques.

MERKEL CELL CARCINOMA

DEFINITION—A malignant mucocutaneous neuroendocrine neoplasm.

CLINICAL FEATURES

EPIDEMIOLOGY

- Very rare (~12 per year in the United States).
- Vulvar tumors account for about 3% of all Merkel cell carcinomas.
- Risk factors include age (>60 years) and sun exposure.

PRESENTATION

- Nonspecific.
- Submucosal nodules or papules.

PROGNOSIS AND TREATMENT

- Poor; even early-stage lesions have a 10% mortality rate.
- Wide local excision with at least 2.5 cm margins and lymphadenectomy or sentinel node sampling.
- Radiation therapy seems to have survival benefit; tumors are chemosensitive, but chemotherapy may not increase survival.

PATHOLOGY

HISTOLOGY

- At low power the tumor is composed of sheets and nodules of cells with a high nuclear-to-cytoplasmic ratio and geographic tumor necrosis.

- The tumor frequently undermines the overlying epithelium.
- At high power the cells are monotonous and undifferentiated with nuclear molding, prominent crush artifact, and a high mitotic index.

IMMUNOPATHOLOGY (INCLUDING IMMUNOHISTOCHEMISTRY)

- Low-molecular-weight keratins (Cam5.2, AEl/AE3), including CK20, are positive in a characteristic dotlike perinuclear pattern.
- Chromogranin and synaptophysin are positive.
- S100 is negative.

MAIN DIFFERENTIAL DIAGNOSIS

- Metastatic pulmonary small cell carcinoma.
- Ewing's sarcoma (primitive neuroectodermal tumor [PNET]).
- Melanoma.
- Lymphoma.

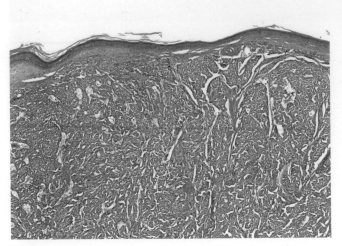

FIGURE 1

Merkel cell carcinoma. Nests of malignant cells filling the dermis. Note the trabecular and nested architecture.

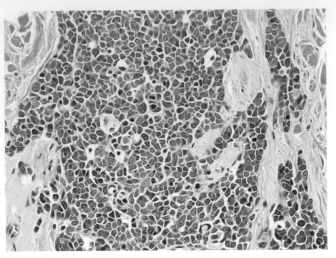

FIGURE 2

Merkel cell carcinoma. Pleomorphic cells with amphophilic cytoplasm, nuclear molding (suggestive of neuroendocrine differentiation).

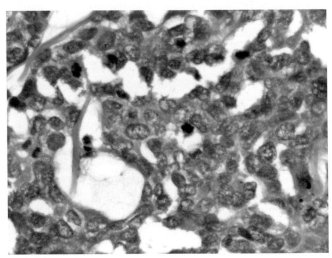

FIGURE 3

Merkel cell carcinoma. Vesicular chromatin with numerous mitotic figures and apoptotic debris.

CLOACOGENIC NEOPLASIA

DEFINITION—"Ectopic," colonic-type neoplasia (adenoma/carcinoma) arising in the vaginal or vulvar mucosa.

CLINICAL FEATURES

EPIDEMIOLOGY

- Origin is in colonic-type epithelium, presumably incorporated into the vaginal or vulvar region following formation of the urorectal septum in early development.
- Another possible scenario is intestinal metaplasia of vaginal adenosis as rare cases have been reported in diethylstilbestrol (DES)–exposed women.
- Typically seen in adults, implying an age-related transformation of colonic-type epithelium to form these neoplasms.

PRESENTATION

- Patients may present with vaginal bleeding or discharge.
- An exophytic or pedunculated polyp is found in the vagina.

PROGNOSIS AND TREATMENT

- Outcome depends on the extent and grade of the disease.
- A favorable outcome is expected for most, although some may recur locally.

PATHOLOGY

HISTOLOGY

- Squamous mucosa is replaced by a lesion closely resembling adenoma with a pseudostratified columnar cell lining with goblet cells.

- Glands may be predominantly tubular, reminiscent of a tubular adenoma, or exhibit prominent villous architecture as seen in villous adenomas.
- Adenocarcinomas arising in either of the above are typically intestinal.

Diagnostic terminology: Cloacogenic polyp, adenoma, and carcinoma.

IMMUNOPATHOLOGY (INCLUDING IMMUNOHISTOCHEMISTRY)

- Tumors are typically CK20 positive and CK7 negative.
- Some studies have demonstrated *O*-acetylated sialomucin, considered a specific marker of large intestinal differentiation.

MAIN DIFFERENTIAL DIAGNOSIS

- Metastatic colonic carcinoma.
- Rectovaginal fistula.

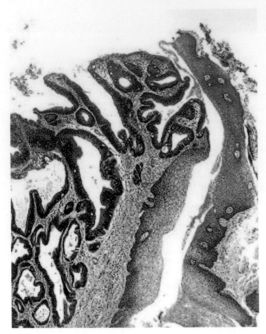

FIGURE 1

Cloacogenic neoplasia of the vagina with merging of normal squamous mucosa *(right)* and a lesion closely resembling a villous adenoma of the colon *(left)*. *(From Crum CP, Nucci MR, Lee KR, editors. Diagnostic Gynecologic and Obstetric Pathology. 2nd ed. Philadelphia: Elsevier; 2011, Fig. 12-17A.)*

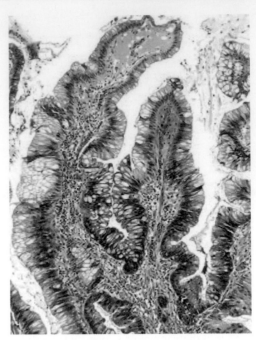

FIGURE 2

Well-differentiated villous architecture in a cloacogenic neoplasm. *(From Crum CP, Nucci MR, Lee KR, editors. Diagnostic Gynecologic and Obstetric Pathology. 2nd ed. Philadelphia: Elsevier; 2011, Fig. 12-17B.)*

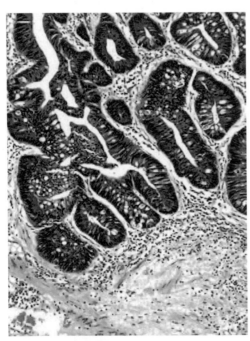

FIGURE 3

Colonic-type glands in a cloacogenic adenoma. *(From Crum CP, Nucci MR, Lee KR, editors. Diagnostic Gynecologic and Obstetric Pathology. 2nd ed. Philadelphia: Elsevier; 2011, Fig. 12-17C.)*

METASTATIC CARCINOMA OF THE VULVA

DEFINITION—Secondary involvement of the vulva by metastatic carcinoma.

CLINICAL FEATURES

EPIDEMIOLOGY

- Rare.
- Accounts for 5% to 8% of vulvar malignancies.

PRESENTATION

- Mass lesion.
- Erythema or other skin changes.

PROGNOSIS AND TREATMENT

- Poor, as metastasis generally suggests late-stage disease.

PATHOLOGY

HISTOLOGY

- Resembles the primary tumor; anogenital, urothelial, breast, lung, and endometrial carcinomas are the most commonly encountered.

- The metastatic carcinoma may form a tumoral mass within the dermis or subcutaneous tissue or may be present as single cells or small nests within lymphatic spaces.

IMMUNOPATHOLOGY (INCLUDING IMMUNOHISTOCHEMISTRY)

- Varies with primary tumor site.
- Urothelial carcinoma is GCDFP negative and CK7 and CK20 positive.

MAIN DIFFERENTIAL DIAGNOSIS

- Paget's disease (particularly with urothelial carcinoma)
- Melanoma. This should be considered for any poorly differentiated epithelioid or spindle cell neoplasm involving the vulva.
- Breast carcinoma arising in ectopic breast tissue.

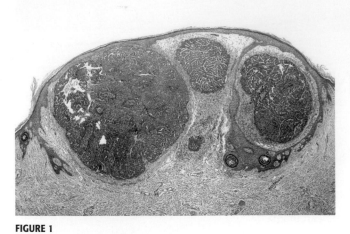

FIGURE 1

Vulvar metastasis. A nodular mass within the dermis. Note the attenuated, uninvolved overlying epidermis.

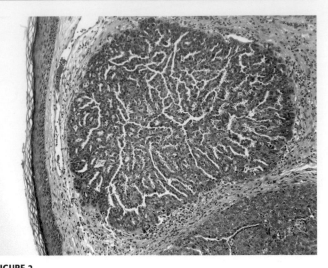

FIGURE 2

Vulvar metastasis. A nodule of metastatic tumor composed of serous carcinoma.

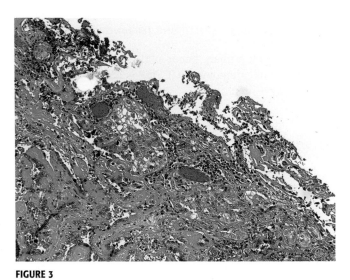

FIGURE 3

Vulvar metastasis. Metastatic clear cell carcinoma with ulceration and loss of the overlying epithelium.

LENTIGO

DEFINITION—Benign pigmented lesion of mucosal surfaces.

CLINICAL FEATURES

EPIDEMIOLOGY

- No distinct demographic associations.
- Increased numbers may be seen in Carney complex.

PRESENTATION

- Most commonly seen as a well-circumscribed, small (<1 cm), flat brown patch, occurring anywhere on genital mucosa.
- Occasionally presents as a large, darkly pigmented, asymmetrical lesion with irregular borders.

PROGNOSIS AND TREATMENT

- Excellent.

PATHOLOGY

HISTOLOGY

- Cytologically benign melanocytes evenly spaced as single cells within the basal layers.

- Mild acanthosis of the epidermis with hyperpigmentation of basal keratinocytes, particularly at the tips of rete ridges.
- Pigment-laden macrophages (melanophages) may be prominent in the papillary dermis.

IMMUNOPATHOLOGY (INCLUDING IMMUNOHISTOCHEMISTRY)

- Noncontributory.

MAIN DIFFERENTIAL DIAGNOSIS

- Lentiginous nevus—enlarged, irregularly spaced melanocytes.

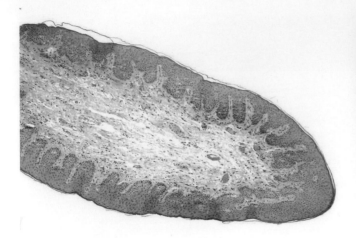

FIGURE 1

Mucosal lentigo. A continuous band of pigment can be seen at low power. Note the absence of visible nests of melanocytes.

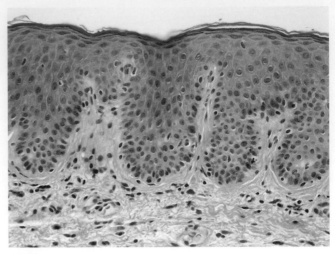

FIGURE 2

Mucosal lentigo. Basal pigmentation, scattered melanocytes, and dermal macrophages with pigment.

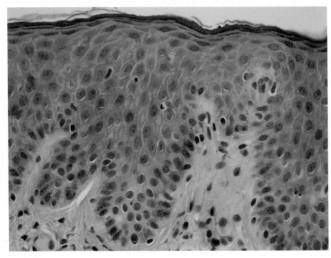

FIGURE 3

Mucosal lentigo. A closer view of the basal pigmentation.

GENITAL-TYPE NEVUS

DEFINITION—A melanocytic proliferation seen in locations with redundant skin, characterized by large junctional melanocyte nests and transepidermal elimination of nests.

CLINICAL FEATURES

EPIDEMIOLOGY

- Uncommon; estimated prevalence of 2.3% in women.
- Young women, most often in the third decade of life.

PRESENTATION

- Most lesions are seen on the labia (majus or minus).
- Seen clinically as small (<1 cm), heavily pigmented, irregular lesions.

PROGNOSIS AND TREATMENT

- Overall prognosis is excellent.
- If significant atypia is present, complete excision is recommended as biologic potential is not well understood.

PATHOLOGY

- May be junctional or compound, symmetrical or asymmetrical, and flat or papillomatous.

- A lentiginous and nested proliferation with characteristically large junctional nests at the sides and tips of the rete with prominent retraction artifact.
- Transepidermal elimination of nests of melanocytes is common (but not epidermal pagetoid spread).
- Only focal atypia should be present.
- Dermal component resembles a typical nevus with basal maturation.

HISTOLOGY

IMMUNOPATHOLOGY (INCLUDING IMMUNOHISTOCHEMISTRY)

- Noncontributory.

MAIN DIFFERENTIAL DIAGNOSIS

- Dysplastic nevus. Look for more pronounced melanocyte atypia at the interface.
- Melanoma.

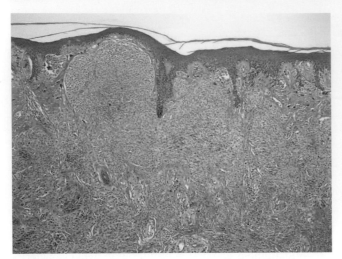

FIGURE 1

Genital-type nevus. Junctional nevus with large nests of melanocytes.

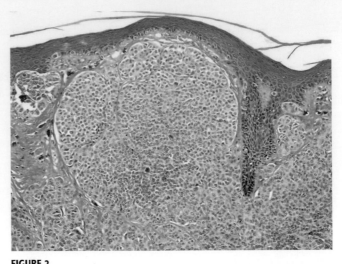

FIGURE 2

Genital-type nevus. Melanocytes composing the nests are regular and lack significant atypia.

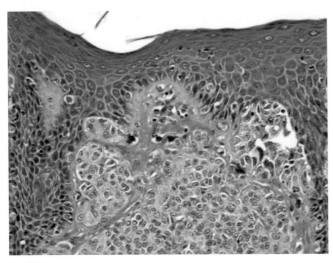

FIGURE 3

Genital-type nevus. Pigment incontinence may be present, especially in a traumatized nevus. Note the lack of atypia and mitotic activity.

DYSPLASTIC NEVUS

DEFINITION—A melanocytic proliferation with architectural, cytologic, and clinical features that are intermediate between those seen in common nevi and melanoma.

CLINICAL FEATURES

EPIDEMIOLOGY

- Patients have a higher risk of melanoma.
- Patients with first-degree relatives who have melanoma have an extremely high risk of developing melanoma (dysplastic nevus syndrome).

PRESENTATION

- Larger than typical nevi and often asymmetrical with irregular borders.

PROGNOSIS AND TREATMENT

- Complete excision is advised.

PATHOLOGY

HISTOLOGY

- Architectural atypia: Variably sized and shaped junctional nests that stream from rete to rete (bridging), a prominent lentiginous growth pattern, and extension of the epidermal component beyond the dermal component (a "shoulder").
- Cytologic atypia: Large nuclei (as compared with adjacent keratinocytes), coarse chromatin, irregular nuclear outlines, and variably prominent nucleoli.
- The pigment is often a gray-brown (dishwater) color.
- Stromal changes include eosinophilic lamellar fibrosis of the papillary dermis.

IMMUNOPATHOLOGY (INCLUDING IMMUNOHISTOCHEMISTRY)

- Noncontributory.

MAIN DIFFERENTIAL DIAGNOSIS

- Melanoma.
- Genital type nevus.

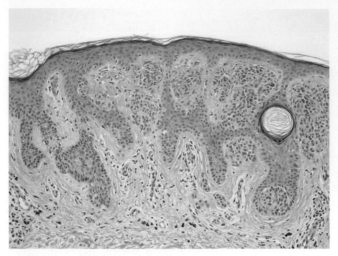

FIGURE 1

Dysplastic nevus. Nests of melanocytes with varying size and shape present in the dermis.

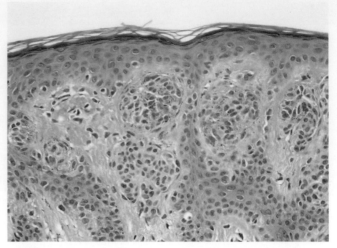

FIGURE 2

Dysplastic nevus. Irregularity of the melanocytes and lamellar fibrosis.

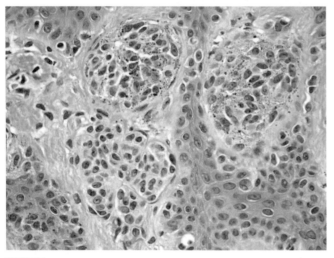

FIGURE 3

Dysplastic nevus. Atypical melanocytes displaying nuclear enlargement and prominent nucleoli. Note the absence of mitotic activity.

MELANOMA

DEFINITION—A highly malignant tumor of dermal melanocytes.

CLINICAL FEATURES

EPIDEMIOLOGY

- Rare.
- Accounts for approximately 3% of all melanomas in women.
- The second most common vulvar malignancy.
- Most often in patients in their sixth decade of life.
- May be more common in patients with a BRCA2 mutation.

PRESENTATION

- A polypoid mass is present in one third of cases.
- Bleeding, ulceration, discomfort, and other nonspecific symptoms may be encountered.
- Flat pigmented lesions are the classic presentation, but amelanotic lesions are not uncommon.
- Labia majora and minora lesions account for approximately 50% of cases, and periclitoral tumors account for another 30%; other sites are less common.

PROGNOSIS AND TREATMENT

- Varies tremendously with extent of disease; Breslow's depth is the single most predictive factor.
- Five-year survival for vulvar melanoma is lower than at nongenital sites, with studies showing a range from 15% to 50%; vaginal melanoma has a 5-year survival of less than 20%.
- Standard treatment includes local excision with 1 to 2 cm margins and sentinel lymph node biopsy.

PATHOLOGY

HISTOLOGY

- The epidermal component is composed of single cells and nests of monotonous, severely atypical melanocytes with irregular chromatin and prominent nucleoli.
- Effacement of the dermal-epidermal junction is common, resulting in a "moth-eaten" appearance.
- The dermal component is most often composed of epithelioid cells with a similar histology to those present in the overlying epidermis and without "maturation."
- Melanoma is known for its variable morphology, and the spectrum is broad; cases range from the epithelioid tumors described earlier to a malignant spindle cell proliferation that can be confused with a sarcomatoid squamous cell carcinoma or a mesenchymal neoplasm.

IMMUNOPATHOLOGY (INCLUDING IMMUNOHISTOCHEMISTRY)

- S100 positive.
- MART1, HMB45, and Melan-A are generally positive but may be lost in poorly differentiated tumors.

MAIN DIFFERENTIAL DIAGNOSIS

- Paget's disease—strongly CK7 positive.
- Squamous cell carcinoma.
- Melanoma in situ.

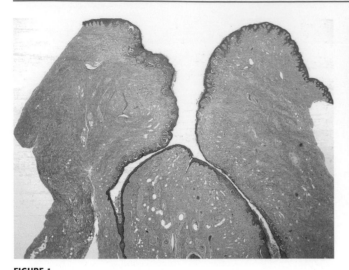

FIGURE 1

Vulvar melanoma. Nests of melanocytes can be seen at low power. Note the bridging of the rete by the theques.

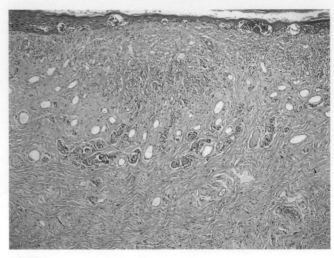

FIGURE 2

Vulvar melanoma. Malignant cells infiltrate into the dermis. There is no maturation of the deep cells when compared with the melanocytes in the junctional component.

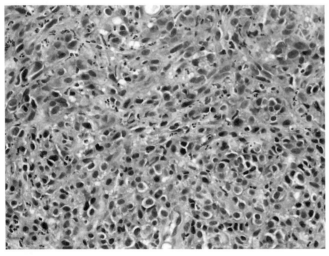

FIGURE 3

Vulvar melanoma. Malignant melanocytes displaying nuclear pleomorphism.

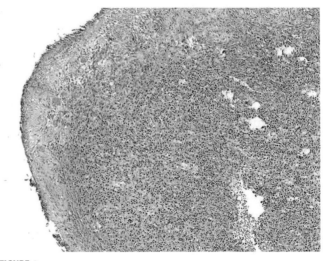

FIGURE 4

Vulvar melanoma. Nodular melanoma composed of sheets of melanocytes.

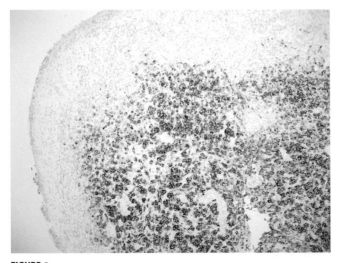

FIGURE 5

Vulvar melanoma. Positive immunohistochemical staining with MART1.

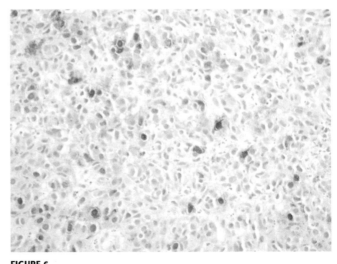

FIGURE 6

Vulvar melanoma. Positive (patchy) staining with S100.

ANGIOMYOFIBROBLASTOMA

DEFINITION—A benign, nonrecurring spindle cell lesion of the vulvovaginal region, characterized by alternating hypercellular and hypocellular areas.

CLINICAL FEATURES

EPIDEMIOLOGY

- Reproductive-age women.
- Uncommon.

PRESENTATION

- Bartholin's gland "cyst," usually smaller than 5 cm.

PROGNOSIS AND TREATMENT

- Excellent.
- There has been one case report of sarcomatous transformation and recurrence.
- Complete excision with negative margins is advised.

PATHOLOGY

HISTOLOGY

- Well circumscribed, with alternating hypercellular and hypocellular areas.

- The stromal cells may be plump and spindled (especially in postmenopausal women) to strikingly epithelioid, and tend to cluster around small capillary-sized vessels.
- Plasmacytoid and multinucleate stromal cells are common.

IMMUNOPATHOLOGY (INCLUDING IMMUNOHISTOCHEMISTRY)

- Desmin positive; smooth muscle actin is variable.

MAIN DIFFERENTIAL DIAGNOSIS

- Aggressive angiomyxoma.
- Asymmetrical vulvar hypertrophy.
- Superficial angiomyxoma.

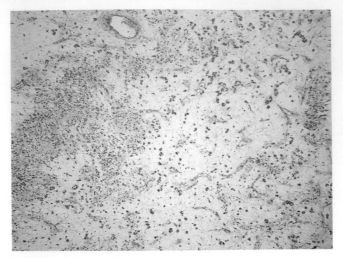

FIGURE 1

Angiomyofibroblastoma. At low power, alternating hypercellular and hypocellular areas can be appreciated. Note the numerous, delicate capillaries present.

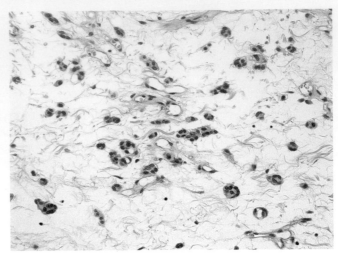

FIGURE 2

Angiomyofibroblastoma. Small, capillary-sized vessels with surrounding clusters of cells with a plasmacytoid appearance. Several multinucleated cells are present.

AGGRESSIVE ANGIOMYXOMA

PITFALL

DEFINITION—A bland, hypocellular, spindle cell lesion of the vulvar/perineal region with a tendency for local infiltration and recurrence.

CLINICAL FEATURES

EPIDEMIOLOGY

- Reproductive-age women in their 30s.
  - Uncommon.

PRESENTATION

- Commonly presents as a labial or Bartholin's gland "cyst."

PROGNOSIS AND TREATMENT

- Nonmetastasizing, but locally destructive.
- Recurrence occurs in 30% to 40% of cases, sometimes years after initial excision.
- Complete excision with negative margins (at least 1 cm).

PATHOLOGY

HISTOLOGY

- Poorly circumscribed, paucicellular neoplasm with inconspicuous infiltration into surrounding soft tissue.
- Bland spindle cells set within a copious myxoid matrix.
- Fibrillary collagen and eosinophilic smooth muscle cells often condense around blood vessels.

IMMUNOPATHOLOGY (INCLUDING IMMUNOHISTOCHEMISTRY)

- Noncontributory.

MAIN DIFFERENTIAL DIAGNOSIS

- Superficial angiomyxoma.
- Angiomyofibroblastoma.

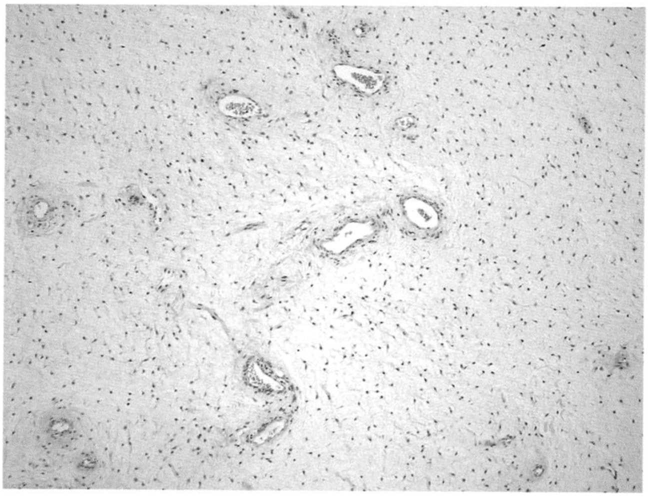

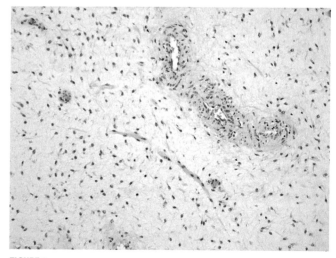

FIGURE 1

Deep aggressive angiomyxoma. Low-power examination reveals a paucicellular, myxoid neoplasm. Note the cellular condensation around the blood vessels.

FIGURE 2

Deep aggressive angiomyxoma. The cells comprising the lesion are small, bland, and spindled. Smooth muscle cells and collagen bundles can be seen condensing around the blood vessel.

SUPERFICIAL ANGIOMYXOMA

DEFINITION—A benign pedunculated myxoid soft tissue neoplasm with a tendency toward local recurrence.

CLINICAL FEATURES

EPIDEMIOLOGY

- Rare.
- Occasionally occurs in the vulva.
- Most frequently seen in reproductive-age women in their 30s.

PRESENTATION

- Solitary, slow-growing, painless polypoid or pedunculated mass.
- Usually less than 5 cm in size.

PROGNOSIS AND TREATMENT

- Complete excision with negative margins.
- Propensity for local recurrence in up to 30% to 40% of cases.

PATHOLOGY

HISTOLOGY

- Well-demarcated and multilobulated superficial angiomyxoma (SAM) is superficial and situated in the subcutis.

- The lobules are strikingly hypocellular and myxoid, with slender stellate spindle cells and thin-walled vessels admixed with polymorphonuclear cells.
- Perivascular hyalinization is not appreciated.
- The tumor cells are small and bland; nuclear atypia is not appreciated.
- Atypical mitotic figures are not seen.
- An epithelial component, usually a squamous-lined cyst, is occasionally present.

IMMUNOPATHOLOGY (INCLUDING IMMUNOHISTOCHEMISTRY)

- Immunohistochemical staining for SMA, desmin, and S100 is negative.

MAIN DIFFERENTIAL DIAGNOSIS

- Deep aggressive angiomyxoma. Deeply situated with the classic vascular pattern.

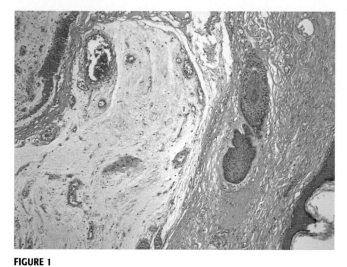

FIGURE 1

SAM. A dermally situated, multilobulated, myxoid mass with well-demarcated borders.

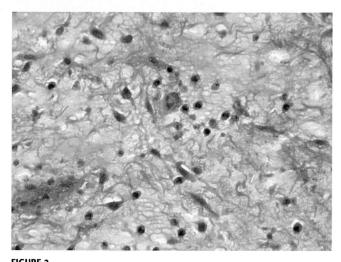

FIGURE 2

SAM. Bland stellate spindle cells set within a myxoid stroma, admixed with neutrophils.

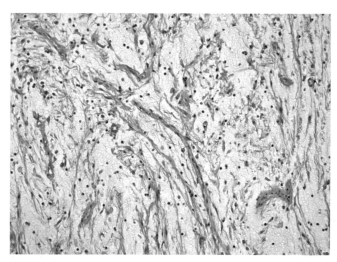

FIGURE 3

SAM. Thin-walled curvilinear vascular structures.

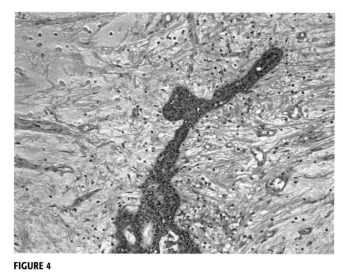

FIGURE 4

SAM. Benign epithelial elements, a squamous-lined cyst, within the tumor.

CELLULAR ANGIOFIBROMA

DEFINITION—A benign subcutaneous neoplasm composed of short fascicles of spindle cells with prominent small, thick-walled, blood vessels.

CLINICAL FEATURES

EPIDEMIOLOGY

- Uncommon.
  - Typically seen in middle-aged women (mean age ~55 years).

PRESENTATION

- Small (<3 cm), painless, subcutaneous vulvovaginal or perineal mass.

PROGNOSIS AND TREATMENT

- Benign.
  - Complete excision is advised as incompletely removed tumors may regrow.

PATHOLOGY

HISTOLOGY

- Well-demarcated proliferation of short fascicles of bland spindle cells with interspersed wispy collagen bundles.

- Prominent vasculature composed of small round vessels with thick, densely hyalinized, eosinophilic walls.
- Entrapped fat or nerve is often present at the periphery.

IMMUNOPATHOLOGY (INCLUDING IMMUNOHISTOCHEMISTRY)

- Variably positive for CD34 and SMA; occasionally desmin positive.
- Negative for S100.

MAIN DIFFERENTIAL DIAGNOSIS

- Solitary fibrous tumor.
  - Angiomyofibroblastoma.
  - Deep aggressive angiomyxoma (when edematous).
- Fibroepithelial stromal polyp—pedunculated, lacks the high vessel density of cellular angiofibroma.

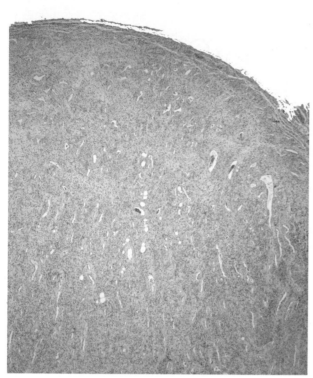

FIGURE 1

Cellular angiofibroma. At low magnification a highly cellular proliferation admixed with numerous small- to medium-sized vessels can be seen.

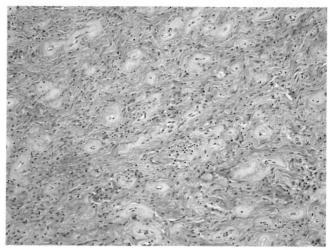

FIGURE 2

Cellular angiofibroma. Fascicles of bland, spindled cells admixed with numerous small vessels with prominent hyalinization.

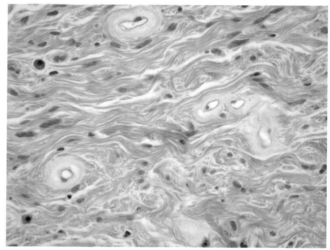

FIGURE 3

Cellular angiofibroma. Bland spindle cells with hyalinized vessels. Note the occasional mast cells.

DERMATOFIBROMA (FIBROUS HISTIOCYTOMA)

DEFINITION—A benign fibrohistiocytic tumor of dermal stroma, composed of spindle cells with a storiform (pinwheel) growth pattern.

CLINICAL FEATURES

EPIDEMIOLOGY

- Occurs in adults.

PRESENTATION

- Papules, plaques, or nodules in the vulva.
- Lesions may be flesh colored or pigmented.

PROGNOSIS AND TREATMENT

- Excellent.
- Excision is adequate treatment.
- For some types (deep, cellular, atypical, aneurysmal), at least marginal excision is advised as these variants are more likely to recur.

PATHOLOGY

HISTOLOGY

- Classical dermatofibroma is a well-circumscribed dermal proliferation of bland spindle cells arranged in a storiform pattern, with trapping of dermal collagen at the edges.
- The overlying epidermis is often hyperplastic (pseudo-epitheliomatous hyperplasia).

IMMUNOPATHOLOGY (INCLUDING IMMUNOHISTOCHEMISTRY)

- CD34 is variable.

MAIN DIFFERENTIAL DIAGNOSIS

- Dermatofibrosarcoma protuberans. Typically more cellular and infiltrates subcutaneous fat.

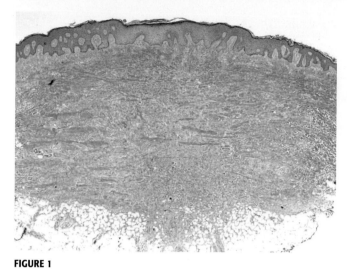

FIGURE 1

Dermatofibroma. A well-circumscribed dermal mass with overlying epidermal (pseudoepitheliomatous) hyperplasia.

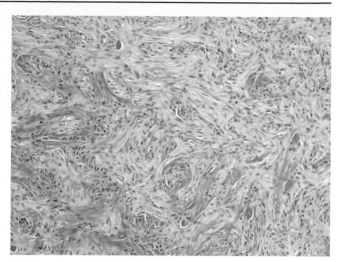

FIGURE 2

Dermatofibroma. Bland, spindled cells with entrapped collagen bundles.

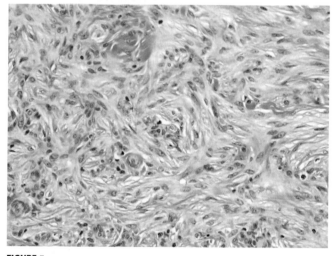

FIGURE 3

Dermatofibroma. Spindle cells arranged in a storiform pattern. Delicate strands of entrapped collagen are present.

DERMATOFIBROSARCOMA PROTUBERANS

DEFINITION—A subcutaneous, locally aggressive spindle cell neoplasm with a storiform growth pattern and honeycomb-like infiltration into adipose tissue.

CLINICAL FEATURES

EPIDEMIOLOGY

- Dermatofibrosarcoma protuberans involving the vulva is rare; however, cases have been reported.

PRESENTATION

- A nodule, plaque, or large multinodular growth in the groin.
- Vulvar lesions are uncommon.

PROGNOSIS AND TREATMENT

- Local recurrence is common; metastases are infrequent.
- Fibrosarcomatous lesions have a higher rate of metastases (up to 15%).
- Complete excision with negative margins is advised.

PATHOLOGY

HISTOLOGY

- A poorly circumscribed mass with a honeycomb pattern of infiltration into subcutaneous adipose tissue.

- A monomorphic, storiform proliferation of spindled cells separated from the overlying atrophic epithelium by a rim of normal stroma (grenz zone).
- Fibrosarcomatous change is identified by its herringbone growth pattern, increased mitotic rate, and hypercellularity.

IMMUNOPATHOLOGY (INCLUDING IMMUNOHISTOCHEMISTRY)

- CD34 is usually diffusely positive.

MAIN DIFFERENTIAL DIAGNOSIS

- Dermatofibroma—less cellular, lacks the deep dermal infiltration into adipose tissue.

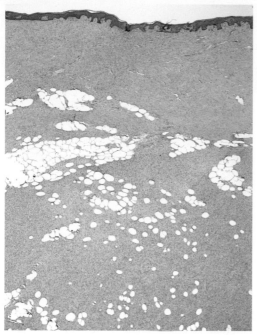

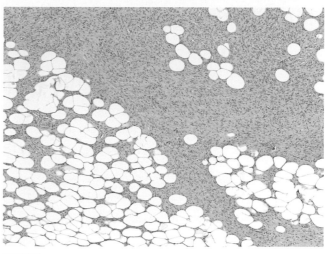

FIGURE 1

Dermatofibrosarcoma protuberans. A poorly circumscribed mass involving the deep dermis and extending into the subcutaneous tissue. Note the absence of pseudoepitheliomatous hyperplasia seen in dermatofibroma and the presence of a grenz zone.

FIGURE 2

Dermatofibrosarcoma protuberans. Infiltration of the spindled cells between fat cells in the subcutaneous tissue creates a honeycomb pattern.

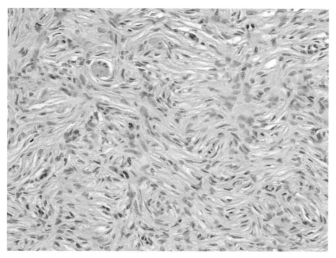

FIGURE 3

Dermatofibrosarcoma protuberans. Bland, spindled cells arranged in a storiform growth pattern.

LOW-GRADE FIBROMYXOID SARCOMA

DEFINITION—A painless, deep-seated, and slow-growing tumor with a deceptively bland histologic appearance and a propensity for local recurrence.

CLINICAL FEATURES

EPIDEMIOLOGY

- Low-grade fibromyxoid sarcoma (LGFMS) is uncommon.
- Most often identified in children and young to middle-aged adults.
- The third and fourth decades of life are the most common age at presentation.

PRESENTATION

- Presents as a slow-growing, painless mass involving the vulva, perineum, or pelvic region.
- May be asymptomatic if deep seated or may present as a palpable mass.

PROGNOSIS AND TREATMENT

- Metastases are uncommon, but local recurrence is frequent.
- Wide local excision is the treatment of choice.

PATHOLOGY

HISTOLOGY

- Grossly, LGFMS ranges in size from 1 to 20 cm, although most are smaller than 10 cm.
- On cut section these tumors are slightly soft, infiltrate into surrounding soft tissues, and are white to yellow with gelatinous glistening areas.

- At low power the tumor is composed of bland spindle cells arranged in alternating hypocellular and hypercellular tongues and nodules.
- The tumor cells are small, with oval to stellate hyperchromatic nuclei, variably prominent small nucleoli, and moderate amounts of indistinct wispy eosinophilic cytoplasm.
- The tumor cells are set in variably fibrous to myxoid-appearing stroma.
- The transitions between the fibrous areas and the myxoid, more hypocellular, areas are abrupt.
- The vasculature is characterized by a proliferation of delicate curvilinear capillary-sized vessels that are most prominent in the myxoid zones.
- Some lesions have prominent collagen rosettes; this pattern was formerly known as "hyalinizing spindle cell tumor with giant rosettes."

IMMUNOPATHOLOGY (INCLUDING IMMUNOHISTOCHEMISTRY)

- Immunohistochemical staining is positive for EMA and MUC4.
- These tumors are characterized cytogenetically by a *FUS/CREB* fusion, which can be detected using a break-apart FISH probe for the *FUS* gene on chromosome 7.

MAIN DIFFERENTIAL DIAGNOSIS

- Nodular fasciitis.
- Deep aggressive angiomyxoma.
- Angiomyofibroblastoma.

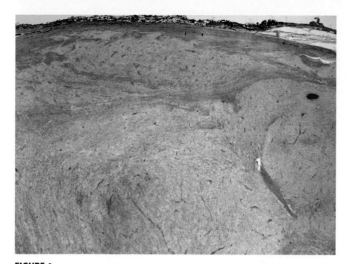

FIGURE 1

LGFMS. Low power showing a spindle cell proliferation with abrupt transition between myxoid and fibrous zones.

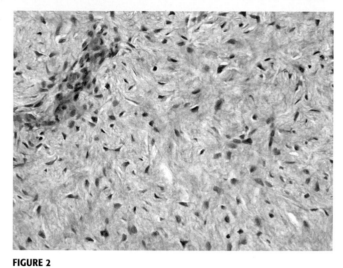

FIGURE 2

LGFMS. Myxoid zone at high power showing bland, oval to stellate tumor cells with indistinct cytoplasm. A small, delicate capillary-sized vessel is present.

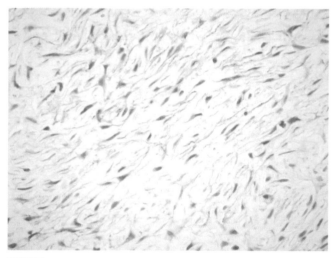

FIGURE 3

LGFMS. Immunohistochemical stain for EMA is positive.

LIPOMA

DEFINITION—A benign adipocytic neoplasm.

CLINICAL FEATURES

EPIDEMIOLOGY

- Rarely encountered in the vulva.

PRESENTATION

- Slow-growing mass in the labium majus.
- Large lesions may be pedunculated.

PROGNOSIS AND TREATMENT

- Excellent.
- Excision is curative.

PATHOLOGY

HISTOLOGY

- Well-circumscribed proliferation of mature adipose tissue.

IMMUNOPATHOLOGY (INCLUDING IMMUNOHISTOCHEMISTRY)

- MDM2 and CDK4 are negative.

MAIN DIFFERENTIAL DIAGNOSIS

- Well-differentiated liposarcoma.

FIGURE 1
Vulvar lipoma. Well-circumscribed mass of mature adipose tissue.

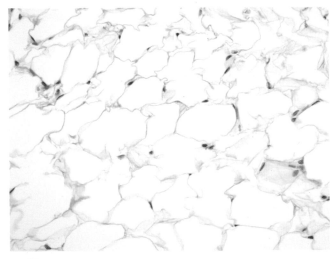

FIGURE 2
Vulvar lipoma. Mature adipocytes. No lipoblasts should be identified.

LIPOSARCOMA

DEFINITION—A malignant neoplasm of adipocytes.

CLINICAL FEATURES

EPIDEMIOLOGY

- Rare.
- Most commonly encountered in middle-aged women.

PRESENTATION

- Vulvar mass or cyst.

PROGNOSIS AND TREATMENT

- If amenable to wide local excision, excellent (in these cases the term *atypical lipomatous tumor* is more appropriate).
- If not completely excised, there is a tendency for destructive local recurrence.
- Distant metastases are extremely rare.

PATHOLOGY

HISTOLOGY

- Well-differentiated liposarcoma is characterized by sheets of adipocytes of varying sizes, cellular fibrous septa containing atypical nuclei, and occasional lipoblasts.

- Occasionally, well-differentiated vulvar liposarcoma may be composed of bland-appearing spindle cells admixed with adipocytes and numerous bivacuolated lipoblasts.
- Dedifferentiated liposarcoma is a spindle cell sarcoma and is recognized by its proximity to a more well-differentiated component.
- Myxoid liposarcoma, as at other sites, is identified by its characteristic thin-walled "chicken-wire" vasculature, mucin pools, and very occasional lipoblasts.

IMMUNOPATHOLOGY (INCLUDING IMMUNOHISTOCHEMISTRY)

- MDM2 and CDK4 are positive in well-differentiated/dedifferentiated liposarcoma.
- Immunohistochemistry is noncontributory for myxoid liposarcoma.

MAIN DIFFERENTIAL DIAGNOSIS

- Lipoma.
- Lipoma with extensive fat necrosis.
- Spindle cell lipoma.
- Angiomyofibroblastoma.

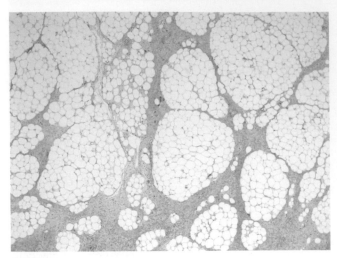

FIGURE 1

Liposarcoma. Nodules of adipose tissue are separated by thick fibrous septa.

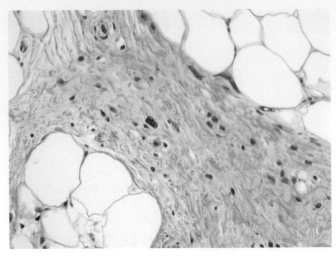

FIGURE 2

Liposarcoma. Atypical stromal cells can be identified within the fibrous bands.

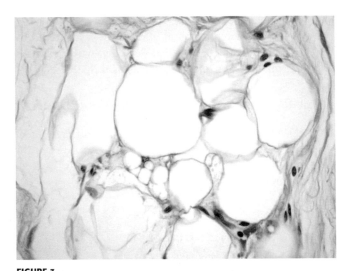

FIGURE 3

Liposarcoma. An example of a lipoblast. Lipoblasts can be identified by the presence of multiple fat vacuoles within the cytoplasm and the distinctive scalloped nuclear contours they create.

SYNOVIAL SARCOMA OF THE VULVA

DEFINITION—A malignant frequently biphasic tumor of soft tissue.

CLINICAL FEATURES

EPIDEMIOLOGY

- Rare.
- Encountered in all age groups, mostly in the second and third decades.
- t(X:18) translocation (representing a fusion of SYT [at 18q11] with either SSX1 or SSX2 [at Xp11]) linked to pathogenesis and prognosis.

PRESENTATION

- Vulvar mass.

PROGNOSIS AND TREATMENT

- Known for high recurrence rate.
- Prognosis depends to some degree on tumor grade, mitotic index, age, size (5-cm cutoff), and resectability.
- Standard is resection if possible; radiation and chemotherapy of uncertain benefit.
- Five-year survival approximately 60%, disease-free survival approximately 30%.
- Adverse outcome linked to older age, high mitotic/proliferative index, monophasic tumors, tumors over 5 cm in diameter, and/or incompletely excised.
- More complex genomes have been linked to adverse outcomes.

PATHOLOGY

HISTOLOGY

- Classic biphasic synovial sarcoma shows a mixture of spindle and epithelial cell components. However, the epithelial component can predominate in the presence of bland-appearing spindled cells.
- Spindle cell component can be rather bland and distinct from, but closely admixed with, the epithelial component.
- Monophasic tumors exhibit spindle cell morphology; epithelial component may be less conspicuous, consisting of eosinophilic cells scattered through the mesenchymal component.
- Myxoid areas may be seen.

IMMUNOPATHOLOGY (INCLUDING IMMUNOHISTOCHEMISTRY)

- PAX8 negative, ER/PR negative.
- TLE-1 strong positivity is highly specific for synovial sarcoma if not exclusive to this tumor.

MAIN DIFFERENTIAL DIAGNOSIS

- Carcinosarcoma—the mesenchymal component will typically be more poorly differentiated; the epithelial component should be PAX8 positive in most cases and TLE-1 negative.
- Endometrioid adenocarcinoma with a spindle cell component—may closely resemble synovial sarcoma. Should be PAX8 positive and TLE-1 negative.
- Spindle cell epithelioma—a benign spindle cell tumor with focal epithelial differentiation. Should be negative for TLE-1.
- Extrarenal Wilms' tumor—this tumor is rarely found in the vulvar region. The epithelial component is typically more primitive in appearance, composed of small tubular structures within blastema.

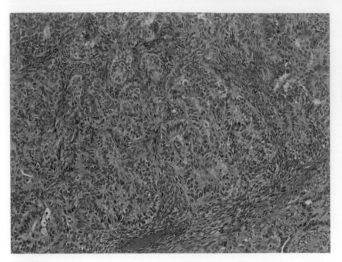

FIGURE 1

Synovial sarcoma. In this field the epithelial component predominates.

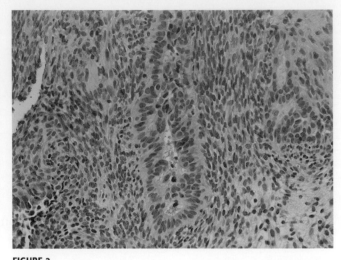

FIGURE 2

Synovial sarcoma. There is a juxtaposed epithelial component *(center)* and adjacent spindle cell component.

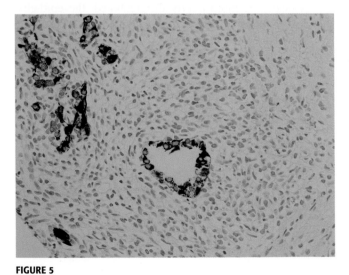

FIGURE 3

Synovial sarcoma. In this field the epithelial nests are more spindled (squamoid) and the mesenchymal component consists of narrow bands of more poorly differentiated spindled cells.

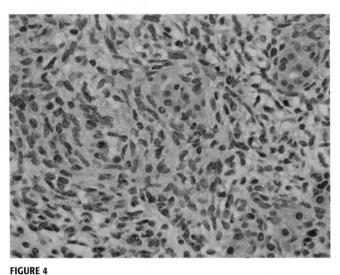

FIGURE 4

This synovial sarcoma is predominantly mesenchymal, with interlacing spindled cells punctuated by a few pink glandlike structures.

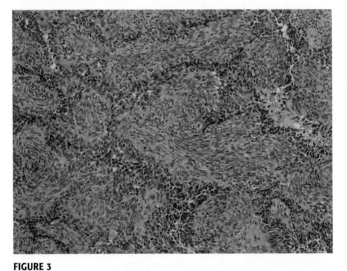

FIGURE 5

An AE1/AE3 immunostain highlights both glandlike and less organized epithelial cells within the sarcomatous stroma.

RHABDOMYOMA

DEFINITION—A solitary, benign, polypoid lesion of the vagina composed of bland rhabdomyoblasts.

CLINICAL FEATURES

EPIDEMIOLOGY

- Middle-aged women.

PRESENTATION

- Solitary polypoid lesion, usually smaller than 3 cm.
- Vagina is the most common site, followed by vulva and cervix.

PROGNOSIS AND TREATMENT

- Excellent.
- Complete excision is curative.

PATHOLOGY

HISTOLOGY

- An irregular and vaguely vascular submucosal proliferation of bland rhabdomyoblasts.
- The rhabdomyoblasts are brightly eosinophilic, spindle to strap shaped, with visible cytoplasmic cross striations.

- Nuclear atypia is absent, and mitotic activity is low.
- Subepithelial condensation (cambium layer) is not present.

IMMUNOPATHOLOGY (INCLUDING IMMUNOHISTOCHEMISTRY)

- Desmin, myogenin, and Myf-4 are positive (skeletal muscle markers).
- S100 is negative, differentiating from a granular cell tumor.

MAIN DIFFERENTIAL DIAGNOSIS

- Embryonal rhabdomyosarcoma—look for smaller, more primitive mesenchymal cells, including a cambium layer.
- Granular cell tumor—typically seen on the vulva. S-100 positive, and often associated with pseudoepitheliomatous hyperplasia.
- Spindle cell epithelioma (mixed tumor)—lacks the prominent eosinophilic cytoplasm and cross-striations of a rhabdomyoma.

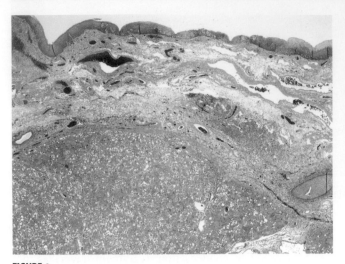

FIGURE 1

Genital rhabdomyoma. Well-circumscribed mass within the submucosa. Note the irregular borders. Brightly eosinophilic cells are evident at low power.

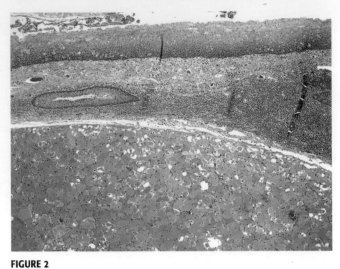

FIGURE 2

Genital rhabdomyoma. Large eosinophilic cells with small nuclei.

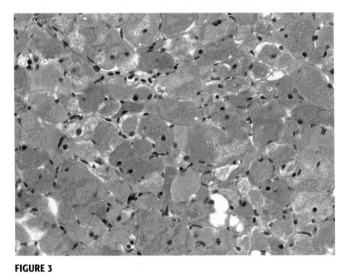

FIGURE 3

Genital rhabdomyoma. Large, polygonal eosinophilic cells with occasional striations. The nuclei are small, round, and regular.

ANGIOKERATOMA

DEFINITION—A discrete vascular ectasia with overlying epidermal hyperplasia.

CLINICAL FEATURES

EPIDEMIOLOGY

- Typically seen in women under age 50.
- Typically sporadic but also associated with Fabry's disease (deficiency of lysosomal alpha-galactosidase).

PRESENTATION

- Generally asymptomatic but may present with bleeding or pain.
- Papular, occasionally warty lesions (<1 cm in size) of the vulva.
- May be solitary or multiple (including angiokeratoma corporis diffusum).

PROGNOSIS AND TREATMENT

- Prognosis is excellent.
- Observation is adequate; if symptomatic, excision or ablation may be required.

PATHOLOGY

HISTOLOGY

- Dilated blood-filled spaces in the papillary dermis, closely apposed to the epidermis.
- The epidermis exhibits prominent acanthosis with hyperkeratosis and occasionally papillomatosis.

IMMUNOPATHOLOGY (INCLUDING IMMUNOHISTOCHEMISTRY)

- Noncontributory.

MAIN DIFFERENTIAL DIAGNOSIS

- Squamous papilloma/condyloma—dilated vascular spaces are not typical in condyloma, and koilocytes are not present in angiokeratoma.
- Hemangioma—should be situated more deeply in the dermis.

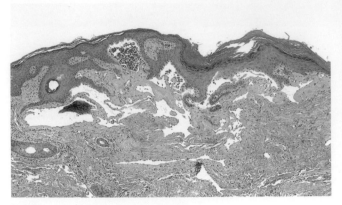

FIGURE 1

Angiokeratoma. Ectatic vessels can be seen in the dermis, several of which contain red blood cells. Even at low power the hyperkeratosis and hypergranulosis are evident.

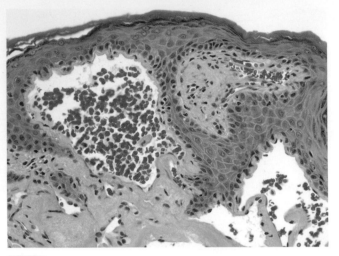

FIGURE 2

Angiokeratoma. Dilated vascular spaces with a bland endothelial lining.

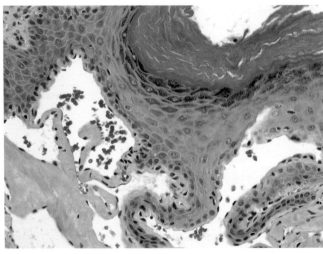

FIGURE 3

Angiokeratoma. Ectatic vascular spaces immediately adjacent to the overlying epidermis, which displays hypergranulosis and hyperkeratosis.

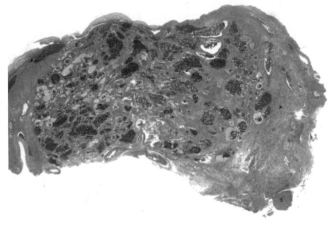

FIGURE 4

Cavernous hemangioma. At low magnification this is a discrete mass-forming lesion in the dermis.

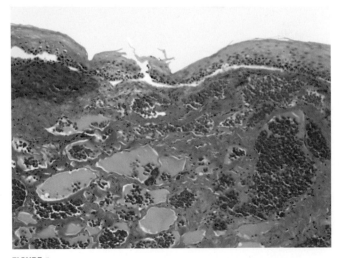

FIGURE 5

Cavernous hemangioma. In contrast to angiokeratoma there is a sharp separation between the epidermis and the lesion.

GRANULAR CELL TUMOR

DEFINITION—A (usually) benign soft tissue tumor of the vulva of presumably neural crest lineage.

CLINICAL FEATURES

EPIDEMIOLOGY

- Uncommon.
- Can occur at any age, with a mean age of presentation of 50 years.
- More common in African-American women.

PRESENTATION

- Present as slow-growing asymptomatic nodules and often found incidentally.
- Vary from 1 to 12 cm in size.

PROGNOSIS AND TREATMENT

- Excision is usually curative.
- Local recurrences are uncommon even in incompletely excised tumors but may be higher in lesions with infiltrative borders.
- Rare malignant tumors reported.

PATHOLOGY

HISTOLOGY

- Located in the subcutis.
- Polygonal cells with abundant eosinophilic granular cytoplasm.

- Centrally located variably hyperchromatic nuclei.
- Pushing or infiltrative borders.
- There can be a distinctive pseudoepitheliomatous hyperplasia of overlying squamous mucosa that can mimic squamous cell carcinoma (PITFALL).

DIAGNOSTIC TERMINOLOGY

- Granular cell tumor (granular cell myoblastoma is no longer used for obvious reasons).

IMMUNOPATHOLOGY (INCLUDING IMMUNOHISTOCHEMISTRY)

- S100 and NSE stains are usually positive; NKI-C3 (lysosomal) is also positive.

MAIN DIFFERENTIAL DIAGNOSIS

- Squamous cell carcinoma, if the pseudoepitheliomatous hyperplasia is prominent.
- Rhabdomyoma—tumor cells will have cross-striations and a more homogeneous eosinophilic versus granular cytoplasm.

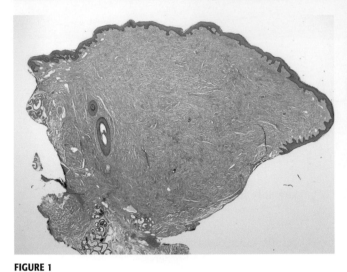

FIGURE 1

Granular cell tumor. At low power this tumor appears as a nondescript soft tissue mass.

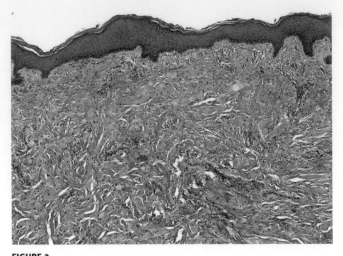

FIGURE 2

Granular cell tumor. At higher magnification the polyhedral cells can be appreciated amid the collagen bundles beneath the surface.

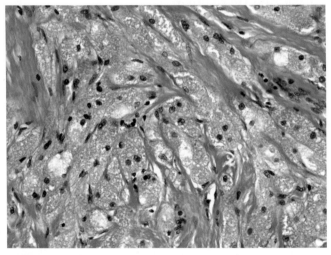

FIGURE 3

Granular cell tumor. At high magnification the prominent granular eosinophilic cytoplasm is evident.

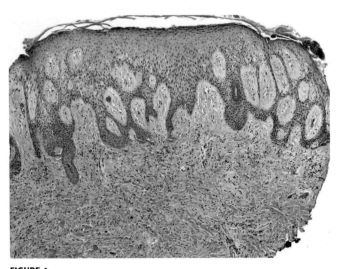

FIGURE 4

Pseudoepitheliomatous hyperplasia overlying a granular cell tumor.

PREPUBERTAL VULVAR FIBROMA

DEFINITION—A rare, benign, spindle cell proliferation that occurs in the vulva of prepubertal women.

CLINICAL FEATURES

EPIDEMIOLOGY

- Rare.
- Prepubertal women, age ranging between 4 and 12 years (median age is 8 years).

PRESENTATION

- Gradual vulvar swelling, resulting in asymmetrical labial enlargement.
- Painless vulvar mass.
- Most commonly affects the labia majora.

PROGNOSIS AND TREATMENT

- This is a benign lesion; controversy exists regarding its classification as a true neoplasm.
- Conservative excision is appropriate treatment.
- If incompletely excised, there is a tendency for recurrence.

PATHOLOGY

HISTOLOGY

- A hypocellular, ill-defined proliferation of bland spindle cells with ovoid nuclei.

- The cells are arranged in a patternless pattern and set within a variably edematous to myxoid to collagenous matrix.
- Small- to medium-sized vessels are scattered throughout the lesion, some with thick walls.
- The lesional cells characteristically infiltrate adjacent adipose tissue, nerve bundles, and adnexal structures.

IMMUNOPATHOLOGY (INCLUDING IMMUNOHISTOCHEMISTRY)

- Positive for CD34.
- SMA, desmin, and S100 are negative.

MAIN DIFFERENTIAL DIAGNOSIS

- Deep aggressive angiomyxoma—these tumors are more deeply situated and have the characteristic myxoid stroma with thick-walled vessels.
- Cellular angiofibroma—well circumscribed, more cellular than prepubertal fibroma.
- Fibroepithelial stromal polyp—typically polypoid, usually a thick-walled central vessel.
- Superficial angiomyxoma—subcutaneous as opposed to submucosal; polypoid.

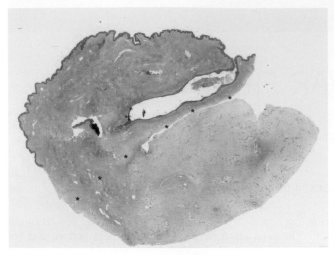

FIGURE 1

Prepubertal vulvar fibroma. This low-power image illustrates an ill-defined submucosal mass (below the *).

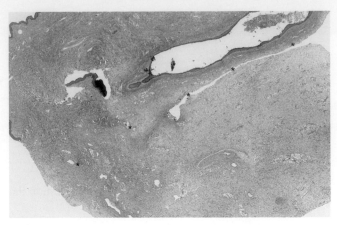

FIGURE 2

Prepubertal vulvar fibroma. At higher magnification the interface between the normal and abnormal stroma is demarcated (*).

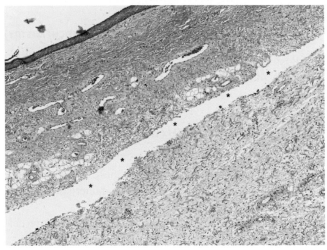

FIGURE 3

Prepubertal vulvar fibroma. At higher magnification the interface between the normal and abnormal stroma is demarcated (*).

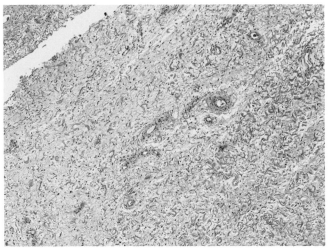

FIGURE 4

Prepubertal vulvar fibroma. Spindled cells with ovoid nuclei set in an edematous, collagenous stroma. Note the small blood vessels.

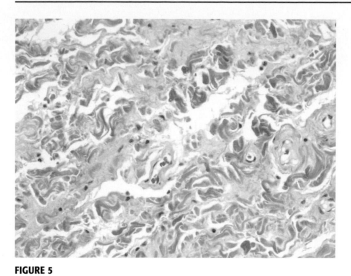

FIGURE 5

Prepubertal vulvar fibroma. Collagenous background with bland spindle cells. Delicate capillary-like vessels are present.

ANAL CONDYLOMA

DEFINITION—A human papillomavirus (HPV)–related exophytic lesion of the perianal skin and anal canal.

CLINICAL FEATURES

EPIDEMIOLOGY

- Associated with low-risk HPV infection (types 6 and 11).
- Increased incidence with immunosuppression, including human immunodeficiency virus (HIV).
- Other risk factors include anal intercourse, other sexually transmitted diseases, and multiple sexual partners.

PRESENTATION

- Seen clinically as pink to gray warty excrescences, sometimes with filiform fronds.

PROGNOSIS AND TREATMENT

- Prognosis is variable; lesions may persist for some time.
- Highly associated with increased risk of subsequent high-grade squamous intraepithelial lesion diagnosis; clinical follow-up is required.
- Treatment options include excision, laser vaporization, and topical antiviral agents.

PATHOLOGY

HISTOLOGY

- The condyloma trifecta includes acanthosis (thickening of the epidermis), papillomatosis (fronds), and koilocy-tosis (viral cytopathic effect). The latter may vary, however, in keratinized mucosa.
- Nuclear atypia is variable but must be confined to the upper layers of epidermis.
- Multiple lesions are frequently present.

IMMUNOPATHOLOGY (INCLUDING IMMUNOHISTOCHEMISTRY)

- Noncontributory.

MAIN DIFFERENTIAL DIAGNOSIS

- High-grade squamous intraepithelial lesion—atypia akin to other high-grade lesions in the vulva or vagina.
- Hemorrhoids—lack the verruciform acanthosis of condyloma.
- Reactive epithelia changes with cytoplasmic halos—minimal atypia present.
- Nonspecific acanthosis—minimal anisokaryosis and no koilocytosis.
- Fibroepithelial stromal polyp–like hemorrhoids—lack the acanthosis and papillomatosis of condyloma.

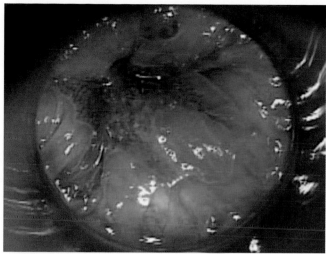

FIGURE 1

Colpophotograph of the anal squamocolumnar junction. *(Courtesy N. Jay and J.M. Berry, UCSF.)*

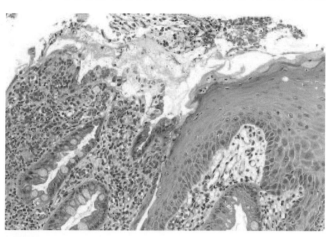

FIGURE 2

Photomicrograph of the squamocolumnar region.

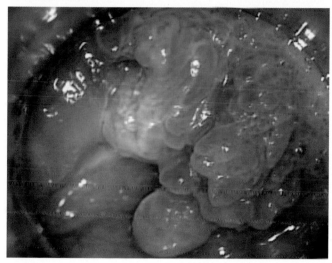

FIGURE 3

Colpophotograph of an exophytic anal condyloma. *(Courtesy N. Jay and J.M. Berry, UCSF.)*

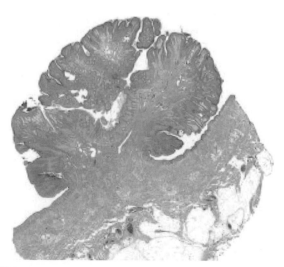

FIGURE 4

Low-power image of an exophytic anal condyloma.

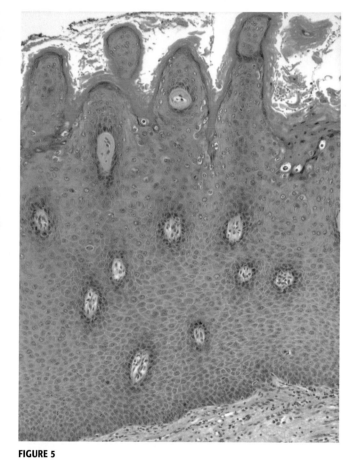

FIGURE 5

Anal condyloma. Acanthosis with small spirelike epithelial projections. Hyperkeratosis is noted throughout. Focal parakeratosis can be identified within the hyperkeratotic layer on the right side. Note the small zone of koilocytotic atypia.

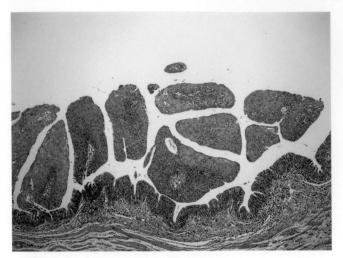

FIGURE 6

Anal condyloma. Papillary-like projections with koilocytic atypia are best seen in the leftmost spire. Note the lack of any cytopathic effect in other areas, a manifestation of lesions that arise in a transitional epithelium.

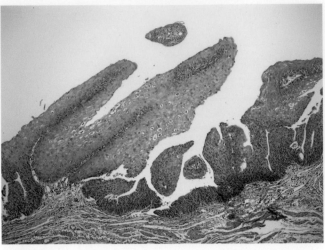

FIGURE 7

Anal condyloma. Fine papillary projections with conspicuous viral cytopathic effect, merging with transitional epithelium on the right. In both Figures 6 and 7 the small papillae with lack of cytopathic effect is similar to that seen with immature condylomas of the cervix arising in immature metaplastic epithelium and similar low-risk HPV infections in the urethra.

ANAL INTRAEPITHELIAL NEOPLASIA II AND III

DEFINITION—A high-grade, human papillomavirus (HPV)–associated, in situ lesion of the squamous anal mucosa.

CLINICAL FEATURES

EPIDEMIOLOGY

- Associated with oncogenic HPV types (16 and 18).
- Increased risk with HPV, human immunodeficiency virus (HIV), anal intercourse, and multiple sexual partners.

PRESENTATION

- May be an incidental finding following an unrelated procedure (such as hemorrhoidectomy).
- Clinical appearance ranges from an inconspicuous smooth or granular flat lesion to a denuded and ulcerated patch.

PROGNOSIS AND TREATMENT

- Natural history is not well understood.
- Regression rates appear low.
- Treatment options include surgical excision (for large lesions), trichloroacetic acid (TCA), and cryotherapy.

PATHOLOGY

HISTOLOGY

- Lesions are characterized by uniform, full-thickness atypia with loss of nuclear polarity.
- Dyskeratosis and frequent mitoses (including atypical forms) are present.
- Parakeratosis with atypical nuclei is often present.
- Lesions often involve skin appendages, especially hair follicles.

IMMUNOPATHOLOGY (INCLUDING IMMUNOHISTOCHEMISTRY)

- Positive for p16.

MAIN DIFFERENTIAL DIAGNOSIS

- Inflamed or reactive epithelium—particularly in the anal transition zone where the native epithleium can appear immature or "transitional."

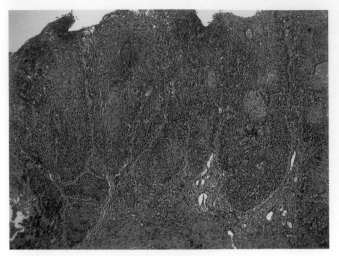

FIGURE 1

Anal intraepithelial neoplasia (AIN) II/III. Acanthotic squamous epithelium with full-thickness loss of maturation and marked cell crowding. Features analogous to those seen in high-grade dysplasia of the vulva, vagina, or cervix.

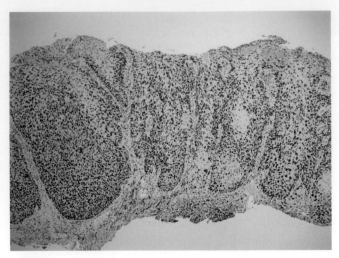

FIGURE 2

AIN II/III. Ki-67 immunostain showing a diffuse increase in labeling, with positive nuclei present in the uppermost epithelial layer.

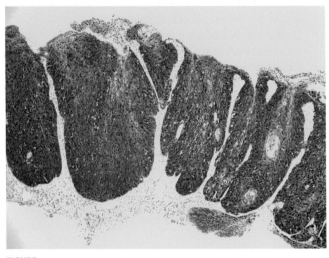

FIGURE 3

AIN II/III. Immunostaining for p16 showing strong, diffuse, nuclear and cytoplasmic positivity.

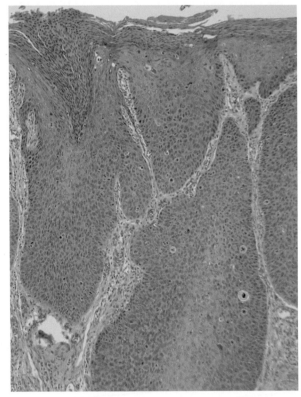

FIGURE 4

II/III. Full-thickness nuclear atypia with numerous apoptotic cells and striking parakeratosis with atypical nuclei.

ANAL CARCINOMA

DEFINITION—Malignant tumors arising from the epithelium of the anal canal.

CLINICAL FEATURES

EPIDEMIOLOGY

- Rare; incidence is estimated at 7 per million women and 9 per million men.
- Incidence is increasing at a rate of approximately 2% a year.
- Squamous cell carcinomas (SCC) account for 80% of cases; risk factors include human papillomavirus (HPV), human immunodeficiency virus (HIV), anal intercourse, and number of sexual partners.
- Adenocarcinomas are much less frequent and account for approximately 20% of tumors.

PRESENTATION

- Often nonspecific and varies with tumor size.
- May present with pruritus, pain, changes in bowel habits, or sensation of a mass.

PROGNOSIS AND TREATMENT

- Overall 5-year survival ranges from 60% to 80% for SCC.
- First-line therapy for SCC is typically chemoradiation; radial resections are reserved for those patients who cannot tolerate other modalities or for salvage therapy.
- Prognosis for SCC varies with tumor stage (including lymph node status) and tumor grade.

PATHOLOGY

HISTOLOGY

- Three major morphologic variants of anal SCC exist: large-cell keratinizing, large-cell nonkeratinizing, and basaloid.

- The large-cell variants are composed of irregularly shaped nests and cords of large cells with pale pink cytoplasm and vesicular nuclei.
- Keratin production may manifest as brightly eosinophilic whorls (pearls) or as single cells with intensely eosinophilic cytoplasm.
- The basaloid (cloacogenic or transitional) variant is characterized by nests of smaller cells with high nuclear-to-cytoplasmic ratios and central necrosis.
- The basaloid nests often exhibit peripheral palisading of nuclei and artifactual retraction from the surrounding stroma.
- An adjacent high-grade intraepithelial squamous lesion is often identified.
- Other rare variants exist, including verrucous carcinoma and anal duct carcinoma.
- Adenocarcinoma of the anal canal is divided into three groups: adenocarcinoma of the anal mucosa, anal gland carcinoma (rare), and adenocarcinoma within a fistula.
- Adenocarcinoma of the anal mucosa has the morphologic appearance of a typical colorectal carcinoma.

IMMUNOPATHOLOGY (INCLUDING IMMUNOHISTOCHEMISTRY)

- SCC may be p16 positive.

MAIN DIFFERENTIAL DIAGNOSIS

- Pseudoepitheliomatous hyperplasia.
- Benign or giant condyloma.
- Basal cell carcinoma.

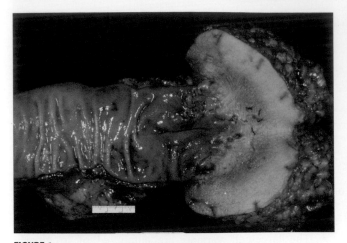

FIGURE 1

Anal carcinoma. A gross photograph showing a 2 cm area of ulceration at the squamocolumnar junction. *(Courtesy Dr. Laura Lamps.)*

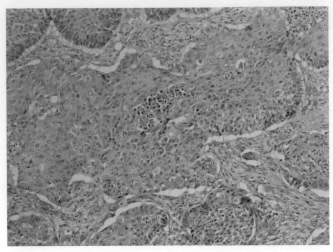

FIGURE 2

Anal carcinoma. Infiltrating nests of SCC with abundant eosinophilic cytoplasm and vesicular nuclei. *(Courtesy Dr. Laura Lamps.)*

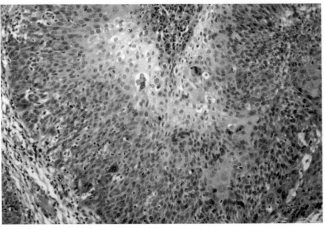

FIGURE 3

Anal carcinoma. SCC with focal dyskeratosis displayed by the occasional brightly eosinophilic cell. Focal, marked pleomorphism can be seen as well. *(Courtesy Dr. Laura Lamps.)*

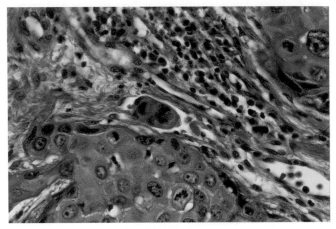

FIGURE 4

Anal carcinoma. A small cluster of dyskeratotic squamous cells within a vascular space. Note the marked increase in cell and nuclear size when compared with the adjacent lymphocytes. *(Courtesy Dr. Laura Lamps.)*

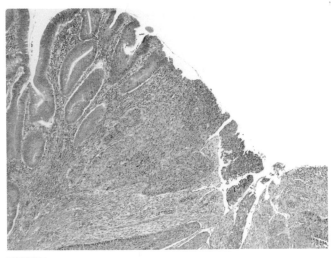

FIGURE 5

Anal carcinoma. Basaloid-type SCC arising adjacent to an area of adenomatous glandular dysplasia. *(Courtesy Dr. Laura Lamps.)*

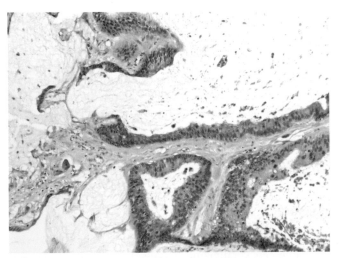

FIGURE 6

Anal carcinoma. Glandular "cloacogenic carcinoma" composed of glands that are identical to those seen in colonic adenocarcinoma. *(Courtesy Dr. Laura Lamps.)*

ANAL PAGET'S DISEASE

DEFINITION—Infiltration of the perianal squamous epithelium by mucin-producing neoplastic cells associated with an anorectal neoplasm. Also called type 2 Paget's disease.

CLINICAL FEATURES

EPIDEMIOLOGY

- Uncommon; represents only 1% to 2% of vulvar malignancies.
- The average age at presentation is 65 years; the majority of patients are over 60 years.

PRESENTATION

- Perianal pruritus is the most common symptom.
- Ill-defined, erythematous plaques on the anus.
- Involved skin may exhibit eczematous changes or ulceration.
- Paget's disease may precede the diagnosis of invasion by months or years.

PROGNOSIS AND TREATMENT

- Wide local excision for noninvasive and either local excision or radical abdominoperitoneal resection for invasive carcinomas.
- Close follow-up is necessary; disease recurs in up to 50% of patients, even with negative margins.
- Ten-year median disease-specific survival for invasive carcinoma. For noninvasive lesions the survival is similar to age-matched controls.
- An associated internal malignancy (e.g., colorectal carcinoma) has been reported in up to 10% to 15% of cases.

PATHOLOGY

HISTOLOGY

- Nests and single cells percolate through the epidermis, frequently extending into adnexal structures.

- The neoplastic cells are large, often with abundant pale blue cytoplasm, large vesicular nuclei, and small conspicuous nucleoli.
- Rarely Paget's cells may form glands within the epidermis.
- A basal keratinocyte is often present between the Paget's cells and the basement membrane.
- Stromal invasion by Paget's cells may be difficult to distinguish from adnexal involvement.

IMMUNOPATHOLOGY (INCLUDING IMMUNOHISTOCHEMISTRY)

- Positive for CK20.
- Negative for CK5/6 (positive in squamous epithelium), S100, p63, CK7, and GCDFP.

MAIN DIFFERENTIAL DIAGNOSIS

- Vulvar or perineal Paget's disease: These are typically CK7 positive.
- Urothelial carcinoma (via direct extension): Typically more poorly differentiated in appearance. Will be both CK7 and CK20 positive.
- Pagetoid vulvar intraepithelial neoplasia: These are rare in the vulva and rarer in the perianal region. Will be p63 positive.
- Melanoma: Will be CK20 negative, Melan-A and MART1 positive.

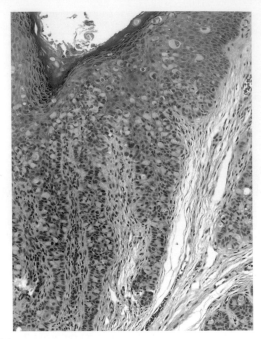

FIGURE 1

Anal Paget's disease. The entire thickness of the epithelium is permeated with neoplastic cells.

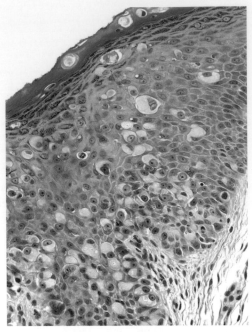

FIGURE 2

Anal Paget's disease. At higher magnification the characteristic Paget's cells with ample cytoplasm are throughout the epithelium.

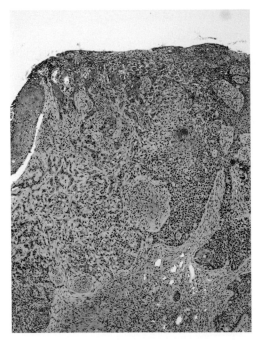

FIGURE 3

Anal Paget's disease. Invasive carcinoma is seen on the left.

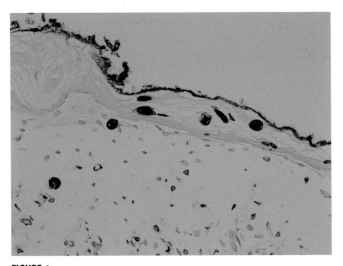

FIGURE 4

Anal Paget's disease. Several Paget's cells are positive for CK20.

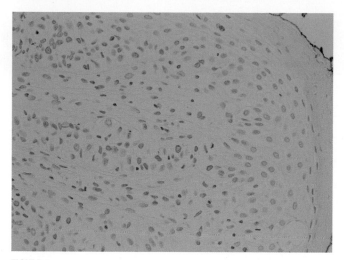

FIGURE 5

Anal Paget's disease. These are typically CK7 negative.

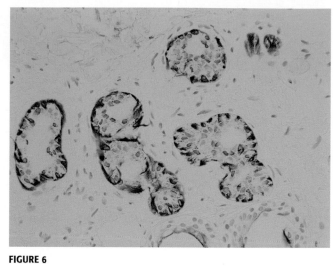

FIGURE 6

Perianal glands are CK7 positive and should not be confused with Paget's cells.

PROLAPSED FALLOPIAN TUBE

DEFINITION—Protrusion of the fallopian tube into the vagina.

CLINICAL FEATURES

EPIDEMIOLOGY

- Occasionally affects women after simple hysterectomy.

PRESENTATION

- May present as a mass in the upper vagina following simple hysterectomy when the tubes are fixed near the vaginal apex. Cases have been reported in laparoscopic procedures where the adnexa are spared. Clinically may appear similar to granulation tissue or recurrent carcinoma (in clinically appropriate setting).

PROGNOSIS AND TREATMENT

- Excellent; excision is curative.

PATHOLOGY

HISTOLOGY

- Typical tubal histology is present. Plica lined with variable amounts of secretory and ciliated cells is present.

Marked acute and chronic inflammation with granulation tissue may be present as well as reactive atypia. In some cases the stroma undergoes an exuberant angiomyofibroblastic response that may mimic a stromal neoplasm. These lesions may be mistaken for adenocarcinoma if the tubal epithelium is not appreciated.

IMMUNOPATHOLOGY (INCLUDING IMMUNOHISTOCHEMISTRY)

- PAX8 staining may be helpful if cilia are not present and there is a concern for a neoplasm that is not müllerian.

MAIN DIFFERENTIAL DIAGNOSIS

- Granulation tissue—This is another sequel to hysterectomy and can mimic prolapsed fallopian tube clinically.
- Recurrent adenocarcinoma (in clinically appropriate setting)—This is usually easily distinguished from prolapsed tube, but the combination of both a prolapsed tube and a prior history of endometrial carcinoma is a recipe for a misdiagnosis.

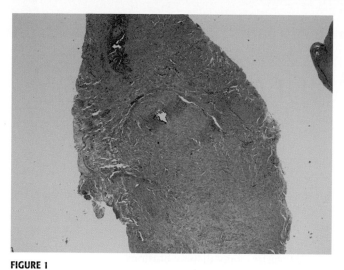

FIGURE 1

A segment of prolapsed tube with a small lumen and surrounding smooth muscle.

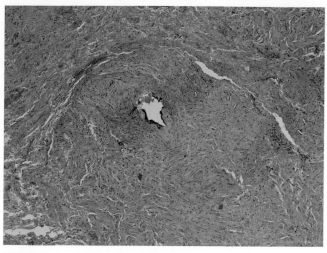

FIGURE 2

Higher magnification showing the lumen and tubal wall.

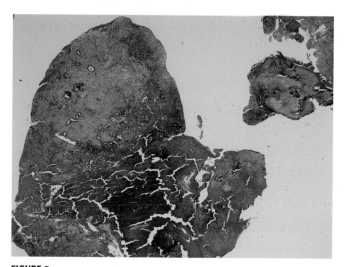

FIGURE 3

Prolapsed fallopian tube. A typical appearance of haphazardly arranged glandlike structures in a fibrotic and inflamed stroma.

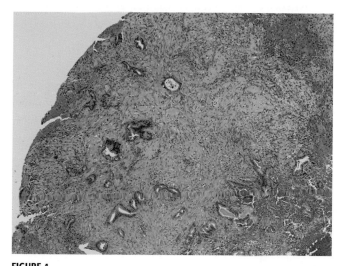

FIGURE 4

Higher magnification of Figure 3. Note the epithelium, being inflamed, may not display evidence of ciliated differentiation, which can make the exclusion of a neoplasm initially difficult.

GRANULATION TISSUE

DEFINITION—A fibrovascular response to injury comprised of small vascular structures, loose stroma, and admixed inflammation.

CLINICAL FEATURES

EPIDEMIOLOGY

- Affects all age groups; vaginal granulation tissue is commonly seen after surgery in the vaginal cuff.

PRESENTATION

- Vaginal granulation tissue presents as a red papule in the upper vagina, adjacent to the sutured vaginal cuff.
- Grossly the lesion may be friable and bleed easily, mimicking recurrent carcinoma.
- Patients may present with vaginal bleeding.

PROGNOSIS and TREATMENT

- Excellent; the lesions are self-limited.
- Simple excision may be considered for large painful lesions.

PATHOLOGY

HISTOLOGY

- Marked inflammation, both acute and chronic, with admixed proliferating vessels and edematous stroma are present in variable proportions.

- The surface may display erosions.
- Reactive atypia may be prominent and mimic neoplastic change.
- As the lesions age, increasing amounts of fibrous tissue will be found.

IMMUNOPATHOLOGY (INCLUDING IMMUNOHISTOCHEMISTRY)

- Noncontributory.

MAIN DIFFERENTIAL DIAGNOSIS

- Carcinoma—this can be a diagnostic problem if squames are trapped within the granulation tissue.

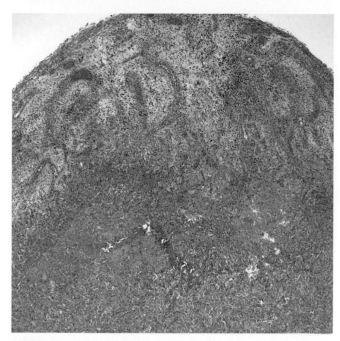

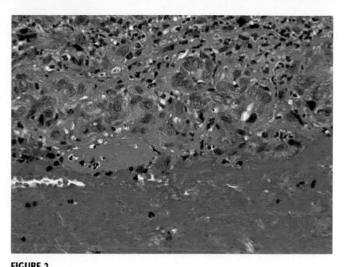

FIGURE 2

Granulation tissue. Admixed inflammatory cells and vascular endothelial cells. The vascular endothelial cells may display reactive atypia that can mimic malignancy.

FIGURE 1

Granulation tissue. Stromal edema, inflammatory cells, and vascular ingrowth can be seen at low power. Note that the surface is denuded.

VAGINAL ADENOSIS

DEFINITION—Congenital glandular differentiation present within the vaginal mucosa.

CLINICAL FEATURES

EPIDEMIOLOGY

- Prior to the use of diethylstilbestrol (DES) and in patients not exposed to DES the incidence of vaginal adenosis was rare. In patients who were exposed to DES the incidence of adenosis approaches one third.

PRESENTATION

- Clinical examination will reveal the presence of red, granular vaginal mucosa. This can be seen in continuity with the cervix. The upper vagina is affected in the vast majority of cases.

PROGNOSIS AND TREATMENT

- There is a small but significant association with DES-associated adenosis and vaginal clear cell carcinoma, which can be seen in 1 in 1000 to 5000 exposed patients. Simple excision is curative.

PATHOLOGY

HISTOLOGY

- The glands comprising adenosis may have differing morphologies including benign endocervical glands, which may be complicated by squamous, tubal, endometrial, and tubal-endometrial metaplasia. Large lesions may rarely contain papillary structures, microglandular change, Arias-Stella effect, and intestinal metaplasia. Varying degrees of glandular atypia may be present.

IMMUNOPATHOLOGY (INCLUDING IMMUNOHISTOCHEMISTRY)

- Noncontributory.

MAIN DIFFERENTIAL DIAGNOSIS

- Endometriosis—this may be particularly difficult to distinguish from adenosis given that the latter often displays tubal-endometrial metaplasia. The presence of separate endocervical-like glands with reserve cells and/or metaplasia supports adenosis.
- Prolapsed fallopian tube—this is another entity that can display bland-appearing "glands" with features of endocervical epithelium. Reserve cells and squamous metaplasia will be absent.
- Mucous cyst of the vagina—this is technically "adenosis" and can undergo squamous metaplasia but is usually an isolated cyst.
- Adenocarcinoma—this can be a concern when there is atypia and criteria used to distinguish clear cell carcinoma or other neoplasms from Arias-Stella effect or reactive changes are applied.

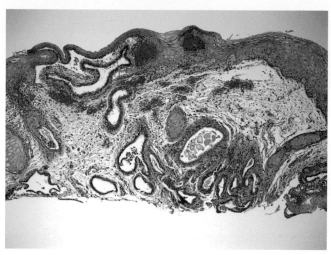

FIGURE 1

Vaginal adenosis. Here a range of columnar epithelial differentiation is seen, mostly tubal-endometrial, but with squamous metaplasia.

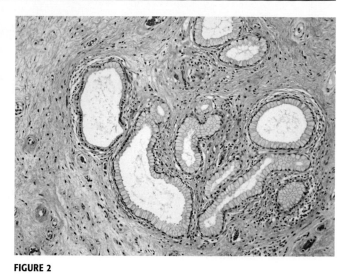

FIGURE 2

Vaginal adenosis. This epithelium is classic endocervical type.

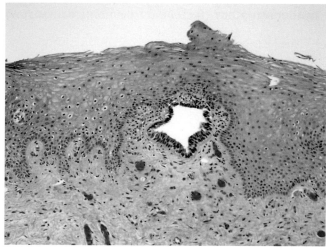

FIGURE 3

Vaginal adenosis. A single tubal-endometrial–type gland beneath squamous metaplasia is virtually identical to stroma-poor endometriosis.

POLYPOID ENDOMETRIOSIS

DEFINITION—A mass-forming, proliferative focus of misplaced endometrial glands and stroma within the vagina.

CLINICAL FEATURES

EPIDEMIOLOGY

- Uncommon; vaginal endometriosis accounts for less than 10% of all endometriosis, with the most common form being traditional endometriosis composed of glands and stroma (as opposed to the mass-forming "polypoid" variety).

PRESENTATION

- Patients present with a mass in the vagina with or without vaginal bleeding.

PROGNOSIS AND TREATMENT

- Excellent; lesions may be cured by excision; however, these lesions do have a small risk of malignant transformation.

PATHOLOGY

HISTOLOGY

- The vaginal mass is composed of variable amounts of endometrial glands and stroma. Rarely lesions may lack or have very rare endometrial glands (stromatosis).

- Hemosiderin deposition (old hemorrhage) may be present within the stroma.
- Because of the mass-forming nature of these lesions, a diagnosis of carcinoma or sarcoma may be entertained; however, endometriosis will lack the malignant stroma and irregular glands of malignant mimics.

IMMUNOPATHOLOGY (INCLUDING IMMUNOHISTOCHEMISTRY)

- Noncontributory.

MAIN DIFFERENTIAL DIAGNOSIS

- Fibrous polyp—will lack the typical endometrial stroma.
- Adenosarcoma—this must always be excluded and will be by the absence of abnormal architecture and stromal condensation. However, rare cases of polypoid endometriosis have been followed by adenosarcoma.

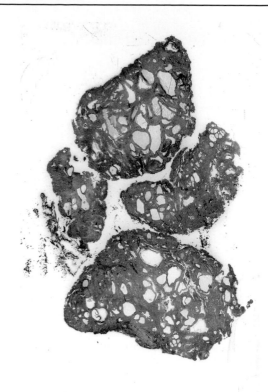

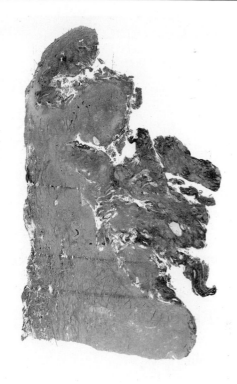

FIGURE 1

Polypoid endometriosis. Polypoid mass of glands and stroma.

FIGURE 2

Polypoid endometriosis. A polypoid mass predominantly composed of stroma with rare interspersed glands.

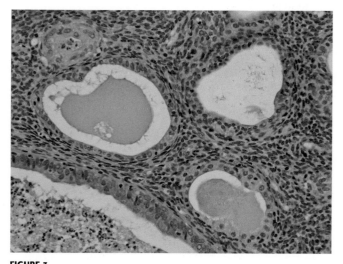

FIGURE 3

Polypoid endometriosis. Close inspection will reveal otherwise normal endometrial glands and stroma in varying amounts.

VAGINAL PAPILLOMATOSIS (RESIDUAL HYMENAL RING)

PITFALL

DEFINITION—Villiform remnants of hymenal ring.

CLINICAL FEATURES

EPIDEMIOLOGY

- Typically seen in young women of reproductive age.
- No symptoms.
- Not related to human papillomavirus (HPV).

PRESENTATION

- In these patients speculum examination of vulvovaginal region leads to their discovery.

PROGNOSIS AND TREATMENT

- Vestibular papillomas do not require treatment.

PATHOLOGY

HISTOLOGY

- Vestibular papillomatosis consists of multiple branching microvillus-like papillae (villiform) analogous to a villiform polyp.
- There is no koilocytosis or atypia.

IMMUNOPATHOLOGY (INCLUDING IMMUNOHISTOCHEMISTRY)

- Not applicable. Will stain weak or negative for Ki-67 and p16.

MAIN DIFFERENTIAL DIAGNOSIS

- Condyloma—exhibits true papillomatosis and koilocytotic atypia.
- White sponge nevus—this is a rare familial lesion of the oral cavity that can be mildly verruciform and involve the vagina.
- Fibroepithelial stromal polyp—typically solitary or few in number, keratinized.

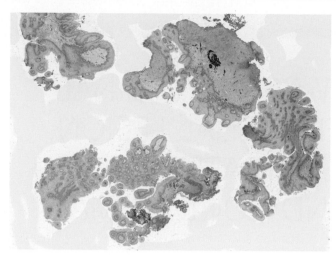

FIGURE 1

Vestibular papilloma. At scanning power multiple fragments of mucosa exhibit a microvillus architecture.

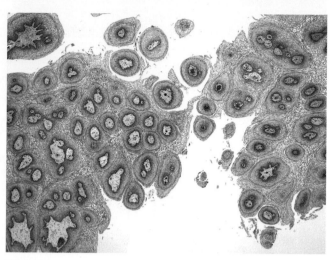

FIGURE 2

Vestibular papilloma. At higher magnification numerous coalescing stromal villi are seen.

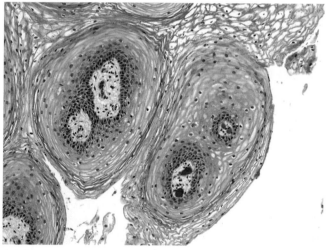

FIGURE 3

Vestibular papilloma. At high magnification there is no evidence of either atypia or coalescing verrucopapillary growth.

LOW-GRADE VAGINAL INTRAEPITHELIAL LESION (VAGINAL INTRAEPITHELIAL NEOPLASIA I AND CONDYLOMA)

DEFINITION—Human papillomavirus (HPV)–related proliferation of the vaginal mucosa.

CLINICAL FEATURES

EPIDEMIOLOGY

- Patients present at a slightly older age than those with cervical dysplasia, with the majority presenting around 40 years of age.
- Sixty-five percent of patients with vaginal intraepithelial lesion (VAIL) have concurrent or prior cervical dysplasia.
- HPV is responsible for the majority of lesions, and predisposing factors include previous cervical intraepithelial neoplasia (CIN), history of previous hysterectomy for dysplasia, history of local radiation therapy, and immunosuppression.

PRESENTATION

- In patients at risk, speculum examination with the intent of discovery of vaginal lesions leads to their discovery in most cases.

PROGNOSIS AND TREATMENT

- The prognosis is excellent; however, the majority of low-grade lesions do not progress.
- Observation is a viable option for most patients.
- If therapy is indicated, topical treatment with fluoro-uracil (5-FU) or laser vaporization may be pursued.
- Excessive treatment can lead to increased morbidity including adhesions and dyspareunia.

PATHOLOGY

HISTOLOGY

LOW-GRADE VAGINAL INTRAEPITHELIAL LESION

- Similar to low-grade cervical lesions, these lesions demonstrate mild atypia in the basal layers with a mild increase in the nuclear density.
- The most conspicuous finding is koilocytotic atypia (including binucleate cells) within the middle to upper third of the epithelium.
- In contrast to condyloma, these flat lesions lack verrucopapillary architecture and may display less acanthosis and parakeratosis. Associated with a range of HPV types including high-risk HPVs.

CONDYLOMA (EXOPHYTIC LOW-GRADE VAIL)

- Exophytic lesions with similar nuclear changes to flat lesions described earlier.
- Condyloma is typically associated with infection by HPV 6 and 11.

VAIL NOT AMENABLE TO PRECISE GRADING

- This category consists of lesions with features of both VAIN1 and VAIN2.
- The basal layer shows more extensive expansion with loss of maturation extending to the middle half of the epithelium.
- Koilocytotic atypia and binucleate cells may be present, although may be decreased in contrast to traditional low-grade lesions.

- Verrucopapillary architecture may or may not be prominent.

IMMUNOPATHOLOGY (INCLUDING IMMUNOHISTOCHEMISTRY)

- Ki-67 (MIB1) immunostaining will highlight superficial keratinocyte nuclei that are actively undergoing DNA turnover in low-grade lesions/condyloma.

MAIN DIFFERENTIAL DIAGNOSIS

- Acantholytic change (prolapse associated).
- Fibrous polyp of the introitus.
- Reactive epithelial changes with pseudokoilocytosis.

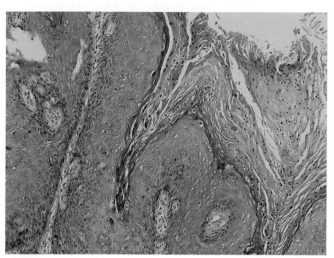

FIGURE 1

Vaginal low-grade squamous intraepithelial lesion. Spirelike hyperkeratosis with parakeratosis. Superficial maturation is present. Note the lack of conspicuous koilocytotic atypia.

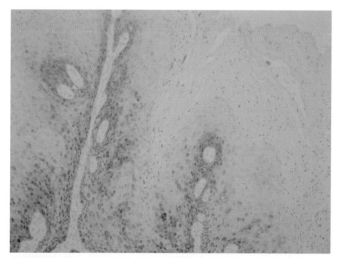

FIGURE 3

Vaginal low-grade squamous intraepithelial lesion difficult to grade. Tangential sectioning of a lesion bordering on a high-grade vaginal squamous intraepithelial lesion. Superficial maturation is present, although not to the extent as in Figures 1 and 2. These lesions are often associated with high-risk HPVs and may be p16 positive, but should be managed with an eye toward a conservative approach that minimizes morbidity.

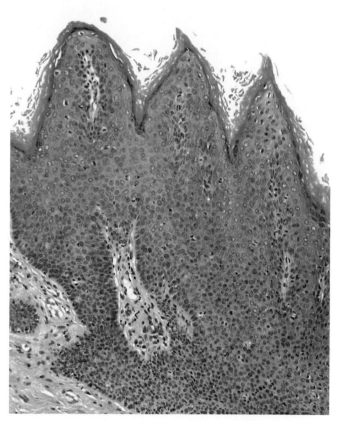

FIGURE 2

Vaginal low-grade squamous intraepithelial lesions/lesions difficult to grade. Immunohistochemical staining for p16 of the case in Figure 1. Note the patchy, basal positivity.

HIGH-GRADE VAGINAL INTRAEPITHELIAL LESION (VAGINAL INTRAEPITHELIAL NEOPLASIA II-III)

DEFINITION—Human papillomavirus (HPV)–related proliferation of the vaginal mucosa that leads to extensive, full-thickness loss of maturation of the vaginal epithelium.

CLINICAL FEATURES

EPIDEMIOLOGY

- Patients present at a slightly older age than those with cervical dysplasia, with the majority presenting around 55 to 57 years of age for high-grade VAIN.
- The advanced age is thought to lead to an increased incidence of invasive disease in this population.
- Sixty-five percent of patients with vaginal intraepithelial lesion (VAIL) have concurrent or prior cervical neoplasia.
- HPV is responsible for the majority of lesions, and predisposing factors include previous cervical intraepithelial neoplasia (CIN), history of previous hysterectomy for dysplasia, history of local radiation therapy, and immunosuppression.

PRESENTATION

- Similar to that of patients with low-grade VAIL.
- Speculum examination with the intent of discovery of vaginal lesions leads to their discovery in most cases.

PROGNOSIS AND TREATMENT

- The prognosis for patients with high-grade VAIL is more guarded than that for those with low-grade dysplasia.

- Around 5% of patients with high-grade VAIL will progress to invasive disease despite close follow-up.
- More aggressive therapy is indicated for high-grade lesions.
- Topical agents (fluorouracil [5-FU]), CO_2 laser therapy, or excision based on the distribution of the lesion may be used.
- Recurrence, ulceration, and scarring may occur.

PATHOLOGY

HISTOLOGY

- Loss of maturation and atypia involving the full thickness of the vaginal epithelium are the hallmark of this lesion.
- Nuclear chromatin is frequently hyperchromatic and coarse.
- Increased mitotic activity with mitoses extending into the upper half of the epithelium is typically present.
- High-grade lesions with papillary architecture (papillary squamous cell carcinoma in situ) have been associated with a risk of concomitant invasion. These lesions are identified by their prominent papillae with fibrovascular cores, full-thickness dysplasia, and lack of stromal invasion.

IMMUNOPATHOLOGY (INCLUDING IMMUNOHISTOCHEMISTRY)

- Ki-67 (MIB1) immunostaining will diffusely highlight superficial keratinocyte nuclei that are actively undergoing DNA turnover.
- Immunostaining with p16 is typically strong and diffusely positive.
- HPV nucleic acid testing is an option, although not usually required.

MAIN DIFFERENTIAL DIAGNOSIS

- Atrophy—more uniform population, low MIB-1 index, p16 negative.
- Radiation effect—p16 negative.
- Reactive changes—p16 negative, but MIB-1 index may be elevated.

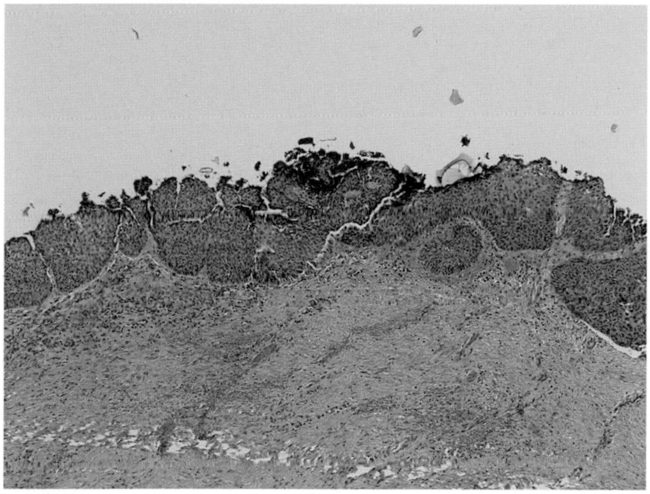

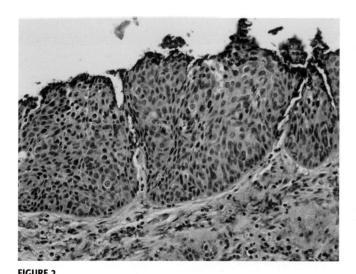

FIGURE 1

High-grade VAIL. Full-thickness loss of maturation evident at low power.

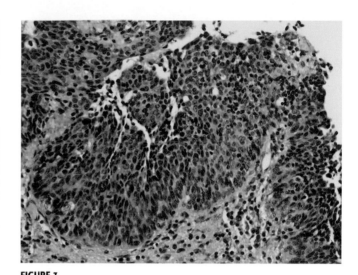

FIGURE 3

High-grade VAIL. Loss of nuclear and cellular maturation extending to the surface of the epithelium.

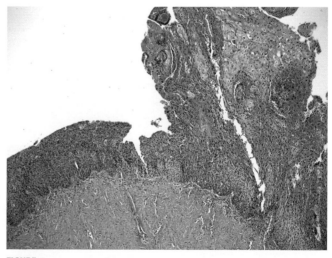

FIGURE 2

High-grade VAIL. Loss of nuclear and cellular maturation extending to the surface of the epithelium.

FIGURE 4

High-grade VAIL. Traditional high-grade VAIL merging with a papillary squamous cell carcinoma in situ. Note the lack of stromal invasion.

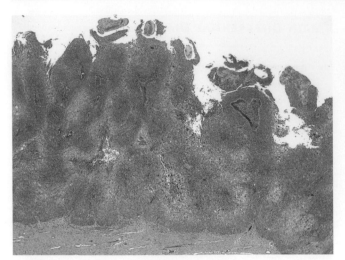

FIGURE 5

High-grade VAIL. Papillary squamous cell carcinoma in situ with numerous fibrovascular cores lined by neoplastic cells. No stromal invasion is present.

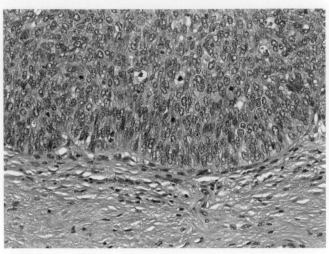

FIGURE 6

High-grade VAIL. The base of a papillary squamous cell carcinoma in situ. Marked nuclear crowding and increased mitotic figures can be seen. No stromal invasion is present.

HIGH-GRADE VAGINAL INTRAEPITHELIAL NEOPLASIA III

DEFINITION—Human papillomavirus (HPV)–related proliferation of the vaginal mucosa that leads to extensive, full-thickness loss of maturation of the vaginal epithelium.

CLINICAL FEATURES

EPIDEMIOLOGY

- Patients present at a slightly older age than those with cervical dysplasia, with the majority presenting around 55 to 57 years of age for high-grade dysplasia.
- The advanced age is thought to lead to an increased incidence of invasive disease in this population.
- Sixty-five percent of patients with vaginal intraepithelial lesion (VAIL) have concurrent or prior cervical high-grade squamous intraepithelial lesion (HSIL).
- HPV is responsible for the majority of lesions, and predisposing factors include previous cervical intraepithelial neoplasia (CIN), history of previous hysterectomy for dysplasia, history of local radiation therapy, and immunosuppression.

PRESENTATION

- Similar to that of patients with low-grade vaginal dysplasia.
- Speculum examination with the intent of discovery of vaginal lesions leads to their discovery in most cases.

PROGNOSIS AND TREATMENT

- The prognosis for patients with high-grade dysplasia is more guarded than that of low-grade dysplasia.
- Around 5% of patients with high-grade dysplasia will progress to invasive disease despite close follow-up.
- More aggressive therapy is indicated for high-grade lesions.
- Topical agents (fluorouracil [5-FU]), CO_2 laser therapy, or excision based on the distribution of the lesion may be used.
- Recurrence, ulceration, and scarring may occur.

PATHOLOGY

HISTOLOGY

- Loss of maturation and atypia involving the full thickness of the vaginal epithelium are the hallmark of this lesion.
- Nuclear chromatin is frequently hyperchromatic and coarse.
- Increased mitotic activity with mitoses extending into the upper half of the epithelium is typically present.
- High-grade lesions with papillary architecture (papillary squamous cell carcinoma in situ) have been associated with a risk of concomitant invasion. These lesions are identified by their prominent papillae with fibrovascular cores, full-thickness dysplasia, and lack of stromal invasion.

IMMUNOPATHOLOGY (INCLUDING IMMUNOHISTOCHEMISTRY)

- Ki-67 (MIB1) immunostaining will diffusely highlight superficial keratinocyte nuclei that are actively undergoing DNA turnover.
- Immunostaining with p16 is typically strong and diffusely positive.
- HPV nucleic acid testing is an option, although not usually required.

MAIN DIFFERENTIAL DIAGNOSIS

- Atrophy—distinguished by a uniform population of immature keratinocytes with bland chromatin; however, some cases show atypia. MIB1 and p16 stains are helpful in occasional cases.

- Radiation effect—this is typically characterized by nuclear enlargement, opaque chromatin, and preservation of a low nuclear-to-cytoplasmic (N/C) ratio. As in atrophy, special stains will exclude HSIL.

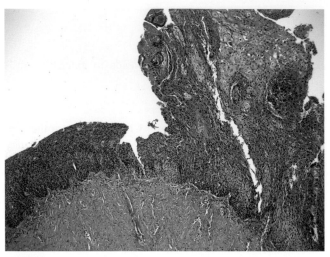

FIGURE 1

High-grade VAIL. At low power the lesion can show variable thickness ranging from flat to focally exophytic.

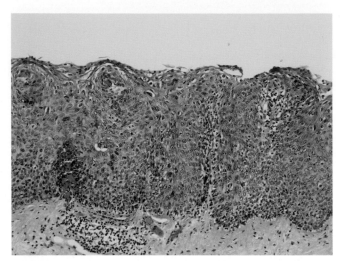

FIGURE 3

High-grade VAIL. A highly cellular epithelium with high N/C ratio and slight surface maturation.

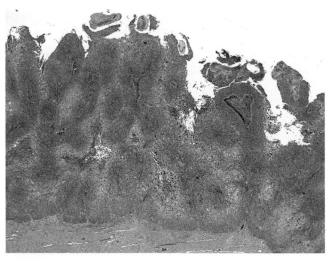

FIGURE 2

High-grade VAIL. At low power the lesion can show variable thickness ranging from flat to focally exophytic.

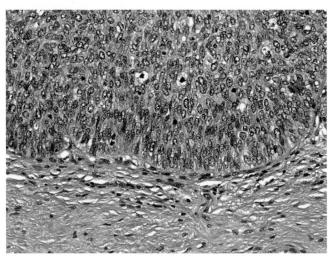

FIGURE 4

High-grade VAIL. Note high nuclear density and numerous mitotic figures.

RADIATION-INDUCED ATROPHY

DEFINITION—Iatrogenically induced atrophic changes seen in the vaginal mucosa following radiation therapy.

CLINICAL FEATURES

EPIDEMIOLOGY

- Common occurrence following radiation therapy.

PRESENTATION

- Patients experience pain and vaginal itching and dryness, similar to that seen in atrophic vaginitis.
- Colposcopic examination reveals thinned, friable vaginal mucosa with loss of the rugae. Lack of glycogenization leads to poor uptake of Lugol's solution.
- Irregular vessels may be visible, mimicking intraepithelial neoplasia.

PROGNOSIS AND TREATMENT

- Radiation-induced atrophic changes tend to be chronic with significant morbidity.

PATHOLOGY

HISTOLOGY

- Marked reactive changes including cytoplasmic vacuolization, cytomegaly and nucleomegaly, and multinucleation may be present.

- Keys to recognizing these changes as reactive include preservation of the nuclear-to-cytoplasmic ratio and homogeneous, sometimes smudgy nuclear chromatin.
- Vascular changes consisting of fibrosis and thrombosis are occasionally seen.

IMMUNOPATHOLOGY (INCLUDING IMMUNOHISTOCHEMISTRY)

- Noncontributory. p53 immunostaining can be increased following therapy.

MAIN DIFFERENTIAL DIAGNOSIS

- Atrophic vaginitis.
- Reactive changes secondary to other irritating stimuli.

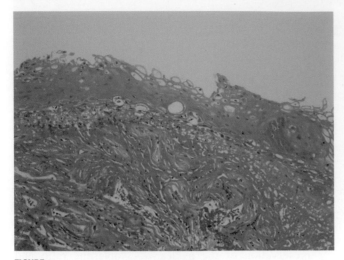

FIGURE 1

Radiation-induced vaginal atrophy. Thinned mucosa with loss of glycogen.

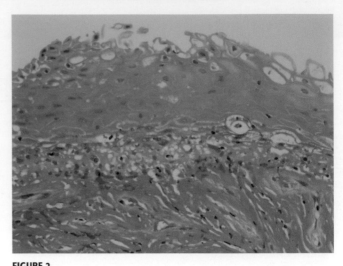

FIGURE 2

Radiation-induced vaginal atrophy. Occasional cytoplasmic vacuoles can be seen.

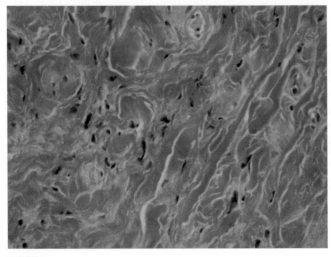

FIGURE 3

Radiation-induced vaginal atrophy. Underlying vaginal stroma with fibrosis and irregular, atypical stromal cells.

PAPILLARY SQUAMOUS CARCINOMA

DEFINITION—A malignant neoplasm of the vagina comprised of squamous epithelial cells with prominent papillary architecture.

CLINICAL FEATURES

EPIDEMIOLOGY

- Associated with high-risk human papillomavirus (HPV) infection and may follow preexisting cervical intraepithelial or invasive neoplasia.
- Usually older women, in the sixth to ninth decades.

PRESENTATION

- Patients typically present with abnormal bleeding, especially following intercourse.
- Patients may also present with pain or a clinically identifiable mass lesion.
- Presents clinically as an exophytic mass near the apex of the vagina.

PROGNOSIS AND TREATMENT

- Many lesions are superficial and can be treated by local excision.
- Radical therapy may be required for deeply invasive lesions.
- Brachytherapy in cases that cannot be resected.
- Generally a favorable outcome, particularly for localized lesions.

PATHOLOGY

HISTOLOGY

- Papillary/exophytic architecture.
- Polarized neoplastic epithelium overlying stromal cores, ranging from squamous (similar to high-grade squamous intraepithelial lesions [HSIL]) to a transitional appearance.
- Invasion may be particularly difficult to confirm if underlying stroma at the base of the tumor is not appreciated. For this reason, a diagnosis of "papillary HSIL with complex architecture" might also be made in some smaller samples, with the proviso that invasion must be excluded.

IMMUNOPATHOLOGY (INCLUDING IMMUNOHISTOCHEMISTRY)

- Positive for CK7 and p63.
- Diffusely positive for p16ink4.
- Negative for CK20.

MAIN DIFFERENTIAL DIAGNOSIS

- Verrucopapillary HSIL—overlaps with this entity, but extensive frankly exophytic lesions are usually classified as carcinomas irrespective of whether invasion can be demonstrated, albeit with a caveat that depth of invasion cannot be determined.
- Occasional primitive basaloid carcinomas—these are typically not papillary.
- Transitional cell carcinoma of urothelial origin—will be CK20 positive.
- Metastatic uterine or extrauterine papillary (serous) carcinoma—might mimic a squamotransitional lesion if poorly differentiated and will be p16ink4 positive, but also p53 positive.

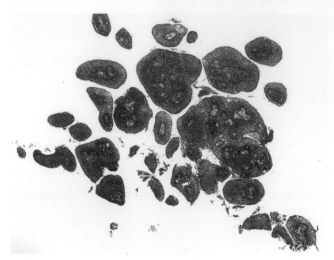

FIGURE 1

Papillary squamotransitional cell carcinoma (STCC) of the vagina. A typical biopsy showing free-floating papillae lined by neoplastic squamous epithelium.

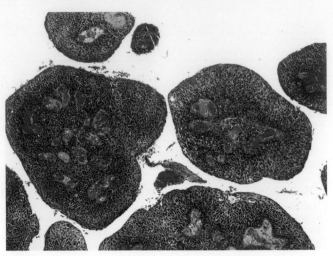

FIGURE 2

STCC. At higher magnification the papillae of STCC exhibit the typical lining, composed of a polarized high-grade neoplastic squamous epithelium. "Transitional" features may be seen, but the immunophenotype is typically squamous.

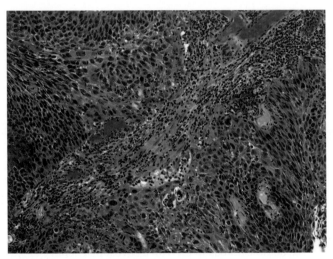

FIGURE 3

An occasional papilla may reveal stroma with features suggesting early invasion, including cytoplasmic maturation and loss of polarity at the lesional-stromal interface. However, ascertaining the true extent of the lesion will invariably require excision of the lesion with margins, if clinically possible.

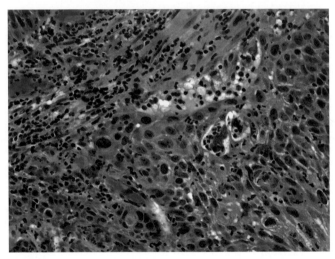

FIGURE 4

Higher magnification of a focus suggesting stromal invasion.

CLEAR-CELL ADENOCARCINOMA

DEFINITION—An uncommon primary adenocarcinoma of the vagina, associated with in utero exposure to synthetic estrogen.

CLINICAL FEATURES

EPIDEMIOLOGY

- Rare, except in women who were exposed to diethylstilbestrol (DES) in utero.
- The risk in DES-exposed women is estimated to be between 1:1000 and 1:5000 individuals.
- The peak age at diagnosis for DES-exposed women is 20, and it is rarely seen in women over 40.
- In non–DES-exposed women, the age at presentation is usually in the seventh or eighth decade of life; however, the age distribution seems to be bimodal, with a smaller group presenting around the time of menarche.

PRESENTATION

- Vaginal bleeding or discharge.
- Often a visible vaginal (or cervical) mass or ulceration is present, usually centered on the anterior wall in the upper one third of the vagina.

PROGNOSIS AND TREATMENT

- Prognosis is closely tied to stage; most patients present with early (stage I or II) disease.

PATHOLOGY

HISTOLOGY

- Clear-cell adenocarcinoma of the vagina has the microscopic appearance of clear-cell adenocarcinomas found elsewhere in the genital tract of women.

- These tumors are characterized by polyhedral cells with optically clear (to eosinophilic) cytoplasm and strikingly atypical pleomorphic nuclei.
- The cells may be arranged in solid sheets, or forming tubules, cysts, or papillary structures with hyaline stromal changes.
- When seen lining spaces, the cells are typically present as a single layer and often have a "hobnail" appearance.

IMMUNOPATHOLOGY (INCLUDING IMMUNOHISTOCHEMISTRY)

- Noncontributory in most primary cases.
- PAX8, HINF1-β, and Napsin-A staining might be helpful in confirming an origin in a primary clear-cell carcinoma of the genital tract.

MAIN DIFFERENTIAL DIAGNOSIS

- Endometrioid adenocarcinoma with secretory differentiation—nuclear atypia, hobnail patterns, and hyaline stromal changes are helpful. Squamous metaplasia argues against this diagnosis.
- Arias-Stella effect—this will typically be found within adenosis or endocervix and not as a separate lesion.

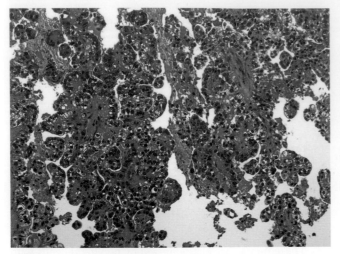

FIGURE 1

Vaginal clear-cell carcinoma. Cells are eosinophilic and only focally clear. Note the hyaline change to the stroma.

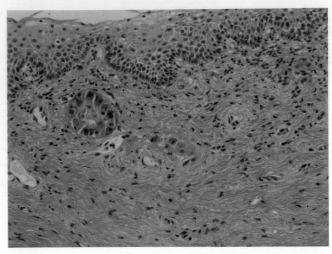

FIGURE 2

Metastatic clear-cell carcinoma of the vagina. Markedly atypical cells are present, several of which are in a lymphatic space *(center)*.

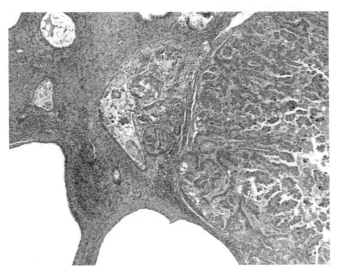

FIGURE 3

Metastatic clear-cell carcinoma of the vagina. The tumor in Figure 2 is derived from this clear cell carcinoma of the endometrium with a prominent papillary architecture and hobnail cells.

METASTATIC ADENOCARCINOMA

DEFINITION—Epithelial malignancies that metastasize to the vagina.

CLINICAL FEATURES

EPIDEMIOLOGY

- Patients with a primary carcinoma of another site.
- The vast majority are of endometrial origin.
- Over 90% of adenocarcinomas identified in the vagina are metastatic.

PRESENTATION

- Vaginal mass, nodularity, or epithelial irregularity.
- Vaginal bleeding.

PROGNOSIS AND TREATMENT

- Varies with the specific primary tumor.

PATHOLOGY

HISTOLOGY

- Endometrioid endometrial adenocarcinoma.
- Uterine or pelvic serous carcinoma.

- Carcinosarcoma.
- Renal cell carcinoma.
- Urothelial carcinoma.
- Breast carcinoma.
- Colorectal adenocarcinoma.

IMMUNOPATHOLOGY (INCLUDING IMMUNOHISTOCHEMISTRY)

- Varies with the suspected primary tumor.

MAIN DIFFERENTIAL DIAGNOSIS

- Adenocarcinoma arising in endometriosis.
- Clear cell adenocarcinoma of the vagina.

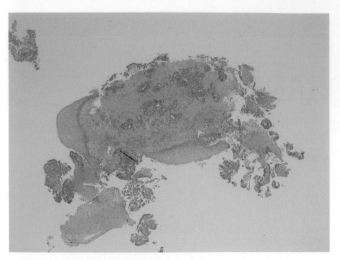

FIGURE 1

Carcinoma metastatic to the vagina. Metastatic endometrioid endometrial adenocarcinoma. Note the extensive stromal involvement and normal overlying epithelium.

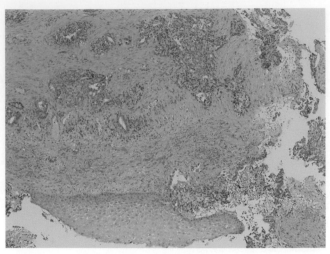

FIGURE 2

Carcinoma metastatic to the vagina. Metastatic endometrioid endometrial adenocarcinoma with squamous morular metaplasia.

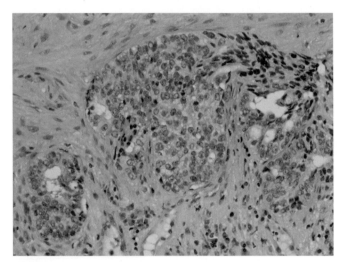

FIGURE 3

Carcinoma metastatic to the vagina. Metastatic endometrioid endometrial adenocarcinoma.

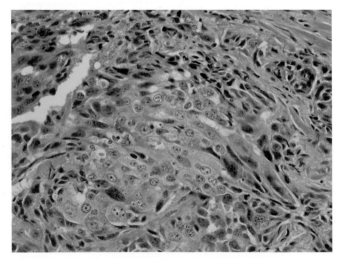

FIGURE 4

Carcinoma metastatic to the vagina. Metastatic breast carcinoma. Note the single file lines of cells.

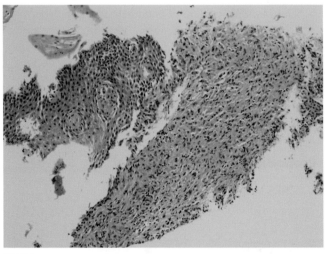

FIGURE 5

Carcinoma metastatic to the vagina. Metastatic serous carcinoma displaying prominent nuclear pleomorphism.

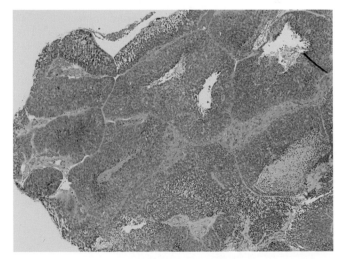

FIGURE 6

Carcinoma metastatic to the vagina. Metastatic rectal carcinoma.

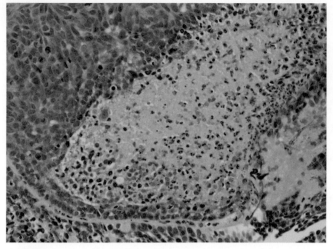

FIGURE 7

Carcinoma metastatic to the vagina. Metastatic rectal carcinoma with necrosis.

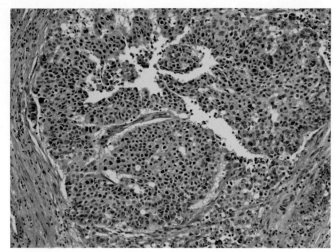

FIGURE 8

Carcinoma metastatic to the vagina. Metastatic transitional cell carcinoma.

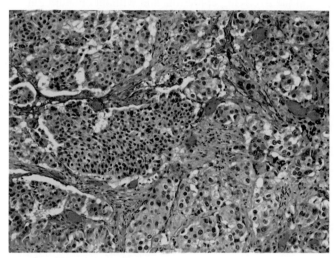

FIGURE 9

Carcinoma metastatic to the vagina. Metastatic transitional cell carcinoma. Note the focal nuclear streaming near the center of the image.

MELANOMA

DEFINITION—A very aggressive malignant tumor of dermal melanocytes arising in the vagina.

CLINICAL FEATURES

EPIDEMIOLOGY

- Uncommon but not rare.
- Typically seen in postmenopausal women.
- May be more common in patients with a BRCA2 mutation.

PRESENTATION

- Vaginal bleeding or discharge.
- A palpable mass may or may not be present.
- The most common location is the lower one third of the vagina.

PROGNOSIS AND TREATMENT

- Poor; these tumors are more aggressive than cutaneous or vulvar melanomas.
- Deep invasion and extensive superficial spread of the tumor are particularly problematic.
- Five-year survival ranges from 5% to 20% depending on the study.
- Radical surgery and adjuvant chemoradiation are the standard treatments, but these tumors have a poor response rate and some studies have shown that wide local excision has a similar survival rate.

PATHOLOGY

HISTOLOGY

- The epidermal component is composed of single cells and nests of monotonous, severely atypical melanocytes with irregular chromatin and prominent nucleoli.

- Effacement of the epithelial-stromal junction is common, resulting in a "moth-eaten" appearance.
- The stromal component is most often composed of epithelioid cells with a similar histology to those present in the overlying epidermis and without "maturation."
- Melanoma is known for its variable morphology, and the spectrum is broad; cases range from the epithelioid tumors described earlier to a malignant spindle cell proliferation that can be confused with a sarcomatoid squamous cell carcinoma or a mesenchymal neoplasm (PITFALL).
- Melanin pigment is variably present.

IMMUNOPATHOLOGY (INCLUDING IMMUNOHISTOCHEMISTRY)

- S100 positive.
- MART1, HMB45, and Melan-A are generally positive but may be lost in poorly differentiated tumors.

MAIN DIFFERENTIAL DIAGNOSIS

- Squamous cell carcinoma.
- Poorly differentiated carcinomas.
- Sarcomas.

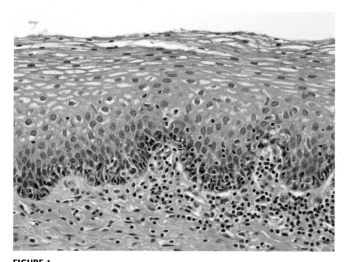

FIGURE 1

Vaginal melanoma. Vaginal epithelium with numerous atypical melanocytes is seen in the basal layer.

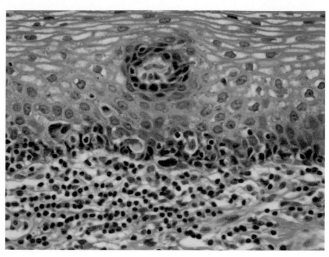

FIGURE 2

Vaginal melanoma. Marked melanocytic atypia.

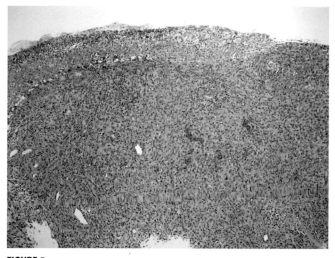

FIGURE 3

Vaginal melanoma. An ill-defined mass of atypical cells is present. Note the superficial ulceration.

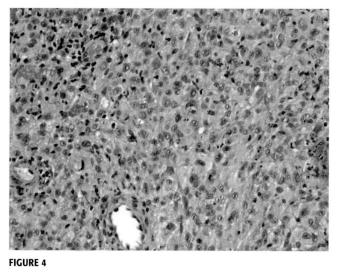

FIGURE 4

Vaginal melanoma. High-power examination of Figure 3 demonstrates marked nuclear atypia, prominent nucleoli, and rare pigment.

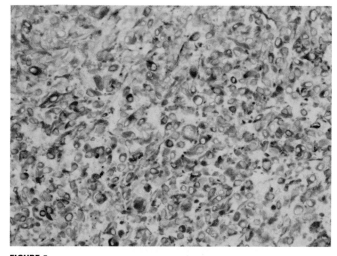

FIGURE 5

Vaginal melanoma. Positive immunohistochemical staining for Melan-A.

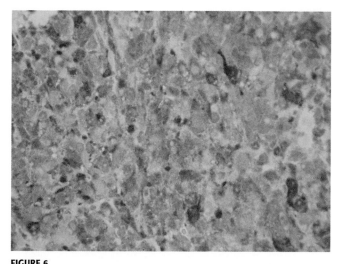

FIGURE 6

Vaginal melanoma. Positive immunohistochemical staining for S100.

SPINDLE CELL EPITHELIOMA

DEFINITION—A benign vaginal tumor composed of keratin-positive stromal cells.

CLINICAL FEATURES

EPIDEMIOLOGY

- Uncommon.
- Seen in a wide age range (20 to 80 years), with a mean age of 40 years.

PRESENTATION

- Submucosal vaginal mass, often located near the hymenal ring.
- Often discovered incidentally during routine gynecologic examination.

PROGNOSIS AND TREATMENT

- Excellent; this is a benign tumor.
- Recurrence has been reported, so complete surgical excision is advised.

PATHOLOGY

HISTOLOGY

- A well-circumscribed, but unencapsulated, proliferation of spindled cells ranging from 1 to 9 cm in size.
- The predominant cell type is a bland spindle cell with round-to-oval nuclei and scant amounts of eosinophilic-to-pale cytoplasm.

- The spindled cells are variably arranged as nests or sheets, often with focally corded or reticular architecture.
- Mitoses are infrequent.
- Minor epithelial elements are occasionally identified; they can consist of glandular or squamous epithelium or squamous morula.
- If present, the glandular epithelium is typically cuboidal to low columnar with periodic acid–Schiff (PAS)–positive, diastase-sensitive luminal secretions.

IMMUNOPATHOLOGY (INCLUDING IMMUNOHISTOCHEMISTRY)

- Stroma-like cells are positive for AE1/AE3, and sometimes for CK7 or CK20.
- Stroma-like cells are positive for CD10; SMA, desmin, and caldesmon are variably positive.
- Both the stromal and epithelial components are frequently positive for ER and PR.
- S100 is negative in both components.

MAIN DIFFERENTIAL DIAGNOSIS

- Smooth muscle neoplasms—contrasting epithelial and spindled cell differentiation helps to distinguish spindle cell epithelioma.

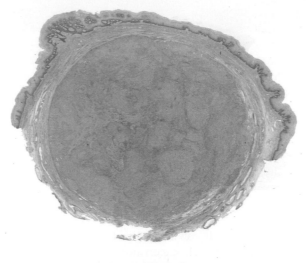

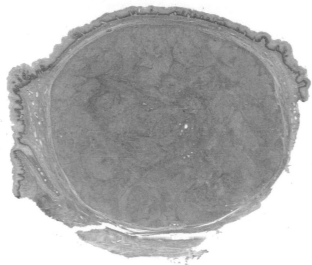

FIGURE 1

Spindle cell epithelioma. Two low-power images of well-circumscribed mass underlying the vaginal epithelium.

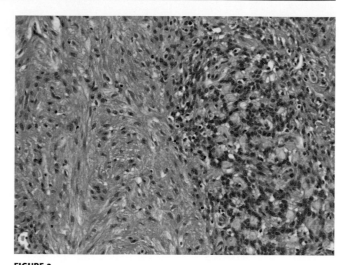

FIGURE 2

Spindle cell epithelioma. Bland spindle cells admixed with nodules of glandular structures composed of low cuboidal epithelium.

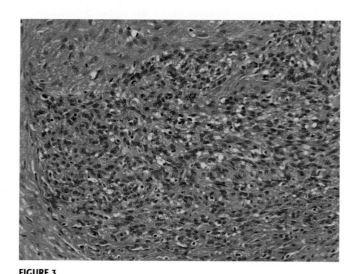

FIGURE 3

Spindle cell epithelioma. Bland spindle cells forming a fascicle, note the lack of atypia and mitotic activity.

EMBRYONAL RHABDOMYOSARCOMA

DEFINITION—A malignancy of skeletal muscle presenting as a polypoid vaginal mass in young girls.

CLINICAL FEATURES

EPIDEMIOLOGY

- Uncommon.
- Usually seen in females under the age of 5 years.

PRESENTATION

- A bulky, polypoid vaginal mass that can resemble a cluster of grapes (botryoid).
- Vaginal bleeding may be the presenting symptom.

PROGNOSIS AND TREATMENT

- Prognosis is good in contrast to other subtypes of rhabdomyosarcoma.
- Surgical excision with chemotherapy and radiation is the standard of care.

PATHOLOGY

HISTOLOGY

- The low-power architecture is composed of exophytic, polypoid papillary structures.
- The subepithelial condensation of cells (the so-called cambium layer) is characteristic.
- Rhabdomyoblasts, which compose the cambium layer, are characterized by a high nuclear-to-cytoplasmic ratio and prominent brightly eosinophilic (rhabdoid) cytoplasmic inclusions.
- Cytoplasmic striations can be identified in a subset of cells with elongated cytoplasm (strap cells).
- The deceptively bland stromal core of the polypoid projections is composed of a loose fibromyxoid tissue, often containing inflammatory cells.

IMMUNOPATHOLOGY (INCLUDING IMMUNOHISTOCHEMISTRY)

- Skeletal muscle markers are positive (Myf-4 and MyoD1).

MAIN DIFFERENTIAL DIAGNOSIS

- Fibroepithelial stromal polyp—lacks the rhabdoid cells or cambium layer.
- Adenosarcoma—spindled cells admixed with glands.

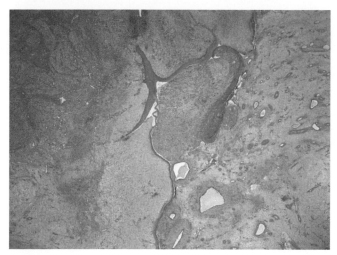

FIGURE 1

Embryonal rhabdomyosarcoma. Polypoid projections of tumor can be seen underlying the vaginal squamous epithelium. Subepithelial condensation of the cells (cambium layer) is apparent at low power.

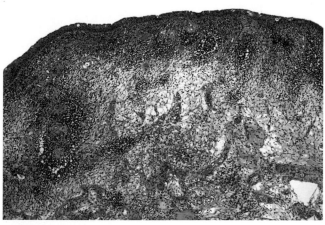

FIGURE 2

Embryonal rhabdomyosarcoma. Vaginal epithelium with a distinctive cambium layer.

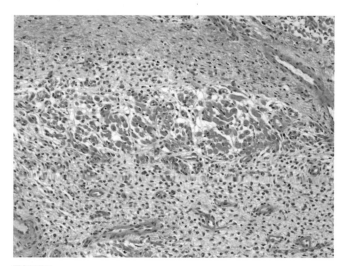

FIGURE 3

Embryonal rhabdomyosarcoma. Rhabdomyoblasts with abundant, brightly eosinophilic cytoplasm.

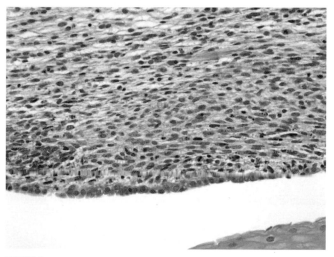

FIGURE 4

Embryonal rhabdomyosarcoma. A cambium layer with only rare rhabdomyoblasts, best seen in the upper half of the photo.

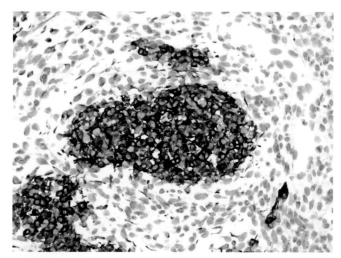

FIGURE 5

Embryonal rhabdomyosarcoma. Positive immunohistochemical staining for desmin.

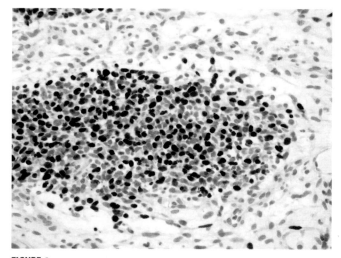

FIGURE 6

Embryonal rhabdomyosarcoma. Positive immunohistochemical staining for myogenin.

Cervix

EXOPHYTIC LOW-GRADE SQUAMOUS INTRAEPITHELIAL LESION

DEFINITION AND TERMINOLOGY

- An exophytic cervical condyloma represents an infection of the mature ectocervical or metaplastic cervical transformation zone epithelium by human papillomavirus (HPV) type 6 or 11 (low-cancer-risk subtypes).
- The most appropriate term is low-grade squamous intraepithelial lesion (LSIL).

CLINICAL FEATURES

EPIDEMIOLOGY

- Reproductive-age, sexually active women.

PRESENTATION

- Papanicolaou smear typically classified as atypical squamous cells of undetermined significance (ASCUS) or LSIL.
- Colposcopic abnormality, typically an exophytic lesion on the cervix.

PROGNOSIS AND TREATMENT

- Clinicians can opt to treat exophytic condyloma patients in one of two ways: cryoablation or follow-up.
- Conservative management is the rule, with attention to periodic follow-up. Large lesions may require ablation.
- Patients infected with HPV 6 or 11 are not directly at risk for cancer, but having HPV places them at risk of infection with the other strains that predispose to cancer.

PATHOLOGY

HISTOLOGY

- Exophytic LSILs are characterized by a mature squamous epithelium with verruciform architecture, acanthosis (epidermal hyperplasia or thickening), and parakeratosis (retention of nuclei at the epithelial surface).

- A mildly increased nuclear density is present in the surface epithelium.
  - An increased nuclear-to-cytoplasmic ratio is seen.
  - Koilocytotic atypia with perinuclear halos, irregular nuclear membranes, and enlarged single or binucleate forms is seen in the upper epithelial layers.
  - Only mild atypia is present in the lower epithelial layers.

IMMUNOHISTOCHEMISTRY

- Ki-67 expression is mild to moderate, with staining in the upper epithelial layers particularly in areas of viral cytopathic effect.
- p16ink4 expression is negative or patchy, the latter being the most prominent in maturing cell cytoplasm with variable nuclear staining. This is the classic pattern seen in low-risk HPV types and is very helpful in distinguishing this entity from papillary high-grade squamous intraepithelial lesions (HSILs) or papillary squamous carcinomas.

DIFFERENTIAL DIAGNOSIS AND PITFALLS

- The most common pitfall is reactive epithelial changes.
- Rarely, well-differentiated squamous carcinomas will manifest with koilocytosis.
- Exophytic condylomas may coexist with HSILs, but the two entities are caused by two distinct HPV types. Always exclude HSIL and ensure that the cytologic diagnosis matches the histology. An HSIL will manifest with strong p16 staining unlike condyloma. If HSIL is suspected on cytology, further sampling is indicated.

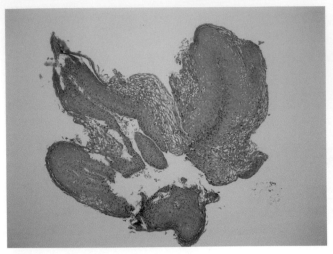

FIGURE 1
Exophytic LSIL. At low power the characteristic verruciform architecture and acanthosis are apparent. A suggestion of koilocytic forms is visible at this power.

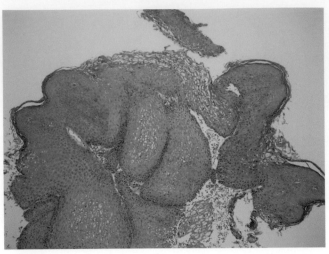

FIGURE 2
Exophytic LSIL. An example with prominent acanthosis. Mildly increased nuclear density toward the surface of the epithelium can already be appreciated at this power.

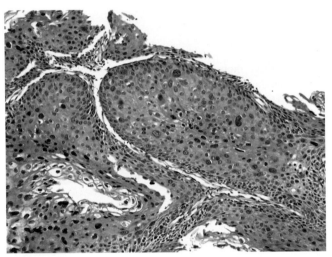

FIGURE 3
Exophytic LSIL. At higher power, scattered atypical cells with enlarged, irregular nuclei are present. Mild nuclear atypia is seen in the basal layers of the epithelium. There is an increased density of nuclei at the epithelial surface.

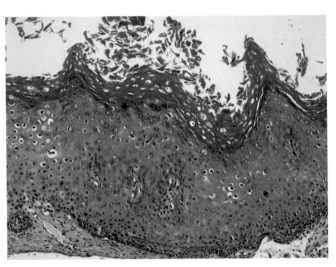

FIGURE 4
Exophytic LSIL. This example has prominent hyperkeratosis in addition to the parakeratosis. Abundant koilocytic forms are present. There is only focal mild nuclear atypia in the basal layers of the epithelium.

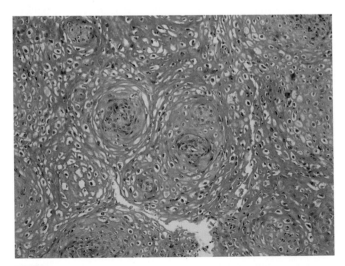

FIGURE 5
Exophytic LSIL. Koilocytes with prominent perinuclear halos and irregular nuclear membranes are present.

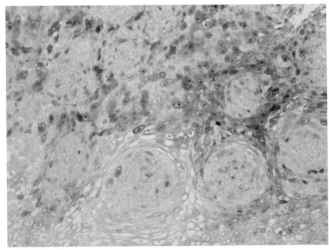

FIGURE 6
Exophytic LSIL. p16 immunostain corresponding to the hematoxylin and eosin (H&E) seen in Figure 5. A typical p16 staining pattern for low-risk HPV infections. There is patchy positivity, especially in the more superficial layers of the epithelium. Rare nuclear positivity is noted, and cytoplasmic positivity is more apparent.

LOW-GRADE SQUAMOUS INTRAEPITHELIAL LESION (FLAT CONDYLOMA/CERVICAL INTRAEPITHELIAL NEOPLASIA I)

DEFINITION—An infection of the mature ectocervical and/or metaplastic cervical transformation zone epithelium by human papillomavirus (HPV).

CLINICAL FEATURES

EPIDEMIOLOGY

- Most commonly seen in sexually active, reproductive-age women.
- Can be diagnosed in any age group.
- Flat low-grade squamous intraepithelial lesions (LSILs) can be caused by either low- or high-risk HPV subtypes. Approximately one-half of ectocervical/metaplastic (squamocolumnar [SC] junction–negative) lesions contain high-risk HPVs in contrast to nearly all SC junction–positive lesions.

PRESENTATION

- Typically identified on screening Pap smears with a diagnosis of atypical squamous cells of undetermined significance (ASCUS) or LSIL.
- Colposcopic examination may display a sessile cervical lesion or may only appear as a white area following the application of acetic acid (acetowhite epithelium).

PROGNOSIS AND TREATMENT

- These are low-grade lesions, and as such have a good prognosis. SC junction–negative lesions have been shown to rarely be followed by a diagnosis of high-grade squamous intraepithelial lesion (HSIL). Lesions in the SC junction may have a higher HSIL outcome, but this appears to be minimized if the diagnosis of LSIL is agreed on by multiple observers.
- Treatment may consist of either follow-up alone or cryoablation.

- A 1-year follow-up is usual in most patients as the vast majority of these lesions will regress on their own.
- A persistent biopsy diagnosis of LSIL may require consideration of treatment rather than follow-up alone.

PATHOLOGY

HISTOLOGY

The biopsy appearance of a flat LSIL varies depending on where the lesion is located, and these appearances will be described separately.

- *LSIL in mature squamous epithelium:*
  - The most notable features are preserved epithelial maturation and nuclear polarity with a subtle expansion of the basal third of the epithelium, combined with conspicuous atypia in the superficial layers.
  - This superficial cell atypia may consist of binucleated or multinucleated cells, nuclear hyperchromasia, and/or nuclear enlargement, often with irregular nuclear membranes.
  - The nuclear-to-cytoplasmic ratio is, in general, preserved in these lesions.
  - The cells in the lower portions of the epithelium are bland, uniform, and have minimal or no nuclear atypia.
- *LSIL in immature squamous epithelium (transition zone, squamous metaplasia):*
  - This appearance is more common for lesions in the SC junction. In these areas the degree of maturation is less apparent than in mature squamous epithelium,

but it is still present, and there is only minimal nuclear overlapping.

- The upper epithelial layers are notable for increased nuclear density, and less prominent koilocytic changes may be seen in mature squamous epithelium.
- The nuclei are very uniform, but mitotic activity is minimal to low, and the nuclei are not hyperchromatic.

- *LSIL in cytologic preparations (Pap test):*
  - Intermediate and superficial cells with nuclear enlargement at least 2.5× to 3× larger than normal intermediate cells, nuclear hyperchromasia, and slightly irregular nuclear borders.
  - Binucleate koilocytes with enlarged hyperchromatic nuclei and sharply defined cytoplasmic halos may be present, but are not required.
  - Binucleation alone is not sufficient for a diagnosis of LSIL.
  - The amount of cytoplasm in low-grade lesions is abundant, and an increase in the nuclear-to-cytoplasmic ratio should not be appreciated.

IMMUNOPATHOLOGY (INCLUDING IMMUNOHISTOCHEMISTRY)

- Ki-67 expression is mild to moderate, with some staining in the upper epithelial layers.

- p16 expression is variable, but will be linear and continuous (i.e., positive) in up to 70% of cases, particularly if in the SC junction. In our experience the p16 immunostain does not have a significant impact on outcome (i.e., HSIL risk) if the lesion is indisputably an LSIL by histologic examination.
- It is critical to note that p16 staining is not a reliable marker to distinguish a low-grade lesion from a high-grade lesion without taking into consideration the histologic features.

MAIN DIFFERENTIAL DIAGNOSIS

- Reactive epithelial changes (may contain surface atypia or cytoplasmic halos).
- High-grade squamous intraepithelial lesions with focal surface maturation.
  - Well-differentiated squamous cell carcinoma (superficial biopsy).

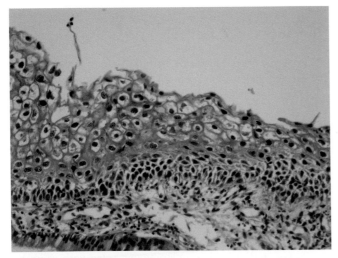

FIGURE 1
Classic example of an LSIL in mature metaplastic squamous epithelium. There is abrupt maturation with some increased density of nuclei toward the surface with clear if not striking nuclear atypia. The surface cells are hyperchromatic, with irregular nuclear membranes. The basal layers are bland and lack atypia.

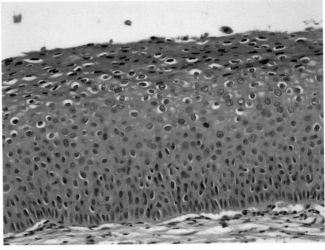

FIGURE 2
This variant of metaplastic LSIL has an expanded zone of parabasal cells with uniform differentiation and preserved polarity. Note the absence of any conspicuous nuclear enlargement in the lower epithelium. Both nuclear contour and chromasia in this region are rather uniform.

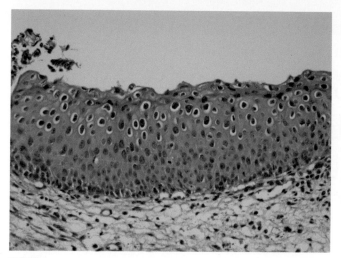

FIGURE 3

An LSIL from the region of the SC junction. This is similar to Figures 1 and 2, with some expansion of the less mature cells, but without appreciable atypia.

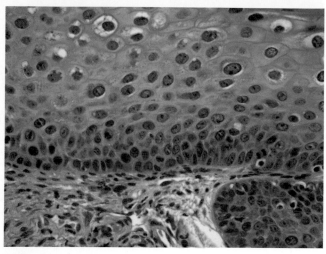

FIGURE 4

A closer view of basal and parabasal cells in an LSIL. Note this compartment, which is responsible for cell replenishment, does not display the more conspicuous nuclear chromatin and size differences characteristic of cervical intraepithelial neoplasia 2 (CIN2) (HSIL).

HIGH-GRADE SQUAMOUS INTRAEPITHELIAL LESION (CERVICAL INTRAEPITHELIAL NEOPLASIA II AND III)

DEFINITION AND TERMINOLOGY

- A precancerous lesion arising at the cervical squamocolumnar (SC) junction that displays near full-thickness atypia and variable maturation of the neoplastic epithelium.
- Should be associated *always* with high-risk human papillomaviruses (HPVs) and with HPV16 in 40% to 60% of cases depending on the cytologic presentation.

CLINICAL FEATURES

EPIDEMIOLOGY

- Reproductive-age, sexually active women.

PRESENTATION

- Papanicolaou smear typically classified as low-grade squamous intraepithelial lesion (LSIL), high-grade squamous intraepithelial lesion (HSIL), or atypical squamous cells of undetermined significance (ASCUS).
- Colposcopic abnormality, typically acetowhite epithelium at the SC junction.

PROGNOSIS AND TREATMENT

- From 40% to 60% of CIN2 have been described to resolve spontaneously in up to 3 years in young women. Resolution of cervical intraepithelial neoplasia III (CIN3) is much less.
- Small risk of concurrent carcinoma (less than 1%) in women under age 25.
- Long-term risk of progression to carcinoma estimated at 5% for CIN2 and 12% for CIN3. Estimates based on untreated women followed for long periods of time are higher.
- Typically treated by cone biopsy or loop electrosurgical excision procedure (LEEP). Cryotherapy used previously and still appropriate if the entire lesion can be visualized (CIN2). Recurrence rates depend on whether excision margins are free of disease; usually less than 10%.
- In young women (under age 25) with CIN2 there is the option of follow-up with a repeat exam in 6 months in hopes the lesion will regress, permitting the patient to preserve cervical anatomy and lower the risk of future pregnancy complications that could occur following a cone biopsy. However, this is contingent on full visualization of the lesion, absence of any areas suspicious for invasion, and cervical cytology that is concordant. Continued follow-up is always needed to ensure resolution.

PATHOLOGY

HISTOLOGY

- High nuclear density throughout the epithelium with nuclear overlap.
- Relatively more conspicuous atypia in the lower epithelial layers distinguishes CIN2 from CIN1 (LSIL).
- Variations in both nuclear size and staining and contour and chromasia.
  - An increased nuclear-to-cytoplasmic ratio in lower epithelial layers.
  - Surface maturation, with koilocytosis, can be seen in CIN2, but the cells usually display greater degrees of nuclear enlargement and atypia.
- Atypical parakeratosis.

IMMUNOHISTOCHEMISTRY

- Diffuse linear p16ink4 staining. If the diagnosis of CIN2 is made with certainty, a p16ink4 can be used to *confirm the presence of an HPV-associated lesion. Reliance on the p16ink4 stain solely to make the diagnosis of CIN2 is not recommended by these authors.*
- High Ki-67 nuclear staining index (>50%), in all layers.
- Strong krt7 and arg2 staining is typical of these lesions arising in the SC junction.

DIFFERENTIAL DIAGNOSIS AND PITFALLS

- Reactive epithelial changes—the most common pitfall (prominent nucleoli, negative or patchy p16 staining).

- Superficial biopsy of a carcinoma.
- LSIL, tangentially sectioned.
- LSILs associated with low-risk HPVs will show weak or patchy p16 staining.
- LSILs associated with high-risk HPVs on the ectocervix often manifest with weak or negative krt7 and arg2 staining.
- LSILs arising in the SC junction have a high frequency of association with high-risk HPVs and are strongly p16 positive. *They can only be distinguished from CIN2 by histology given the common HPV types and p16 staining pattern.*

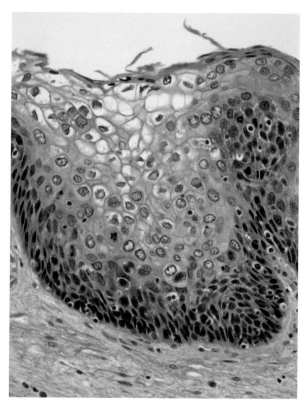

FIGURE 1
HSIL (CIN2). Conspicuous maturation but prominent parabasal atypia.

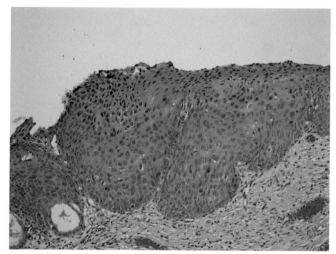

FIGURE 2
HSIL (CIN2), keratinizing.

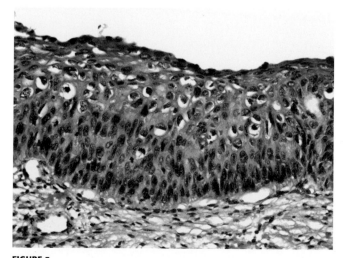

FIGURE 3
HSIL (CIN2) with slight maturation

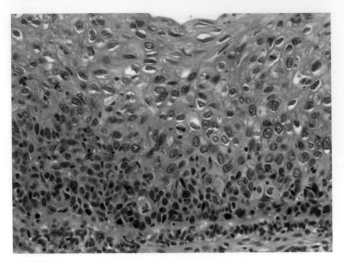

FIGURE 4

HSIL (CIN2) with koilocytosis. Note the parabasal atypia.

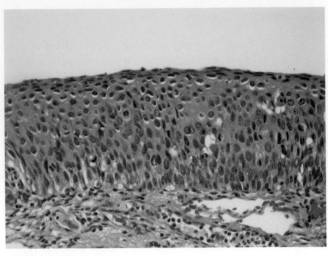

FIGURE 5

HSIL (CIN2). A less abrupt transition from immature to mature in this CIN2.

LOW-GRADE SQUAMOUS INTRAEPITHELIAL LESION (GIANT CONDYLOMA)

PITFALL

DEFINITION—A variant of condyloma that presents as a grossly enlarged mass and appears to replace or cover the cervix and/or distal vagina.

CLINICAL FEATURES

EPIDEMIOLOGY

- Sexually active, reproductive-age women.
- Uncommon.

PRESENTATION

- A Pap smear diagnosis of atypical squamous cells of undetermined significance (ASCUS), low-grade squamous intraepithelial lesions (LSIL), or occasionally high-grade squamous intraepithelial lesions (HSIL).
- A conspicuous verruciform or fungating mass detected on digital and speculum exam in the distal vagina/ectocervix.

PROGNOSIS AND TREATMENT

- Conservative removal, cryotherapy, and/or laser ablation.

PATHOLOGY

HISTOLOGY

- Giant condyloma is characterized by mildly atypical immature metaplastic epithelium with papillary architecture.
- The papillae are thin and slender (filiform), not verrucous and blunt like the papillae seen in condyloma acuminata.

- A mild increase in nuclear density can be appreciated, as can a mildly increased nuclear-to-cytoplasmic ratio.
- The nuclei are well spaced and do not overlap each other.
- The cell borders can be prominent.
- Koilocytic changes are minimal or absent in these lesions.
- Overlying columnar cell layers may be preserved.

IMMUNOHISTOCHEMISTRY

- Ki-67 expression is mild to moderate, and staining in the upper epithelial layers is low due to lack of viral cytopathic effect.
- p16ink4 expression is negative or patchy, the latter being most prominent in maturing cell cytoplasm with variable nuclear staining. This is the classic pattern seen in low-risk human papillomavirus (HPV) types and is very helpful in distinguishing this entity from most HSILs or papillary squamous carcinomas.

DIFFERENTIAL DIAGNOSIS AND PITFALLS

- The major pitfall is misclassifying this entity as a verrucous carcinoma. The latter can be excluded if any of the following are found, including cytopathic effect and extension into crypt epithelium. It is very important to exclude a large condyloma and use a diagnosis of verrucous carcinoma in any well-differentiated exophytic lesion of the cervix in a young woman.
- Papillary carcinoma is easily distinguished by more poorly differentiated epithelium and strong diffuse p16 immunostaining.

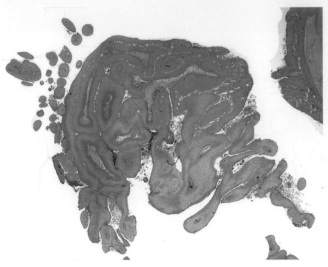

FIGURE 1

LSIL (giant condyloma). Low-power image of a large cervical condyloma. Note the relatively slender, filiform papillae.

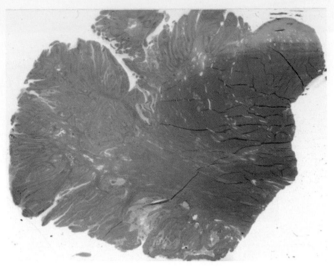

FIGURE 2

LSIL (giant condyloma). This lesion has a broader base.

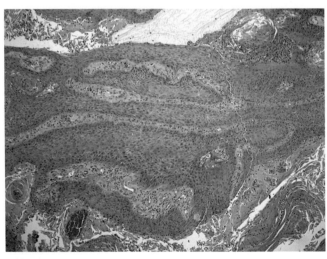

FIGURE 3

LSIL (giant condyloma). Extension into crypts supports the diagnosis of an intraepithelial lesion versus verrucous carcinoma.

LOW-GRADE SQUAMOUS INTRAEPITHELIAL LESION (IMMATURE CONDYLOMA)

DEFINITION—Immature condyloma represents an infection of the immature metaplastic cervical transformation zone epithelium by human papillomavirus (HPV) type 6 or 11. Also variably called squamous papilloma or papillary immature metaplasia; the most appropriate term is low-grade squamous intraepithelial lesion (LSIL) (immature condyloma).

CLINICAL FEATURES

EPIDEMIOLOGY

- Reproductive age, sexually active women.

PRESENTATION

- Papanicolaou smears are typically classified as atypical squamous cells of undetermined significance (ASCUS), as LSIL, or occasionally as high-grade squamous intraepithelial lesions (HSIL).
- The colposcopic abnormality typically presents as an exophytic or discrete cerebriform lesion on the cervix corresponding to the papillary metaplastic epithelium.

PROGNOSIS AND TREATMENT

- Clinicians can opt to treat immature condyloma patients in two ways: cryoablation or follow-up.
- Conservative management should only be done for patients with favorable biopsy, Papanicolaou smear, and colposcopy results who can ensure close follow-up.
- Patients infected with HPV 6 or 11 are not directly at risk for cancer, but having HPV places them at risk of infection with the other strains that predispose to cancer.

PATHOLOGY

HISTOLOGY

- The histologic features of immature exophytic LSIL represent a spectrum of changes.
- At low power these lesions exhibit prominent papillary growth composed of small, filiform papillae.
- Notably there is minimal to no epithelial maturation toward the surface of the papillae.
- The cells are uniform and bland, with only mildly increased nuclear-to-cytoplasmic ratios, and minimal nuclear crowding.
- Nuclear atypia, if present, is mild.
- Koilocytes are not present, and often the overlying columnar epithelial cells are preserved.

IMMUNOHISTOCHEMISTRY

- Ki-67 expression is low to moderate, with sparing of the upper epithelial layers.
- p16 staining is negative or patchy.

DIFFERENTIAL DIAGNOSIS AND PITFALLS

- Condyloma acuminatum—this is an acceptable diagnosis but might not be suspected in the absence of cytopathic effect.
- Papillary carcinoma in situ—if the mitotic rate is high or there is any appreciable nuclear overlap or loss of the monotonous uniform nuclei with nucleoli, consider this diagnosis. A strong diffuse p16 stain and a high MIB1 index will characterize this lesion versus immature condyloma.
- Papillary carcinoma—it must be excluded if the diagnosis of papillary carcinoma in situ is made.

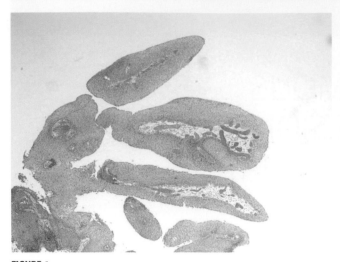

FIGURE 1

Immature condyloma (LSIL). Note the papillary architecture at low-power magnification.

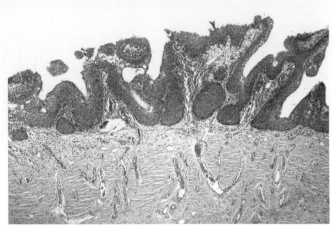

FIGURE 2

Immature condyloma. Note the papillary architecture at low-power magnification.

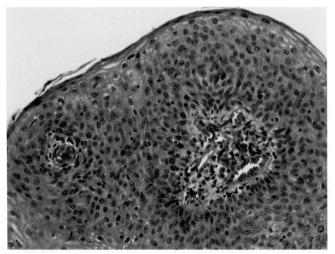

FIGURE 3

Immature condyloma. Immature condyloma at high magnification. Note the relatively high nuclear density; however, the cell population, while immature, is uniform, with regular nuclear spacing. There is a low mitotic index.

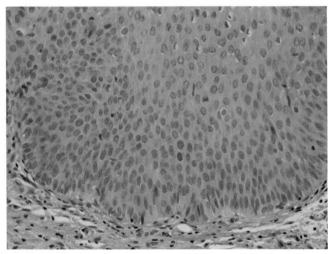

FIGURE 4

Immature condyloma. At higher power, again note the bland, uniform, slightly crowded nuclei. There is minimal nuclear atypia and overlapping.

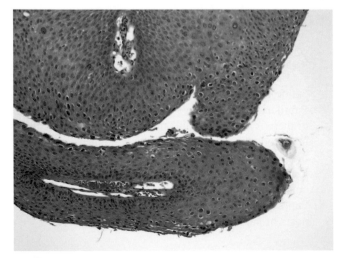

FIGURE 5

Immature condyloma. Note the lack of significant koilocytic change.

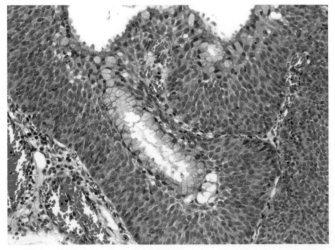

FIGURE 6

Immature condyloma. Immature metaplastic cells undermining columnar epithelium. Note the high cell density in contrast to normal metaplastic epithelium.

MIXED-PATTERN SQUAMOUS INTRAEPITHELIAL LESION (LOW- AND HIGH-GRADE SQUAMOUS INTRAEPITHELIAL LESIONS)

DEFINITION—The presence of two different human papillomavirus (HPV)–type specific lesions in the same specimen.

CLINICAL FEATURES

EPIDEMIOLOGY

- Reproductive-age, sexually active women, in the vulva or anal region may be associated with immunosuppression but not specific for this condition.

PRESENTATION

- Papanicolaou smear typically classified as atypical squamous cells of undetermined significance (ASCUS), low-grade squamous intraepithelial lesion (LSIL), or high-grade squamous intraepithelial lesion (HSIL).
- Colposcopic or gross abnormality, typical for squamous intraepithelial lesion (SIL).

PROGNOSIS AND TREATMENT

- Management is directed toward the more severe lesion.
- Treatment of any underlying predisposing factors.

PATHOLOGY

HISTOLOGY

Three scenarios in which both LSIL and HSIL are encountered are as follows:
- Coexisting condyloma or LSIL of the vulva or anus and HSIL (vulvar intraepithelial neoplasia II/III) or anal intraepithelial neoplasia (AIN II/III).

- Coexisting LSIL of the cervix and either HSIL or adenocarcinoma in situ.
- Coexisting immature condyloma (LSIL) and HSIL.
- The two lesions will either be juxtaposed or in separate biopsy specimens.

IMMUNOHISTOCHEMISTRY

- Ki-67 and p16ink4 expression will often define two different processes. HPV testing is not usually employed but will reveal two different HPV types.

DIFFERENTIAL DIAGNOSIS

- A spectrum of atypia is often present in SIL, such that a small focus of LSIL might be seen in continuity with HSIL. In our experience these are usually a manifestation of a single HPV infection and contrast with the presence of two distinctly different lesions (often separated or in separate biopsies) that typify a double infection.

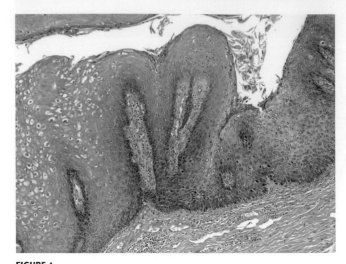

FIGURE 1

Mixed pattern SIL(s). This condyloma of the anal canal *(left)* merges abruptly with a higher-grade lesion (AIN 2 and 3) *(right)*.

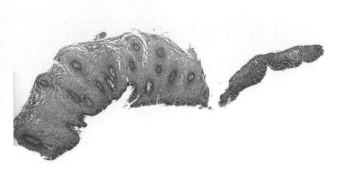

FIGURE 2

Mixed pattern SIL(s). This cervical biopsy contains both HSIL *(right)* and LSIL (condyloma, *left*).

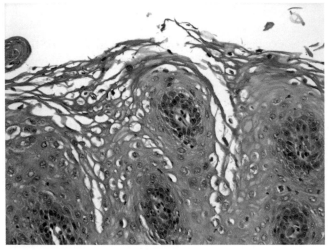

FIGURE 3

Higher magnification of the condyloma in Figure 2.

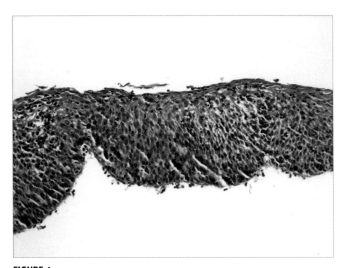

FIGURE 4

Higher magnification of the HSIL in Figure 2.

ATROPHY INCLUDING SQUAMOUS INTRAEPITHELIAL LESION IN ATROPHY

DEFINITION—Any one of the spectrum of alterations within the cervical epithelium of postmenopausal women, including squamous intraepithelial lesions (SILs).

CLINICAL FEATURES

EPIDEMIOLOGY

- Occurs predominantly in postmenopausal women.
- Also can be seen in any low-estrogen state (postpartum, breast-feeding).

PRESENTATION

- Typically detected on routine Pap smear analysis.
- Misinterpretation of atrophy for neoplasia can lead to colposcopy and biopsy.
- In some instances, atypia may be striking and mimic squamous cell carcinoma.

PROGNOSIS AND TREATMENT

- Excellent prognosis; this is a benign condition.
- The management of atypical atrophy often involves a trial of vaginal estrogen cream. This will usually resolve the atrophy and normalize the vaginal cytology.

PATHOLOGY

HISTOLOGY

- **Atrophy**
  - Histologic features of atrophy include hyperchromasia and elongated nuclei with occasional grooves (transitional metaplasia).
- Chromatin is usually finely distributed.
  - Mitotic activity is not typically present, but occasional mitoses may be found if there are inflammation and repair.
  - The nuclei are uniform throughout the epithelial compartment.
- **"Mature" Atrophy**
  - The surface shows some features of maturation including a decrease in nuclear size relative to the amount of cytoplasm.
  - Variable amounts of glycogenated epithelium are present, resulting in pseudokoilocytosis.
  - The basal layer is typically distinct and not thickened.
- **Atypical Atrophy**
  - Occasional cases have enlarged, atypical nuclei with or without partial maturation.
  - These cases are distinguished from SIL by the lack of appreciable mitotic activity, the presence of conspicuous intercellular bridging, and widely spaced nuclei.

IMMUNOPATHOLOGY (INCLUDING IMMUNOHISTOCHEMISTRY)

- The Ki-67 labeling index is not increased.
- In some cases, patchy cytoplasmic p16 positivity is noted.

MAIN DIFFERENTIAL DIAGNOSIS

- High-grade SILs (cervical intraepithelial neoplasia [CIN] III).

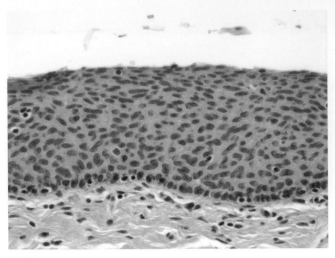

FIGURE 1

Cervical atrophy. This typical example of atrophy shows uniform, somewhat hyperchromatic, nuclei evenly distributed throughout the thickness of the sample. The nuclei are elongated, with occasional grooves. Maturation toward the surface is not present. Mitoses are not identified.

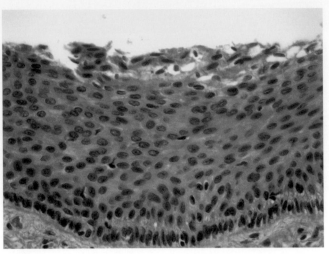

FIGURE 2

Cervical atrophy. A classical example of cervical atrophy. The basal nuclei are small, and the cells above that layer are uniformly hyperchromatic with elongated grooved nuclei. Nuclear atypia in the superficial layers is not present. Mitotic figures are not seen.

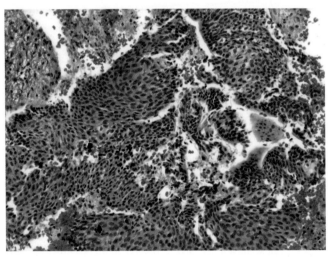

FIGURE 3

Cervical atrophy. In this curettage specimen, many fragments of atrophic cervical epithelium are present. The cells are uniform, hyperchromatic, elongated, and bland. Mitoses are not seen.

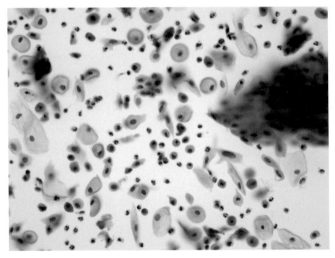

FIGURE 4

Benign atrophy in a cervical cytologic preparation. The variable nuclear size and dyskeratosis might mislead the cytopathologist. When uncertain, the pathologist should recommend a trial of intravaginal estrogen followed by a repeat cytology.

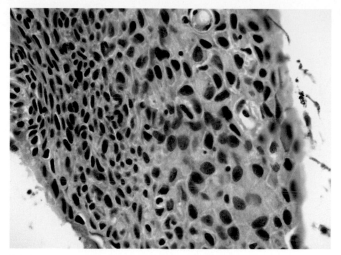

FIGURE 5

Cervical atrophy. A detached fragment of atypical atrophy. The nuclei are hyperchromatic, and some are enlarged and atypical. Features favoring a diagnosis of atrophy include the prominent intracellular bridges and the complete lack of mitotic activity.

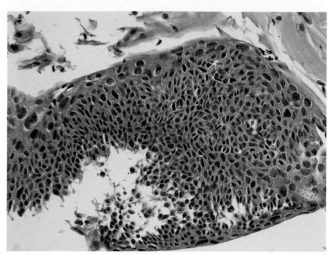

FIGURE 6

SIL occurring in atrophic changes. Note the focal discrete nuclear atypia. This biopsy specimen was strongly positive for p16.

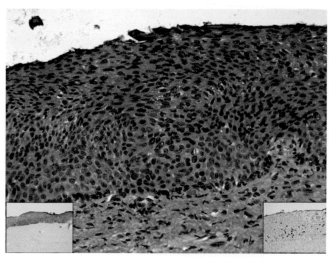

FIGURE 7

A rather subtle SIL associated with atrophy and not amenable to precise grading. p16 *(left inset)* and MIB1 staining *(right inset)* are increased.

MINOR p16-POSITIVE METAPLASTIC ATYPIAS

DEFINITION—Immature metaplastic or reserve cell proliferations with mild atypia and strong p16 immunostaining.

CLINICAL FEATURES

EPIDEMIOLOGY

- Reproductive-age women.
- Inconsistent human papillomavirus (HPV) association.
- Typically present with atypical squamous cells of undetermined significance (ASCUS) cervical smear.

PRESENTATION

- Variable, some acetowhite epithelium on colposcopy.

PROGNOSIS AND TREATMENT

- Limited follow-up at present to determine the risk of high-grade squamous intraepithelial lesion (HSIL) outcome.
- No data supporting this as a significant cancer precursor but some are likely an early form of SIL and more followup is needed.
- Managed by follow-up with reevaluation of the cervix.

CYTOPATHOLOGY

- Commonly ASCUS.

HISTOLOGY

- Immature metaplastic phenotype or basal proliferation with columnar differentiation.
- Uniform epithelial stratification with some cytoplasmic differentiation.
- Low level of anisokaryosis.

- Slightly higher nuclear density in all epithelial layers with some reduction near the surface.

IMMUNOPATHOLOGY (INCLUDING IMMUNOHISTOCHEMISTRY)

- p16ink4—diffusely positive.
- MIB1—less than 50% of the cells and typically confined to basal layers.
- Positive for squamocolumnar junction markers (CK7).

MAIN DIFFERENTIAL DIAGNOSIS

- Reactive or immature metaplasia—this entity will usually demonstrate more pronounced drop in cell density near the surface relative to immature low-grade squamous intraepithelial lesion (LSIL) with cytoplasmic maturation.
- Immature metaplastic squamous intraepithelial lesion (SIL)—higher nuclear density and nuclear-to-cytoplasmic (N/C) ratio, lack of uniform nuclear spacing, less distinct cytoplasmic borders, some syncytial groupings of surface nuclei, and "microheterogeneity" in nuclear size. Increase in MIB1 index in addition to being strongly p16 positive.
- This entity will pose some difficulty in management under the current guidelines for managing SIL in the laboratory. Some pathologists might interpret this process as reactive or low grade in nature, and manage with follow-up. However, if the pathologist is concerned about HSIL, the use of a p16 immunostain (which will be positive) might prompt treatment with cone biopsy or loop electrosurgical excision procedure (LEEP). In younger women, depending on the setting, management with a repeat exam in 6 months or LEEP might be performed.

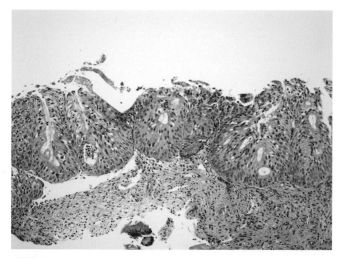

FIGURE 1

Mildly atypical immature metaplasia with columnar differentiation. Note the low nuclear density overall and the presence of mucin in the upper epithelial layers.

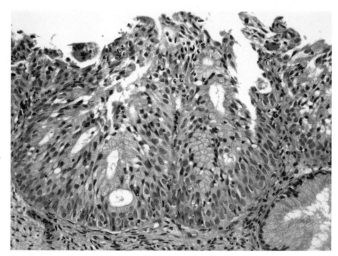

FIGURE 2

Higher magnification of Figure 1. Note the lack of appreciable atypia.

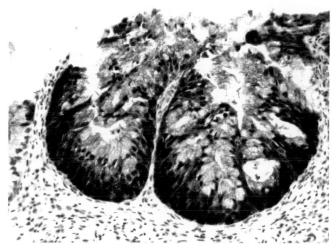

FIGURE 3

The p16 immunostain is intense, likely due to the immaturity of the epithelium.

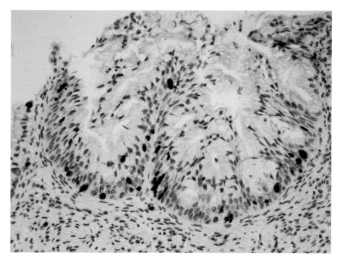

FIGURE 4

The MIB1 index is low despite the high p16 staining index.

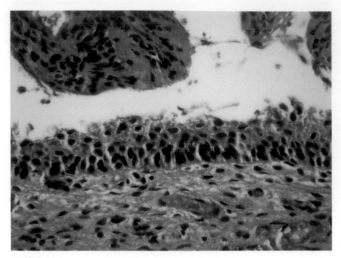

FIGURE 5

Mildly atypical immature metaplasia. The population is uniform with surface differentiation.

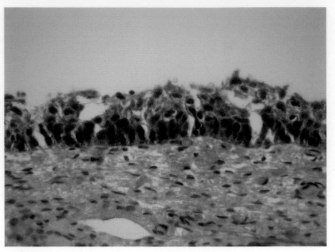

FIGURE 6

The p16, as in the prior case, is strongly positive.

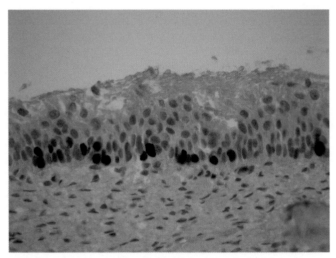

FIGURE 7

The MIB1 index is very low. This speaks against a diagnosis of HSIL and is of note given that some recent studies have not detected HPV in these lesions. Nevertheless, the possibility that these may be very early SILs in metaplastic epithelium must be considered.

SQUAMOUS INTRAEPITHELIAL LESION, NOT AMENABLE TO PRECISE GRADING (QSIL)

DEFINITION—A squamous intraepithelial lesion not amenable to precise grading (QSIL) that demonstrates features seen in both low-grade squamous intraepithelial lesion (LSIL) and high-grade squamous intraepithelial lesion (HSIL).

CLINICAL FEATURES

EPIDEMIOLOGY

- Typically encountered in reproductive-age women with atypical squamous cells of undetermined significance (ASCUS) or squamous intraepithelial lesion (SIL) on cervical cytology.

PRESENTATION

- The vast majority of lesions are first identified by routine screening with Pap smears.
- The pathologist is usually faced with two scenarios:
  1. The level of atypia is intermediate between cervical intraepithelial neoplasias 1 (CIN1) and 2 (CIN2).
  2. The lesion is immature (metaplastic), and there is a disparity between the degree of immaturity and level of cytologic atypia. This includes some cases that arise in microglandular change.

PROGNOSIS AND TREATMENT

- These lesions usually generate some disagreement in terms of grade, with some observers classifying them as LSIL and others opting for HSIL.
- In general, if there is agreement that the lesion does not fulfill the criteria for HSIL, the odds of HSIL on follow-up are low. If there is agreement on CIN2, the frequency of spontaneous resolution within 6 months is still approximately 40% and may be higher in young women under age 25.
- The fundamental question that should be asked by the pathologist when he or she examines the biopsy specimen is whether the patient should be managed by observation with a repeat exam or an ablative or excisional procedure. Given the high rate or resolution of many

SILs including CIN2, management options thus include either cryotherapy/loop electrosurgical excision procedure (LEEP) taking into account the cytologic and colposcopic findings or follow-up exam in approximately 6 months.

PATHOLOGY

HISTOLOGY

- Lesions with intermediate levels of atypia may exhibit:
  Increased parabasal cellularity
  Increased mitotic activity
  Abnormal mitotic figures
- Lesions with a disparity between level of atypia and degree of maturity exhibit:
  A metaplastic phenotype
  Persistently high nuclear density in the upper epithelial layers
  Uniform nuclear spacing
  Mild to moderate increase in the nuclear chromatin
  Absence of marked nuclear pleomorphism or coarse chromatin
- SIL associated with microglandular change:
  Lesions associated with microglandular change can be identified by their lobular architecture at low power that resembles squamous metaplasia.
  The cells are often immature and display cytoplasmic maturation with minimal crowding of the nuclei.
  The nuclei themselves are typically enlarged with occasional multinucleation.
  These lesions are frequently associated with high-risk HPV and may be diagnosed as mentioned earlier; however, the clinical impression (colposcopic) and cytologic findings should be considered.

255

IMMUNOPATHOLOGY (INCLUDING IMMUNOHISTOCHEMISTRY)

- These lesions are typically strongly p16 positive.
- Staining for squamocolumnar (SC) junction markers (CK7) will usually be strong.

MAIN DIFFERENTIAL DIAGNOSIS

- HSIL (CIN2 and CIN3)—This lesion will generate a higher level of agreement for HSIL due to greater nuclear overlap, irregularity in nuclear morphology, and more complex chromatin patterns, including abnormal mitoses.
- Atrophy or immature metaplasia with reactive changes. Both will be p16 negative. Reactive changes might display nuclear enlargement, but the chromatin is usually open with nucleoli.

DIAGNOSTIC TERMINOLOGY: *Squamous intraepithelial lesion, not amenable to precise grading (CIN1 and CIN2)*, with the proviso that management options include ablation/excision and observation with a repeat exam in approximately 6 months, or as clinically appropriate.

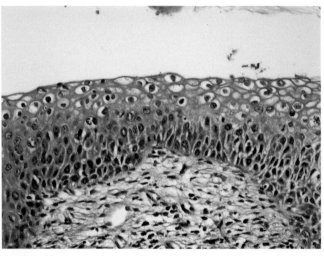

FIGURE 1

"QSIL" (SIL, not amenable to precise grading). There is increased nuclear chromasia and crowding in the lower third of the epithelium. This would often be classified as LSIL or QSIL, depending on the pathologist.

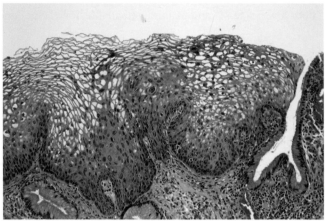

FIGURE 3

SIL, not amenable to precise grading (or QSIL). The overall architecture is that of an LSIL, but there is some increased parabasal atypia and a prominent abnormal mitosis in the center.

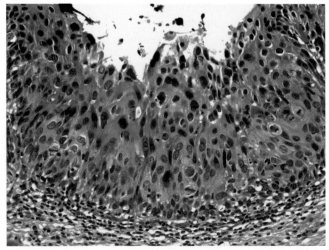

FIGURE 2

SIL, not amenable to precise grading (or QSIL). The cell growth appears somewhat disorganized with mitotic activity, but note the low nuclear-to-cytoplasmic (N/C) ratio, numerous multinucleated cells, and rather bland chromatin.

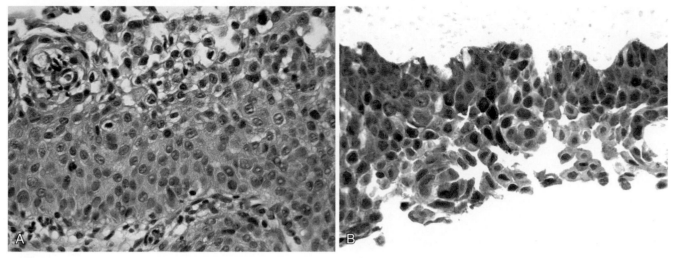

FIGURE 4

SIL, not amenable to precise grading (or QSIL). (**A**) Note the rather high nuclear density with rounded nuclei in the superficial layers of this metaplastic epithelium, yet the nuclei are uniform and do not overlap. (**B**) The lesion stains strongly for p16.

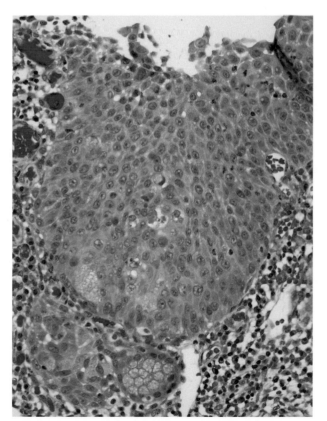

FIGURE 5

SIL, not amenable to precise grading (or QSIL). This is similar to the lesion in Figure 4, displaying a high nuclear density from base to surface. Both this and the prior lesion might be interpreted as reactive metaplasia by some given the lack of marked atypia. Others might prefer to classify them as "SIL in metaplasia, favor LSIL." Irrespective of the choice of words in the diagnosis, these lesions do not fit into the current concept of LSIL and HSIL as illustrated in most texts. Both are probably best managed by a repeat exam in approximately 6 months if more worrisome features are not seen on colposcopic exam.

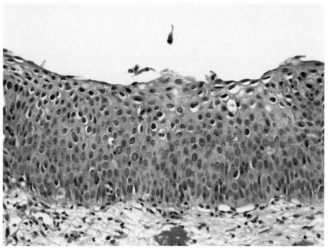

FIGURE 6

SIL, not amenable to precise grading (or QSIL). Another SC junction SIL that was variably classified as CIN1 and CIN2 by multiple observers. Note there is some nuclear overlap in the lower third of the epithelium, but there seems to be an orderly transition to differentiation without the more striking abnormalities in chromatin that typify HSIL.

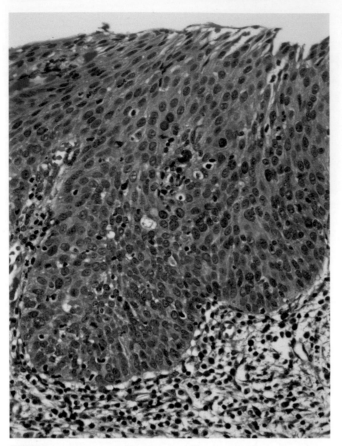

FIGURE 7

QSIL or HSIL? This metaplastic proliferation shows in addition a greater degree of nuclear overlap and hyperchromasia. Nucleoli are less conspicuous. In this case the pathologist will most likely render a diagnosis of HSIL.

SUPERFICIALLY INVASIVE SQUAMOUS CELL CARCINOMA

DEFINITION—Early invasive squamous cell carcinoma (SCC) measuring no more than 3 mm in depth in the biopsy or conization specimen.

CLINICAL FEATURES

EPIDEMIOLOGY

- Associated with high-risk human papillomavirus (HPV) infection and preexisting cervical intraepithelial neoplasia.
- Will be found in approximately 1:200 cone biopsies of high-grade squamous intraepithelial lesion (HSIL).
- Can be found at any age; median age around 35 to 40 years.

PRESENTATION

- Patients are often asymptomatic and are being evaluated for an abnormal cervical cytology.
- The cytologic findings may be atypical squamous cells of undetermined significance (ASCUS), HSIL, or malignant cells.
- Some patients typically present with abnormal bleeding, especially following intercourse.

PROGNOSIS AND TREATMENT

- Small lesions have an excellent outcome with conservative management (cold knife cone), provided that the lesion is less than 7 mm in length and there is no capillary lymphatic space invasion, with 5-year survival of 99% for stage IA1 lesions.
- Hysterectomy is the treatment of choice for those not desiring to preserve fertility.
- If lymphovascular invasion or deep stromal invasion (beyond 3 mm) is discovered, radical hysterectomy or trachelectomy (or large conization) will usually be performed as clinically appropriate.
- Risk of lymph node metastases increases from a few percent for lesions under 3 mm to over 5% for invasion over 3 mm.

HISTOLOGY

Several well-defined criteria must be applied to accurately diagnose stromal invasion:

- A desmoplastic stromal response.
- Blurring of the epithelial-stromal interface with loss of polarity of the cells at the epithelial-stromal border.
- Irregular or jagged stromal-epithelial interfaces.
- "Pseudocrypt" involvement with variable amounts of retraction artifact and occasional areas of central necrosis.
- Complex or reduplicated layers of epithelium with no intervening stroma.
- Abnormal keratinization of deep epithelial cells.
- Epithelial budding into the stroma, and single cells or clusters of small cells below the epithelial-stromal interface (early stromal invasion).
- A desmoplastic response can often be seen surrounding the aforementioned features.

In all cases of superficially invasive SCC a depth of invasion, horizontal extent, and the number of foci of invasion should be reported.

In cases of early superficial invasion the presence or absence of capillary-lymphatic space invasion should always be noted. If tumor is in spaces but the pathologist is unsure that they signify vascular invasion, it should be noted.

In biopsies the diagnosis of superficially invasive carcinoma should be made with caution and only if there is sufficient tissue to recognize the lesion as superficial. If the entire biopsy contains tumor, it should be stated as such and the dimensions of the biopsy given.

PREFERRED DIAGNOSTIC TERM: Superficially invasive SCC (*well, moderately, poorly*) differentiated, measuring (specify) _____mm in length by (specify) _____mm in depth. Lymphovascular space involvement is present/absent. Margins are free of invasive carcinoma (closest margin is (specify) _____mm).

IMMUNOPATHOLOGY (INCLUDING IMMUNOHISTOCHEMISTRY)

- Generally noncontributory excepting stains to verify capillary endothelium. Superficial carcinoma of the cervix is almost universally positive for pan-cytokeratins, CK7, and p63 immunostains, but these are rarely needed.

MAIN DIFFERENTIAL DIAGNOSIS

- Tangentially sectioned epithelium.
- Displaced epithelium due to previous procedures.
- Marked inflammation in cervical intraepithelial neoplasia (CIN) with blurring of the epithelial-stromal interface.
- Gland (crypt) involvement (can be tangentially sectioned).
- Prominent endothelial cells.

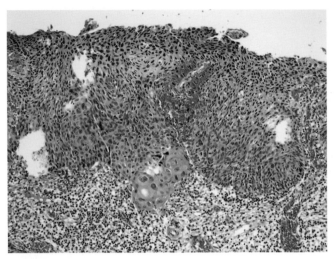

FIGURE 1

Early budding invasion. An invasive tongue *(center)* demonstrates loss of polarity and cytoplasmic differentiation.

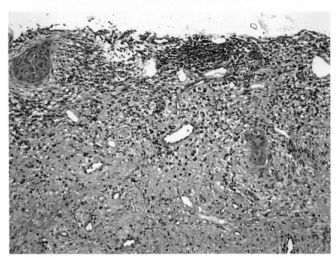

FIGURE 3

Subtle superficial invasion. The surface is eroded. Note the small nests of invasive carcinoma with stromal reaction.

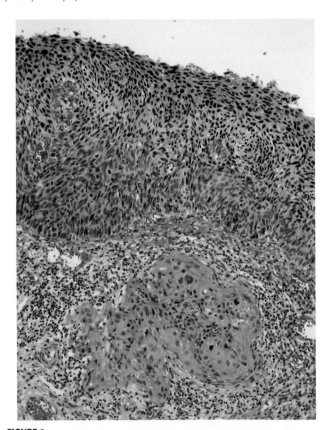

FIGURE 2

The same case as Figure 1 with superficial invasion.

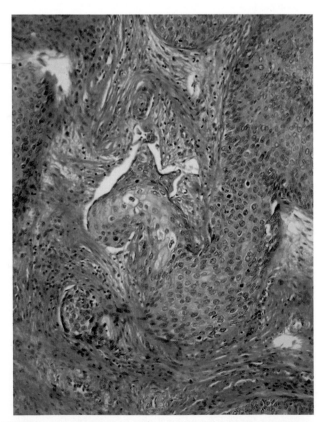

FIGURE 4

Another invasive tongue of epithelium. The complexity of this protruding neoplastic epithelium is inconsistent with crypt involvement.

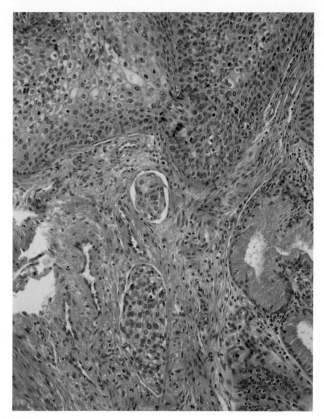

FIGURE 5

Lymphovascular invasion with rounded tumor nests in small sharply defined spaces devoid of stromal reaction.

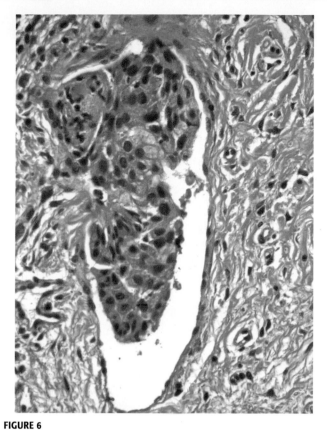

FIGURE 6

Pseudovascular invasion with detached fragments in a space. This can occur with injection of anesthetic or during specimen processing.

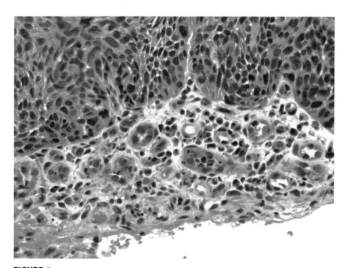

FIGURE 7

Pseudoinvasion in the form of prominent subepithelial capillaries with endothelial hyperplasia.

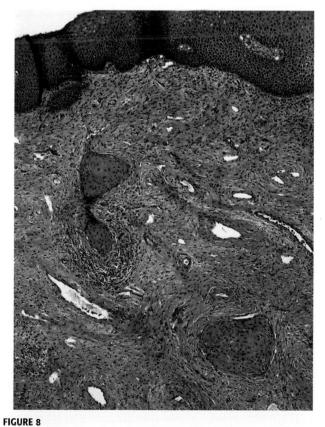

FIGURE 8

Pseudoinvasion created by prior biopsy that buried the epithelium in the superficial stroma.

CONVENTIONAL SQUAMOUS CELL CARCINOMA

DEFINITION—A malignant neoplasm of the cervix comprised of squamous epithelial cells. Variants include large-cell keratinizing, large-cell nonkeratinizing, and small-cell nonkeratinizing squamous cell carcinoma (SCC), as well as papillary SCC.

CLINICAL FEATURES

EPIDEMIOLOGY

- Associated with high-risk human papillomavirus (HPV) infection and preexisting cervical intraepithelial neoplasia.
- The progression rate from a high-grade squamous intraepithelial lesion to invasive squamous cell carcinoma in a patient undergoing close follow-up is less than 1%.
- The majority of patients that present with SCC are those who have not undergone regular screening with Pap smears.
- Historically the incidence is dropping, and a larger percentage are presenting at lower stage. In 2010, 11,800 women developed cervical cancer in the United States and 3,900 died of the disease.

PRESENTATION

- Patients typically present with abnormal bleeding, especially following intercourse.
- Patients may also present with pain or a clinically identifiable mass lesion.

PROGNOSIS AND TREATMENT

- Small lesions have an excellent outcome with conservative management (cold knife cone\trachelectomy), with 5-year survival between 97% and 99% for stage IA lesions.
- Radical hysterectomy is the treatment of choice in patients not desiring to preserve fertility. Patients with high risk factors reported on their final pathology will receive adjuvant chemotherapy and/or radiation therapy.
- If lymphovascular invasion or deep stromal invasion is present, lymph node dissection may be undertaken.

- Patients with stage IIB and above tumors are treated with concurrent chemotherapy and radiation therapy.
- Five-year survival rates rapidly decrease to 80% (stage IB), 65% (stage II), 33% to 39% (stage III), and 9% to 17% for stage IV disease.
- Outcome is not dictated by lesion grade or subtype within this spectrum of common variants.

PATHOLOGY

HISTOLOGY

Large-cell keratinizing (well-differentiated) SCC

- Uncommon, characterized by mild to moderate nuclear atypia and prominent keratinization.

Large-cell nonkeratinizing (moderately or poorly differentiated) SCC

- Most common variant, with moderate to marked atypia, presenting sheets of squamous cells with focal keratinization. Mucin droplets often present.

Small-cell nonkeratinizing (poorly differentiated) SCC

- Sharply demarcated nests of basal-type carcinoma cells with minimal keratinization.
- Some differentiation with features of large-cell nonkeratinizing carcinoma may be seen.

Papillary squamotransitional carcinoma

- This variant overlaps with papillary forms of high-grade squamous intraepithelial lesion (HSIL) and usually presents on biopsy with irregular fragments of papillary or frondlike neoplasia without associated stroma and with complex reduplication of epithelial layers without intervening stroma. The diagnosis of invasion may not be possible without further sampling.

Cytologic features of SCC

- Several features have been identified in cytologic preparations associated with invasive disease:
  - Tumor diathesis composed of cellular, necroinflammatory debris (may be absent on liquid-based preparations).
  - Large, abnormally keratinized cells, frequently with "ink black" nuclei.
  - Large groups of hyperchromatic cells that may resemble endometrial or endocervical cells.
  - Enlarged, atypically shaped squamous cells that are frequently keratinized.

IMMUNOPATHOLOGY (INCLUDING IMMUNOHISTOCHEMISTRY)

- SCC of the cervix is almost universally positive for pan-cytokeratins, CK7, and p63 immunostains.

MAIN DIFFERENTIAL DIAGNOSIS

- Tangentially sectioned HSIL, displaced epithelium due to previous procedures and marked inflammation in cervical intraepithelial neoplasia (CIN) with blurring of the epithelial-stromal interface, and gland (crypt) involvement are more relevant to the differential diagnosis of early invasion.
- Poorly differentiated adenocarcinoma or adenosquamous carcinoma—these are the most common mimics and best separated by p63 immunostains.
- Sarcomatoid (spindled) SCC and lymphoepithelial-like SCC are discussed elsewhere.
- Melanoma—rare in the cervix (versus vagina) but must always be considered with undifferentiated large-cell tumors. The presence of melanin pigment and immunostains for CK7 and HMB45 will aid in making this distinction.
- Basaloid carcinoma of the cervix—rare variant with unique pattern of basaloid cell growth with no appreciable squamous differentiation.
- Adenoid basal carcinoma of the cervix—a rare variant with not only squamous but also basal and adenoid differentiation. This mixture of patterns will distinguish it from a conventional cervical SCC.
- Neuroendocrine carcinomas of the cervix—distinguished by the absence or near absence of squamous differentiation (some tumors can be admixed with SCC or adenocarcinoma), discohesive growth, minimal inflammatory response, and positivity with neuroendocrine markers.

- Cervical involvement by, or sampling of, poorly differentiated endometrial carcinoma—these are typically heterogeneous for p16ink4 staining, vimentin positive, and HPV negative.

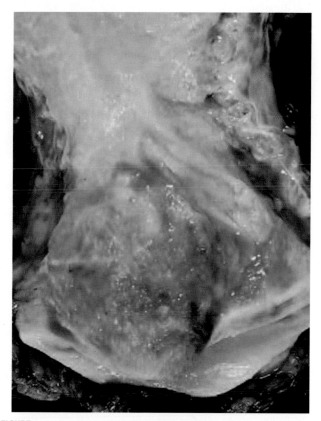

FIGURE 1

A small carcinoma forms a disc-shaped erosion at the squamocolumnar junction *(at left)*.

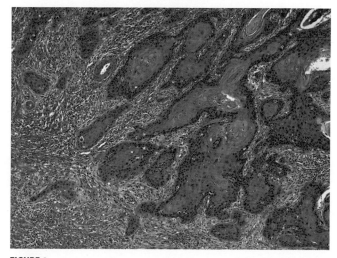

FIGURE 2

Large-cell keratinizing or well-differentiated cervical SCC. Note the prominent keratinization and mild atypia. This is a rare variant in the cervix as opposed to the vulva.

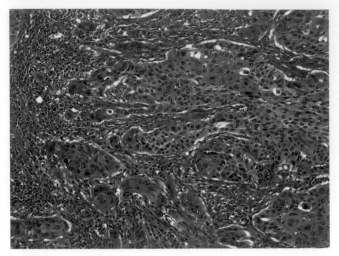

FIGURE 3

Large-cell nonkeratinizing or moderately differentiated SCC. This is by far the most common variant of cervical SCC. Keratinization is not conspicuous but can be present. Cells tend to be large and grow in sheets.

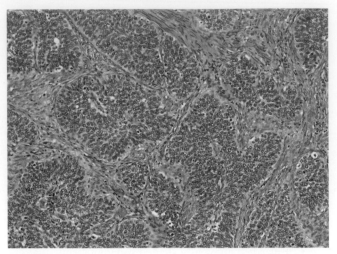

FIGURE 4

Small-cell nonkeratinizing or poorly differentiated SCC. Like the well-differentiated variant, this is relatively uncommon. Note the uniform sheetlike growth and preserved tumor cell cohesion.

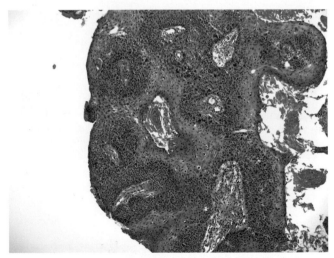

FIGURE 5

Papillary squamotransitional SCC. A typical presentation in curettings consists of poorly formed squamous neoplasia arranged in confluent papillae.

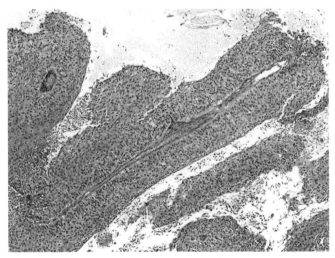

FIGURE 6

Papillary squamotransitional SCC. A particularly "transitional" appearance. Note that invasion cannot be assessed in this field.

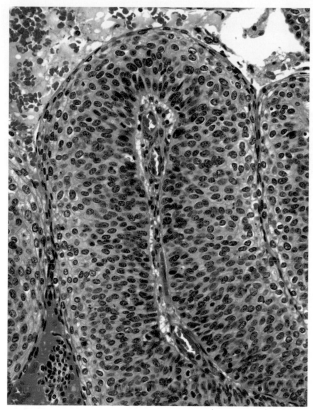

FIGURE 7

Papillary squamotransitional SCC. The lining cells show preserved polarity and cannot be distinguished from HSIL. The latter is excluded by confirming stromal invasion.

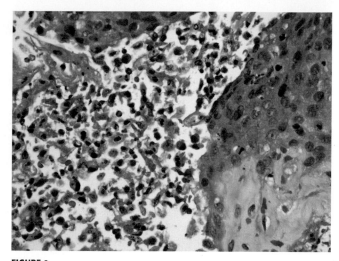

FIGURE 8

Exfoliated keratinized tumor cells from cervical SCC.

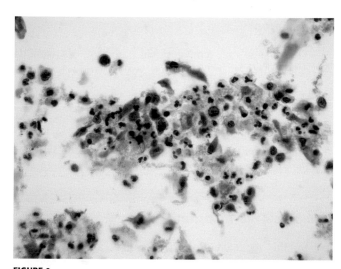

FIGURE 9

Pap smear showing cells identical to those in Figure 8 (same case).

PSEUDOCRYPT INVOLVEMENT BY SQUAMOUS CELL CARCINOMA

DEFINITION—A specific pattern of invasive carcinoma that either mimics crypt involvement or combines crypt involvement with invasion, thus mimicking noninvasive carcinoma.

CLINICAL FEATURES

EPIDEMIOLOGY

- The same as conventional invasive squamous carcinoma.

PRESENTATION

- Typically encountered on examination of a cone biopsy for high-grade squamous intraepithelial lesion (HSIL).
- Patients may also present with a clinically identifiable mass lesion.

PROGNOSIS AND TREATMENT

- Similar to conventional carcinoma, and depends on lesion size, depth of invasion, and status of regional lymph nodes.

PATHOLOGY

HISTOLOGY

- Tumor arranged in large discrete nests closely resembling crypt involvement.
- Cryptlike growths display irregular outlines and vary in caliber.
- Intense inflammatory response in adjacent stroma.
- Subtle irregularity in the epithelial-stromal interface with loss of polarity and/or budding invasion.
- Necrotic keratin debris in the centers of the pseudocrypts.
- Variable desmoplastic response in the adjacent stroma.

IMMUNOPATHOLOGY (INCLUDING IMMUNOHISTOCHEMISTRY)

- Keratin immunostains might highlight the irregularity in the interface.

MAIN DIFFERENTIAL DIAGNOSIS

- Crypt involvement by HSIL. The presence of normal columnar epithelium is helpful but not necessary. Preserved epithelial polarity, minimal interface inflammation.
- Adenoid basal carcinoma of the cervix. The squamous component of this tumor can closely mimic crypt involvement and when seen alone the pathologist must both exclude crypt involvement and recognize the possibility that the tumor is an adenoid basal carcinoma, which has minimal risk of metastases.

REPORTING TERMINOLOGY

Typically classified as invasive squamous cell carcinoma. If the only invasion appears to be coming from a crypt, the pathologist should report two measurements: the distance of the invasive nest from the crypt and the distance of the invasion from the highest epithelial stromal interface.

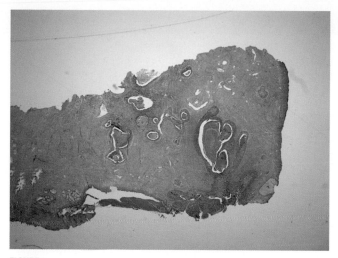

FIGURE 1

Pseudocrypt pattern of invasive squamous carcinoma. Note the irregular distribution of pseudocrypts with deep involvement.

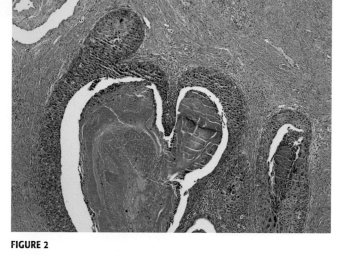

FIGURE 2

Pseudocrypt pattern of invasive squamous carcinoma. The irregular pattern on the left is characteristic of invasive carcinoma.

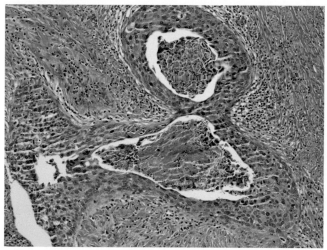

FIGURE 3

Pseudocrypt pattern of invasive squamous carcinoma. The "crypts" exhibit an anastomosing pattern not typical of normal crypt involvement.

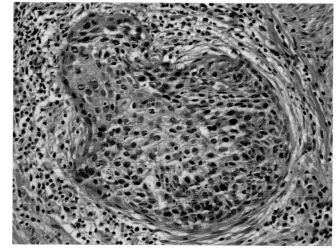

FIGURE 4

Pseudocrypt pattern of invasive squamous carcinoma. Note the desmoplastic response.

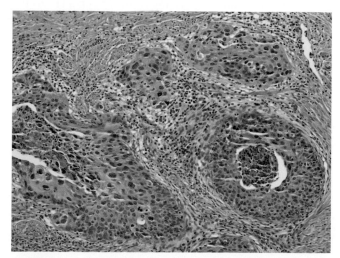

FIGURES 5

Pseudocrypt pattern of invasive squamous carcinoma. Here the irregular epithelial stromal interface and loss of polarity are obvious.

LYMPHOEPITHELIAL-LIKE SQUAMOUS CARCINOMA

DEFINITION—A poorly differentiated nonkeratinizing squamous carcinoma with prominent lymphocytic infiltrates.

CLINICAL FEATURES

EPIDEMIOLOGY

- A malignant cervical neoplasm.
- Most prevalent in the fourth to sixth decades of life.
- Human papillomavirus (HPV) testing of a few cases has been negative; thus its relationship to HPV is unclear.
- Unrelated to Epstein-Barr virus infection.

PRESENTATION

- Patients may present with abnormal bloody or blood-tinged cervical discharge.
- Patients may be asymptomatic or present with signs and symptoms of lower genital tract or abdominal spread of tumor.
- Detected on Pap smear screening.

PROGNOSIS AND TREATMENT

- Treated as any cervical cancer, according to stage.
- Prognosis may be better than the typical squamous carcinoma, but there are too few cases in the literature to confirm this.

PATHOLOGY

HISTOLOGY

- A hallmark of this tumor is ill-defined nests of epithelioid cells within a prominent inflammatory stroma.
- The infiltrate is predominantly lymphocytes with plasma cells and eosinophils.
- Morphologically resembles the nasopharyngeal tumor by the same name.

IMMUNOPATHOLOGY (INCLUDING IMMUNOHISTOCHEMISTRY)

- LCA stains will discriminate the lymphoid from epithelial cells.
- Epithelial cells are strongly p63 and p16ink4 positive.

MAIN DIFFERENTIAL DIAGNOSIS

- Severe inflammatory changes or lymphoma in the cervix—p63 or keratin stains will highlight the epithelial cells.

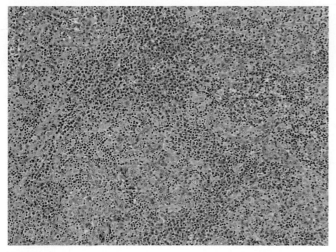

FIGURE 1

Lymphoepithelial-like cervical squamous carcinoma. At low power the ill-defined epithelial nests blend with the background lymphoplasmacytic infiltrate.

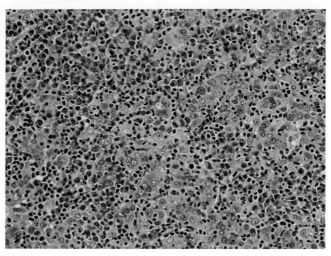

FIGURE 2

At higher magnification the epithelial cells are more easily distinguished.

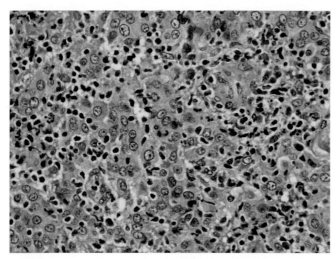

FIGURE 3

This field contains predominantly epithelial cells.

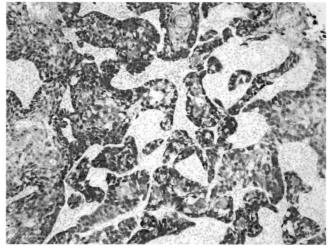

FIGURE 4

p16ink4 immunostaining is diffuse and strong in the epithelial tumor cells.

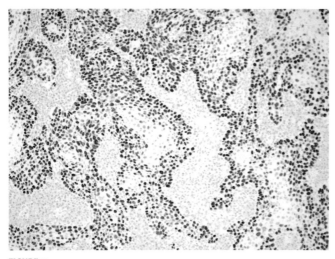

FIGURE 5

The tumor cells are strongly p63 positive, characteristic of a squamous carcinoma.

SUPERFICIAL (EARLY) ADENOCARCINOMA IN SITU

DEFINITION—A subtle pattern of endocervical adenocarcinoma in situ (AIS) which is frequently mistaken for reactive epithelial change.

CLINICAL FEATURES

EPIDEMIOLOGY

- Young women; mean age at diagnosis is early 20s.
- Human papillomavirus (HPV) associated.

PRESENTATION

- Abnormal Pap.
- Incidental, diagnosed during workup for a squamous intraepithelial lesion (SIL).

PROGNOSIS AND TREATMENT

- Same as for conventional AIS.

PATHOLOGY

HISTOLOGY

- At low power these lesions are present as discrete foci only in the superficial epithelium, making them easy to overlook.

- At high power they are characterized by nuclear hyperchromasia and stratification; mitotic activity and apoptosis are not as prominent as in conventional patterns of AIS.
- These discrete lesions lack the ciliated surface cells typical of benign endocervical epithelium.

IMMUNOPATHOLOGY (INCLUDING IMMUNOHISTOCHEMISTRY)

- Positive for p16 (diffuse) and Ki-67 (diffuse).

MAIN DIFFERENTIAL DIAGNOSIS

- Reactive epithelial changes or tubal metaplasia. Either can appear discrete. The former can exhibit a high proliferative index but is p16 negative. Problematic cases of tubal metaplasia will stain heterogeneous with p16.

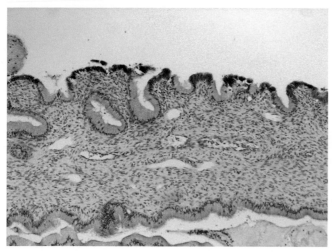

FIGURE 1

Superficial cervical AIS. At low power, foci of hyperchromatic glandular epithelial cells are present at the surface of the biopsy specimen. The cells deeper in the glands appear unremarkable.

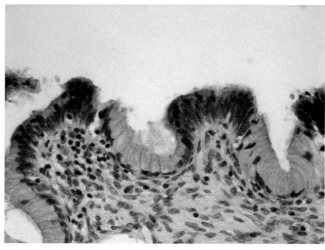

FIGURE 2

Superficial cervical AIS. Higher power of the lesion seen in Figure 1. The cells are stratified, are hyperchromatic, and lack the usual component of mucin. Apical mitoses are also present, although they are not prominent in this image.

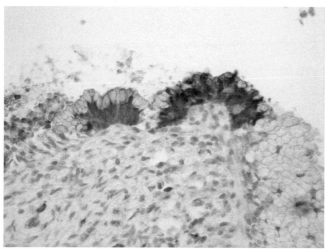

FIGURE 3

Superficial cervical AIS. p16 stain for the area seen in Figure 2. The hyperchromatic stratified cells are strongly and diffusely positive for p16. The bland-appearing epithelial cells are negative.

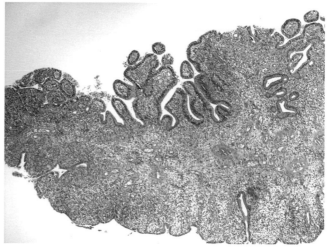

FIGURE 4

Superficial cervical AIS. In this endocervical polyp the AIS cells line the surface of the polyp on the superior half of the image. This can easily be mistaken for reactive change. The hyperchromatic-appearing cells are stratified, and apical mitoses can be identified.

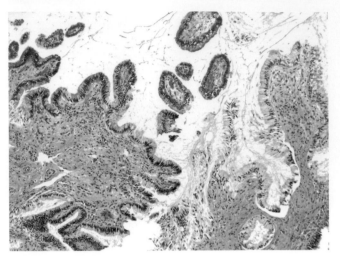

FIGURE 5

Superficial cervical AIS. AIS is seen on the left, in contrast to the normal endocervical cells on the right. Without the contrast, the cells on the left can easily be confused with a reactive process.

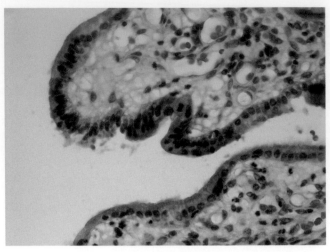

FIGURE 6

Superficial cervical AIS. In this subtle example the AIS cells are at the center and center-left. There is subtle nuclear stratification. A p16 stain was strongly positive in this area.

CONVENTIONAL ADENOCARCINOMA IN SITU

DEFINITION—Precursor lesion to invasive endocervical adenocarcinoma.

CLINICAL FEATURES

EPIDEMIOLOGY

- Average age at diagnosis is 38 years.
- Human papillomavirus (HPV) related (>90%), especially types 16 and 18 in roughly equal proportion.
- About half of cases have a concurrent squamous intraepithelial lesion (SIL).
- Positive association with oral contraceptive use, although a potential mechanism is unclear.

PRESENTATION

- Abnormal Pap smear (atypical glandular cells of undetermined significance [AGUS]), although Pap smears have an overall low sensitivity for glandular lesions.
- Abnormal examination at the time of colposcopy in 75% of cases.
- Often diagnosed concurrently with an in situ squamous lesion at the time of colposcopy for a cytologic diagnosis of SIL.

PROGNOSIS AND TREATMENT

- Cervical cone biopsy (usually cold knife cone) is the standard treatment.
- Up to 45% of patients with negative margins at the time of cone biopsy have residual or recurrent disease at subsequent hysterectomy.
- Other studies have reported that 13% of patients with negative margins at the time of cone biopsy go on to develop recurrent adenocarcinoma in situ (AIS), and rarely, invasive adenocarcinoma.
- Rare variants are associated with endometrial, tubal, or ovarian involvement. These tend to be extensive lesions that may spread by direct extension to other locations in the reproductive tract. However, they seem to have a good prognosis.

PATHOLOGY

HISTOLOGY

- At low power, AIS is usually near the squamocolumnar junction but can be found more deeply situated in the endocervix.
- The diagnostic criteria include the presence of epithelial cell crowding (nuclear stratification, tufting), moderate hyperchromasia, and mitotic figures.
- Other features that may aid in diagnosis include apoptotic bodies, which are found in the basal epithelium in 70% of cases, and architectural changes such as cribriforming, or papillae.
- Luminal eosinophilia with suspended mitoses is also a feature, albeit somewhat nonspecific.
- Architectural abnormalities may be florid, but this feature alone does not warrant a diagnosis of invasive adenocarcinoma, even in the presence of surrounding inflammation.
- Histologic variants (often present with conventional AIS) include:

  Endometrioid AIS, which is characterized by marked nuclear stratification and minimal amounts of cytoplasm, and therefore bears a resemblance to endometrial epithelium.

  Unusual variants, including intestinal or gastric (pyloric) AIS and stratified AIS, are discussed in other chapters.

  Tubal AIS is exceedingly rare; diagnostic features of AIS must be unequivocal as the vast majority of ciliated lesions in the cervix are benign.

- If seen on a cytologic preparation, AIS presents as clusters of hyperchromatic cells with the following features suggestive of glandular differentiation: (1) columnar cells with basally oriented nuclei and pale cytoplasm, (2) cellular feathering or radial projection of the nuclei around the periphery of the cellular clusters, and (3) glandlike structures or rosettes.

273

IMMUNOPATHOLOGY (INCLUDING IMMUNOHISTOCHEMISTRY)

- Positive for p16 (diffuse) and Ki-67 (usually exceeding 50% of neoplastic cell nuclei).

proliferative index but will exhibit patchy p16 immunostaining.
- Early invasive endocervical adenocarcinoma. Florid variants of AIS may be difficult to distinguish from invasion but have an excellent prognosis.

MAIN DIFFERENTIAL DIAGNOSIS

- Reactive epithelial changes (tubal metaplasia, Arias-Stella reaction, cervicitis)—these may have a high

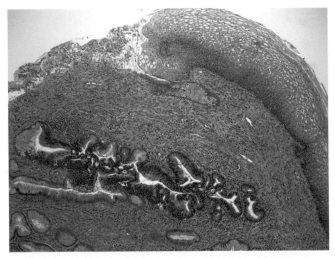

FIGURE 1

Conventional AIS. Low-power examination shows a hyperchromatic population of glandular cells in the transition zone of the cervix. Squamous epithelium is to the right and benign glandular epithelium to the left.

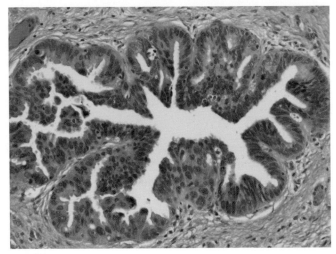

FIGURE 3

Conventional AIS. In addition to nuclear stratification and "tufting," the cells in this example of AIS show a prominent papillary and micropapillary growth pattern.

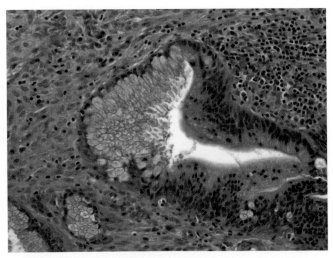

FIGURE 2

Conventional AIS. High-power examination reveals pseudostratified glandular epithelial cells with apical mitoses. These changes are seen in contrast to the background benign endocervical epithelium on the left, which has basally positioned nuclei with abundant mucinous cytoplasm.

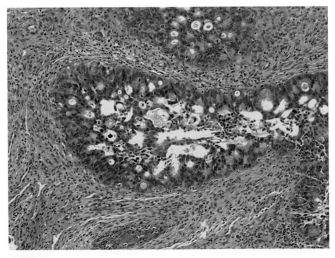

FIGURE 4

Conventional AIS. In this example the nuclear stratification is somewhat obscured by the microacinar growth pattern of the cells.

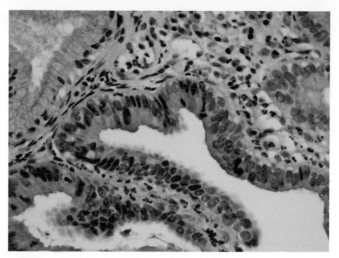

FIGURE 5

Conventional AIS. There is subtle nuclear stratification and rare apical mitoses in this example, but the changes contrast to normal epithelium in the upper left.

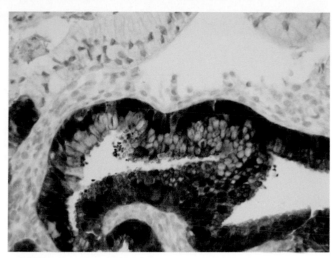

FIGURE 6

Conventional AIS. The corresponding p16 immunohistochemical stain for the biopsy seen in Figure 5. The atypical appearing endocervical cells are diffusely positive (nuclear and cytoplasmic) for p16. The background normal epithelium is entirely negative.

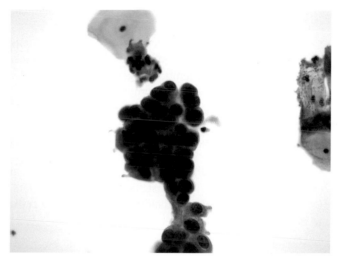

FIGURE 7

AIS on a Pap smear. A hyperchromatic cluster of atypical glandular cells is present.

STRATIFIED ADENOCARCINOMA IN SITU

DEFINITION—A stratified mucin-producing intraepithelial lesion with prominent columnar cell differentiation (also called stratified adenocarcinoma in situ [AIS]).

CLINICAL FEATURES

EPIDEMIOLOGY

- Young women, most ranging in age from 20 to 40 years.
- High-risk human papillomavirus (HPV) associated.

PRESENTATION

- Abnormal Pap, atypical squamous cells of undetermined significance (ASCUS), atypical glandular cells of undetermined significance (AGUS), AIS, and high-grade squamous intraepithelial lesion (HSIL).
- Diagnosed during workup for a squamous intraepithelial lesion (SIL).

PROGNOSIS AND TREATMENT

- Same as for conventional AIS.
- Some of these lesions are associated with invasion. The latter might occur more frequently in these precursors relative to conventional HSIL.

PATHOLOGY

HISTOLOGY

- These are high-grade intraepithelial lesions with prominent columnar differentiation. They are emblematic of the bridge between squamous and columnar differentiation and are sometimes classified as adenosquamous carcinomas in situ.
- Some may have basal cells with prominent squamous features blending with superficial columnar cell differentiation with mucin-containing vacuoles in the middle or superficial epithelial layers (i.e., HSIL with columnar differentiation).
- Many do not contain conspicuous basal squamous cells and are composed entirely of cells with mucin vacuoles, the latter in a honeycomb arrangement throughout the epithelium. These are aptly termed stratified adenocarcinomas in situ.

IMMUNOPATHOLOGY (INCLUDING IMMUNOHISTOCHEMISTRY)

- Positive for p16 (diffuse) and Ki-67 (diffuse); mucin stains are positive in at least the mid to upper layers. Importantly, all layers, including mucin positive cells, are p16 positive.

MAIN DIFFERENTIAL DIAGNOSIS

- Low-grade squamous intraepithelial lesion (LSIL) or mild metaplastic atypia with columnar differentiation—the nuclear density is lower and the lesion more closely resembles a benign metaplasia with mucin vacuoles. Low proliferative index, but a diffusely positive p16 staining distribution.
- Metaplastic HSIL—these lesions can have a slight columnar appearance since they may occupy crypts and undermine normal columnar cells.

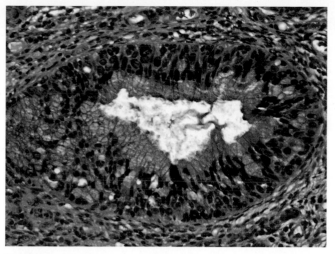

FIGURE 1

HSIL with superficial columnar differentiation. This lesion undergoes a transition from a basal squamous phenotype to columnar differentiation on the surface.

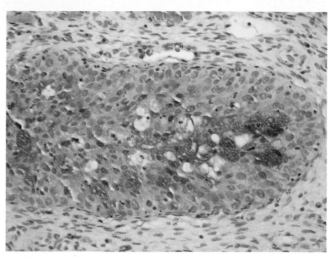

FIGURE 2

The case in Figure 1 displays superficial mucin positivity only.

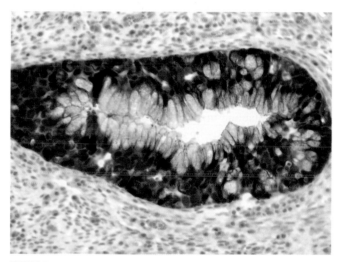

FIGURE 3

The case in Figure 1 contains diffuse p16 staining, in keeping with the fact that the entire process, including the columnar differentiation, is neoplastic.

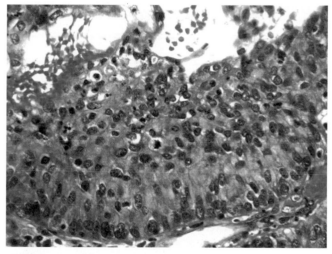

FIGURE 4

Stratified adenocarcinoma in situ. Note the vacuoles extend to the basal cells. There is no evidence of squamous differentiation.

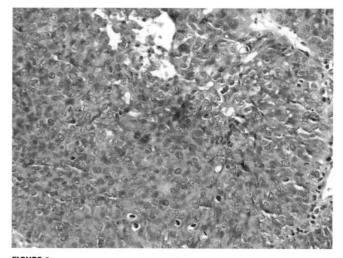

FIGURE 5

The biopsy specimen from the case in Figure 4 is diffusely positive for mucin, signifying scant if any squamous differentiation.

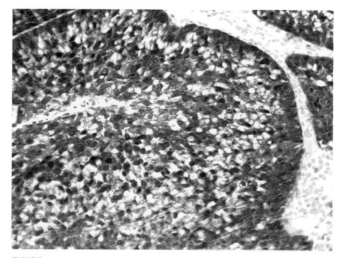

FIGURE 6

Like the prior case (Figures 1-3), the p16 staining is diffuse, underscoring the neoplastic character of the columnar differentiation.

INTESTINAL VARIANT OF ADENOCARCINOMA IN SITU

■ **Brooke E. Howitt, MD**

DEFINITION—A distinct subset of adenocarcinoma in situ (AIS) with intestinal differentiation.

CLINICAL FEATURES

EPIDEMIOLOGY

- Average age at diagnosis is 45 years (about 10 years older than conventional AIS).
- Human papillomavirus (HPV) detected in approximately 66%.

PRESENTATION

- Detected by an abnormal cervical cytology.

PROGNOSIS AND TREATMENT

- Standard therapy is cone biopsy or loop electrosurgical excision procedure (LEEP) if preservation of fertility is desired.
- Hysterectomy is recommended if not, due to the potential risk of multifocal disease or risk of recurrence despite negative margins.

PATHOLOGY

HISTOLOGY

- The lesion histology is punctuated by features of conventional AIS, such as hyperchromasia, apoptosis, and increased mitotic activity.

- Prominent cytoplasmic vacuoles are typical of goblet cell intestinal differentiation.

IMMUNOPATHOLOGY (INCLUDING IMMUNOHISTOCHEMISTRY)

- p16—will stain a proportion of these lesions strongly, but may be weak or unremarkable.
- Ki-67—staining index is usually over 50% in conventional AIS but may be less conspicuous in the intestinal variant.
- HPV testing—may be negative in up to one third of cases.

MAIN DIFFERENTIAL DIAGNOSIS

- Goblet cell differentiation, even in the absence of atypia, should prompt a search for ACIS.
- Gastric differentiation should also be distinguished, and is associated with lobular hyperplasias and rarely minimal deviation adenocarcinomas.

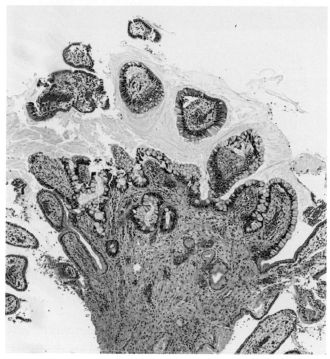

FIGURE 1

Intestinal AIS of the cervix. Note the normal mucosa at the far right and left. The center of the image is punctuated by hyperchromatic columnar epithelium with prominent vacuoles.

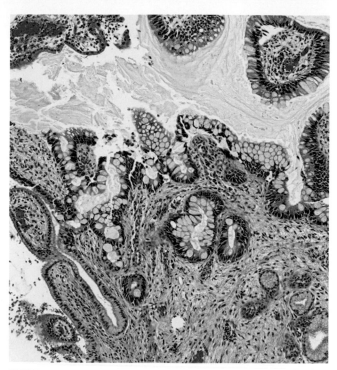

FIGURE 2

Intestinal AIS. Note the sharp transition from normal to neoplastic epithelium.

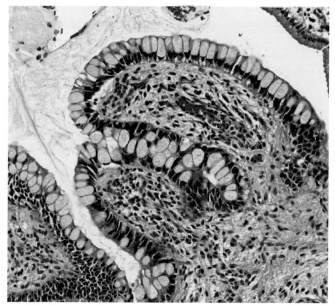

FIGURE 3

Intestinal AIS. At high magnification this field demonstrates uninterrupted goblet cells.

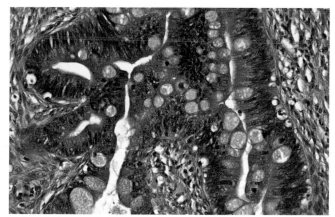

FIGURE 4

Intestinal AIS. Numerous apoptotic bodies are seen near the base of the epithelium. Mitoses are not conspicuous and are not a critical parameter for the diagnosis.

CERVICAL ENDOMETRIOSIS

DEFINITION—Ectopic endometrial glands and stroma (endometriosis) or endometrial stroma in isolation (stromatosis).

CLINICAL FEATURES

EPIDEMIOLOGY

- Endometriosis is common.
- Seen across all ages and demographic groups.
- Often follows punch or cone biopsy presumably because endometrial tissue colonizes the exposed stroma.

PRESENTATION

- In reproductive-age women, fluctuations in hormone levels lead to symptoms such as pain or abnormal bleeding.
- Many patients are asymptomatic.
- Pap smears may detect glandular cells.
- Pigmented lesion on the cervix.

PROGNOSIS AND TREATMENT

- The prognosis is favorable, and generally, no treatment is needed.
- Severe cases of endometriosis may require surgery or hormonal therapy.
- Rare cases of endometrioid carcinoma arising in endometriosis have been known to occur.

PATHOLOGY

HISTOLOGY

- Well-developed examples are similar to endometriosis at other sites and have both endometrial glands and stroma, often with evidence of old bleeding in the form of hemosiderin deposition.
- The endometrial stromal component may be attenuated or blend imperceptibly with cervical stroma.
- Occasional cases may consist solely of endometrial glands closely apposed to cervical stroma.
- In cases with little to no stroma, care must be taken to distinguish the glands from those seen in endocervical adenocarcinoma in situ (AIS), as both display stratified nuclei and mitotic activity.
- Endometriotic glands are uniformly spaced and have less nuclear hyperchromasia and pleomorphism than their AIS counterparts.
- The presence of old hemorrhage is helpful in cases of endometriosis.
- Following cone biopsy, squamous overgrowth may occur.

IMMUNOPATHOLOGY (INCLUDING IMMUNOHISTOCHEMISTRY)

- CD10 can stain endometrial stroma.
- Reticulin stains endometrial stroma in a pericellular fashion.
- Endometrial stroma is red on a trichrome stain, whereas cervical stroma is blue (due to the higher levels of collagen in the cervical stroma).
- Endometrioid glands stain positive for ER and heterogeneous for p16.

MAIN DIFFERENTIAL DIAGNOSIS

- Cervical adenocarcinoma, endometrioid type—intense p16 staining.
- Cervical AIS—this can be excluded if the pathologist is reasonably familiar with endometrioid gland histology. AISs have hyperchromatic glands, mucin production, suspended mitoses, and often a rather dense eosinophilic apical cytoplasm. Atypia alone is less helpful, since tubal metaplasia often exhibits a pleomorphic appearance due to the mixture of ciliated and nonciliated cells. p16 staining will also be intense.
- Metastatic low-grade endometrial endometrioid adenocarcinoma—two mimics including superficially situated "drop metastases" and mesonephric-like metastases from endometrial adenocarcinomas can pose a diagnostic problem (discussed elsewhere). However, neither matches the morphology of normal endometrial glands, which typify endometriosis, even in the absence of stroma.

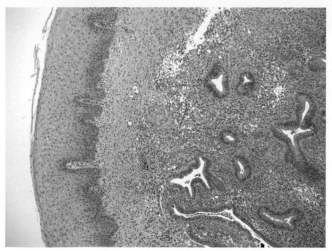

FIGURE 1

Cervical endometriosis. Low power reveals the presence of endometrioid glands and stroma centered in the cervical stroma, deep to the ectocervical squamous epithelium. The background cervical stroma is pink, with small spindled cells. The endometrioid stroma is darker, with larger spindled to ovoid nuclei. There is some evidence of recent hemorrhage, which is likely just procedural.

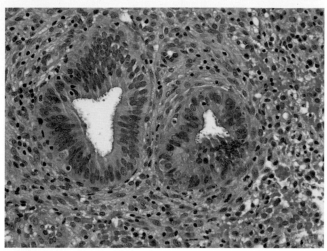

FIGURE 2

Cervical endometriosis. Higher-power examination reveals glands with typical endometrioid histology with large elongated stratified nuclei. The endometrioid stroma is loose, with large plump nuclei and scattered mononuclear lymphocytes. Mitoses in the epithelium and stroma are often identified. Rare clusters of pigment consistent with hemosiderin are present in this example.

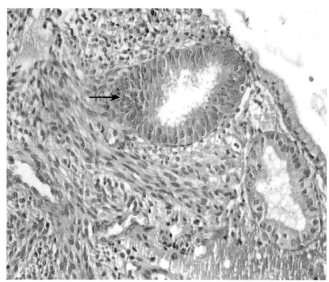

FIGURE 3

A focus of stroma-poor endometriosis (or tubal-endometrioid metaplasia). A mitotic figure is present *(arrow)*.

PREGNANCY-RELATED CHANGES IN THE CERVIX

DEFINITION—Hormonally driven benign morphologic alteration of the endocervical epithelium, most commonly associated with pregnancy or the recent postpartum state.

CLINICAL FEATURES

EPIDEMIOLOGY

- Endocervical Arias-Stella effect may be seen in up to 50% of extensively examined gravid cervices.
- Occasionally a rare, focal finding in nonpregnant women.

PRESENTATION

- Incidental finding at the time of cervical sampling.

PROGNOSIS AND TREATMENT

- Excellent; no treatment is required.

PATHOLOGY

HISTOLOGY

- Cells with Arias-Stella effect exhibit marked cytomegaly and protrude into lumina in a striking tufted or hobnail pattern.
- The cytoplasm is abundant, is eosinophilic to clear, and occasionally has extensive basal vacuole formation.
- Eosinophilic inclusions may be noted.
- Nuclear changes are variable and include atypia with smudged, vacuolated, or clear nuclei.
- Mitotic figures are very rare.
- The extent of these changes is variable and may involve all the glands within a given specimen, a single gland, or a portion of one gland.

- A generally unreported consequence of pregnancy is basal vacuoles seen as discrete round vacuoles at the epithelial-stromal interface. This is not of clinical importance but is distinctly pregnancy related.

IMMUNOPATHOLOGY (INCLUDING IMMUNOHISTOCHEMISTRY)

- Ki-67 labeling index is low.
- p16 and p53 stains may be positive but are usually patchy.

MAIN DIFFERENTIAL DIAGNOSIS

- Clear-cell adenocarcinoma—this usually presents as an expansile lesion and a slightly higher N/C ratio.
- Endocervical adenocarcinoma in situ (both conventional and intestinal types)—these typically exhibit more complex architecture and are readily distinguished by the strong p16 immunostaining.
- Intramucosal metastases from an endometrial or upper genital tract high-grade serous carcinoma—this can occur but typically the nuclear-to-cytoplasmic (N/C) ratio is higher, and the cells are strongly p53 positive.
- Radiation effect—this can also cause nuclear atypia with an Arias-Stella effect–like appearance. The cells will usually exhibit degenerative changes with smudged or ground-glass chromatin and a lower N/C ratio.

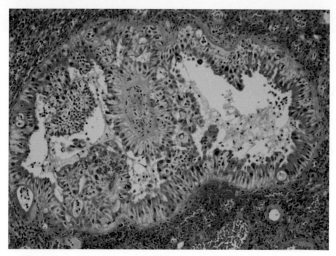

FIGURE 1

Hypersecretory changes in the cervical columnar epithelium in pregnancy. This is not technically Arias-Stella effect but is an accentuation of secretory activity with basal vacuoles, also a feature of pregnancy.

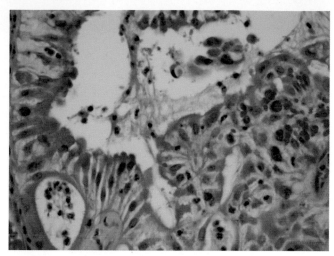

FIGURE 2

Hypersecretory changes in the cervical columnar epithelium in pregnancy. At higher magnification these vacuoles span the entire length of the cell.

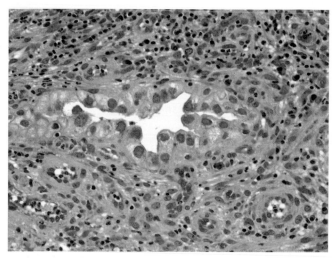

FIGURE 3

Cervical Arias-Stella effect. This crypt shows the characteristic single layer of epithelial cells with nuclear enlargement and cytoplasmic vacuoles.

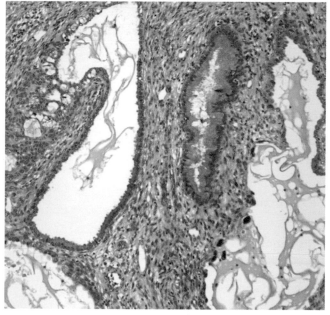

FIGURE 4

Arias-Stella effect in a cervical polyp. Note the hyperchromatic nuclei lining the crypt at the lower right of the image.

REACTIVE ATYPIAS IN THE ENDOCERVIX

DEFINITION—A multinucleated endocervical cell atypia commonly associated with chronic inflammation.

CLINICAL FEATURES

EPIDEMIOLOGY

- Relatively common, occasionally pronounced.
- Typically reproductive age, but can occur at any age.

PRESENTATION

- Incidental finding.

PROGNOSIS AND TREATMENT

- Not pathologic.

PATHOLOGY

HISTOLOGY

- Typically, multinucleated endocervical cells with ground-glass or amphophilic cytoplasm.

- Some cases are not multinucleated and will simply display hyperchromatic nuclei with variable enlargement.
- Homogeneous chromatin.
- Usually intermittent, but can be focally prominent.

IMMUNOPATHOLOGY (INCLUDING IMMUNOHISTOCHEMISTRY)

- Noncontributory except if excluding viral inclusions.

MAIN DIFFERENTIAL DIAGNOSIS

- Viral inclusions—denser and characteristic of cytomegalovirus (CMV) or herpes simplex virus (HSV). Usually not as polynucleated.
- Adenocarcinoma in situ—these are usually not polynucleated but rarely can be in which case the other features of adenocarcinoma in situ will be appreciated.
- Arias-Stella effect—usually not polynucleated and exhibits a denser hyperchromatic nucleus.

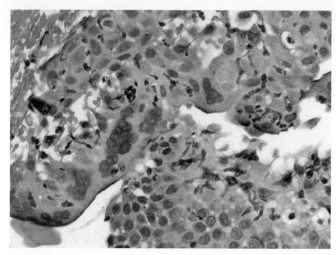

FIGURE 1

Classic reactive endocervical cell atypia with multinucleation and amphophilic cytoplasm.

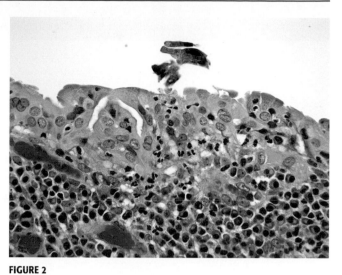

FIGURE 2

Another example of endocervical cell atypia overlying granulation tissue. Note the similarity to Figure 1, although there is less multinucleation.

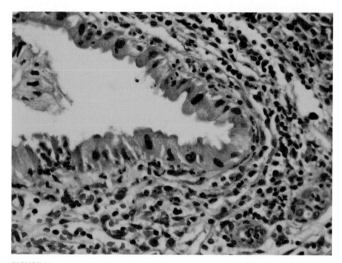

FIGURE 3

Focal reactive atypia in endocervical crypts manifesting as nuclear hyperchromasia only.

RADIATION ATYPIAS

DEFINITION—Changes seen in the cervical-vaginal epithelium following radiation therapy.

CLINICAL FEATURES

EPIDEMIOLOGY

- A common finding in tissue samples following radiation therapy to the genital area.

PRESENTATION

- Often seen in conjunction with radiation-induced atrophy of the vaginal canal epithelium.
- Presenting symptoms include vaginal itching, dryness, and pain, which often lead to colposcopic examination.

PROGNOSIS AND TREATMENT

- Radiation effect of the cervix/vagina tends to be chronic, and significant morbidity can be attributed to both vaginal and cervical involvement.

PATHOLOGY

HISTOLOGY

- Ectocervical/vaginal, endocervical, stromal, and endothelial cells can be affected.
- Cytomegaly with nuclear enlargement, irregular nuclear membranes, and hyperchromasia are most commonly seen; however, the nuclear chromatin is indistinct and has a smooth "smudgy" consistency, which is different from the coarse chromatin seen in dysplastic cells.
- Despite the marked atypia, there is a noticeable lack of mitotic activity and nuclear crowding.

- Abundant cytoplasm is present, resulting in a low nuclear-to-cytoplasmic (N/C) ratio despite the frequently impressive nuclear enlargement.
- Preservation of nuclear spacing should be present.
- Degenerative changes, such as cytoplasmic vacuoles, may or may not be prominent.
- Associated radiation necrosis of the underlying stroma may be present.

IMMUNOPATHOLOGY (INCLUDING IMMUNOHISTOCHEMISTRY)

- Ki-67 is negative in radiation changes.
- p16 is negative in radiation changes.
- p53 might be positive, which can cause some diagnostic confusion.

MAIN DIFFERENTIAL DIAGNOSIS

- Adenocarcinoma in situ—should exhibit increased proliferative activity, higher nuclear density, mitotic figures, and so forth.
- Arias-Stella effect—similar, but can be distinguished by history.
- Clear-cell carcinoma—usually greater hyperchromasia and higher N/C ratio.
- Squamous intraepithelial neoplasia—usually will demonstrate a higher nuclear density and increased N/C ratio.
- Recurrent squamous carcinoma or adenocarcinoma—nuclear features more pronounced, with enlargement, hyperchromasia, and prominent nucleoli.

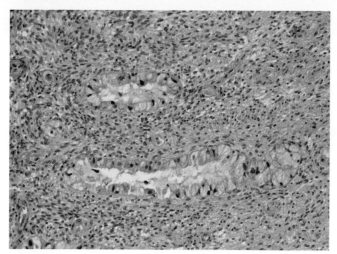

FIGURE 1

Radiation atypia. At medium power, scattered epithelial cells appear enlarged, hyperchromatic, and stand out from the background epithelium.

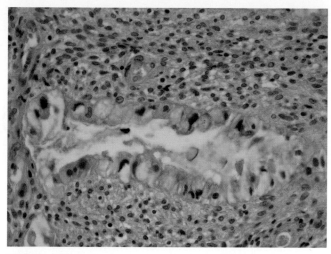

FIGURE 2

Radiation atypia. At higher power the hyperchromatic cells have normal N/C ratios and smooth, "smudgy" chromatin. Mitotic activity is not present.

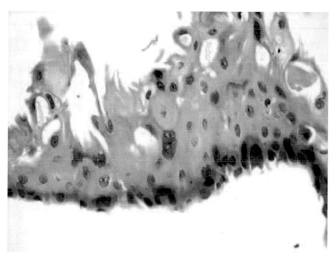

FIGURE 3

Radiation atypia. This vaginal squamous epithelium demonstrates the characteristic nuclear enlargement, low N/C ratio, and absence of coarse chromatin. Note also some cells are degenerated (apoptotic, center). *(Kindelberger DW, Crum CP: Diagnostic Gynecologic and Obstetric Pathology, Philadelphia, 2011, Saunders, Figure 11-6.)*

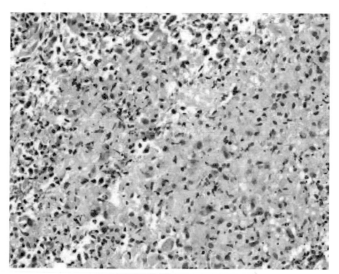

FIGURE 4

Radiation necrosis of the underlying stroma. *(Kindelberger DW, Crum CP: Diagnostic Gynecologic and Obstetric Pathology, Philadelphia, 2011, Saunders, Figure 11-7.)*

VILLOGLANDULAR ADENOCARCINOMA OF THE CERVIX

DEFINITION—A well-differentiated adenocarcinoma with a major exophytic and villoglandular component.

CLINICAL FEATURES

EPIDEMIOLOGY

- Wide age range (third to seventh decades) with a mean age of 38 years.
- Human papillomavirus (HPV) associated.

PRESENTATION

- Most common symptom is abnormal vaginal bleeding (75%).
- Occasionally diagnosed on abnormal cervical cytology.
- Two thirds present in the International Federation of Gynecology and Obstetrics (FIGO) stage IB.

PROGNOSIS AND TREATMENT

- Standard treatment as for any cervical epithelial malignancy.
- Lymph node metastases occur in less than 10% of patients.
- Overall good prognosis although it is stage dependent.
- Disease-free 5-year survival of 75%.
- Should not be viewed as a distinct entity in terms of behavior inasmuch as some tumors may be quite invasive.

PATHOLOGY

HISTOLOGY

- A distinctive feature of this tumor is a uniform branching, papillary, and interconnecting stromal network lined by a moderately atypical epithelium reminiscent of endometrial lining.

- Growth is predominantly exophytic and endophytic. Further sampling will be needed in some cases to ascertain the extent of invasion.
- Invasion may be pushing or infiltrative and may not be readily evaluable in a small superficial biopsy.

IMMUNOPATHOLOGY (INCLUDING IMMUNOHISTOCHEMISTRY)

- May be helpful in cases where the origin of the tumor is uncertain including small biopsies.
- Strong p16 immunopositivity.

MAIN DIFFERENTIAL DIAGNOSIS

- Florid endocervical adenocarcinoma in situ—adenocarcinoma in situ can be exuberant, involving papillae or microglandular change. These variants usually do not display the prominent dense supporting stroma.

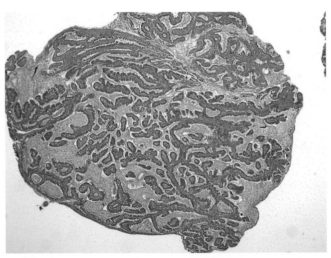

FIGURE 1

Villoglandular adenocarcinoma of the cervix. A typical superficial biopsy displays only the exophytic portion.

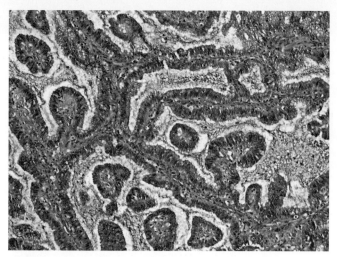

FIGURE 2

Higher magnification displays the regular network of stromal support.

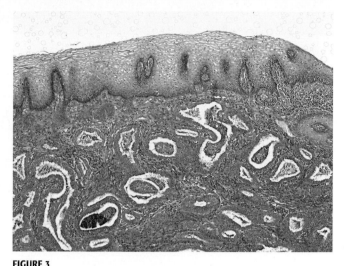

FIGURE 3

A blunt invasion of the underlying stroma is characteristic of many of these villoglandular carcinomas.

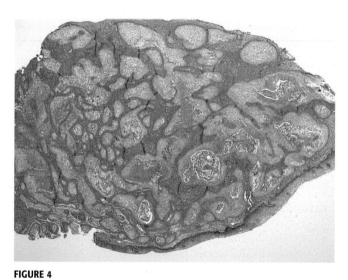

FIGURE 4

Rarely a nested pattern of squamous metaplasia will be seen. This is consistent with replacement of some of the neoplastic glandular epithelium by squamous metaplasia, a rare event in an untreated cervix.

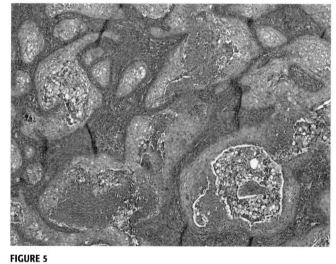

FIGURE 5

At higher magnification note how the squamous epithelium has populated the tracts previously occupied by the glandular lesion.

SUPERFICIALLY INVASIVE ENDOCERVICAL ADENOCARCINOMA

DEFINITION—Early-stage invasive endocervical adenocarcinoma.

CLINICAL FEATURES

EPIDEMIOLOGY

- Average age at diagnosis is early 40s.
- Human papillomavirus (HPV) associated.

PRESENTATION

- Lack of a clinically visible lesion is a component of the definition of early invasive carcinoma.

PROGNOSIS AND TREATMENT

- Largely depends on the patient's desire for future child-bearing, treatment ranging from cone biopsy alone to radical hysterectomy with pelvic lymph node dissection (most common). No consensus for appropriate treatment exists.
- Stage IA1 (cervical stromal invasion <3 mm) has a 1.5% risk of pelvic lymph node metastases.
- Stage IA2 (cervical stromal invasion 3 to 5 mm) has a slightly higher risk of lymph node spread.
- The presence or absence of lymphovascular space involvement is not included in the staging criteria. However, it will influence management in most institutions.

PATHOLOGY

HISTOLOGY

- For a diagnosis of early invasive endocervical adenocarcinoma, the microscopic area of invasion does not exceed 7 mm in the greatest linear dimension and does not exceed 5 mm of cervical stromal invasion (see preceding section).
- The diagnosis is not reliable when there is any question of where in situ disease stops and invasion begins. For this reason, large expansile lesions resembling adenocarcinoma in situ (AIS) are not likely to be resolved. It is best achieved with infiltrative disease with a distinct transition from in situ to invasion.
- Exophytic growth must be evaluated separately.
- A diagnosis of early invasive adenocarcinoma should not be made on small biopsy specimens; the possibility may be suggested but a conclusive diagnosis must be reserved for larger samples, such as cervical cone biopsy.

IMMUNOPATHOLOGY (INCLUDING IMMUNOHISTOCHEMISTRY)

- Not helpful for distinguishing early invasive disease from an in situ lesion; however, p16 may be helpful in determining the extent of neoplastic epithelium.

MAIN DIFFERENTIAL DIAGNOSIS

- Endocervical adenocarcinoma in situ involving microglandular change.

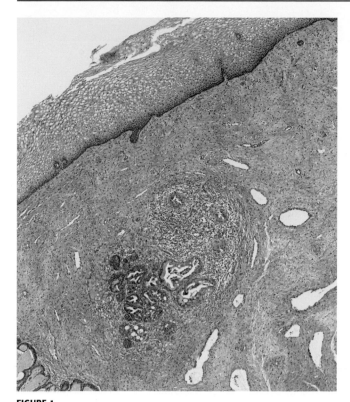

FIGURE 1

Early endocervical adenocarcinoma. An irregular nest of poorly oriented glands and inflammatory cells lies just beneath the normal mucosa.

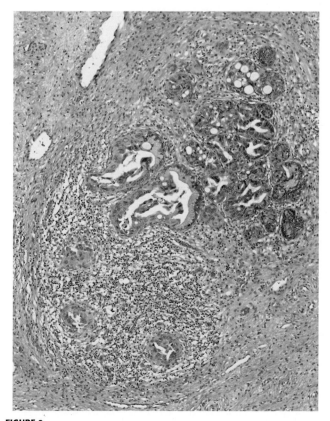

FIGURE 2

Early endocervical adenocarcinoma. Higher magnification of the focus in Figure 1.

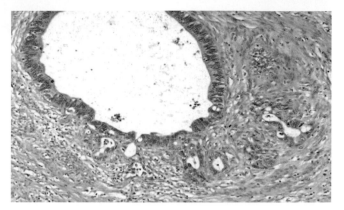

FIGURE 3

Early endocervical adenocarcinoma. Small poorly formed buds of neoplastic epithelium radiate from an involved crypt.

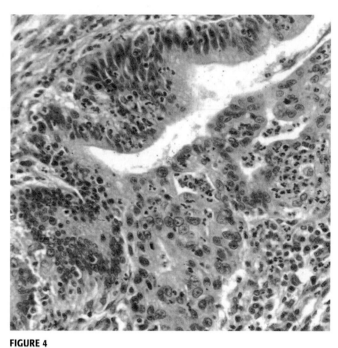

FIGURE 4

Early endocervical adenocarcinoma. In this field a small, solid, unoriented cell outgrowth is present at the bottom of a crypt.

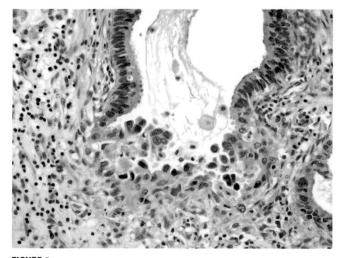

FIGURE 5

Early endocervical adenocarcinoma. In this focus the base of the crypt has dissolved, with complete loss of epithelial polarity.

EXTENSIVE ADENOCARCINOMA IN SITU VS INVASION

DEFINITION—A florid pattern of endocervical adenocarcinoma in situ (AIS) that mimics invasive adenocarcinoma.

CLINICAL FEATURES

EPIDEMIOLOGY

- The same as for conventional AIS.

PRESENTATION

- The same as for conventional AIS.

PROGNOSIS AND TREATMENT

- The same as for conventional AIS, depending on the level of suspicion for invasive cancer.
- Because of the difficulty of separating this entity from early invasive adenocarcinoma, occasional cases will be associated with endometrial or even ovarian involvement. Cases requiring multiple cone biopsies should raise a "red flag" for this risk.

PATHOLOGY

HISTOLOGY

- At low power these lesions are extensive and involve the native endocervical glands and even endocervical polyps.
- The epithelial architecture may be simple or complex (cribriforming, papillary).

- AIS may extensively involve endocervical glands circumferentially and extend into the high endocervix, but this alone is not sufficient for a diagnosis of invasion.
- At low power a smooth, lobulated appearance is seen around the glands, and at high power the eosinophilic basement membrane is present.
- Acute or chronic inflammation may be present surrounding the involved glands.
- In general, AIS replaces native endocervical epithelium and may expand the gland tracts, but does not extend more deeply into the cervical stroma than do adjacent normal endocervical glands.
- The depth of extension into the surrounding stroma compared with normal glands may be difficult to assess in the presence of a very diffuse process.

IMMUNOPATHOLOGY (INCLUDING IMMUNOHISTOCHEMISTRY)

- Noncontributory.
- As in other examples of AIS, p16 will be diffusely positive, but this finding does not help differentiate the lesion from invasive adenocarcinoma.

MAIN DIFFERENTIAL DIAGNOSIS

- Early invasive endocervical adenocarcinoma—this lesion also may have an expansile growth pattern, but the conformation of the glands is more irregular (un-cryptlike) and some stromal response is usually present.

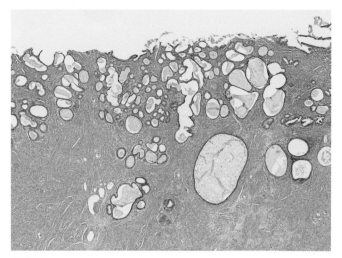

FIGURE 1

Extensive AIS. This field is not particularly difficult. Despite the relatively deep glands, the architecture is uniform.

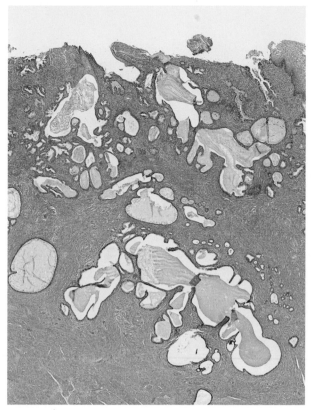

FIGURE 2

Extensive AIS. These glands (crypts) extend much more deeply into the cervical stroma. Note the lobular contour.

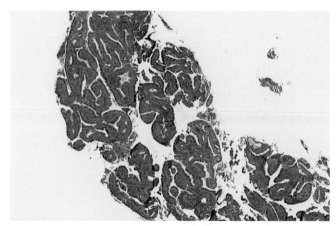

FIGURE 3

Extensive AIS in curettings. The glands interdigitate with nondesmoplastic stroma. This could be either an exophytic component of AIS or part of a villoglandular adenocarcinoma. Importantly the diagnosis of invasive adenocarcinoma should not be made based on this pattern in the curetting alone. If uncertain, the pathologist should recommend a cone biopsy.

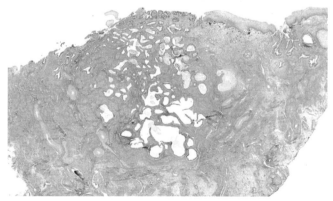

FIGURE 4

A particularly deep AIS with lobular contour. The distinction from invasive carcinoma becomes particularly difficult. Nonetheless, in the absence of stromal response the risk of lymph node metastases is considered extremely low.

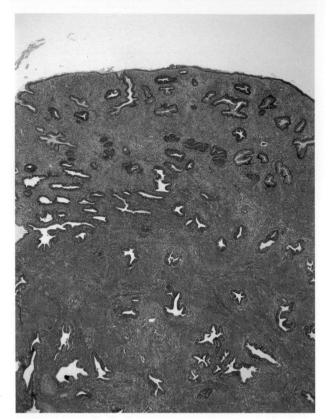

FIGURE 5

Invasive well-differentiated adenocarcinoma. Note the more widely distributed single neoplastic glands and the absence of a more lobulated contour as seen in Figures 1, 2, and 4.

INFILTRATIVE ENDOCERVICAL ADENOCARCINOMA

DEFINITION—Invasive adenocarcinoma originating in the endocervix.

CLINICAL FEATURES

EPIDEMIOLOGY

- Average age at diagnosis is early 40s.
- Human papillomavirus (HPV) associated.
- A positive association with oral contraceptive use has been noted, but the mechanism is not understood.
- Not associated with tobacco use.

PRESENTATION

- Abnormal Pap smear, although this is an unusual presentation.
- Vaginal bleeding or a sensation of pelvic pressure and/or pain.
- Rarely abnormal pelvic exam with a visible cervical mass or a "barrel" cervix.

PROGNOSIS AND TREATMENT

- Treatment typically includes hysterectomy and pelvic lymph node dissection for early-stage tumors, with adjuvant chemotherapy and/or radiation therapy if there are high-risk factors on the final pathology. Patients with stage IIB or above tumors are treated with concurrent chemotherapy and radiation therapy, often followed by extra fascial hysterectomy.
- Traditionally thought to have worse prognosis than squamous cell carcinoma of the cervix, but outcomes are similar when adjusted for tumor size. However, patients with an adenocarcinoma with nodal metastases definitely have a worse prognosis.
- Ovarian metastases occur in 5% of patients.
- A wide variety of histologic variants have been described, but their presence does not affect prognosis. Carcinomas with a serous pattern of cytology and growth must be viewed carefully as they could signify "drop metastases" from a uterine or upper genital tract carcinoma.

PATHOLOGY

HISTOLOGY

- Invasive endocervical adenocarcinomas are those with invasive foci greater than 7 mm in the greatest linear dimension, and/or invasion more than 5 mm into the cervical stroma.
- If the invasion is less than this, the lesion is termed "early endocervical adenocarcinoma."
- Usual endocervical adenocarcinoma is often associated with residual adenocarcinoma in situ (AIS) and resembles benign endocervical glands.
- The tumor cells are usually columnar and can be mucinous, eosinophilic, or a combination of both; a number of histologic variants exist and are described separately.
- The low-power architecture and pattern of invasion are variable.
- Infiltrative invasion is characterized by individual cells and irregularly shaped glands permeating through the cervical stroma.
- Expansile invasion is notable for its large, smooth-contoured nests of cells resembling AIS. These nests extend more deeply into the cervical stroma than do normal background glands.
- Exophytic invasion is characterized by tumor growth into the endocervical canal; the bulk of tumor is present as polypoid mass.
- On cytologic examination variable numbers of hyperchromatic cellular groups can be identified. The groups may show architectural disarray and loss of the normal honeycomb pattern seen in normal endocervical cells.
- The presence of large groups and papillary clusters in a cytologic preparation suggests an invasive process over AIS.
- When compared with cells representing AIS, invasive cells are frequently larger. The cytoplasm may display vacuoles and be pale to eosinophilic. Mitoses may be

identified, and the nuclear chromatin may be vesicular to coarse and darkly stained.

IMMUNOPATHOLOGY (INCLUDING IMMUNOHISTOCHEMISTRY)

- Positive for Keratin 7 and p16 (in most cases).

- Early invasive endocervical adenocarcinoma.
- Florid benign microglandular change.

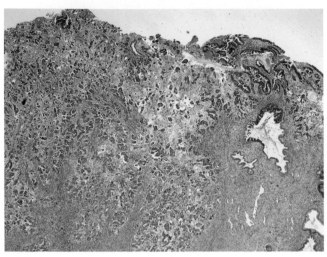

FIGURE 1

Endocervical adenocarcinoma. At low power the endocervix is partially effaced by a malignant appearing proliferation of cells. Residual AIS is noted on the right side of the image, suggesting that this represents an invasive endocervical adenocarcinoma (even at low power).

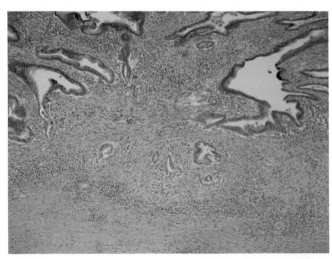

FIGURE 3

Endocervical adenocarcinoma. At low power an expansile proliferation of hyperchromatic glands is present in the endocervix. The overall growth pattern could be consistent with expansile invasion, but areas of stromal reaction and desmoplasia toward the edges suggest that classical infiltrative invasion is also present.

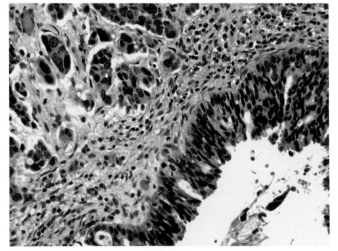

FIGURE 2

Endocervical adenocarcinoma. At high power the invasive adenocarcinoma on the left is sharply contrasted with AIS on the right. The cells of invasive carcinoma are noticeably larger, atypical, and pleomorphic.

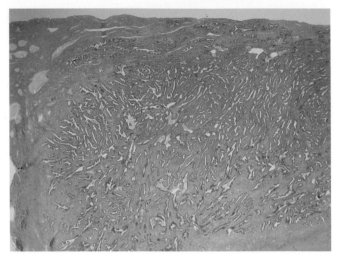

FIGURE 4

Endocervical adenocarcinoma. At low power, hyperchromatic glands involved by AIS are present in the top portion of the image. Small, irregularly shaped infiltrative invasive glands are present in the lower center, accompanied by inflammation and a stromal response.

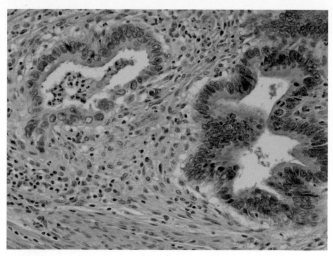

FIGURE 5

Endocervical adenocarcinoma. An invasive gland of endocervical adenocarcinoma is on the left, compared with AIS on the right side of the image. The invasive gland has more brightly eosinophilic cytoplasm and no longer has stratified nuclei. Inflammation and stromal changes suggestive of a desmoplastic response are present.

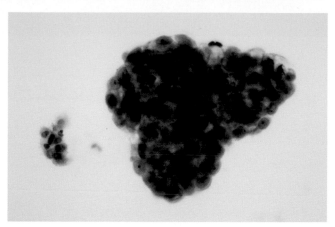

FIGURE 6

Endocervical adenocarcinoma in a Pap smear. A large cluster of hyperchromatic cells with enlarged nuclei and prominent nucleoli. A cluster of benign cells is seen on the left.

CLEAR-CELL CARCINOMA OF THE CERVIX

DEFINITION—A unique, typically HPV-negative adenocarcinoma that has been associated with prenatal diethylstilbestrol exposure.

CLINICAL FEATURES

EPIDEMIOLOGY

- Rare.
- Historically linked to diethylstilbestrol (DES) exposure in utero.
- Sporadic occurrences now much more frequent than DES-related cases.
- Wide age range, with a mean age of 45 to 50 years, but case reports include occurrences in children and adolescents.

PRESENTATION

- Abnormal Pap smear.
- Cervical abnormality on physical exam, often described as a "fullness" of the cervix.
- Vaginal bleeding due to cervical ulceration.

PROGNOSIS AND TREATMENT

- Standard treatment includes total abdominal hysterectomy and pelvic lymph node dissection.
- Adjuvant chemotherapy and/or radiation therapy for patients with high-risk features.
- Studies regarding prognosis are conflicting; some report equivalent outcomes with conventional cervical adenocarcinoma, whereas others report a much more aggressive disease course.

PATHOLOGY

HISTOLOGY

- Cervical clear-cell carcinoma has a similar histologic appearance to clear-cell carcinomas found elsewhere in the gynecologic tract.

- The low-power appearance is characterized by a predominantly endophytic growth pattern involving the deep cervical stroma.
- Tumor cells may be arranged in glands, papillae, solid sheets, or a tubulocystic pattern; often more than one pattern can be identified.
- At higher power, lining cells protrude into the lumina and spaces in a characteristic "hobnail" fashion.
- Pink hyaline stromal cores are characteristic when a papillary growth pattern is present.
- Tumor cells classically have a clear, glycogen-rich cytoplasm, but not infrequently the cytoplasm may appear more eosinophilic.

IMMUNOPATHOLOGY (INCLUDING IMMUNOHISTOCHEMISTRY)

- Noncontributory.

MAIN DIFFERENTIAL DIAGNOSIS

- Benign microglandular hyperplasia, particularly solid forms, can mimic a clear-cell carcinoma. The presence of reserve cells is often helpful, but the key is to carefully scrutinize the level of atypia and the architecture. Above all, a diagnosis of clear-cell carcinoma in a discrete microacinar proliferation in the cervix in a young woman should be made with great caution.
- Other tumors can present with clear cytoplasm, including metastatic renal cell carcinoma, yolk sac tumors, and clear-cell adenosquamous carcinoma. However, the classic tubulocystic and papillary architecture of clear-cell carcinoma combined with the presentation should exclude these other entities.

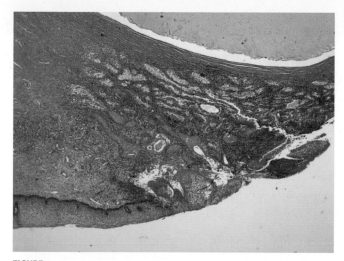

FIGURE 1

Cervical clear-cell carcinoma. This lesion is near the squamocolumnar junction.

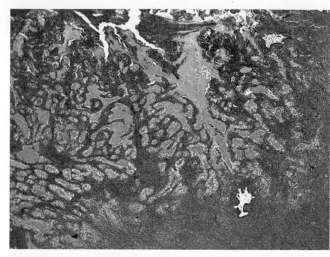

FIGURE 2

Cervical clear-cell carcinoma. An expansile, mostly exophytic lesion.

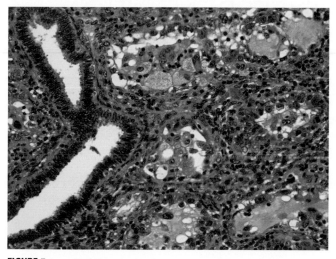

FIGURE 3

Cervical clear-cell carcinoma. Note the juxtaposition of the neoplastic epithelium and a focus of tubuloendometrial metaplasia.

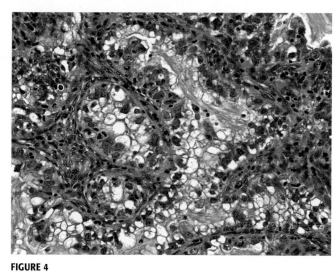

FIGURE 4

Clear-cell carcinoma. Tubulocystic glands are lined by cuboidal cells with enlarged nuclei and focally prominent nucleoli.

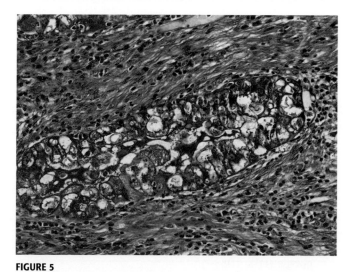

FIGURE 5

Clear-cell carcinoma. There is abundant periodic acid–Schiff (PAS)–positive, diastase-sensitive material (glycogen).

ATYPICAL LOBULAR ENDOCERVICAL GLANDULAR HYPERPLASIA AND INVASIVE (MINIMAL DEVIATION) ADENOCARCINOMA OF THE CERVIX WITH GASTRIC DIFFERENTIATION

DEFINITION—A deceptively bland-appearing mucinous adenocarcinoma of the cervix. Atypical lobular endocervical glandular hyperplasia (ALGH) is considered a potential precursor to minimal deviation adenocarcinoma (MDA).

CLINICAL FEATURES

EPIDEMIOLOGY

- Uncommon.
- *Not* associated with human papillomavirus (HPV).
- Reproductive-age women; mean age at diagnosis is 42 years.
- Associated with Peutz-Jeghers syndrome (10% to 15% of cases).

PRESENTATION

- Vaginal bleeding and/or discharge.
- Firm, indurated cervix (barrel cervix).
- Some cases are associated with ovarian mucinous carcinomas (both primary and metastatic).

PROGNOSIS AND TREATMENT

- Possibly because of false-negative biopsies, this entity is often diagnosed at high stage.
- Worse prognosis than usual-type adenocarcinoma, with a reported overall survival rate of less than 30% based on the literature.
- Treatment includes resection, chemotherapy, and radiation.

PATHOLOGY

HISTOLOGY

MINIMAL DEVIATION ADENOCARCINOMA
- The low-power histology is characterized by irregularly shaped endocervical glands invading deeply into the cervical stroma.
- Glands typically extend into the outer third of the cervical wall and can be seen adjacent to large vessels.
- A loss of the overall lobular architecture of the cervical glands is notable.
- At least some invasive glands are associated with a desmoplastic stromal response.
- Nuclear atypia should be found at least focally, although in some cases this can be remarkably subtle.
- Produces neutral mucins and gastric mucous cell phenotype (HIK 1083+).
- In small biopsies look for association with large vessels, variation in gland size and shape, particularly small

glands that appear deeply situated. This tumor can be missed in limited samples (PITFALL).

ATYPICAL LOBULAR ENDOCERVICAL GLANDULAR HYPERPLASIA

- Often associated with MDA.
- Nuclear enlargement, irregular nuclear contour, nucleoli, mitoses, apoptosis, epithelial infolding with papillary projections.

IMMUNOPATHOLOGY (INCLUDING IMMUNOHISTOCHEMISTRY)

- Generally noncontributory, but PAX2 may be negative.
- Positive for gastric markers HIK1083 and MUC6.

MAIN DIFFERENTIAL DIAGNOSIS

- Benign endocervical hyperplasia—both laminar and lobular hyperplasias may exhibit deep or irregular glands, but the lining of both is usually uniform and the variation from gland to gland is much less than that seen in minimal deviation adenocarcinomas.
- Endocervical adenomyoma.
- Usual mucinous endocervical adenocarcinoma.

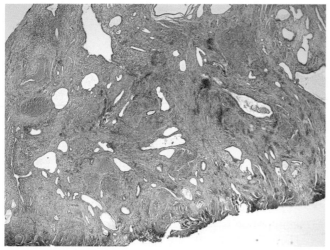

FIGURE 1

Minimal deviation adenocarcinoma. Low-power image of cervix showing a proliferation of bland-appearing but somewhat irregularly shaped glands extending deep into the cervical stroma. A desmoplastic stromal response is not seen here. There is a loss of the normal lobular configuration of endocervical glands, with some single, elongated glands present.

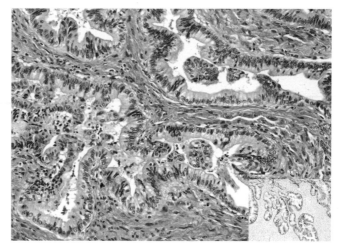

FIGURE 3

ALGH. Note the epithelial infolding with some atypia. Strong MUC6 staining *(inset)* is present.

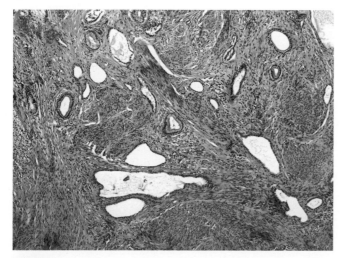

FIGURE 2

At higher magnification an irregular arrangement of otherwise bland-appearing glands can be seen.

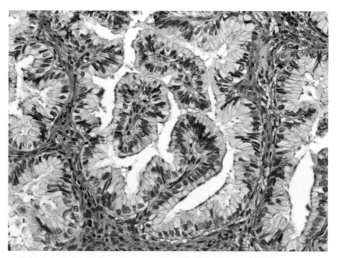

FIGURE 4

Another focus of LEGH with some mild nuclear hyperchromasia.

"SEROUS" CARCINOMA OF THE CERVIX

DEFINITION—A carcinoma resembling an upper genital tract serous carcinoma but originating in the cervix and usually human papillomavirus (HPV) related.

CLINICAL FEATURES

EPIDEMIOLOGY

- Rare.
- There is a distinctly bimodal age distribution; most patients are under age 45, but there is a second smaller peak after age 65.
- As a rule of thumb, for cases in older women a metastasis from the endometrium, tube, or ovary should be excluded.

PRESENTATION

- Abnormal vaginal bleeding or discharge.
- Abnormal Pap smear.
- Physical exam is highly variable; most cases reveal an exophytic polypoid mass, although often no abnormality is identified.

PROGNOSIS AND TREATMENT

- Primary cervical cancers treated as any adenocarcinoma.
- Cases in older women should be worked up to exclude a metastasis.
- In general, treatment includes radical hysterectomy with pelvic lymphadenectomy and/or chemotherapy and radiation therapy.
- Early (stage I) tumors have a prognosis similar to that of usual endocervical adenocarcinoma.
- Later stage (II or III) tumors tend to be rapidly fatal and have a very low 5-year survival rate.

PATHOLOGY

HISTOLOGY

- Histologic features in cervical serous carcinoma are similar to serous carcinomas of the endometrium and pelvis.
- At low power the tumor has a complex papillary and branching architecture, with characteristic cracks and crevices (a fjordlike appearance); a solid growth pattern may be apparent in deeper areas.
- At high power, complex epithelial budding with nuclear stratification is seen.
- The individual cells are markedly atypical and have high nuclear-to-cytoplasmic ratios, prominent nucleoli, and frequent mitotic figures.
- This histologic pattern (serous adenocarcinoma) may also be associated with areas of more typical, well-differentiated adenocarcinoma, which solidifies the cervical origin but does not affect prognosis.

IMMUNOPATHOLOGY (INCLUDING IMMUNOHISTOCHEMISTRY)

- Primary carcinomas are usually p53 negative (heterogenous staining as opposed to very strong or completely absent staining), but not all are. Strong p16 staining will be seen in both primary and metastatic serous carcinomas.
- Usually positive in situ hybridization for HPV.

DIAGNOSTIC TERMINOLOGY: Poorly differentiated adenocarcinoma with a caveat if a metastatic serous carcinoma is suspected. In a young woman an unqualified diagnosis of "serous carcinoma" in the cervix should not be made as it might confuse the clinician. If the term is introduced, it should be emphasized that this is a variant of cervical adenocarcinoma and should be treated as such.

MAIN DIFFERENTIAL DIAGNOSIS

• Metastatic uterine or pelvic serous carcinoma.

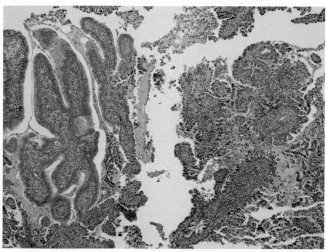

FIGURE 1

Cervical adenocarcinoma with serous histology. Lower-power image showing a villoglandular carcinoma on the left merging with a serous component on the right.

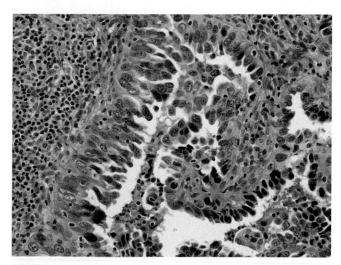

FIGURE 3

Cervical adenocarcinoma with serous histology. The serous component.

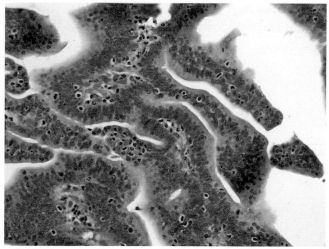

FIGURE 2

Cervical adenocarcinoma with serous histology. The conventional villoglandular component.

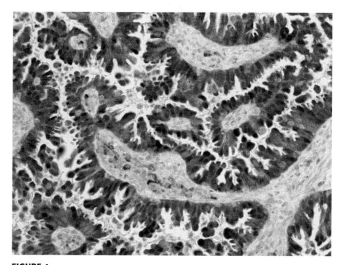

FIGURE 4

Strong p16 staining in the tumor.

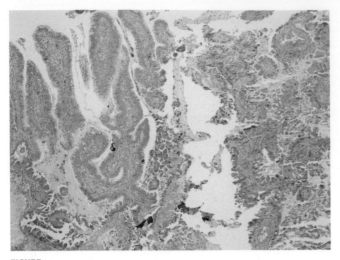

FIGURE 5

p53 staining is weak or heterogenous. However, some of these primary tumors may contain p53 mutations.

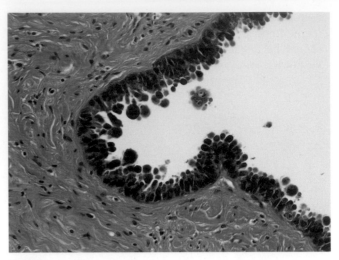

FIGURE 6

Metastatic serous carcinoma to the cervix in an older woman. The tumor occupies crypts and may not invade stroma.

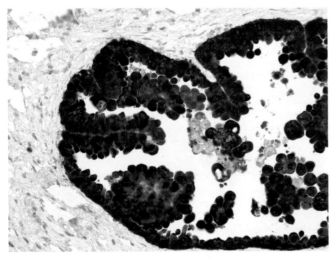

FIGURE 7

Strong p16 staining in a metastatic serous carcinoma to the cervix. This stain will not discriminate primary from metastatic.

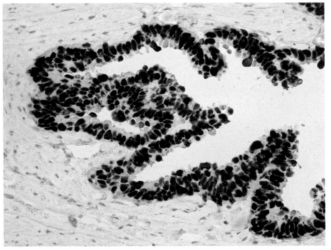

FIGURE 8

Strong p53 staining in a metastatic serous carcinoma to the cervix. Older age and strong p53 staining support a metastatic tumor from the endometrium or upper genital tract.

SIGNET-RING CELL CARCINOMA OF THE CERVIX

DEFINITION—A *rare* variant of invasive adenocarcinoma originating in the endocervix.

CLINICAL FEATURES

EPIDEMIOLOGY

- Limited to case reports.
- Wide age range, but most present in the fourth or fifth decade.
- Human papillomavirus (HPV) associated.
- May be found with other adenocarcinomas such as usual type of adenocarcinoma or neuroendocrine carcinoma (rare cases).

PRESENTATION

- Vaginal bleeding is the most common presenting symptom.
- Occasional cases present with an abnormal Papanicolaou smear.
- Polypoid cervical mass in some.

PROGNOSIS AND TREATMENT

- Treatment typically includes hysterectomy and pelvic lymph node dissection.
- Advanced stage tumors are treated with concurrent chemotherapy and radiation therapy.
- Outcome is similar to other adenocarcinomas and stage dependent.
- Ovarian metastases reported in case reports.

PATHOLOGY

HISTOLOGY

- Typically these tumors will have components that closely resemble the usual types of cervical adenocarcinoma.

- Signet-ring cell differentiation will be present in clusters of typical cells with eccentric nuclei.
- Strong mucicarmine positivity in the signet-ring cells.

IMMUNOPATHOLOGY (INCLUDING IMMUNOHISTOCHEMISTRY)

- Strong Keratin 7 and p16 positivity.
- Variable CDX2 and CEA.
- Negative or weak GCDFP and CK20.

MAIN DIFFERENTIAL DIAGNOSIS

- Metastatic breast carcinoma—a conventional endocervical adenocarcinoma will not be seen. GCDFP may help, but history is important if there is no accompanying endocervical carcinoma.
- Florid benign microglandular change—this could conceivably be confused with a signet-ring cell carcinoma.
- Metastatic gastric carcinoma—this could be impossible to separate on histology alone and would require attention to coexisting conventional adenocarcinoma, and stains for p16.

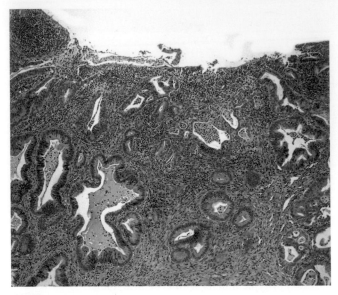

FIGURE 1

Signet-ring cell cervical carcinoma. At low power the dominant pattern is that of a conventional adenocarcinoma of the cervix.

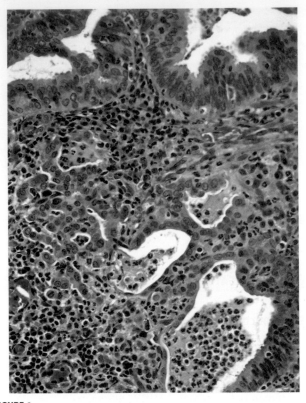

FIGURE 2

Signet-ring cell cervical carcinoma. In this field the glandular pattern *(above)* blends with disaggregated neoplastic epithelium below from which the signet-ring cell pattern will emerge *(below)*.

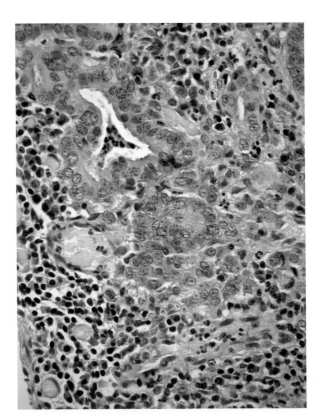

FIGURE 4

Signet-ring cell cervical carcinoma. In another field there is a confluent structureless population of cells forming a pavement with focal mucin droplets.

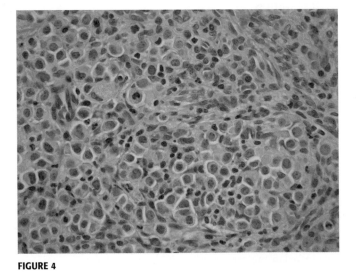

FIGURE 3

Signet-ring cell cervical carcinoma. Mucicarmine staining of the field in Figure 2 reveals positive mucin staining in a few cells in the lower field.

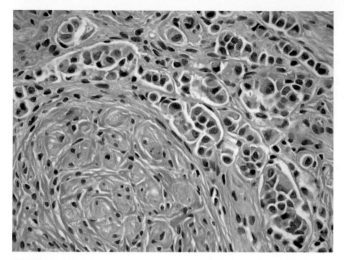

FIGURE 5

Signet-ring cell cervical carcinoma. Classic signet-ring cell differentiation.

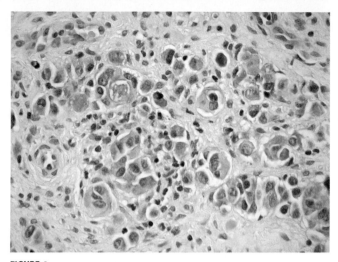

FIGURE 6

Signet-ring cell cervical carcinoma. Strong mucicarmine positivity.

ADENOID BASAL CARCINOMA

DEFINITION—Adenocarcinoma composed of basaloid cells with areas of columnar cell differentiation.

CLINICAL FEATURES

EPIDEMIOLOGY

- Rare; accounts for less than 5% of cervical carcinomas.
- Usually seen in postmenopausal women.
- Human papillomavirus (HPV) associated.
- African-American women are affected more than other ethnicities.

PRESENTATION

- Most often an incidental finding associated with a high-grade squamous in situ lesion.
- Rarely presents as an abnormal Pap smear.

PROGNOSIS AND TREATMENT

- Excellent when present as a pure adenoid basal carcinoma (ABC) lesion.
- Atypia in the basaloid cells does not alter outcome.
- No recurrences or metastases have been reported in tumors without additional components.

PATHOLOGY

HISTOLOGY

- This lesion is nearly always underlying a typical high-grade squamous in situ lesion.
- Three additional patterns, or components, can be present within the cervical stroma:
  1. Discrete nests of squamoid cells with variable nuclear atypia and pleomorphism, low nuclear-to-cytoplasmic ratio, and a prominent peripheral rim of basal cells.
  2. Small, discrete well-demarcated infiltrating nests composed of basaloid cells with focal cystic change.
  3. Foci of columnar differentiation within small, infiltrating basaloid nests.
- A desmoplastic reaction is notably absent.
- The basaloid cells will vary in degree of atypia. Often they appear monotonous, with only mild nuclear atypia, but in some cases a higher mitotic index with nuclear pleomorphism will be seen. The squamous components often have much more prominent nuclear atypia.
- The ABC pattern may sometimes be focally present as a component of a poorly differentiated carcinoma and adequate sampling should be performed to exclude this possibility.
- In particular, an ABC pattern may be seen associated with patterns suggesting basaloid squamous cell carcinoma, carcinosarcoma, or adenoid cystic carcinoma.

PREFERRED DIAGNOSTIC TERM

Adenoid basal carcinoma

Comment (optional): ABC is a rare variant of squamous carcinoma, which is associated with HPV 16 and in its pure form has a favorable outcome without nodal metastases.

IMMUNOPATHOLOGY (INCLUDING IMMUNOHISTOCHEMISTRY)

- Most cases are positive for high-risk HPV, particularly HPV 16.
- p16 immunostaining should be strong.
- Cam 5.2 is positive.

MAIN DIFFERENTIAL DIAGNOSIS

- Adenoid cystic carcinoma—these tumors (if they really exist in the cervix) have additional components including a high-grade gland-forming component.
- Squamous cell carcinoma—these tumors lack the multifaceted picture of ABC.
- Carcinosarcoma—in the cervix rarely can be associated with ABC, but have a prominent spindle cell component.

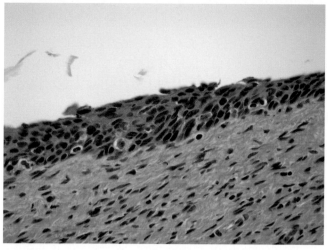

FIGURE 1

ABC. A focus of cervical intraepithelial neoplasia 3 (CIN3) on the surface of the cervix.

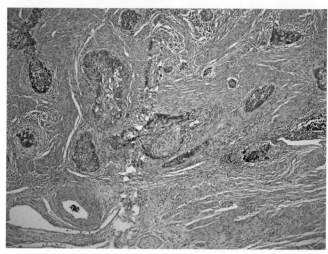

FIGURE 2

A squamoid pattern of infiltration with a combination of squamous differentiation in the center of the invading nest and peripheral basal cells.

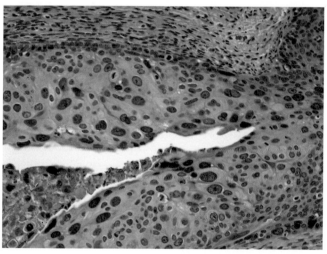

FIGURE 3

Higher magnification showing central squamous differentiation with atypia and a linear row of basal cells at the epithelial-stromal interface *(top)*.

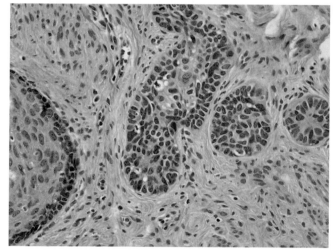

FIGURE 4

A squamous nest *(left)* and small basaloid nests *(right)*.

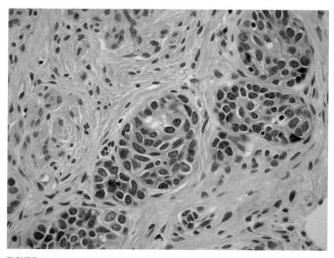

FIGURE 5

These basaloid nests display a hint of columnar differentiation.

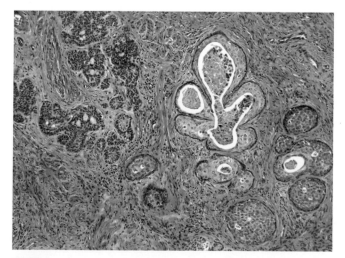

FIGURE 6

Squamoid nests *(right)* and basaloid nests *(left)* of tumor. The latter also shows acinar (adenoid) differentiation.

MESONEPHRIC REMNANTS

DEFINITION—Embryologic remnants of mesonephric differentiation found in the gynecologic tract.

CLINICAL FEATURES

EPIDEMIOLOGY

- Mesonephric remnants may be identified in up to one fifth of well-sampled cervices.
- No age or demographic predilection has been identified.

PRESENTATION

- Noted incidentally at the time of cervical sampling.

PROGNOSIS AND TREATMENT

- Excellent; no treatment is required.

PATHOLOGY

HISTOLOGY

- Mesonephric remnants are small glandular structures that are typically found in the lateral cervical walls.
- The lining cells are small and cuboidal and lack cilia.
- A dense, eosinophilic intraluminal material is commonly present.

- Multiple clusters of glands may be seen in which case the diagnosis of mesonephric hyperplasia is justified (see differential diagnosis).

IMMUNOPATHOLOGY (INCLUDING IMMUNOHISTOCHEMISTRY)

- PAX2 is strongly positive in mesonephric remnants and mesonephric hyperplasia.

MAIN DIFFERENTIAL DIAGNOSIS

- Endocervical adenocarcinoma—this is not usually a difficult distinction.
- Metastatic endometrial carcinoma—this may closely mimic mesonephric remnants when present in a format of tubular glands. The lining epithelium should demonstrate atypia, albeit subtle, and the distribution will be more haphazard than mesonephric remnants. Moreover, the gland outlines are typically more variable and not exclusively tubular.
- Mesonephric "hyperplasia" versus carcinoma—if the remnants are extensive, the term mesonephric hyperplasia might be entertained, but does not increase the risk of an adverse outcome. However, a careful search for a transition to confluent glands or more striking atypia should be made, and these changes would indicate a coexisting carcinoma.

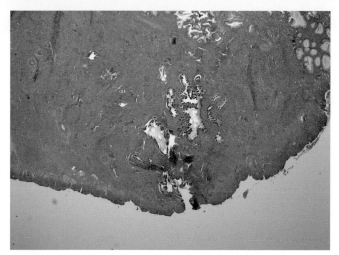

FIGURE 1

Mesonephric remnants in the cervix. Low power reveals the presence of additional glandular structures deep to the usual endocervical glands.

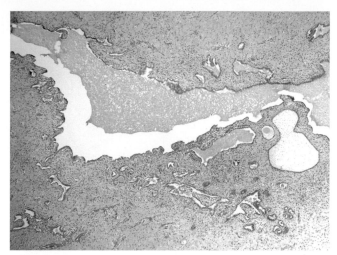

FIGURE 2

Mesonephric remnants in the cervix. In this example small glands appear to emanate from a dilated duct.

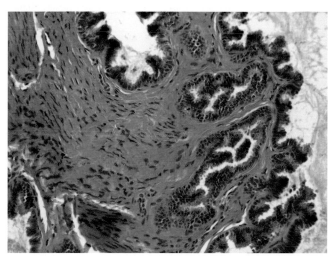

FIGURE 3

Mesonephric remnants in the cervix. At high power the cells comprising the remnants are relatively small and cuboidal. Cilia are not seen. Nuclear atypia is absent. Areas of eosinophilic intraluminal secretions are present.

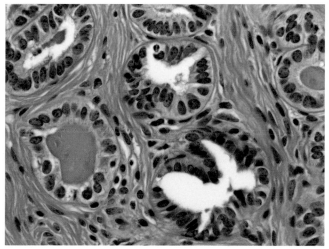

FIGURE 4

Mesonephric remnants of the cervix. Note the intraluminal eosinophilic material.

MESONEPHRIC CARCINOMA

DEFINITION—A carcinoma derived from mesonephric remnants located in the lateral walls of the uterine cervix.

CLINICAL FEATURES

EPIDEMIOLOGY

- Very rare.
- The mean age at presentation is early 50s.

PRESENTATION

- Abnormal vaginal bleeding.
- Barrel-shaped cervix or a symptomatic cervical mass.

PROGNOSIS AND TREATMENT

- Prognosis is uncertain due to the rarity of this tumor; some reports suggest that it may be an indolent tumor with potential for late recurrence.

PATHOLOGY

HISTOLOGY

- On gross examination, if a discrete mass is present, it is located at the lateral cervical wall.
- The histologic patterns are remarkably variable and may resemble a wide variety of other tumors including carcinomas, malignant mixed müllerian tumor (MMMT), and uterine tumors resembling an ovarian sex cord tumor (UTROSCT).
- Although rare, the histologic patterns seen in this tumor have been well documented and a wide variety of patterns have been described, including tubular, ductal, retiform, and solid.
- Glandlike spaces and intraluminal eosinophilic hyaline secretions are present in all of the histologic patterns.

- The tumor cells are mild to moderately pleomorphic and hyperchromatic, with variably prominent nucleoli.
- The architectural pattern may be solid, with only occasional glandlike spaces, or may be composed of round, variously sized ductlike spaces lined by columnar cells.
- The so-called tubular pattern is identified by the presence of innumerable small, tightly packed gland structures that are lined by flattened to cuboidal epithelial cells; the retiform pattern is similar except that the glandlike spaces are narrow and slitlike.
- Intraluminal papillary projections can be seen in any of the patterns.
- Sex cord–like tumors are composed of cells with minimal amounts of cytoplasm and are arranged in single-file lines of cells.
- The mitotic count is highly variable and can be markedly elevated.
- Occasional heterologous elements, such as cartilage, have been noted.

IMMUNOPATHOLOGY (INCLUDING IMMUNOHISTOCHEMISTRY)

- Positive for Keratin 7, EMA, calretinin, and GATA3.
- Negative for Keratin 20, ER, PR, and WT1.

MAIN DIFFERENTIAL DIAGNOSIS

- Florid mesonephric hyperplasia—this distinction is a matter of degree.
- Metastatic endometrioid adenocarcinoma—this neoplasm can involve the cervix in a unique and subtle pattern in which the glands are uniform, deeply situated, and cytologically bland, resembling mesonephric remnants or mesonephric hyperplasia.

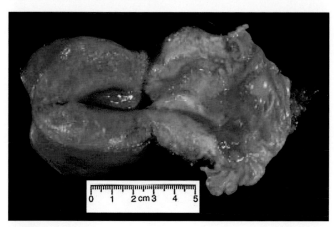

FIGURE 1

Mesonephric carcinoma. In this gross photograph the opened cervix *(right)* is diffusely expanded, with a narrowing at the endocervical-uterine junction. This explains the reported cases of "failure to progress" during labor, as occurred in the patient prior to diagnosis.

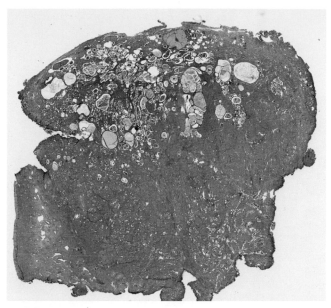

FIGURE 2

Mesonephric carcinoma associated with mesonephric hyperplasia. A classic scanning power appearance of this tumor, with mesonephric remnants in the lower half of the image becoming more cystic and crowded as they approach the lumen.

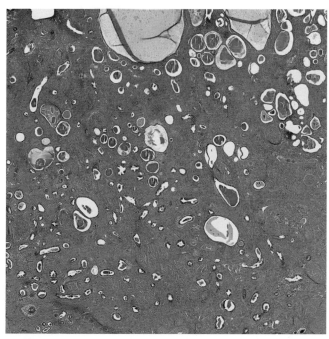

FIGURE 3

Mesonephric hyperplasia. This part of the tumor is identical to mesonephric hyperplasia.

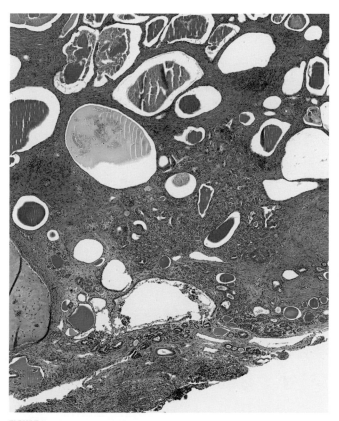

FIGURE 4

Near the endocervical canal the tumor transforms, with a malignant appearing cluster of neoplastic glands. These glands can resemble sex cords or endometrioid carcinoma.

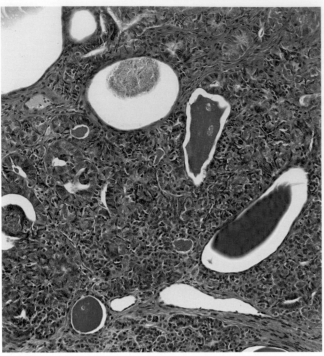

FIGURE 5

Higher magnification of the malignant appearing cluster of neoplastic glands. These glands can resemble sex cords or endometrioid carcinoma.

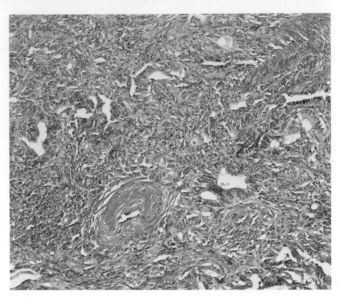

FIGURE 6

Focal spindle cell differentiation in a mesonephric carcinoma. This can be confused with carcinosarcoma or Wilms' tumor of the uterus.

PROSTATIC METAPLASIA OF THE CERVIX

DEFINITION—The histologic appearance of large prostatic duct–like tissue within the cervical stroma.

CLINICAL FEATURES

EPIDEMIOLOGY

- Prostatic metaplasia is a rare (or possibly under-reported) process.
- There is no age predilection.

PRESENTATION

- Prostatic metaplasia is an incidental finding at the time of cervical biopsy or hysterectomy.
- There are no gross findings.

PROGNOSIS AND TREATMENT

- The prognosis is excellent as this process is not associated with neoplasia.
- No treatment is required.

PATHOLOGY

HISTOLOGY

- Microscopically, prostatic metaplasia consists of glands with the appearance of large prostatic ducts set within cervical stroma.
- The nests of glands are well circumscribed and have an identifiable population of reserve cells at the periphery.
- The cells composing the glands consist of cuboidal to columnar mucinous cells with small, bland, uniform nuclei.

- Squamous metaplasia is common.
- The squamous cells within the center are also bland, but these cells typically have clear cytoplasm.

IMMUNOPATHOLOGY (INCLUDING IMMUNOHISTOCHEMISTRY)

- Prostate-specific antigen (PSA) and prostate-specific acid phosphatase (PSAP) are positive in the areas of metaplasia.
- p16ink4 staining will be weak or negative, distinguishing this from either adenoid basal carcinoma (ABC) or adenosquamous carcinoma in situ.

DIAGNOSTIC TERMINOLOGY

- Prostatic metaplasia (benign).

MAIN DIFFERENTIAL DIAGNOSIS

- Adenoid basal carcinomas (ABCs) share with prostatic metaplasia a mixture of immature squamous cells and columnar differentiation as well as an impression of an accentuated perimeter cell layer. However, the situation of the columnar cell acini within the squamous nests or just inside (rather than outside of) the basal layer of squamous is unique to prostatic metaplasia. They are negative or weakly positive for p16ink4 in contrast to ABCs.
- Adenosquamous carcinomas in situ exhibit conspicuous atypia plus strong staining for p16ink4.

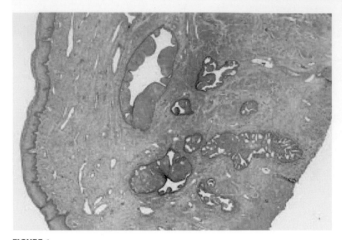

FIGURE 1

Cervical prostatic metaplasia. This focus is rather deeply situated.

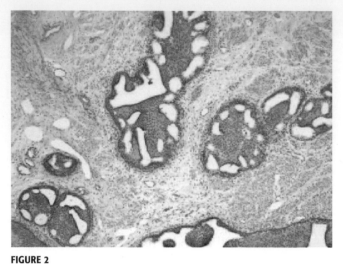

FIGURE 2

Cervical prostatic metaplasia. On higher power, well circumscribed nests squamous epithelium with glandular elements are present within stroma. Note the resemblance to morular metaplasia, where a collar of incomplete acinar architecture merges with central squamous differentiation.

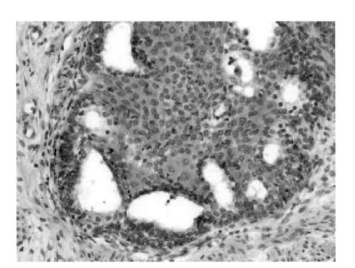

FIGURE 3

At higher magnification, showing the juxtaposition of small columnar acini and bland squamous epithelium.

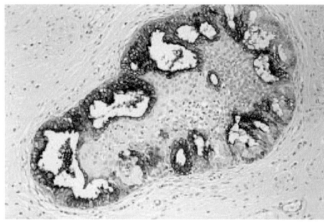

FIGURE 4

Cervical prostatic metaplasia immunostained for prostatic acid phosphatase. Such strong staining is confirmatory, but this biomarker will not always be positive.

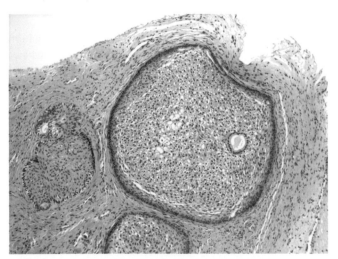

FIGURE 5

Intrasquamous columnar cell acini at low and higher magnifications. This pattern is virtually pathognomonic of prostatic metaplasia.

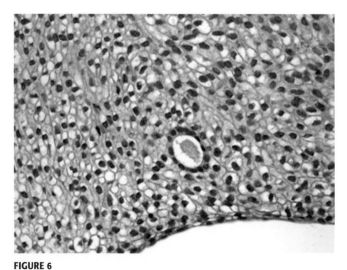

FIGURE 6

Higher magnification of an intrasquamous acinar structure.

ENDOCERVICAL GLANDULAR HYPERPLASIA

DEFINITION—An increase in the number of endocervical glands. May be idiopathic or secondary to increased hormonal stimulation. Some atypical hyperplasias may be associated with minimal deviation adenocarcinomas and Peutz-Jeghers syndrome (see page 300).

CLINICAL FEATURES

EPIDEMIOLOGY

- Usually seen in reproductive-age women as an incidental finding.

PRESENTATION

- Most patients are asymptomatic and have non–mass-forming lesions.
- One third of patients present with a mass-forming lesion, either with or without clinical symptoms (e.g., pain, bleeding).
- Endocervical glandular hyperplasia, when severe, may be clinically mistaken for a malignant process.

PROGNOSIS AND TREATMENT

- The prognosis is excellent as this is a benign lesion.
- No treatment is typically undertaken, except in cases requiring symptomatic relief.

PATHOLOGY

HISTOLOGY

- **Lobular glandular hyperplasia**
  - An increase in small- to medium-sized glands that maintain a lobular profile.
  - Often, a centrally located, large gland can been identified at low power.
  - The glandular proliferation is usually limited to the inner half of the cervical wall and is sharply demarcated from the cervical stroma.
  - The epithelial cells lining the glands are columnar mucinous cells that have a pyloric gland phenotype.
- **Diffuse laminar glandular hyperplasia**
  - A proliferation of glands similar to the lobular type; however, the glands extend to the same depth within the cervical stroma.
  - The hyperplastic glands involve the entire circumference of the cervix.
  - There is an unusually sharp interface between the glands and the stroma.
  - The glands maintain a round or tubular profile with occasional branching.
  - Inflammation may be present and is typically more prominent in the deeper aspect.
  - Nuclear atypia should be minimal to absent.

IMMUNOPATHOLOGY (INCLUDING IMMUNOHISTOCHEMISTRY)

- p16 is negative. Lobular endocervical hyperplasia may stain for gastric mucins (MUC6) but staining is normally not necessary.

MAIN DIFFERENTIAL DIAGNOSIS

- Endocervical adenocarcinoma.
  - Minimal deviation endocervical adenocarcinoma (adenoma malignum; see page 300).
  - Atypical lobular endocervical glandular hyperplasia (see page 300).

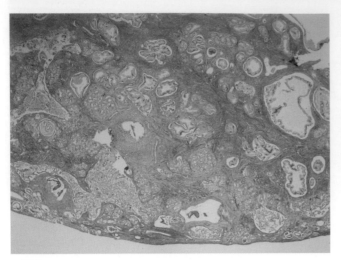

FIGURE 1

Endocervical glandular hyperplasia. Diffuse laminar hyperplasia involving the entire circumference and depth of the cervical stroma. The groups of glands maintain an overall lobular architecture.

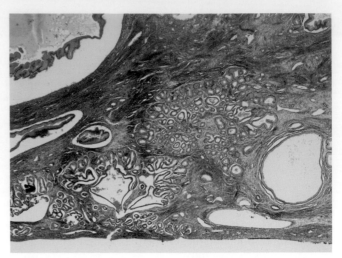

FIGURE 2

Endocervical glandular hyperplasia. The glands are in lobular groups and are tubular with only rare branching glands. A central, larger gland can be seen in some of the groups.

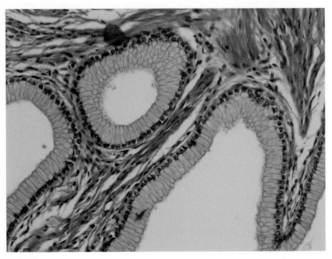

FIGURE 3

Endocervical glandular hyperplasia. At higher power the pyloric (gastric) phenotype of the glands can be seen. Note the lack of nuclear atypia and mitotic activity.

METASTATIC SEROUS CARCINOMA TO THE CERVIX

DEFINITION—Serous carcinoma originating from the upper genital tract involving the cervix (drop metastasis).

CLINICAL FEATURES

EPIDEMIOLOGY

- Uncommon.
- Women in their 60s to 70s.

PRESENTATION

- Abnormal vaginal bleeding.
- May be present as a clinically identifiable mass or abnormal cervix.
- May be clinically occult and identified only on endocervical brushings.

PROGNOSIS AND TREATMENT

- Poor.
- Treatment is based on tumor stage and may include surgery and/or chemoradiation.
- Workup to determine primary tumor site is the standard of care.

- Features that favor a metastatic carcinoma include high nuclear grade and complex architecture (papillae).

IMMUNOPATHOLOGY (INCLUDING IMMUNOHISTOCHEMISTRY)

- Positive for p16, p53 (strong, diffuse), and CK7.
- Negative for human papillomavirus (HPV).

MAIN DIFFERENTIAL DIAGNOSIS

- Primary serous carcinoma of the cervix. These women are usually younger and a more conventional cervical adenocarcinoma is also present.
- Adenocarcinoma in situ. These can be difficult. A p53 stain (will be negative in AIS) is helpful.
- High-grade squamous intraepithelial lesion. Rarely may be mimicked by a metastatic carcinoma.

PATHOLOGY

HISTOLOGY

- These tumors are histologically similar to the primary tumor and composed of large pleomorphic cells with vesicular nuclei and prominent nucleoli.
- Neoplastic cells may be present only on the surface, replacing normal cervical epithelium, may form an exophytic mass lesion, or may diffusely invade the cervical stroma.
- Similar to the architecture of the primary tumor, the cells may be arranged in sheets (with characteristic cracks and crevices) or may form papillae and micropapillae.

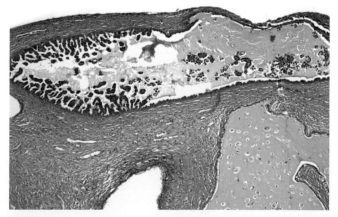

FIGURE 1

Metastatic serous carcinoma to the cervix. Low-power image showing neoplastic papillary epithelium lining mucous cyst.

319

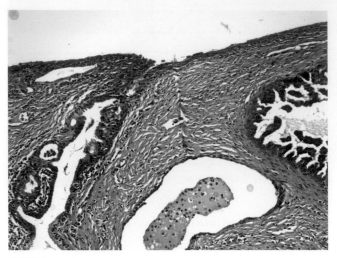

FIGURE 2

Metastatic serous carcinoma to the cervix. At higher power the normal mucosa *(left)* is opposite the involved mucous cyst *(right)*.

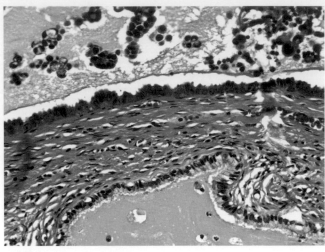

FIGURE 3

Metastatic serous carcinoma to the cervix. At higher magnification the cyst contains free-floating papillae. Note the rather subtle neoplastic epithelium seen here as a cuboidal epithelium with a high nuclear-to-cytoplasmic (N/C) ratio.

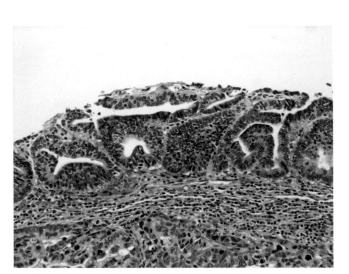

FIGURE 4

In this metastatic focus the glands somewhat resemble a primary glandular neoplasm of the cervix.

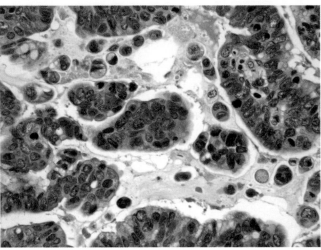

FIGURE 5

The detached fragments are clearly serous in morphology.

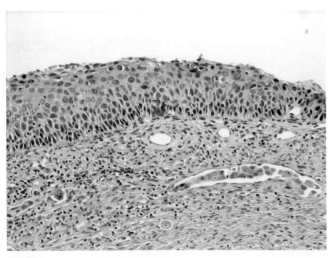

FIGURE 6

Metastatic serous carcinoma in superficial lymphatics. Is that a high-grade squamous intraepithelial lesion (HSIL) above or a metastatic serous carcinoma mimicking an HSIL? Likely the latter!

METASTATIC ENDOMETRIOID CARCINOMA TO THE CERVIX

DEFINITION—Endometrial adenocarcinoma which has spread caudally to involve the cervix.

CLINICAL FEATURES

EPIDEMIOLOGY

- Varies with the subtype of endometrial adenocarcinoma.

PRESENTATION

- May be identified clinically as a prolapsing cervical mass or as an abnormally firm endocervical canal.
- May be identified at the time of frozen section or upon opening the uterus (tumor grossly extends past the lower uterine segment to the cervix).
- May be identified in routine histologic sections of cervix or in an outpatient cervical biopsy.
- Patients are typically over age 50.

PROGNOSIS AND TREATMENT

- Endocervical *stromal* involvement by endometrial adenocarcinoma increases tumor stage (to stage II).
- Replacement of the endocervical glandular epithelium by carcinoma does not increase tumor stage.
- Involvement of endocervical glands by tumor does not increase tumor stage.
- Overall prognosis and treatment plan is dependent on the characteristics of the primary tumor.

PATHOLOGY

HISTOLOGY

- Tumor involvement may be contiguous with the endometrial mass or may be a discrete focus (drop metastasis).

- The histology varies with tumor subtype (endometrioid, clear cell, mucinous) and may be well or poorly differentiated.
- Features that favor a metastatic endometrioid carcinoma include low-grade nuclei, bland mucinous glands, well-differentiated squamous metaplasia, and lack of concurrent cervical adenocarcinoma in situ.
- Uterine sampling (endometrial biopsy or curettage) is required for complete evaluation of the potential primary site.

IMMUNOPATHOLOGY (INCLUDING IMMUNOHISTOCHEMISTRY)

- The same as the primary uterine tumor, and varies slightly with subtype.
- A panel of stains is sometimes used to distinguish a cervical (p16+, CEA+, vimentin–, ER/PR–) from an endometrial (p16–, CEA–, vimentin+, ER/PR+) primary adenocarcinoma in biopsy samples; however, a degree of skepticism must be employed when interpreting the results as there is significant overlap between the two tumor groups.

MAIN DIFFERENTIAL DIAGNOSIS

- Primary endocervical adenocarcinoma. Look for intense p16 staining, at least moderate nuclear atypia, apical mitoses.
- Adenocarcinoma arising out of cervical endometriosis.

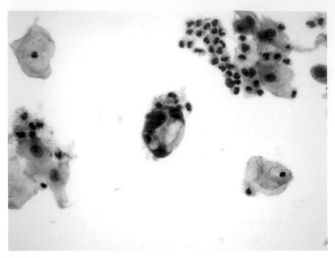

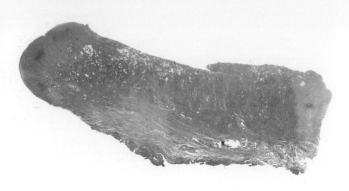

FIGURE 2

Metastatic endometrial adenocarcinoma involving the cervix. This low-power view of the cervix depicts a confluent arrangement of delicate glands mimicking mesonephric hyperplasia or endocervical tunnel clusters.

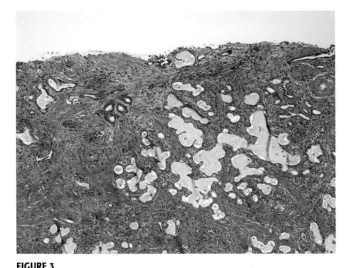

FIGURE 1

Endometrial adenocarcinoma involving the cervix. A single neoplastic cell is seen in the cervical cytology.

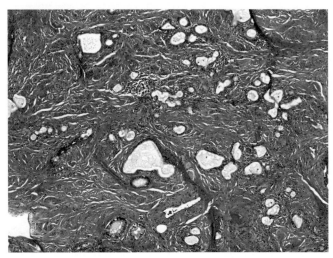

FIGURE 3

Metastatic endometrial adenocarcinoma involving the cervix. This could be confused with tunnel clusters.

FIGURE 4

Metastatic endometrial adenocarcinoma involving the cervix. A key feature here is the lack of gland crowding.

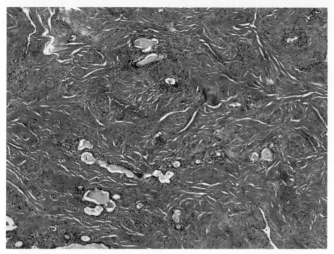

FIGURE 5

Metastatic endometrial adenocarcinoma involving the cervix. Note here the resemblance to mesonephric remnants.

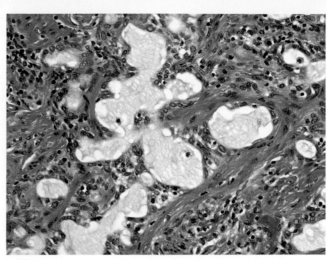

FIGURE 6

Metastatic endometrial adenocarcinoma involving the cervix. At higher magnification the neoplastic glands are deceptively bland appearing. The key is to distinguish them from benign endocervix or mesonephric remnants.

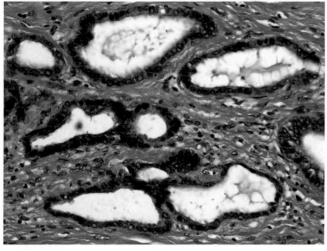

FIGURE 7

Metastatic endometrial adenocarcinoma involving the cervix. Note the lining of the neoplastic glands is a single cell layer in this case, which can be deceptive.

ATYPICAL ENDOCERVICAL POLYP

■ **Brooke E. Howitt, MD**

DEFINITION—An endocervical polyp with an atypical epithelial-stromal proliferation that resembles adenosarcoma but is not diagnostic.

CLINICAL FEATURES

EPIDEMIOLOGY

- Uncommon but will be encountered.
- No predisposing factors have been identified.

PRESENTATION

- Patients present with a cervical polyp or mass.
- Most often asymptomatic, with a polyp identified on routine exam.
- May present with spotting.

PROGNOSIS AND TREATMENT

- Atypical polyps are benign and so have an excellent prognosis,
- Excision of the polyp or mass is required for diagnosis and is also the treatment of choice.
- A small subset of endocervical adenosarcomas are misclassified as polyps initially; thus any atypical polyp should be monitored for regrowth.

PATHOLOGY

HISTOLOGY

- Adenosarcoma-like polyps display some architectural resemblance to low-grade adenosarcoma.
- The most common feature is the presence of irregularly shaped glands with occasional cleftlike, branching spaces that are reminiscent of phyllodes tumor of the breast.
- These irregular glands are best appreciated at low power.
- The area of concern typically occupies only a portion of the polyp.
- High-power examination reveals a notable lack of significant mitotic activity that is usually less than 2 per 10 high powered (400×) fields.
- Periglandular stromal condensation (cuffing) is present to some degree, but there should be minimal or no stromal atypia or nuclear crowding.

IMMUNOPATHOLOGY (INCLUDING IMMUNOHISTOCHEMISTRY)

- Noncontributory.

MAIN DIFFERENTIAL DIAGNOSIS

- Endocervical polyp—typical polyps present no problem given the lack of stromal hypercellularity.
- Low-grade endocervical adenosarcoma—these should have conspicuous nuclear atypia in the periglandular stroma, manifested primarily by nuclear crowding, coupled with mitotic activity.
- Prolapsed endometrial polyp—these can appear atypical, but the classic periglandular cuffing is not seen.
- Adenomyoma—the key to this diagnosis is the presence of smooth muscle fascicles between the endocervical crypts.

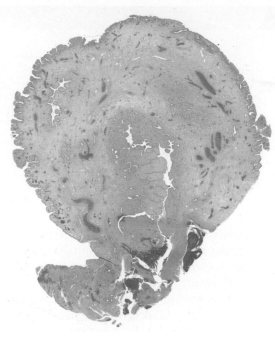

FIGURE 1

Atypical endocervical polyp. Low-power examination shows a cervical polyp with a central focus of leaflike architecture. This is a typical presentation. It could be argued that this is an "early" adenosarcoma arising in a polyp; however, the implication is the same, which is a lesion at low risk for recurrence once excised.

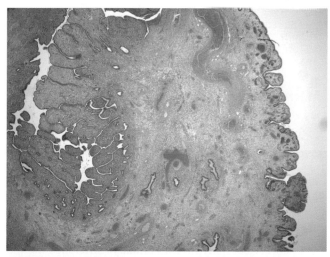

FIGURE 2

Atypical endocervical polyp. At higher magnification there is focal leaflike arrangement of epithelial fronds.

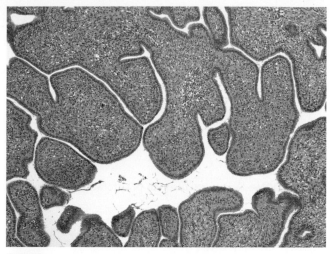

FIGURE 3

Atypical endocervical polyp. At higher magnification there is a leaflike arrangement of epithelial fronds.

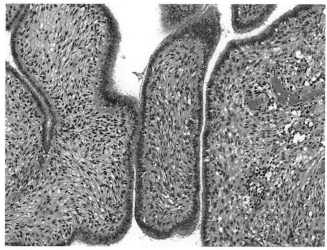

FIGURE 4

Atypical endocervical polyp. At moderate power there is minimal subepithelial stromal condensation seen.

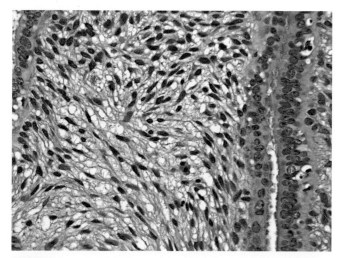

FIGURE 5

Atypical endocervical polyp. At high magnification there is minimal stromal cell atypia.

ADENOMYOMA OF THE CERVIX

DEFINITION—A benign, discrete proliferation of smooth muscle stroma and endocervical glands.

CLINICAL FEATURES

EPIDEMIOLOGY

- Adenomyomas and polypoid adenomyomas of the cervix are rare.
- The majority of these lesions occur within the uterine cavity, not at the cervix.
- The mean age at diagnosis is 40 years.

PRESENTATION

- Pedunculated or sessile-based cervical masses.
- May be identified as a polyp at routine screening, or patients may report vaginal spotting or complain of symptoms related to mass effect (such as pressure).

PROGNOSIS AND TREATMENT

- Excision of the mass to establish diagnosis is common.
- Cervical adenomyomas have an excellent prognosis, and once completely excised, no further treatment is warranted.
- Incompletely excised lesions may recur locally.

PATHOLOGY

HISTOLOGY

- By definition, adenomyomas are composed of benign glandular elements admixed with smooth muscle–type stroma.

- The glands are lined by bland endocervical cells and may exhibit focally prominent cystic change.
- Clusters of glands have a lobular profile at low power; a stromal reaction should not be present.
- The well-circumscribed, lobular glands are important in distinguishing sessile adenomyomas from the histologically similar minimal deviation adenocarcinoma of the cervix (adenoma malignum).

IMMUNOPATHOLOGY (INCLUDING IMMUNOHISTOCHEMISTRY)

- Endocervical adenomyomas typically stain positive for PAX2. The majority of endocervical adenocarcinomas (particularly adenoma malignum) are negative for PAX2.
- The stroma should be positive for smooth muscle markers (SMA).

MAIN DIFFERENTIAL DIAGNOSIS

- Adenoma malignum variant of endocervical adenocarcinoma: Gland architecture is more complex and rambling rather than tightly arranged as in adenomyoma. Gland epithelium and outlines will appear more complex. Look for a lobular arrangement of glands with a defined smooth muscle–type stroma in the adenomyoma.
- Endocervical polyp: The primary difference is the stromal smooth muscle differentiation in the adenomyoma.
- Adenosarcoma or atypical polyp: Demonstrate both irregular intraglandular polypoid growth and subepithelial stromal condensation.

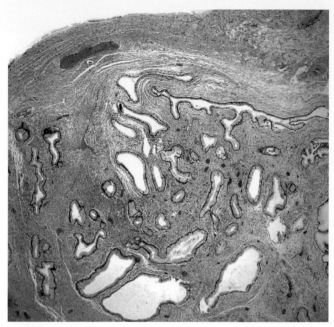

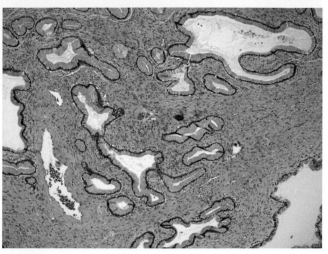

FIGURE 2

Cervical adenomyoma. High-power examination shows bland endocervical epithelium without nuclear atypia. Nuclear stratification and apical mitoses are not seen. The stroma is pink and smooth muscle–like without a desmoplastic reaction.

FIGURE 1

Cervical adenomyoma. Low-power examination shows a somewhat discrete, nodular proliferation of endocervical epithelium and myomatous stroma. The glands/crypts are arranged in lobules. A desmoplastic stromal response is not present.

MICROGLANDULAR HYPERPLASIA OF THE CERVIX

DEFINITION—A proliferation of specialized cuboidal cells derived from the squamocolumnar junction that gives rise to reserve cells, squamous metaplasia, and can harbor squamous intraepithelial lesions (SILs).

CLINICAL FEATURES

EPIDEMIOLOGY

- Most commonly occurs in young women with an uncertain relationship to hormones.
- Occasionally occurs in women not receiving hormonal therapy, as well as postmenopausal women.
- Likely a proliferation of multipotential squamocolumnar junction–type cells.

PRESENTATION

- Typically incidental at the time of cervical sampling.
- Large lesions may form masses and present with a friable cervix, which may simulate polyps or neoplasia.

PROGNOSIS AND TREATMENT

- Excellent; no treatment is required but can harbor SIL.

PATHOLOGY

HISTOLOGY

- In early forms, low-power evaluation will show an increased number of keratin 7–positive acini lined by cuboidal cells with a well-defined, lobular contour.
- More florid lesions will display loss of intervening stroma with back-to-back acini and cysts. In some forms, acini will be absent and the cuboidal cells will form a near-solid array.
- The cells comprising the glands are bland with cytoplasmic vacuoles, both subnuclear and supranuclear.
- Abundant neutrophilic inflammation is typically present, but apoptotic cells are not typically seen.
- Eosinophilic luminal mucin is often noted.

- The proliferative index is low.
- In more advanced lesions, p63 and krt5 are induced, found first in the acini and later in subcolumnar reserve cells that arise from acini.
- In advanced forms the reserve cells undergo expansion to form metaplasia, and the cuboidal surface cells evolve into mature columnar cells.
- Several variants have been described (hobnailed cells, signet-ring cells, solid pattern, and trabecular patterns) and may lead to diagnostic confusion; however, close attention to the cellular and nuclear morphology should lead to the correct diagnosis.
- SILs can occasionally arise in some cases of microglandular change, seen as an expansion of atypical reserve cells.

IMMUNOPATHOLOGY (INCLUDING IMMUNOHISTOCHEMISTRY)

- Keratin 7 is strongly positive in the acini.
- p63 and krt5 are positive in endocervical reserve cells and immature metaplasia.
- CEA is negative.
- p16 is negative or patchy in distribution.

MAIN DIFFERENTIAL DIAGNOSIS

- Endocervical adenocarcinoma (in situ) can be confused with this entity! However, cellular atypia is usually conspicuous. p16ink4 and MIB1 staining will be markedly increased.
- Clear-cell adenocarcinoma of the cervix does not display reserve cells. Moreover, the nuclei are larger and uniform appearing.
- Endometrial adenocarcinoma (low grade, mucinous type) can present with small groups of microacini and is one of the more difficult distinctions. However, the microacini tend to have a "soft" appearance with less sharply defined vacuoles, and often with minimal intervening stroma.

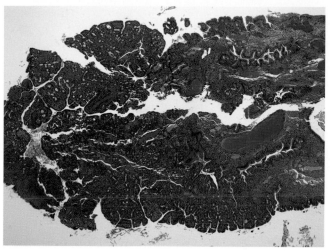

FIGURE 1

Microglandular change. Low-power image showing a polypoid proliferation of epithelial cells. The cells are arranged in a solid pattern, but nuclear atypia, mitotic activity, and nuclear stratification are not seen.

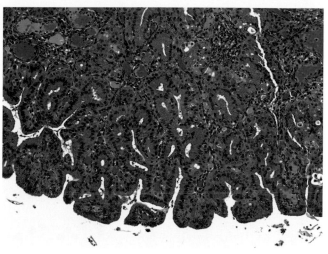

FIGURE 2

Microglandular change. At higher magnification regular acini are seen. Reserve cells are inconspicuous.

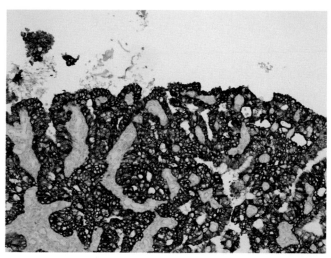

FIGURE 3

Microglandular change. These lesions stain strongly for CK7, a marker of squamocolumnar junction cells and most prominent in immature low-columnar cells.

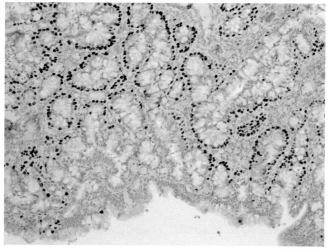

FIGURE 4

p63 highlights reserve cells in microglandular change.

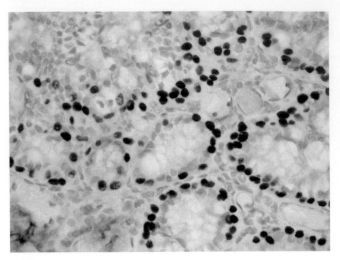

FIGURE 5

At higher magnification p63-positive acini merge with acini in which the reserve cells have segregated beneath the lining cells.

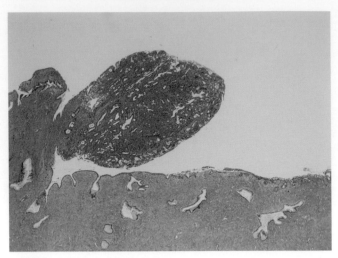

FIGURE 6

Endocervical polyp mimicking a carcinoma due to prominent glandular proliferation.

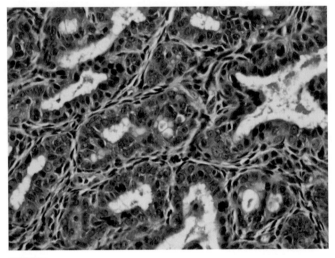

FIGURE 7

Higher magnification of the case in Figure 6. The glands may appear worrisome at first but in this case are associated with a distinct reserve cell layer.

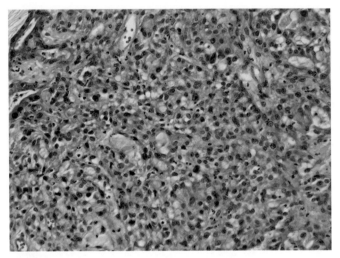

FIGURE 8

An uncommon variant of microglandular change in which the acini are not well formed. This pattern can be more difficult to distinguish from adenocarcinoma.

ADENOSARCOMA OF THE CERVIX

■ Brooke E. Howitt, MD

DEFINITION—A bi-patterned low-grade malignancy composed of neoplastic stroma admixed with benign but architecturally unique epithelial elements.

CLINICAL FEATURES

EPIDEMIOLOGY

- Extremely rare; accounts for less than 2% of all müllerian adenosarcomas.
- Average age at presentation is 31 years, with an age range from 11 to 65 years.
- One third of patients are under the age of 15.

PRESENTATION

- Vaginal bleeding is most often the presenting symptom.
- Physical exam often reveals a mass protruding through the cervical os, mimicking a benign endocervical polyp.
- Polyp/mass size is variable and ranges from less than 1 cm to 5 cm.

PROGNOSIS AND TREATMENT

- Prognosis is good, and linked to depth of invasion.
- Up to one third recur, but recurrences are typically locoregional (pelvic).
- Hysterectomy with close clinical observation is the treatment of choice; however, some, particularly those with very bland histology or those particularly polypoid, may be treated with excision alone and close monitoring of the cervix for regrowth.
- Oophorectomy is traditionally performed, but in young women with small or noninvasive lesions some may defer oophorectomy.
- Rare cases exhibit frankly malignant behavior.

PATHOLOGY

HISTOLOGY

- In classic cases the low-power appearance is reminiscent of a phyllodes tumor of the breast, with broad, leaf-shaped stromal proliferations protruding into glandular lumina.
- The glandular spaces may be dilated or slitlike and are distorted by the stromal proliferation, which is often most prominent immediately adjacent to the glands (cuffing).
- The neoplastic stromal cells are spindled, with moderate nuclear-to-cytoplasmic ratios, mild nuclear atypia, and easily identifiable mitoses (>2/10 hpf). Stromal atypia is a cardinal sign of adenosarcoma and most important in distinguishing it from an atypical polyp or adenomyomatous polyp.
- Glandular epithelium often shows altered differentiation, such as ciliated or endometrioid type epithelium.
- Heterologous elements, such as skeletal muscle or cartilage, are occasionally seen, although well-defined myomatous stroma is not consistent with this diagnosis.

IMMUNOPATHOLOGY (INCLUDING IMMUNOHISTOCHEMISTRY)

- Noncontributory.

MAIN DIFFERENTIAL DIAGNOSIS

- Benign endocervical (atypical) polyp—these usually exhibit stromal condensation and some albeit rather minimal phyllodes-like glandular architecture. They should be devoid of conspicuous stromal atypia.
- Adenomyoma—this tumor will exhibit conspicuous myomatous differentiation.
- Adenosarcoma arising in endometriosis and uterine adenosarcomas metastatic to the cervix are other considerations but can usually be distinguished clinically or by mode of presentation.
- Rare cervical polyps can display bizarre symplastic-like nuclei, but do not otherwise resemble adenosarcoma.
- Embryonal rhabdomyosarcoma—subepithelial cambium layer but no excess benign glands. Typically vaginal in location.

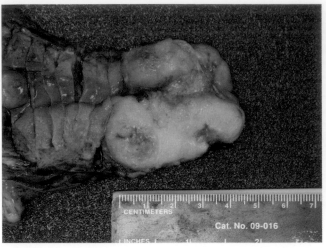

FIGURE 1

Cervical adenosarcoma. Gross examination shows a fleshy mass located in the endocervix and extending nearly to the lower uterine segment. In this example the upper portion of the mass is vaguely polypoid, while other areas are invasive into the cervical stroma.

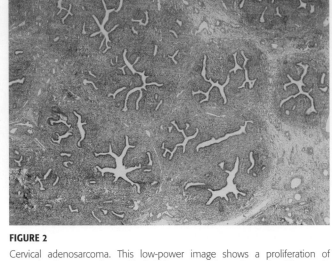

FIGURE 2

Cervical adenosarcoma. This low-power image shows a proliferation of stromal cells surrounding epithelial elements and creating polypoid, vaguely leaflike architecture within the glandular spaces. Periglandular cuffing is prominent.

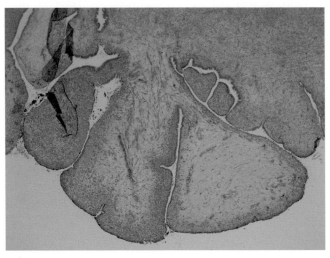

FIGURE 3

Cervical adenosarcoma. Low power of this lesion is characterized by the presence of large, broad leaflike structures. Stromal cuffing or condensation just beneath the epithelium is prominent.

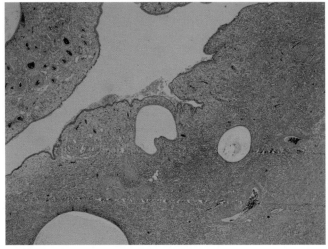

FIGURE 4

Cervical adenosarcoma. This lesion is characterized by dilated, distending glandular structures. Stromal cuffing is subtle, but present.

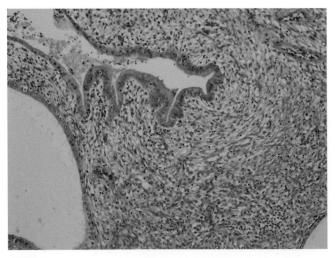

FIGURE 5

Cervical adenosarcoma. High-power examination confirms the benign histology of the epithelial elements. There are small intraluminal polypoid projections. The stromal cells are densely arranged adjacent to the epithelium, with mild nuclear atypia. Mitoses are subtle and infrequent in this example.

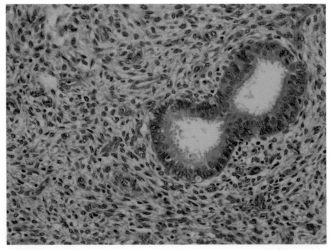

FIGURE 6

Cervical adenosarcoma. The glands in this high-power image are dilated and exhibit altered differentiation (cilia). The stromal cells have mild nuclear atypia, and mitoses are not easily identified.

CERVICAL SCHWANNOMA

DEFINITION—A generally benign, peripheral nerve sheath tumor.

CLINICAL FEATURES

EPIDEMIOLOGY

- Rare, limited to occasional case reports.
- Most reported cases—benign and malignant—occur in the third to eighth decades.

PRESENTATION

- Vaginal bleeding in many cases.
- May be asymptomatic, detected on routine examination.
- Well-circumscribed cervical mass, usually less than 5 cm.
- Red to gray-white on sectioning.

PROGNOSIS AND TREATMENT

- Excisional therapy is usually adequate.
- Malignant lesions can be cured by excision but occasional recurrences have been reported.

PATHOLOGY

HISTOLOGY

- Spindle cell proliferation.
- Nuclear pallisading.
- Thick-walled hyalinized blood vessels.

IMMUNOPATHOLOGY (INCLUDING IMMUNOHISTOCHEMISTRY)

- Positive for S-100, vimentin.
- Negative for neurofilament protein (NFP), CD34, desmin, actin, chromogranin, synaptophysin, and melanoma markers (MART-1, MelanA, HMB-45).

MAIN DIFFERENTIAL DIAGNOSIS

- Neurofibroma—CD34 and NFP positive.
- Desmoplastic melanoma—positive for melanoma markers.
- Leiomyoma or angiomyomfibroblastoma—negative for S100.

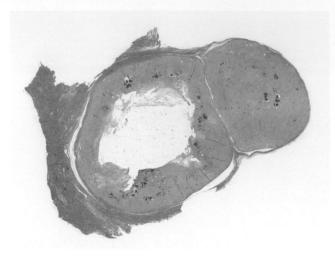

FIGURE 1

Cervical schwannoma. Note the well circumscribed appearance at low magnification.

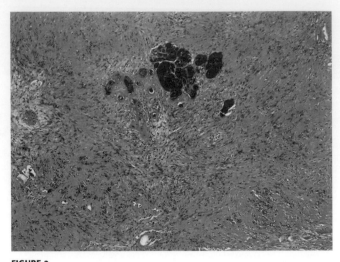

FIGURE 2

Cervical schwannoma. At medium power the pallisaded nuclei and thick-walled vessels can be seen.

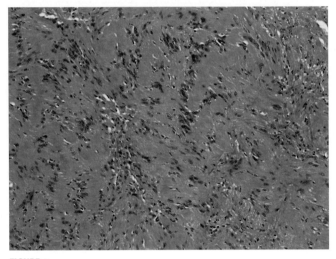

FIGURE 3

Cervical schwannoma. Higher magnification of the pallisaded nuclei.

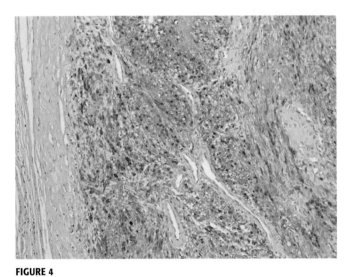

FIGURE 4

Cervical schwannoma. There is strong staining for S-100.

GLIAL POLYP OF THE CERVIX

DEFINITION—A polyp of the cervix composed of mature glial tissue.

CLINICAL FEATURES

EPIDEMIOLOGY

- Extremely rare.
- Signifies retained glial tissue from a prior pregnancy based on genetic studies.
- Reproductive age group.

PRESENTATION

- Pedunculated or sessile-based cervical masses.
- May be identified as a polyp at routine screening, or patients may report vaginal spotting or complain of symptoms related to mass effect (such as pressure).
- Typically there is a history of pregnancy or spontaneous abortion.

PROGNOSIS AND TREATMENT

- Excision of the mass is curative.

PATHOLOGY

HISTOLOGY

- The polyp consists of glial tissue in a connective tissue matrix.
- Erosion and granulation tissue may also be present.
- Typical features of glial tissue are present, and the glia is sharply demarcated.

IMMUNOPATHOLOGY (INCLUDING IMMUNOHISTOCHEMISTRY)

- Positive for GFAP and S100.

MAIN DIFFERENTIAL DIAGNOSIS

- Schwannoma—this tumor exhibits the characteristic interlaced spindled cells in contrast to the more monotonous array of glia.

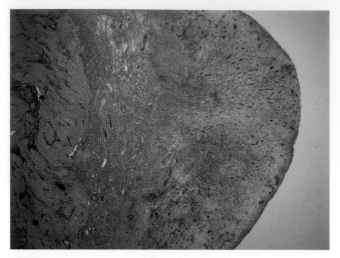

FIGURE 1

Glial polyp of the cervix. At low magnification the glial tissue is seen in the stromal *(left)* and deep to a layer of granulation tissue.

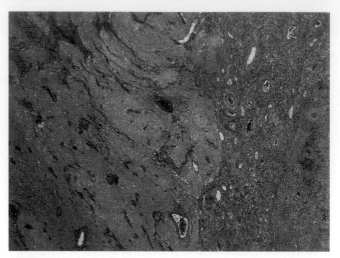

FIGURE 2

Glial polyp of the cervix. At higher magnification the glia is juxtaposed with a vascular stroma.

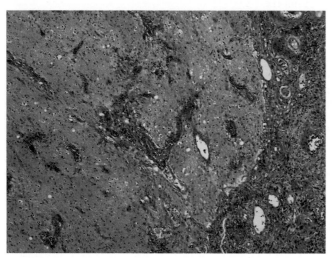

FIGURE 3

At higher magnifications the monotonous array of mature glial cells can be seen within a slightly fibrillar matrix.

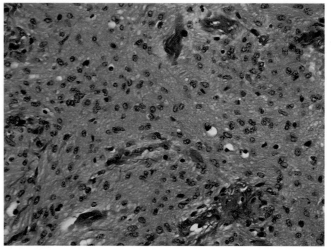

FIGURE 4

At higher magnifications the normal-appearing mature glial cells can be appreciated.

Uterus

DYSFUNCTIONAL UTERINE BLEEDING (EARLY OR MID-CYCLE BREAKDOWN)

DEFINITION—Bleeding that occurs in the absence of ovulation and is not associated with an endometrial structural abnormality or other visible cause (fibroid or polyp).

CLINICAL FEATURES

EPIDEMIOLOGY

- Dysfunctional uterine bleeding (DUB) is common, more frequently seen near menopause.
- Based on histology, the pattern suggests failed follicle and/or the absence of progression to the luteal phase with mid or early cycle shedding.

PRESENTATION

- Patients present with unexplained uterine bleeding in premenopause.

PROGNOSIS AND TREATMENT

- DUB is benign but not associated with a visible cause that can be corrected surgically.
- Management is symptomatic with resampling if bleeding persists or recurs.
- In adolescents, workup and correction of coagulation disturbance as appropriate.

PATHOLOGY

HISTOLOGY

- The pattern is that of a mid-cycle breakdown, with tubular glands and diffuse stromal breakdown.

- Mitoses may or may not be seen depending on interval from cessation of estrogen output and breakdown.
- Relatively normal-appearing luteal phase endometrium may also be seen if there is an extrinsic (coagulopathy) or other cause for bleeding.

IMMUNOPATHOLOGY (INCLUDING IMMUNOHISTOCHEMISTRY)

- Noncontributory.

MAIN DIFFERENTIAL DIAGNOSIS/ASSOCIATED CONDITIONS

- Persistent follicle and benign hyperplasia—cystic glands will be seen.
- Follicular inadequacy and coagulopathy are other potential causes of mid-cycle bleeding.
- A short course of estrogen with withdrawal will produce the same pattern.

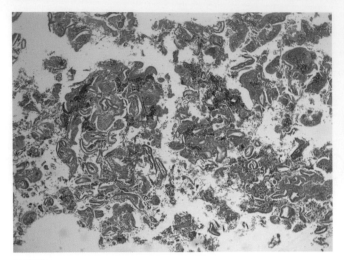

FIGURE 1

DUB. Here is a typical pattern of dysfunctional bleeding, with mostly stromal breakdown and scattered glands and surface epithelium.

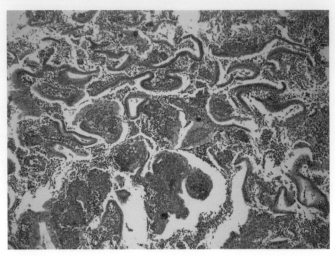

FIGURE 2

DUB. At higher magnification the recognizable glands are nondescript and admixed with stromal breakdown. A similar pattern could be produced by a short course of progestins followed by withdrawal.

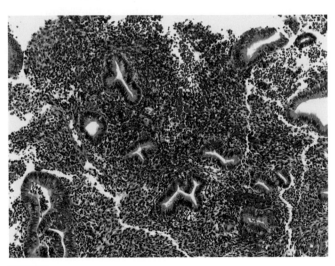

FIGURE 3

DUB. Another example, with proliferative-type glands admixed with a diffuse pattern of stromal breakdown. Note there is evidence of neither persistent follicle (which would produce cystic glands) nor ovulation (which would produce a pseudodecidualized stroma).

BREAKDOWN MIMICKING NEOPLASIA

DEFINITION—Scheduled menstrual breakdown and abnormal stromal breakdown histologically mimicking adenocarcinoma.

CLINICAL FEATURES

EPIDEMIOLOGY

- The presence of stromal breakdown within an endometrial biopsy is relatively common; fortunately, however, extensive breakdown, mimicking neoplasia, is relatively uncommon.

PRESENTATION

- Patients typically present with abnormal uterine bleeding and are biopsied.
- More typically encountered with unscheduled (anovulatory) bleeding due to the prominent repair and irregular breakdown pattern seen in such cases.

PROGNOSIS AND TREATMENT

- Breakdown and menstruation are normal and carry no adverse prognosis.
- If identified correctly, no treatment is warranted, whereas misdiagnosis may lead to unnecessary surgery.

PATHOLOGY

HISTOLOGY

- Glands may appear crowded due to loss of intervening stroma.

- Aggregates of degenerating stroma may form hyperchromatic, cellular balls and cords, which can simulate poorly differentiated carcinoma.
- Papillary surface (repair) changes may be associated with stromal breakdown and lead to the misdiagnosis of malignancy.
- Alternatively, fragments of carcinoma with loss of architecture may resemble stromal breakdown.

IMMUNOPATHOLOGY (INCLUDING IMMUNOHISTOCHEMISTRY)

- Negative staining for p53 and decreased staining for Ki-67 may be helpful in cases in which serous carcinoma is a concern.

MAIN DIFFERENTIAL DIAGNOSIS

- Adenocarcinoma—the key to this diagnosis is a careful scrutiny of the epithelium, which if neoplastic can be distinguished from necrotic stroma. In rare cases in which small fragments of tumor from either a serous or neuroendocrine carcinoma are encountered, special stains (p53, p16) might be helpful.
- Curettage or procedural artifacts such as telescoping artifact, exfoliation artifact.

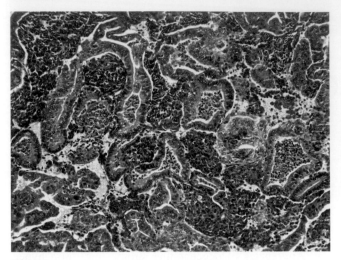

FIGURE 1

Breakdown and menstruation mimicking malignancy. Strips of endometrial glandular epithelium and stromal "blue balls."

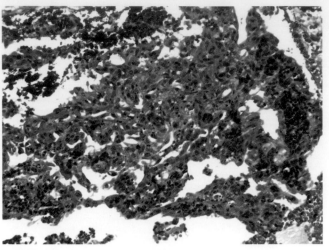

FIGURE 2

Breakdown and menstruation mimicking malignancy. Superficial repair type epithelium with small punched out spaces mimicking carcinoma. Note the stromal breakdown on the right.

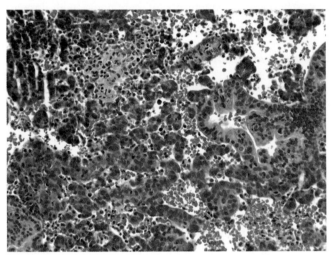

FIGURE 3

Breakdown and menstruation mimicking malignancy. Strips of menstrual endometrium forming cords, which can mimic malignancy.

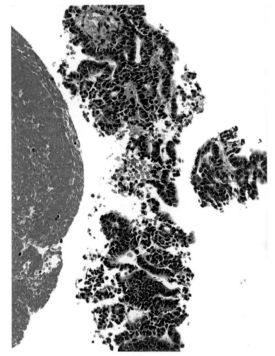

FIGURE 4

Fragments of endometrial adenocarcinoma simulating menstrual endometrium. *(From Crum CP, Nucci MR, Lee KR, editors: Diagnostic Gynecologic and Obstetric Pathology, ed 2, Philadelphia, 2011, Elsevier.)*

ANOVULATORY ENDOMETRIUM WITH PERSISTENT FOLLICLE

DEFINITION—Alterations in the endometrium due to lack of ovulation and estrogenic effects of a persistent follicle.

CLINICAL FEATURES

EPIDEMIOLOGY

- Most commonly seen at or around menopause with failed ovulation and persistent follicle.
- Common in polycystic ovarian syndrome (PCOS).
- Abnormal uterine bleeding in the fourth or fifth decade is the most common presenting sign.
- Can be mimicked by excessive estrogen administration post menopause.

PRESENTATION

- Unscheduled bleeding.
- Signs of PCOS may be present in younger women.

PROGNOSIS AND TREATMENT

- Usually uneventful in the fifth decade, with bleeding ceasing at menopause.
- Anovulatory bleeding occurring with increased levels of estrogen may lead to benign hyperplasia if estrogen levels are persistently elevated.
- Treatment ranges from clinical follow-up to hormonal therapy.
- Risk of subsequent endometrial cancer estimated at 1%.

PATHOLOGY

HISTOLOGY

- Proliferative endometrium with mitotic figures but may vary as a function of timing of endometrial sampling (during or after cessation of estrogenic stimulation).

- The most pronounced finding is that of uniformly distributed glands with cystic dilatation.
- Glandular karyorrhexis, breakdown, thrombi, repair, and tubal metaplasia will often be present.
- Useful diagnostic terms for this include "altered endometrium with alterations in gland architecture consistent with anovulation" and "disordered proliferative endometrium."

IMMUNOPATHOLOGY (INCLUDING IMMUNOHISTOCHEMISTRY)

- Noncontributory.

RECOMMENDED DIAGNOSTIC TERMINOLOGY

- Anovulatory-pattern endometrium.
- Proliferative endometrium with alterations in gland architecture consistent with delayed or absent ovulation.
- Disordered proliferative endometrium is another term commonly used albeit less informative.

MAIN DIFFERENTIAL DIAGNOSIS

- Endometrial polyps often display cystic glands but can be recognized by polyp stroma.
- Benign hyperplasia is an exaggerated form of anovulatory change, with slightly higher gland density and undulating gland contours with outpouchings (mouse ears).
- Endometrial intraepithelial neoplasia (atypical hyperplasia) is a clonal expansion of crowded glands that differ in appearance from the background endometrium.
- Basalis or lower uterine segment may display cystic glands as well.

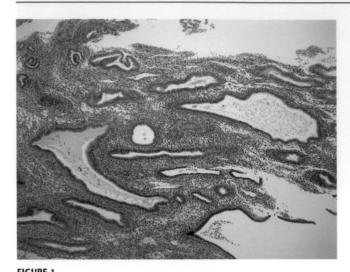

FIGURE 1

Anovulatory endometrium with persistent follicle. Irregularly regular glands with cystic dilatation.

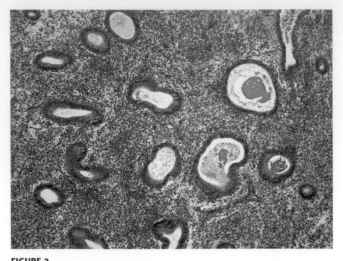

FIGURE 2

Anovulatory endometrium. Variable gland size is the norm. Glands tend to be relatively round without undulating borders.

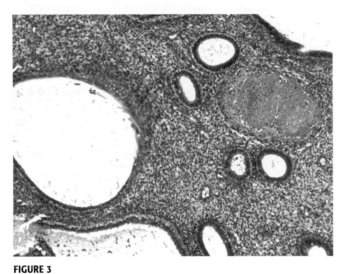

FIGURE 3

Anovulatory endometrium with fibrin thrombi. Gland karyorrhexis will also be common.

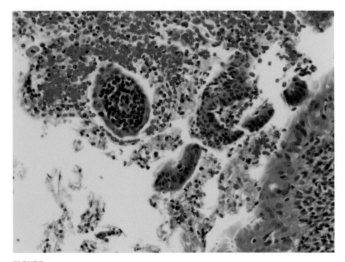

FIGURE 4

Anovulatory endometrium. Reparative epithelial changes adjacent to focal stromal breakdown.

BENIGN ENDOMETRIAL HYPERPLASIA

DEFINITION—An exaggerated response to unopposed estrogen but lacking the features of endometrial intraepithelial neoplasia (EIN) (atypical hyperplasia).

CLINICAL FEATURES

EPIDEMIOLOGY

- Most commonly seen at or around menopause with failed ovulation and persistent follicle.
- Common in polycystic ovarian syndrome (PCOS).
- Abnormal uterine bleeding in the fourth or fifth decade is the most common presenting sign.
- Can be mimicked by estrogen administration post menopause.

PRESENTATION

- Unscheduled bleeding.
- Signs of PCOS may be present in younger women.

PROGNOSIS AND TREATMENT

- Usually uneventful in the fifth decade, with bleeding ceasing at menopause.
- Anovulatory bleeding occurring with increased levels of estrogen may lead to benign hyperplasia if estrogen levels are persistently elevated.
- Treatment ranges from clinical follow-up to hormonal therapy. Repeat sampling is indicated if clinical circumstances (recurrent bleeding, evidence of an endometrial lesion) dictate.
- Risk of subsequent endometrial cancer estimated at 1%.

PATHOLOGY

HISTOLOGY

- Proliferative endometrium with mitotic figures but may vary as a function of timing of endometrial sampling (during or after cessation of estrogenic stimulation).

- The most pronounced finding is that of uniformly distributed glands with cystic dilatation and groups of glands with irregular contours or outpouchings (ears).
- Glandular karyorrhexis, breakdown, thrombi, repair, and tubal metaplasia will often be present.

RECOMMENDED DIAGNOSTIC TERMINOLOGY

- Benign hyperplasia.
- Note: This pattern reflects unopposed estrogen, but there is no evidence of neoplasia (EIN). Repeat sampling is advised if there are clinical concerns (e.g., recurrent bleeding and other abnormal uterine findings).

IMMUNOPATHOLOGY (INCLUDING IMMUNOHISTOCHEMISTRY)

- Noncontributory.

MAIN DIFFERENTIAL DIAGNOSIS

- Endometrial polyps often display cystic glands but can be recognized by stromal changes. The adjacent endometrium will not contain cystic glands.
- In contrast to the usual changes of persistent follicle, benign hyperplasia is an exaggerated form of anovulatory change, with slightly higher gland density.
- EIN (atypical hyperplasia) is a clonal expansion of crowded glands that differ in appearance from the background endometrium.

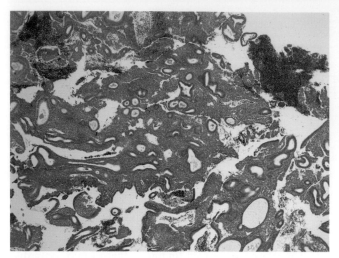

FIGURE 1

Benign hyperplasia at low magnification. Note the relatively high gland density.

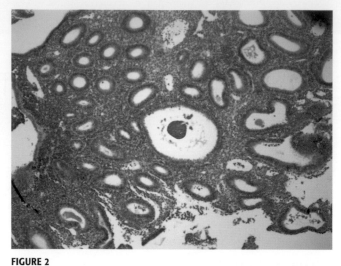

FIGURE 2

Benign hyperplasia at medium magnification. Scattered cystic glands are present.

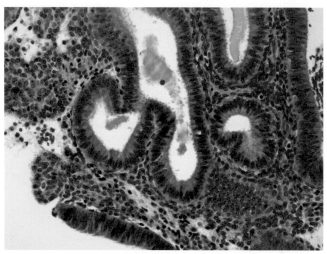

FIGURE 3

Benign hyperplasia. Note the outpouching with "ears" projecting from glands.

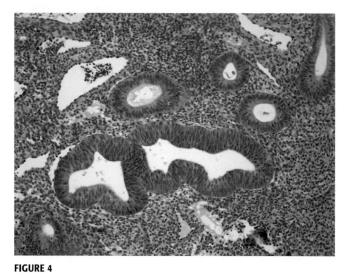

FIGURE 4

Benign hyperplasia. A cluster of glands with more prominent pseudostratification creating some contrast with the other glands. However, other than this there is little difference in cytology between the glands and there is no discrete outgrowth of crowded cytologically altered glands, as seen in EIN.

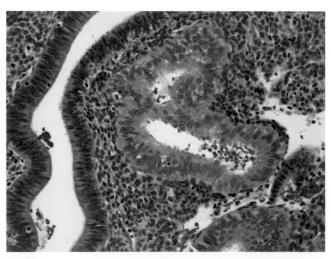

FIGURE 5

Benign hyperplasia. Note the single gland with tubal metaplasia.

TELESCOPING ARTIFACTS MIMICKING NEOPLASIA

DEFINITION—Artifactual compression of glands during the biopsy process.

CLINICAL FEATURES

EPIDEMIOLOGY

- Telescoping artifact is common and can be identified in a large proportion of endometrial biopsies.

PRESENTATION

- Telescoping artifact is an incidental finding, usually during histologic examination of a sample due to abnormal uterine bleeding.

PROGNOSIS AND TREATMENT

- Gland compression is an artifact and no treatment is required.
- Failure to recognize telescoping artifact may lead to the erroneous diagnosis of endometrial intraepithelial neoplasia (EIN) and further, unnecessary treatment.

PATHOLOGY

HISTOLOGY

- Telescoping of proliferative glands leads to back-to-back glands with little intervening stroma.

- Lack of stroma or stromal fragmentation and hemorrhage are useful clues in ruling out true gland crowding.
- Glandular epithelium is pulled into the lumen causing enlargement of the gland with redundancy of the epithelium.
- Folding of the epithelium may lead to pseudopapillary structures.
- This artifact is also common in the early secretory phase.

IMMUNOPATHOLOGY (INCLUDING IMMUNOHISTOCHEMISTRY)

- Noncontributory.

MAIN DIFFERENTIAL DIAGNOSIS

- EIN or well-differentiated carcinoma—these two lesions are characterized by closely arranged glands with altered cytology. The glands in telescoping artifact are typically no different in appearance from the surrounding epithelium.
- Secretory hyperplasia or EIN—this entity will display an altered epithelium, usually with prominent pseudostratification or some atypia (see secretory EIN). Telescoping artifacts in early secretory endometrium will not appreciably alter the cytology of the lining epithelium.

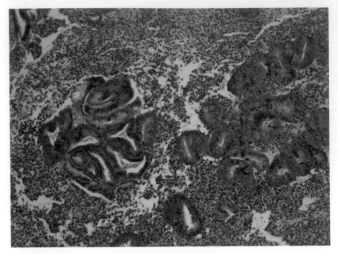

FIGURE 1

Telescoping artifact. Glands on the left are compressed within one gland tract; those on the right are compressed longitudinally.

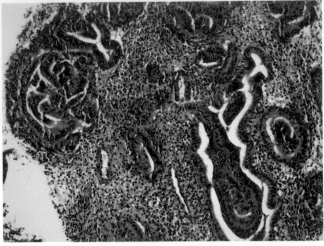

FIGURE 2

Telescoping artifact. Large glands with redundant epithelium. Note that the telescoped gland is at the edge of the tissue fragment.

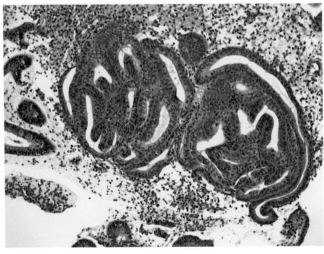

FIGURE 3

Telescoping artifact. Gland in gland formation with pseudopapillae. Stromal fragmentation is readily apparent.

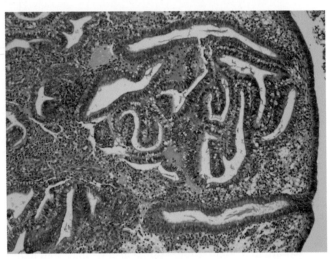

FIGURE 4

Telescoping or compression artifact in secretory endometrium can cause conspicuous crowding. Note the normal appearance of the glandular epithelium.

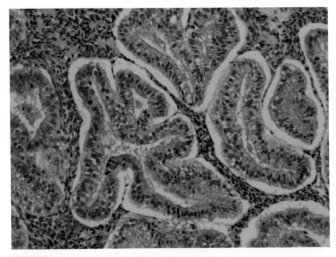

FIGURE 5

Telescoping or compression artifact in early secretory endometrium is common.

MIXED-PATTERN ENDOMETRIUM

DEFINITION—Endometrium with both secretory and proliferative pattern glands.

CLINICAL FEATURES

EPIDEMIOLOGY

- True mixed-pattern endometrium is relatively uncommon and can be attributed to four likely causes:
  1. Hormonal imbalance (therapy)
  2. Irregular ovulation
  3. Defects in follicle development
  4. Clonal lesions
- The most common cause of a mixed pattern is hormonal imbalance secondary to therapy or assisted reproduction.

PRESENTATION

- Typically found at the time of endometrial sampling for abnormal uterine bleeding.
- May be discovered in biopsies utilized in fertility workups.

PROGNOSIS AND TREATMENT

- Mixed-pattern endometrium is benign and carries no adverse prognosis.
- Hormone therapy may be used to attempt to restore normal ovulation.

PATHOLOGY

HISTOLOGY

- Mixture due to hormonal therapy presents with cystically dilated, tubular glands and prominent stromal changes (pseudodecidualization).

- Cases of irregular ovulation (anovulation followed by ovulation) lead to glands with a marked discrepancy in size. Stromal edema is typically present, and the glands may display secretory features. Cystic dilation and tubal metaplasia are typically present.
- Mixture in the presence of a follicular failure shows quiescent, tubular glands persisting into the secretory phase.
- Clonal causes of a mixed pattern may be identified by the presence of two physiologic states of endometrium in close apposition. The histology is variable, but may consist of a population of stratified glands with (or without) mitotic activity or a "lagging secretory phase."

IMMUNOPATHOLOGY (INCLUDING IMMUNOHISTOCHEMISTRY)

- Noncontributory.

MAIN DIFFERENTIAL DIAGNOSIS

- Hormonal effect—hormonal treatment often will produce a mixed pattern, including cystic endometrial glands and the illusion of polyp, and must be taken into account when considering this diagnosis.
- Follicular dysfunction—this is a generic term for midcycle bleeding that occurs without a clear cause (dysfunctional bleeding). The glands will appear tubular but may lack mitoses after cessation of estrogen stimulation, thus giving the appearance of a mixed pattern.
- Luteal phase defect—this term implies delayed secretory maturation (early for stated date) but presumably a normal morphology.
- Clonal evolution (endometrial intraepithelial neoplasia [EIN])—when a component of the mixed pattern consists of crowded glands with altered cytology, EIN must be excluded.

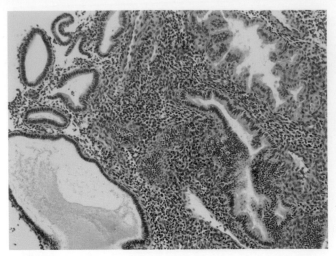

FIGURE 1

Mixed-pattern endometrium. Anovulatory endometrium showing a diversity of secretory maturation varying from hypersecretory *(center)* to less so *(left)*.

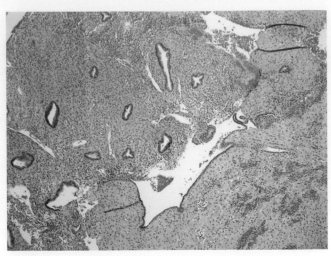

FIGURE 2

Mixed-pattern endometrium. Hormonally treated endometrium with quiescent tubular (proliferative pattern) glands set in a pseudodecidualized stroma.

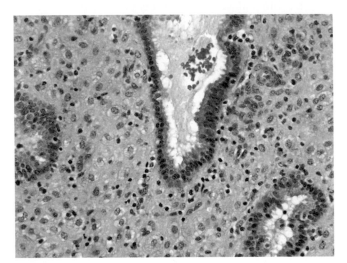

FIGURE 3

Mixed-pattern endometrium. Higher magnification of the case shown in Figure 2 shows the prominent pseudodecidualized stroma.

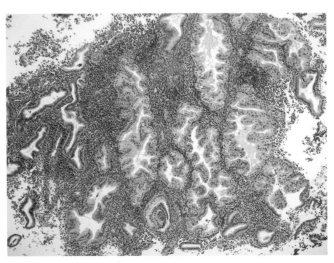

FIGURE 4

Mixed-pattern endometrium. A "clonal mixed pattern" showing secretory glands *(bottom)* and a population of glands with pseudostratification above. This implies that one or more mutations occurred in a clone that led to a difference in response to progestins.

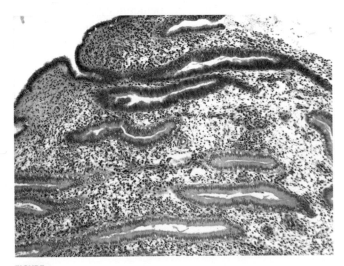

FIGURE 5

Anovulation with superimposed progestin therapy or ovulation. In this scenario, glands have become cystic due to persistent estrogen stimulation, followed by ovulation or progestin therapy. The latter imparts a superimposed secretory phenotype.

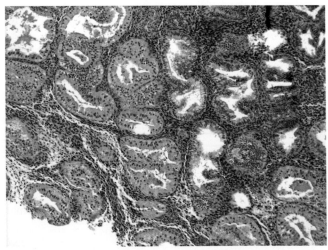

FIGURE 6

"Clonal mixed-pattern" endometrium. In this case a population of eosinophilic glands are situated in the midst of a secretory endometrium. Note the normal distribution of these glands, in keeping with the surrounding secretory glands. These are not always straightforward, and may at times require a follow-up endometrial sampling.

ADENOMYOMATOUS POLYP

DEFINITION—An endometrial polyp composed of benign smooth muscle and glands.

CLINICAL FEATURES

EPIDEMIOLOGY

- Adenomyomatous polyps are a variant of endometrial polyp with smooth muscle differentiation. They are often found in association with conventional polyps.

PRESENTATION

- Patients may be asymptomatic or present with abnormal uterine bleeding.
- Large polyps may prolapse through the cervical os, mimicking malignancy.

PROGNOSIS AND TREATMENT

- Adenomyomatous polyps are benign, and no treatment is warranted other than to manage uterine bleeding.

PATHOLOGY

HISTOLOGY

- Variable amounts of myomatous stroma and endometrial glands are present.

- Glands may display irregular glandular contours.
- The polyp stroma is composed of smooth muscle versus the fibrous stroma that can be seen in typical endometrial polyps.
- No glandular atypia should be present.

IMMUNOPATHOLOGY (INCLUDING IMMUNOHISTOCHEMISTRY)

- The stromal component should be diffusely positive for smooth muscle markers (SMA, Desmin).
- The stromal component of the polyp should be negative for CD10 (endometrial stroma marker) and CD34.

MAIN DIFFERENTIAL DIAGNOSIS

- Endometrial polyp—the stroma lacks the compact bundles of smooth muscle.
- Atypical polypoid adenomyoma (APA)—this is essentially a sessile adenomyomatous polyp with two differences. The first is abnormal gland growth and squamous morules. The second is the smooth muscle differentiation, which is more mature, with conspicuous cytoplasmic differentiation, akin to what would be seen in a leiomyoma.

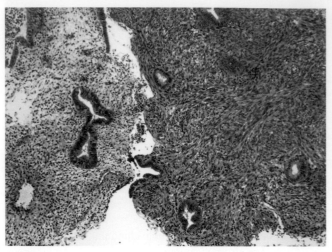

FIGURE 1

Adenomyomatous polyp. Smooth muscle and glands, composing an adeno-myomatous polyp, are seen on the right. Normal endometrium is on the left for comparison.

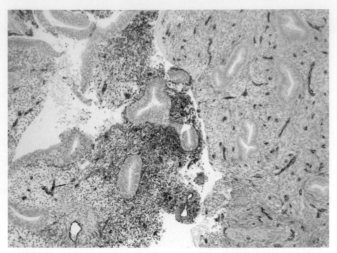

FIGURE 2

Adenomyomatous polyp. Immunostain for CD34 showing positivity in the endometrial stroma and negativity in the polyp.

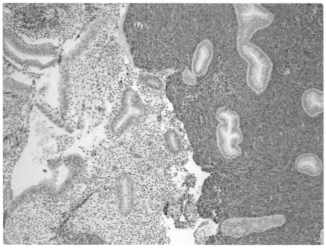

FIGURE 3

Adenomyomatous polyp. Immunostain for SMA showing diffuse positivity in the adenomyomatous polyp.

CHRONIC ENDOMETRITIS

DEFINITION—Chronic inflammatory process within the uterus often associated with infection.

CLINICAL FEATURES

EPIDEMIOLOGY

- Chronic endometritis (CE) is thought to represent an infectious process.
- CE is strongly associated with the presence of pelvic inflammatory disease and acute salpingitis.
- Virtually all organisms described that can cause sexually transmitted diseases have been implicated in CE.
- In young patients the most common cause is infection during a recent pregnancy/delivery.

PRESENTATION

- In all age groups CE is a common cause of abnormal uterine bleeding but is generally seen in the fifth decade.
- Patients may present with obstructive symptoms (concurrent pyometra).
- A large number of patients are asymptomatic other than abnormal bleeding. It is important to emphasize that abnormal bleeding is among the most common signs of chlamydial endometritis, hence the importance of pathologic examination.

PROGNOSIS AND TREATMENT

- CE has a favorable prognosis when treated. It may be idiopathic in older women.
- Treatment usually consists of removal of the inciting agent (if present), such as an intrauterine device (IUD) and antibiotics if indicated.
- Pyometra in postmenopausal women may signal a malignancy, and repeated sampling may be indicated to exclude this possibility.

PATHOLOGY

HISTOLOGY

- Stromal condensation, spindling, and cellularity (attributed to an increased mononuclear cell infiltrate) are typically the easiest to recognize signs of CE.
- Reactive alterations in the normal endometrial glands may be present (typically proliferative phase).
- Lymphoid follicles may be increased in number or easily identifiable.
- Acute inflammatory debris, eosinophilic "repair" epithelium, focal breakdown, and surface squamous metaplasia may be present.
- Plasma cells can be seen within the endometrial stroma, particularly surrounding blood vessels.
- Lymphoid follicles can be seen in normal endometrium and are not diagnostic; likewise, plasma cells may be seen in endometrial polyps, during menstruation, and near submucosal leiomyomas, and by themselves are not diagnostic of CE.

IMMUNOPATHOLOGY (INCLUDING IMMUNOHISTOCHEMISTRY)

- Much is sometimes made of performing special stains for plasma cells. CD138 immunostaining or other stains may be helpful in identifying plasma cells in difficult cases. However, in general, a reasonable search (2 to 3 minutes) should turn up plasma cells if they are in the field of examination.

MAIN DIFFERENTIAL DIAGNOSIS

- Endometrial polyps often display plasma cells, and unless prominent are not classified as CE.
- Stromal breakdown, particularly in late menstrual endometrium, will occasionally display plasma cells.

Menstruation is associated with inflammatory cells, but not plasma cells. Postpartum endometrium will contain lymphocytes and macrophages; the presence of plasma cells warrants a diagnosis of CE.

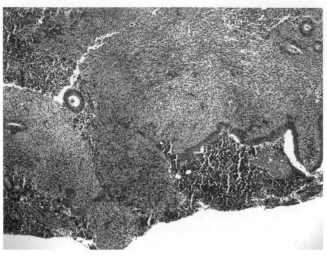

FIGURE 1

CE. Increased stromal cellularity and lymphoid aggregates can be seen at low power.

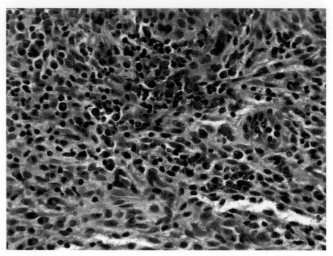

FIGURE 3

CE. Scattered plasma cells can be found, often in the areas surrounding vessels or near breakdown and hemorrhage.

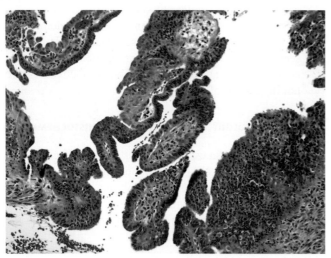

FIGURE 2

CE. The surface endometrium may display reactive, repair-type epithelial changes.

PSEUDOACTINOMYCOTIC RADIATE GRANULES

DEFINITION—Granular material that may be found in association with intrauterine devices.

CLINICAL FEATURES

EPIDEMIOLOGY

- The finding of granular material associated with intrauterine device (IUD) use is not uncommon, happening in slightly less than 10% of patients.
- To date, no microbial association has been made with pseudoactinomycotic radiate granules (PAMRAGs).

PRESENTATION

- Patients may be asymptomatic or may be experiencing adverse symptoms from IUD use (prompting removal).

PROGNOSIS AND TREATMENT

- PAMRAGs are not associated with microbial organisms, and no treatment is needed.
- Misdiagnosis of a PAMRAG as a sulfur granule (actinomycotic granule) may lead to unnecessary treatment.

PATHOLOGY

HISTOLOGY

- PAMRAGs typically demonstrate radiant filamentous structures with blunted ends.
- The majority of PAMRAGs have a glassy, coarse eosinophilic appearance.

IMMUNOPATHOLOGY (INCLUDING IMMUNOHISTOCHEMISTRY)

- Special stains for organisms will be negative.
- Cultures of the IUD will be negative.

MAIN DIFFERENTIAL DIAGNOSIS

- Actinomycosis—here the fine detail of the organisms can be appreciated.

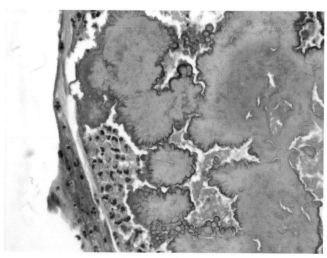

FIGURE 1

PAMRAG. Acellular, eosinophilic material with blunted ends characterizes this deposit, which is virtually exclusive to endometria with IUDs.

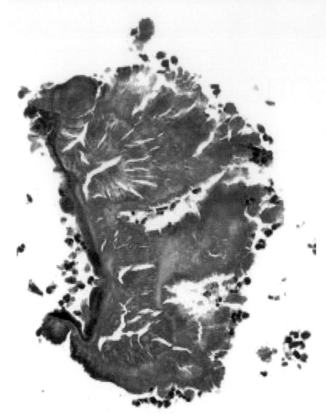

FIGURE 2

PAMRAG. *(From Crum CP, Nucci MR, Lee KR, editors: Diagnostic Gynecologic and Obstetric Pathology, ed 2, Philadelphia, 2011, Elsevier, Figure 16-30C.)*

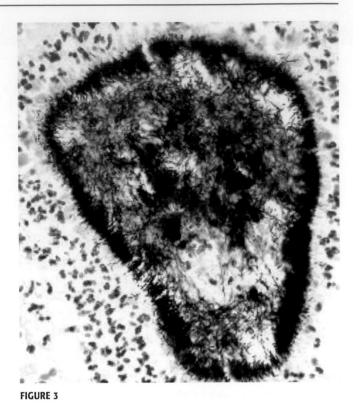

FIGURE 3

Actinomycosis for comparison. *(From Crum CP, Nucci MR, Lee KR, editors: Diagnostic Gynecologic and Obstetric Pathology, ed 2, Philadelphia, 2011, Elsevier, Figure 16-30B.)*

PYOMETRA

DEFINITION—Extensive necroinflammatory debris within the uterine cavity.

CLINICAL FEATURES

EPIDEMIOLOGY

- Overall rare (0.1% to 0.5% of women) but more commonly occurs in postmenopausal women.
- Associated with a wide range of disorders, including cervical stenosis, leiomyomata, retained IUD, and prior radiotherapy. There is a small but significant risk (5% to 10%) of associated malignancy

PRESENTATION

- Patients may be asymptomatic or present with abdominal pain with or without spotting. Additional symptoms/findings include nausea and uterine enlargement.

PROGNOSIS AND TREATMENT

- Management is based on either treating the infection or malignancy or hysterectomy. Resampling may be necessary if malignancy is a concern.

PATHOLOGY

HISTOLOGY

- Sampling reveals abundant neutrophilic inflammation, fragments of necrotic tissue, and superficial endometrium with features of repair.

IMMUNOPATHOLOGY (INCLUDING IMMUNOHISTOCHEMISTRY)

- Noncontributory.

MAIN DIFFERENTIAL DIAGNOSIS

- Endometrial carcinoma (must be ruled out). The most common conundrum is distinguishing reactive epithelial changes from malignant epithelium.

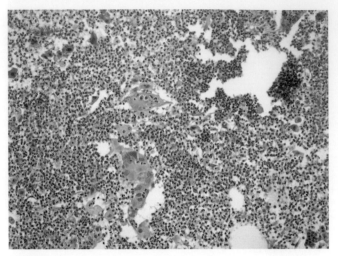

FIGURE 1

Pyometra. Sheets of neutrophils and scattered reactive, atypical epithelial cells.

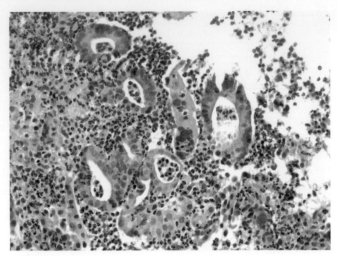

FIGURE 2

Pyometra. Reactive atypia may be marked.

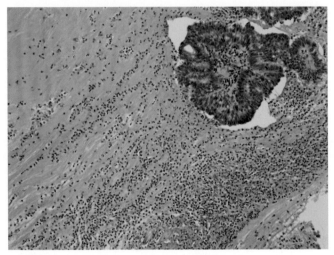

FIGURE 3

Pyometra. A dense neutrophilic infiltrate, note the adenocarcinoma in the upper right.

TUBERCULAR ENDOMETRITIS

DEFINITION—Infection of the uterus (endometrium) by *Mycobacterium tuberculosis*.

CLINICAL FEATURES

EPIDEMIOLOGY

- Involvement of the uterus by tuberculosis (TB) is exceedingly rare, due to modern treatment.
- Patients with uterine involvement often have systemic (or miliary) disease.
- Uterine involvement is most commonly seen in immunocompromised patients.

PRESENTATION

- Patients may present with systemic symptoms of illness.
- Abnormal uterine bleeding is common.

PROGNOSIS AND TREATMENT

- Prognosis is variable based on the immunologic state of the patient and the extent of their infection.
- Multiple-drug cocktails are typically used to treat systemic TB infection.
- Severe cases of granulomatous endometritis may require hysterectomy.

PATHOLOGY

HISTOLOGY

- Caseating granulomas may be identified in the endometrium or myometrium.

- The granuloma is composed of a central necrotic core, surrounded by multinucleated giant cells, lymphocytes, plasma cells, and histiocytes.
- Characteristic viral inclusions suggestive of cytomegalovirus or herpes should be sought for and be absent.

IMMUNOPATHOLOGY (INCLUDING IMMUNOHISTOCHEMISTRY)

- Special stains (AFB) are required for visualization of the mycobacteria.
- Corresponding PPD (skin test) may be helpful.

MAIN DIFFERENTIAL DIAGNOSIS

- Sarcoid—this may closely mimic TB. Granulomas should be nonnecrotic; however, special stains and other tests to exclude TB may be needed as clinically appropriate.
- Granulomatous endometritis following ablation—clinical history and other features of ablation (tissue necrosis) should be present.
- Microbial infections (cytomegalovirus, herpes virus, toxoplasmosis, schistosomiasis) should be excluded in the appropriate clinical setting.

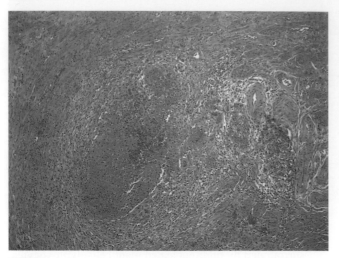

FIGURE 1

Uterine TB. A granuloma with a necrotic core surrounded by a mononuclear cell infiltrate.

FIGURE 2

Uterine TB. A dense rim of lymphohistiocytic inflammation can be seen surrounding the necrotic core *(right)*. *(Courtesy Matthew R. Lindberg, M.D.)*

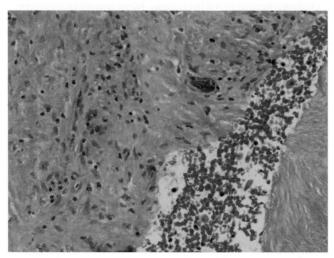

FIGURE 3

Uterine TB. Multinucleated giant cell and surrounding lymphohistiocytic inflammation. *(Courtesy Matthew R. Lindberg, M.D.)*

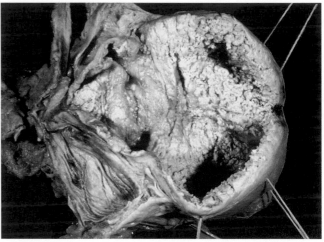

FIGURE 4

Gross pathology of endometrial tuberculosis with caseous necrosis filling the endometrial cavity. *(From Crum CP, Nucci MR, Lee KR, editors: Diagnostic Gynecologic and Obstetric Pathology, ed 2, Philadelphia, 2011, Elsevier.)*

SUBMUCOSAL LEIOMYOMA

DEFINITION—Attenuation of the functionalis due to compressing smooth muscle tumor.

CLINICAL FEATURES

EPIDEMIOLOGY

- Similar to uterine leiomyomas.
- Frequently associated with uterine polyps.

PRESENTATION

- Abnormal uterine bleeding is the most common presenting symptom.
- History of uterine leiomyomata.
- Appearance of a polyp on ultrasound or hysteroscopy.

PROGNOSIS AND TREATMENT

- Predicated on size and extent of bleeding.
- Hysteroscopic-guided removal is the preferred approach.

PATHOLOGY

HISTOLOGY

- The endometrial specimen contains a proliferative- or secretory-phase endometrium, with strips of surface functionalis showing a paucity of glands (aglandular functionalis).
- Reactive stromal changes with old hemorrhage may also be encountered if there has been prior endometrial injury with bleeding.

- Fragments of submucosal leiomyoma may or may not be present.

IMMUNOPATHOLOGY (INCLUDING IMMUNOHISTOCHEMISTRY)

- Noncontributory.

DIAGNOSTIC TERMINOLOGY

- Strips of aglandular functionalis, see comment.
- Comment: This finding is not diagnostic but can be seen with submucosal leiomyoma.

MAIN DIFFERENTIAL DIAGNOSIS

- Endometrial polyp—these may display aglandular functionalis.
- Progestin therapy—aglandular functionalis may be seen. For this reason, a diagnosis of possible submucosal leiomyoma should not be made in the setting of progestin therapy.
- Hormone replacement therapy, tamoxifen therapy, or menopausal endometrium—any scant endometrial sample will exhibit functionalis without glands.
- Endometrial stromal tumor—another cause of aglandular functionalis. Look for stromal cellularity and atypia.

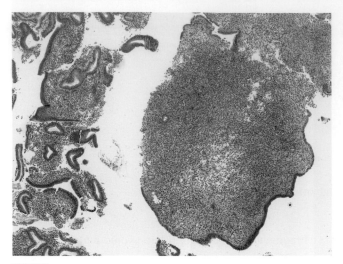

FIGURE 1

Strip of aglandular functionalis next to normal-appearing endometrium.

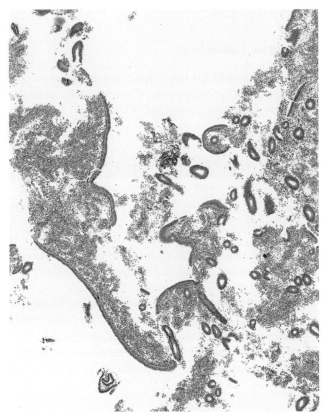

FIGURE 2

A strip of aglandular functionalis with proliferative endometrium on the right. This suggests a submucosal leiomyoma may be nearby.

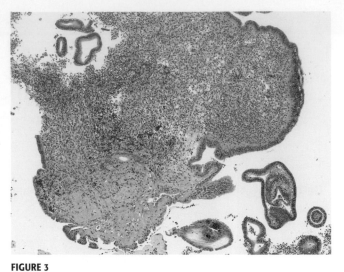

FIGURE 3

This fragment of aglandular functionalis displays some ischemic changes *(lower left)*.

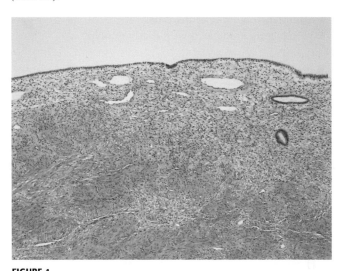

FIGURE 4

Leiomyoma-endometrial interface showing attenuated functionalis with few glands.

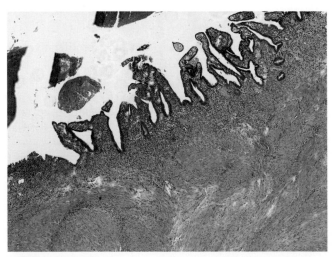

FIGURE 5

A fragment of endomyometrium with a submucosal leiomyoma. Note the unusual villiform reparative surface changes in the attenuated endometrium.

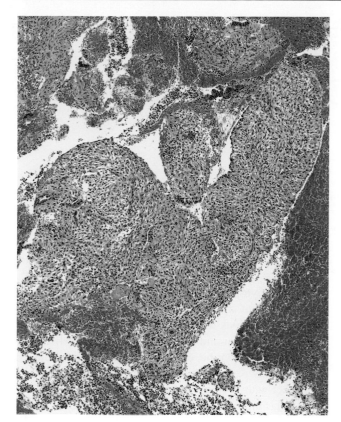

FIGURE 6

A fragment of aglandular functionalis associated with progestin therapy. This does not exclude a submucosal leiomyoma, but the latter cannot be confirmed on histology alone if the progestin has been administered for a prolonged period of time.

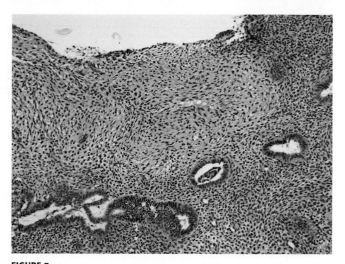

FIGURE 7

Aglandular functionalis associated with polyp.

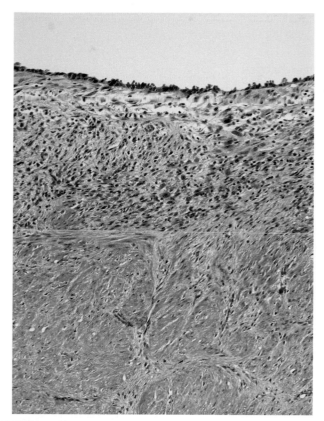

FIGURE 8

A thin strip of stromal sarcoma on the surface of a curetting fragment mimicking aglandular functionalis.

EXFOLIATION ARTIFACT

DEFINITION—A preservation artifact in the endometrial epithelium leading to epithelial discohesion and exfoliation.

CLINICAL FEATURES

EPIDEMIOLOGY

- Exfoliation artifact has been noted in association with hysteroscopic biopsies secondary to fluid instillation during the procedure.

PRESENTATION

- Found incidentally at the time of histologic examination of the endometrial tissue.

PROGNOSIS AND TREATMENT

- Exfoliation artifact carries no adverse outcome and requires no treatment.

PATHOLOGY

HISTOLOGY

- Superficial endometrial epithelium shows disaggregation, which leads to pseudomicropapillary clusters of epithelial cells protruding into the lumen.
- Occasionally the cells become "hobnailed" and mimic serous or clear-cell carcinoma. They may also mimic secretory epithelium due to the appearance of a nonlayered epithelium (due to exfoliated cells). However, the presence of mitoses will confirm the diagnosis of a proliferative-phase endometrium.
- The adjacent stroma typically reinforces the diagnosis, showing various degrees of preservation artifact, with indistinct nuclei and loosely disaggregated cells.
- Malignancy can be excluded based on the adjacent degenerative changes in the stroma, blending of the artifact with normal adjacent glands, a low nuclear-to-cytoplasmic ratio, and the absence of nuclear atypia.

IMMUNOPATHOLOGY (INCLUDING IMMUNOHISTOCHEMISTRY)

- A negative p53 stain may be helpful in cases in which serous carcinoma is a concern and should be normal.

MAIN DIFFERENTIAL DIAGNOSIS

- Secretory endometrium—some exfoliation artifacts in proliferative-phase endometrium will mimic secretory endometrium, but the presence of mitoses will distinguish.
- Clear-cell or serous carcinoma—these entities might be expected with prominent hobnail patterns due to disaggregation of the epithelial cells; however, with exfoliation artifact there should be no atypia.

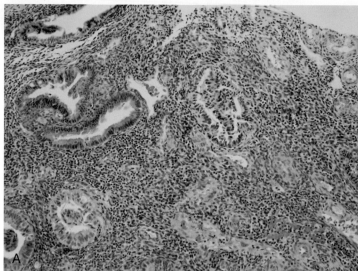
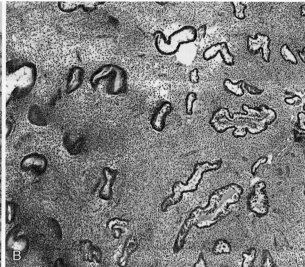

FIGURE 1A AND 1B

Exfoliation artifact. These lower-power images of the endometrium show a transition from well preserved glands to poorly preserved glands and stroma with disaggregated epithelial cells in the gland lumens. Note how in 1B the proliferative glands on the right appear secretory.

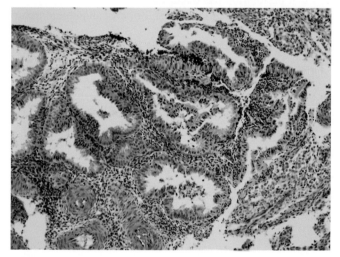
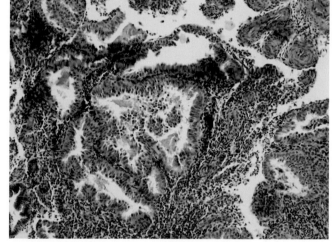

FIGURE 2

Exfoliation artifact. A cluster of endometrial glands with exfoliative epithelium. Note the somewhat poorly preserved stroma with mildly disaggregated cells and lightly staining nuclei.

FIGURE 3

Exfoliation artifact. Higher-power image of proliferative endometrium with luminal exfoliation.

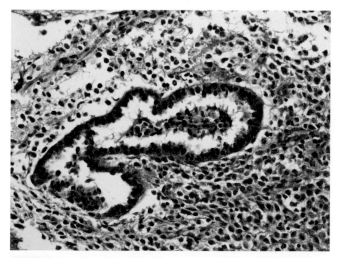
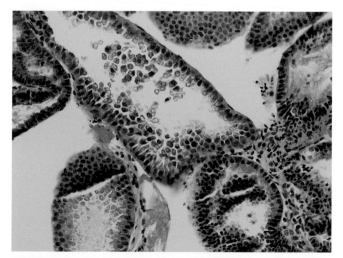

FIGURE 4

Exfoliation artifact in proliferative endometrium. Note the resemblance to secretory-phase endometrium.

FIGURE 5

Exfoliation artifact. The exfoliated cells in this gland exhibit a hobnail appearance and could be confused with serous intraepithelial carcinoma.

PERFORATION

DEFINITION—Perforation of the uterus, usually during endometrial sampling.

CLINICAL FEATURES

EPIDEMIOLOGY

- Perforation is a rare complication of endometrial sampling.

PRESENTATION

- Clinical suspicion of perforation may or may not be present.
- Pathologic evidence of perforation may be the first sign.
- Patients may be asymptomatic (usually) or present with an "acute abdomen."

PROGNOSIS AND TREATMENT

- The prognosis is variable.
- Cases with perforation range from asymptomatic to surgical emergencies.
- Repair of the defect or hysterectomy may be indicated based on severity.

PATHOLOGY

HISTOLOGY

- Typically the presence of adipose tissue is the indication that perforation has occurred.
- Occasionally bladder, bowel, or other abdominal tissue may be identified.

IMMUNOPATHOLOGY (INCLUDING IMMUNOHISTOCHEMISTRY)

- S100 will be positive in adipose tissue, differentiating adipose tissue from fatlike spaces in blood clot.

MAIN DIFFERENTIAL DIAGNOSIS

- Blood clot with artifactual fatlike spaces.

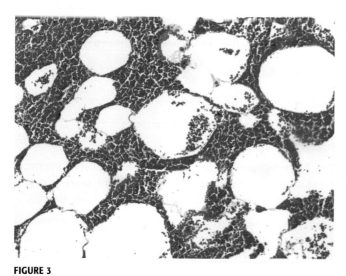

FIGURE 1

Uterine perforation. Adipose tissue adjacent to an endometrial polyp.

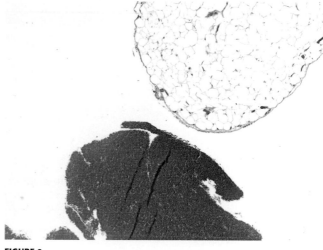

FIGURE 2

Uterine perforation. Blood clot and adipose tissue.

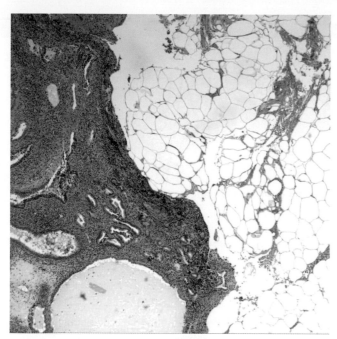

FIGURE 3

Blood clot as a mimic of uterine perforation. The lack of adipocyte nuclei is helpful in identifying fatlike spaces. Note the variability in size and shape of the spaces.

ABLATION ARTIFACT

DEFINITION—Morphologic changes secondary to medical therapy that destroys the endometrial lining.

CLINICAL FEATURES

EPIDEMIOLOGY

- Seen in patients who undergo endometrial ablation for dysfunctional uterine bleeding.

PRESENTATION

- Found during sampling of the uterus after ablative therapy.

PROGNOSIS AND TREATMENT

- The most common consequence of ablation is a perplexed pathologist who may not be aware that ablation had been previously attempted. We occasionally see ablation artifact in uteri without a clinical history.
- Occasionally a curetting performed at the time of ablation may show an abnormality, which may lead to hysterectomy and a specimen with ablation artifact.

PATHOLOGY

HISTOLOGY

- Following ablation the endometrial lining becomes necrotic and "devitalized" then hyalinized.
- "Ghosted" endometrial glands may be present.
- Deep endometrial glands (endometrial basalis) may be viable in occasional cases.
- A prominent giant cell reaction may be present.

IMMUNOPATHOLOGY (INCLUDING IMMUNOHISTOCHEMISTRY)

- Noncontributory.

MAIN DIFFERENTIAL DIAGNOSIS

- Necrotic endometrial polyps or submucosal leiomyomas can be impossible to distinguish from necrotic endomyometrium, but the clinical history will be helpful.

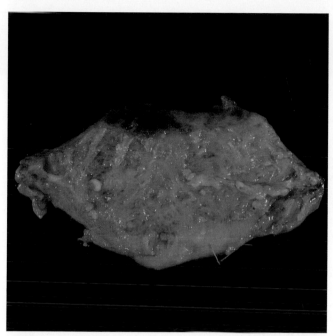

FIGURE 1

Endometrial ablation artifact. Gross image of endometrium and myometrium after ablation. Note the absence of abundant functionalis and the mottled appearance consistent with coexisting hemorrhage.

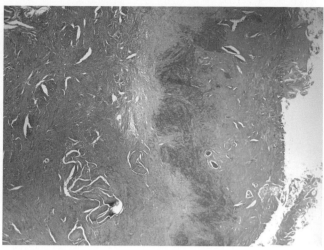

FIGURE 2

Endometrial ablation artifact. Necrosis and extensive hyaline change involving the endometrium.

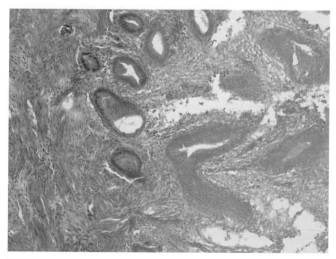

FIGURE 3

Endometrial ablation artifact. Necrotic or "ghosted" endometrial glands on the right. Note the presence of histologically recognizable, deep endometrial glands on the left.

ENDOMETRIAL INTRAEPITHELIAL NEOPLASIA (ATYPICAL HYPERPLASIA)

DEFINITION—A premalignant clonal expansion of altered endometrial glands.

CLINICAL FEATURES

EPIDEMIOLOGY

- Endometrial intraepithelial neoplasia (EIN) is relatively common and carries an increased risk of development of type 1 endometrial adenocarcinoma.
- Women with excess estrogen (whether exogenous or endogenous) are at increased risk.
- Because of the production of excess estrogens, obese women are at an increased risk.
- Patients with hereditary nonpolyposis colorectal cancer (HNPCC) (Lynch syndrome) and Cowden syndrome are at an increased risk.
- Patients taking tamoxifen are at an increased risk of the development of EIN.

PRESENTATION

- Patients typically present with abnormal or postmenopausal uterine bleeding.

PROGNOSIS AND TREATMENT

- EIN carries 46-fold increased risk of concurrent or future adenocarcinoma.
- In women who do not wish to preserve fertility, hysterectomy is the treatment of choice.
- Patients desiring fertility or poor surgical candidates may undergo hormonal therapy with progestins, although some patients may not respond.

PATHOLOGY

HISTOLOGY

- The accurate diagnosis of EIN requires fulfillment of the following histologic criteria:
  1. Area of the glands exceeds that of the endometrial stroma. This does not apply toward cystically dilated, atrophic glands and in glands with squamous morular metaplasia.
  2. Altered cytologic features of the crowded focus of glands. No fixed features defining nuclear atypia are utilized in the diagnosis of EIN; instead, cytologic demarcation of the "atypical" glands from the background "normal" endometrial glands should be sought.
  3. The size of the focus of crowded glands must exceed 1 mm (not including scattered, cytologically altered glands). Lesions failing to meet these criteria are best given a descriptive diagnosis and follow-up is recommended.
  4. The exclusion of benign mimics of EIN (including polyps, metaplasia, endometrial basalis, repair, telescoping, and fragmentation artifact).
  5. The exclusion of low-grade adenocarcinoma.
- Several recognizable patterns of glandular alteration have been described including
  - Intraglandular papillary formations
  - EIN with extensive mucinous differentiation
  - EIN with secretory differentiation
  - EIN with squamous morular metaplasia
  - EIN with eosinophilic or tubal metaplasia

- In cases of suspected EIN arising within an endometrial polyp, comparison with the "background" glands within the polyp is required as all glands in a polyp may be altered compared with the nonpolyp endometrium.

PREFERRED DIAGNOSTIC TERMINOLOGY

- EIN (atypical hyperplasia).

IMMUNOPATHOLOGY (INCLUDING IMMUNOHISTOCHEMISTRY)

- Loss of PTEN and PAX2 has been described in EIN and endometrial adenocarcinoma; however, reliance on these markers over histologic criteria is not recommended.

MAIN DIFFERENTIAL DIAGNOSIS

- Reactive epithelial changes (repair) occur on the endometrial surface and are degenerative in nature. They must be distinguished though from surface growth of an EIN.
- Gland compression or telescoping artifact due to procedure effect. The glands are folded and compressed in the gland tract but are not altered cytologically.
- Benign hyperplasia may show crowding but no discrete cytologically altered population.
- Secretory endometrium can contain crowded glands and mild variations in cytologic appearance. A key discriminator is the normalcy of the secretory maturation as opposed to EIN.
- Endometrial polyps will show some gland heterogeneity and minor gland crowding.
- Endometrial breakdown will push glands together.
- Endometrioid adenocarcinoma must fulfill the criteria including one of the following: loss of gland integrity, papillary architecture, cytologic atypia (beware serous intramucosal [intraepithelial] carcinomas!).
- Gland crowding with altered cytologic can occur in very small foci, in which case a repeat sample is advised.

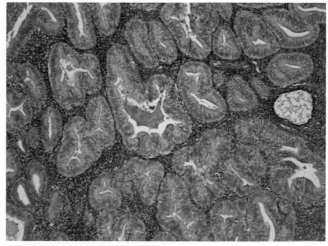

FIGURE 1

EIN. Crowded endometrial glands that are cytologically altered when compared with the cystic gland on the right.

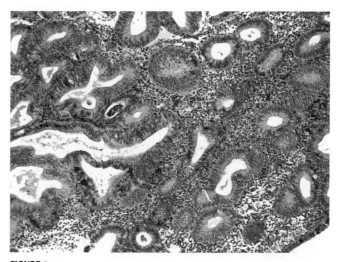

FIGURE 2

EIN. Note the interspersed, cytologically normal glands.

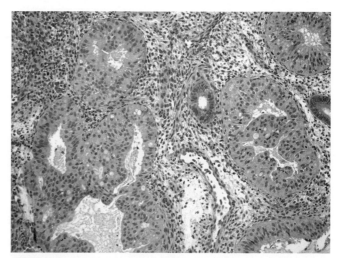

FIGURE 3

EIN. Increased intraglandular complexity justifies the diagnosis of EIN, even in the absence of crowding.

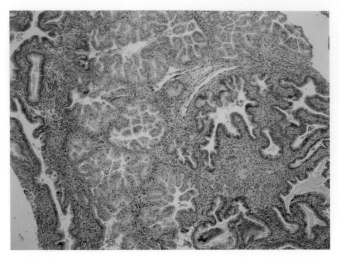

FIGURE 4

EIN. Crowded glands with extensive intraglandular papillae formation. Note the sharp cytologic demarcation between the background and EIN-containing glands.

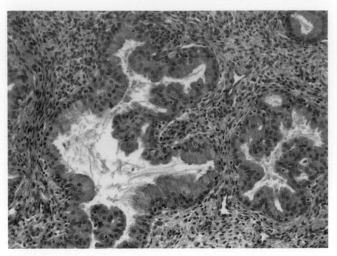

FIGURE 5

EIN. Mucinous metaplasia within EIN. Note the small papillary tufts.

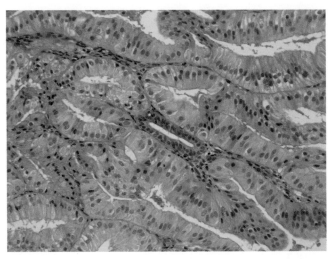

FIGURE 6

EIN. Eosinophilic EIN, with a single, entrapped background gland *(center)*.

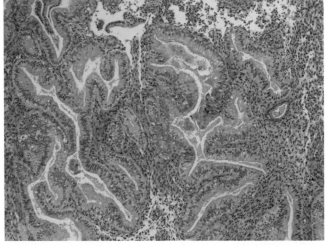

FIGURE 7

EIN. Secretory EIN denoted by scattered cytoplasmic vacuoles. A normal gland can be seen on the right.

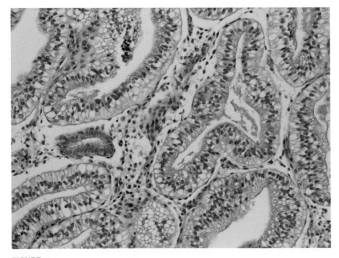

FIGURE 8

EIN. Secretory EIN with extensive vacuole formation.

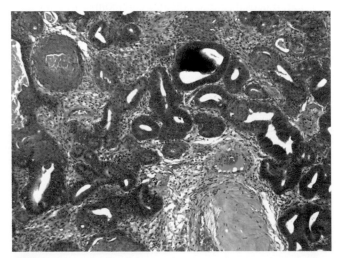

FIGURE 9

EIN. Squamous morular metaplasia within a focus of EIN.

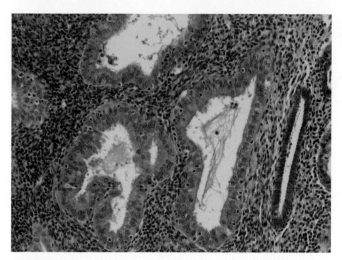

FIGURE 10

EIN. Tubal metaplasia within a focus of EIN. Note the normal gland on the right.

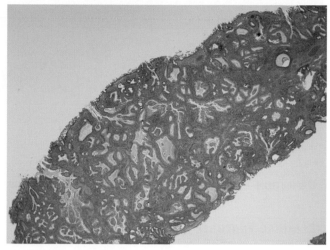

FIGURE 11

EIN. Low-power view of an endometrial polyp containing EIN. Intraglandular papillary tufts are prominent.

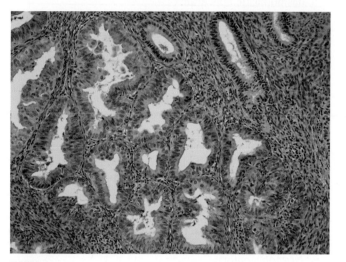

FIGURE 12

EIN. A higher-power view of the polyp in Figure 11. Cytologic demarcation can be seen between the EIN *(left)* and the background glands *(right)*.

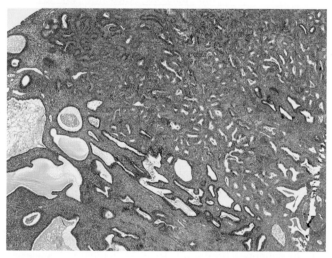

FIGURE 13

Another polyp showing crowded altered glands *(upper)*.

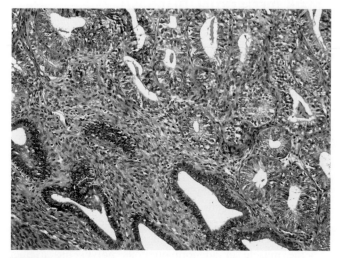

FIGURE 14

Note the sharp contrast between the normal glands *(lower)* and EIN.

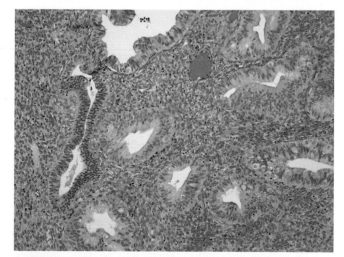

FIGURE 15

Small foci of gland crowding and altered cytology may not fulfill the criteria for EIN, but must be followed with a repeat sample since the risk of EIN on follow-up approaches 25%.

ATYPICAL POLYPOID ADENOMYOMA

DEFINITION—A polypoid neoplasm composed of atypical glands and smooth muscle stroma.

CLINICAL FEATURES

EPIDEMIOLOGY

- Atypical polypoid adenomyomas (APAs) are rare neoplasms.
- Typically seen in the fifth decade.

PRESENTATION

- Patients present with abnormal uterine bleeding or may be asymptomatic.

PROGNOSIS AND TREATMENT

- APAs appear to carry a very low risk of adverse outcome.
- However, they may be difficult at times to distinguish from adenocarcinomas and thus have a guarded prognosis.
- In patients who do not desire hysterectomy, conservative excision has been undertaken with pregnancy outcomes. However, complete removal of these tumors may be difficult because of their sessile nature.

PATHOLOGY

HISTOLOGY

- APAs typically appear as sessile, broad-based polyps. Some may be more pedunculated, others ensconced in the endomyometrium.
- Glands tend to be regular in appearance with mild atypia, consistent with those seen in endometrial intraepithelial neoplasia.
- Well-defined squamous morules are virtually always present and usually abundant and regularly distributed throughout the tumor. There will be rare instances, however, when they will be absent, in which case the distinction between APA and an adenomyomatous polyp may be difficult.

- The glandular complexity may border on well-differentiated adenocarcinoma, and in some cases foci indistinguishable from adenocarcinoma may be present.
- The stroma is a key feature and should be composed of regular fascicles of smooth muscle without a fibrotic or desmoplastic appearance.
- In many cases the smooth muscle stroma may blend imperceptibly with the myometrium.

DIAGNOSTIC TERMINOLOGY

- Atypical polypoid adenomyoma. (Clinician should be made aware that although not considered malignant, APA may nonetheless recur and develop considerable atypia that may make it difficult to distinguish from malignancy. Thus it should be monitored by repeated sampling if preservation of childbearing potential is desired.)

IMMUNOPATHOLOGY (INCLUDING IMMUNOHISTOCHEMISTRY)

- Noncontributory.

MAIN DIFFERENTIAL DIAGNOSIS

- Endometrial intraepithelial neoplasia (atypical hyperplasia) does not exhibit myomatous stroma.
- Well-differentiated adenocarcinoma (with myometrial invasion)—this may be difficult to exclude and if not, should be mentioned in the report.
- Adenomyomas are often encountered in the myometrium. The glands are not atypical, and squamous morules are not seen.
- Adenomyomatous polyps do not typically display squamous morules. They can, however, and the distinction from APA depends somewhat on whether the polyp is pedunculated or sessile. APA also tends to exhibit large well-developed fascicles of smooth muscle, whereas the muscle in adenomyomatous polyps has a finer consistency.

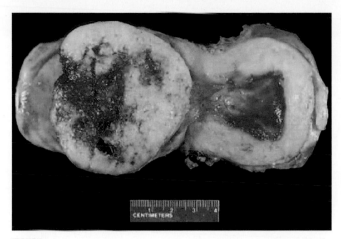

FIGURE 1

APA. A discrete mass in the lower uterine segment occludes the endometrial cavity.

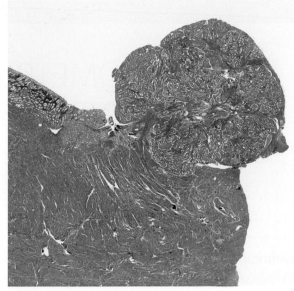

FIGURE 2

APA. This small lesion presents as a polyp.

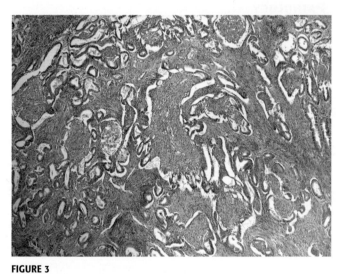

FIGURE 3

APA. Numerous glands with extensive squamous morular metaplasia. Note the smooth muscle stroma.

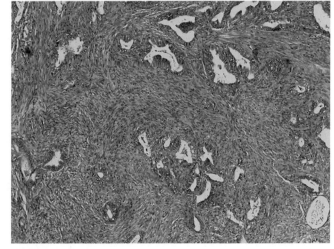

FIGURE 4

APA. Scattered glands separated by well-defined fascicles of smooth muscle. Note the absence of a desmoplastic stromal change.

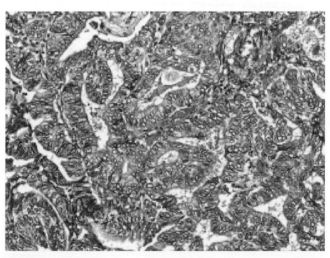

FIGURE 5

Proliferation in an APA may resemble an adenocarcinoma.

ENDOMETRIAL INVOLVEMENT BY ENDOCERVICAL GLANDULAR NEOPLASIA

DEFINITION—Involvement of the endometrium by endocervical glandular neoplasia, either by direct extension or by contamination during sampling.

CLINICAL FEATURES

EPIDEMIOLOGY

- True endometrial involvement (direct extension) by endocervical adenocarcinoma is rare.
- Not uncommonly, endometrial biopsies in patients with endocervical neoplasia may contain fragments of endocervical adenocarcinoma.

PRESENTATION

- Patients present with signs and symptoms of cervical adenocarcinoma, typically abnormal spotting or bleeding and pain.
- Patients may be asymptomatic or present with atypical glandular cells on Pap smear.

PROGNOSIS AND TREATMENT

- True endometrial extension of endocervical adenocarcinoma denotes a higher-stage disease and thus has a more adverse outcome (vs. localized endocervical disease).
- Artifactual contamination of an endometrial biopsy does not increase the surgical stage and is not associated with an adverse outcome.
- Treatment of endocervical adenocarcinoma consists of a radical hysterectomy (or trachelectomy) with or without lymph node dissection.
- Adjuvant therapy may be indicated in advanced cases of invasive carcinoma.

PATHOLOGY

HISTOLOGY

- Tumor fragments will display histologic features similar to those seen in endocervical adenocarcinoma, including pseudostratification, apical mitotic figures, and apoptotic debris.
- The presence of stromal plasma cells may be helpful in indicating a cervical primary.
- Well-defined, crisp, glandular contours are more commonly seen in endocervical primaries, whereas endometrial primaries have less well-defined, punched-out glands.
- Stromal foam cells are more commonly seen in endometrial primaries.

IMMUNOPATHOLOGY (INCLUDING IMMUNOHISTOCHEMISTRY)

- p16 will show strong, diffuse positivity in endocervical adenocarcinoma versus patchy staining in low-grade endometrial adenocarcinoma.
- Vimentin is negative in endocervical adenocarcinoma and positive in a pericellular (piano-key) fashion in endometrial adenocarcinoma.
- ER and PR are diffusely positive in low-grade endometrial adenocarcinoma and typically negative (or only focally positive) in endocervical primaries.
- CEA is positive in cervical lesions and negative in endometrial primaries.

MAIN DIFFERENTIAL DIAGNOSIS

- Low-grade endometrioid adenocarcinoma—this can be distinguished histologically by the more pseudostratified appearance of endometrioid neoplasia and the greater hyperchromasia seen in the endocervical neoplasm, often with coarse chromatin, apical mitoses, and mucin production. A p16 immunostain will be diffusely positive in the endocervical neoplasm.

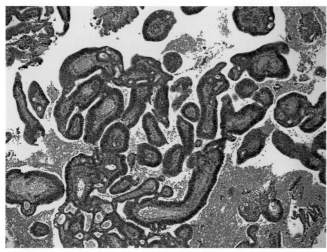

FIGURE 1

Endometrial involvement by endocervical adenocarcinoma. Predominantly papillary growth of endocervical adenocarcinoma in an endometrial biopsy.

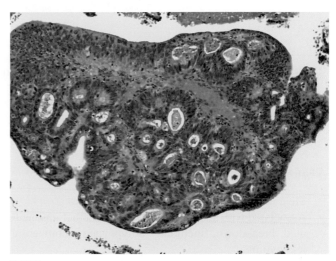

FIGURE 3

Endometrial involvement by endocervical adenocarcinoma. Endocervical adenocarcinoma; note the well-circumscribed, "punched-out," glandular spaces.

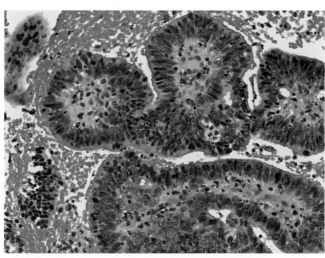

FIGURE 2

Endometrial involvement by endocervical adenocarcinoma. Endocervical adenocarcinoma displaying apical mitoses, pseudostratified nuclei, and apoptotic debris.

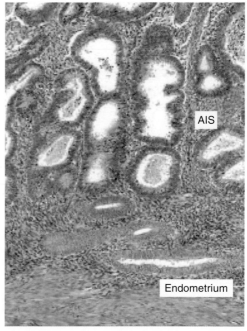

FIGURE 4

Endometrial involvement by adenocarcinoma in situ (AIS). The lesion is in the functionalis, replacing the glands *(left)*. Normal basal endometrium is on the right.

DEGENERATIVE REPAIR

DEFINITION—Degenerative changes of the surface epithelium associated with breakdown and ischemia.

CLINICAL FEATURES

EPIDEMIOLOGY

- Most commonly occurs in the fifth decade.
- Associated with anovulatory bleeding or other unscheduled breakdown, including polyps and submucosal leiomyomas.

PRESENTATION

- Typically in curettings for abnormal uterine bleeding.

PROGNOSIS AND TREATMENT

- Considered benign. Management is predicated on the underlying disturbance.

PATHOLOGY

HISTOLOGY

- Admixed blue clusters of degenerating stroma and epithelium.

- Pseudopapillary architecture, absence of gland differentiation.
- Ill-defined, slit-forming spaces between epithelial cells with a low nuclear-to-cytoplasmic (N/C) ratio.
- Exuberant reparative changes (papillary syncytial metaplasia) occasionally seen.

IMMUNOPATHOLOGY (INCLUDING IMMUNOHISTOCHEMISTRY)

- Noncontributory.

MAIN DIFFERENTIAL DIAGNOSIS

- Endometrial intraepithelial neoplasia (EIN) and adenocarcinoma—both might exhibit some degree of surface or intraglandular papillary changes. The latter should always raise suspicion for malignancy. The surface changes typically will be both multilayered and microacinar in some fashion, too complex for a degenerative or simple proliferative process.
- Proliferative repair—pseudostratification is the rule, with a picture of healthy appearing mucosa. A regenerative rather than degenerative process.

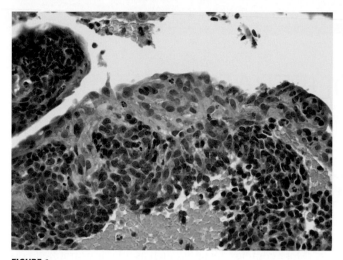

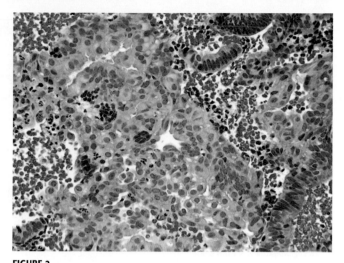

FIGURE 1

Degenerative repair associated with breakdown.

FIGURE 2

Degenerative repair with mild stratified appearance. Note the absence of any true papillary or glandlike architecture.

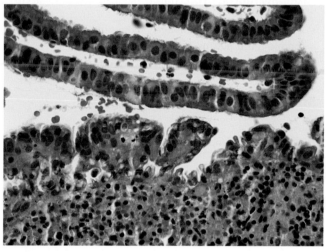

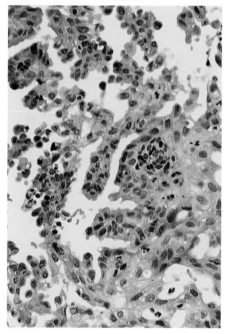

FIGURE 3

Degenerative epithelial changes associated with necrotic polyp.

FIGURE 4

Exaggerated repair (papillary syncytial metaplasia) associated with breakdown.

PROLIFERATIVE REPAIR

DEFINITION—Surface changes in the endometrium associated with breakdown and injury.

CLINICAL FEATURES

EPIDEMIOLOGY

- Most commonly occurs in the fifth decade associated with endometrial breakdown or injury (submucosal leiomyoma or polyp).

PRESENTATION

- Typically abnormal uterine bleeding; however, patients may be asymptomatic.

PROGNOSIS AND TREATMENT

- Considered a benign condition.
- Management is tailored to the underlying cause of the bleeding (submucosal leiomyoma, polyp, altered cycle).

PATHOLOGY

HISTOLOGY

- Surface changes characterized primarily by multilayered epithelium with pseudostratified appearance.

- Tubal or mucinous metaplasia is not uncommon.
- More complex features, such as a highly stratified epithelium or true papillary or microacinar architecture, should not be present, but proliferative repair could coexist with these features in cases of neoplasia.

IMMUNOPATHOLOGY (INCLUDING IMMUNOHISTOCHEMISTRY)

- Noncontributory, although stains for p53 might be employed if serous neoplasia is suspected.

MAIN DIFFERENTIAL DIAGNOSIS

- Endometrial neoplasia—either adenocarcinoma or endometrial intraepithelial neoplasia (EIN) will display more complex surface epithelial architecture.
- Reactive epithelial changes—these will be characterized by nuclear enlargement and some hyperchromasia.

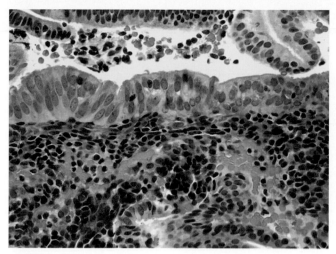

FIGURE 1

Proliferative surface epithelial changes associated with breakdown. Mild changes resemble tubal metaplasia.

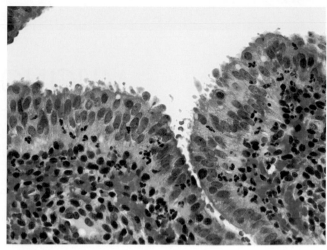

FIGURE 2

Proliferative surface epithelial changes associated with breakdown. Pseudostratified epithelial changes.

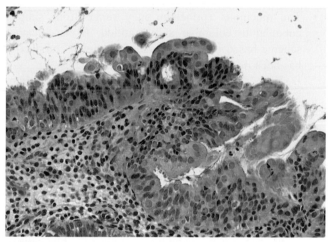

FIGURE 3

Complex "metaplastic" surface changes with stratified appearance and glandlike structures associated with endometrial adenocarcinoma.

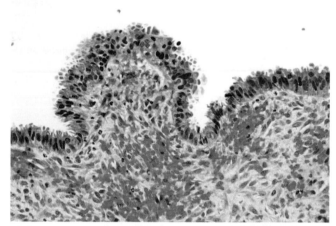

FIGURE 4

Another example of "proliferative repair," possibly overlying a submucosal leiomyoma and bordering on reactive epithelial changes.

MUCINOUS METAPLASIA OF THE ENDOMETRIUM

DEFINITION—Change of the epithelium of the endometrium to a mucinous phenotype.

CLINICAL FEATURES

EPIDEMIOLOGY

- Most commonly occurs in the perimenopausal to post-menopausal years.
- Papillary and microglandular forms are associated with a significantly increased risk of a coexisting endometrioid adenocarcinoma.

PRESENTATION

- Typically abnormal uterine bleeding; however, patients may be asymptomatic.

PROGNOSIS AND TREATMENT

- Simple, nonstratified (or at most tufting) surface mucinous metaplasia is not significantly associated with an increased cancer risk and may be followed up routinely.
- Any intraglandular mucinous epithelium with stratification or tufting should be viewed as a possible endometrial intraepithelial neoplasia (EIN).
- Mucinous metaplasia with well-developed stromal cores or possessing microglandular or microacinar architecture should be treated according to EIN-hyperplasia protocols.
- True *intestinal* mucinous metaplasia (or rarely gastric metaplasia) of the endometrium is rare and may be found in isolation. The risk of malignancy is unknown, and follow-up is required.

PATHOLOGY

HISTOLOGY

- The mucinous epithelium may range from simple, cuboidal to columnar and stratified. A classification scheme based on the amount of epithelial complexity has been described:
  - Type A—cuboidal, endocervical-like epithelium involving the surface of polyps or glands.
  - Type B—mild, increased complexity with pseudo-papillary formations.
  - Type C—cribriform mucinous epithelium or free-floating mucinous epithelium with microglandular or villous architecture (discussed in greater detail under microglandular variants of endometrioid adenocarcinoma in the following).
- A rare variant of intestinal-type mucinous metaplasia has been identified by the presence of goblet cells or intracytoplasmic *O*-acetylated sialomucins (which may be seen in the absence of morphologic evidence of intestinal metaplasia).

IMMUNOPATHOLOGY (INCLUDING IMMUNOHISTOCHEMISTRY)

- Noncontributory.

MAIN DIFFERENTIAL DIAGNOSIS

- Endocervical microglandular hyperplasia—look for reserve cells, cervical stroma, etc.

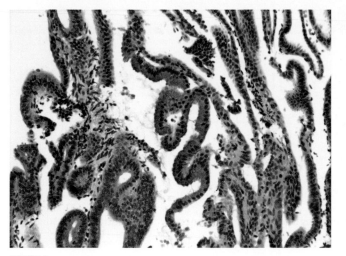

FIGURE 1

Mucinous metaplasia. Type A mucinous metaplasia consisting of a single layer of mucinous epithelium. This does not require further action.

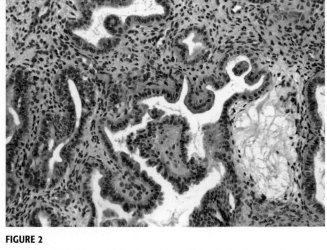

FIGURE 2

An endometrial polyp with focal mucinous differentiation in a papillary structure (Type B mucinous metaplasia). These changes can be managed with a follow-up office endometrial sampling if there are clinical concerns.

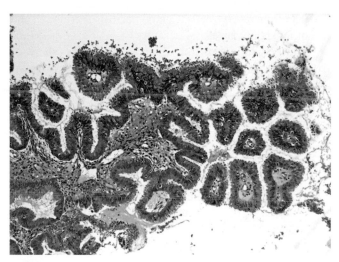

FIGURE 3

Mucinous metaplasia. Increased complexity with small papillae. This should be managed with follow-up sampling to exclude EIN or a subtle adenocarcinoma.

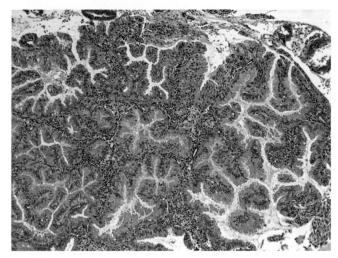

FIGURE 4

Mucinous metaplasia. True papillae with mucinous metaplasia in the background of an endometrial polyp. Followup sampling is needed.

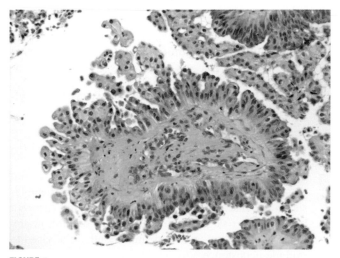

FIGURE 5

Mucinous differentiation. This surface change is associated with an obvious papillary structure with a stromal core. This requires close follow-up with repeat sampling to exclude neoplasia.

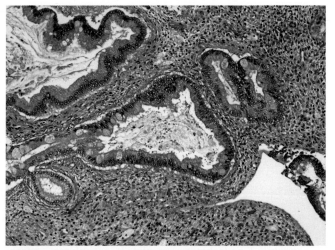

FIGURE 6

Mucinous metaplasia. A rare example of intestinal-type mucinous metaplasia displaying occasional goblet cells. This may be benign but should be followed with repeat sampling to exclude neoplasia.

SQUAMOUS AND MORULAR METAPLASIA

DEFINITION—Partial or complete replacement of an endometrial gland tract by a generally nonkeratinizing squamous metaplasia.

CLINICAL FEATURES

PATHOGENESIS

- Squamous morules are seen at all ages, mostly in the fifth decade.
- Can be isolated, associated with minor gland proliferations, seen with endometrial intraepithelial neoplasia (EIN) and cancers.

PRESENTATION

- Patients may be asymptomatic or present with abnormal uterine bleeding.
- Commonly seen in association with otherwise normal-appearing cyclic endometrium.

PROGNOSIS AND TREATMENT

- Risk of developing an adenocarcinoma with isolated morules or morules accompanied by mild gland proliferations is low (less than 5%). High rate of resolution on follow-up sampling.
- Risk of carcinoma increases to 20% when morules are associated with EIN.
- Treatment ranges from repeat sampling when EIN is not present to hysterectomy or hormonal therapy when EIN is present.

PATHOLOGY

HISTOLOGY

- Morules consist of well-demarcated if somewhat irregularly shaped aggregates of uniform nonkeratinizing squamoid cells having an almost granuloma appearance. They typically are found in the center of (or entirely replace) glands and unlike conventional cervical squamous metaplasia appear often to arise by direct transdifferentiation from glandular epithelium rather than from reserve cells. Central necrosis is common and of no significance.
- Morules fall into four general categories short of adenocarcinoma:
  1. Isolated morules without appreciable glandular proliferation. These carry a low risk of progression and are managed by a follow-up sampling.
  2. Morules associated with mild glandular proliferation. In contrast to EIN, these glands do not differ appreciably from the surrounding proliferative endometrium. The glands may form a ringlet or garland around the morule. Like the first category the risk of carcinoma on follow-up is no more than 5%.
  3. Morules associated with EIN, with a 20% or higher risk of adenocarcinoma.
  4. Confluent morular metaplasia without visible EIN or adenocarcinoma. These can be diagnostically confusing, and a careful search for EIN is necessary. However, if not present, they are simply designated as extensive morular metaplasia.

IMMUNOPATHOLOGY (INCLUDING IMMUNOHISTOCHEMISTRY)

- Squamous metaplasia shows some positivity for p63.
- Morules are hormonally inert, as shown by their typically negative staining for ER and PR.

DIAGNOSTIC TERMINOLOGY

- Morular metaplasia (if isolated or accompanied by mild gland proliferation) with a comment: Morular metaplasia, in the absence of EIN, often resolves and carries a low (~5%) risk of adenocarcinoma on follow-up. However, a follow-up sample in 6 months is advised to exclude persistence.
- EIN with morular metaplasia (if associated with EIN).

Main Differential Diagnosis

- Other forms of squamous metaplasia associated with chronic endometritis (morular metaplasia may be associated with plasma cells).
- Endometrial adenocarcinoma with squamous metaplasia. If bizarre keratinization is seen, this must be excluded.

- Squamous carcinoma or high-grade adenocarcinoma with a predominantly squamous component is usually easily distinguished. Nevertheless, any squamous differentiation on the surface of the endometrium requires excluding this entity, inasmuch as even the most malignant squamous lesions can harbor deceptively benign foci.
- Occasionally, cohesive clusters of macrophages will mimic morules.

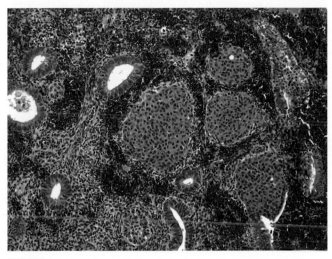

FIGURE 1

Isolated squamous morules. These often resolve on follow-up.

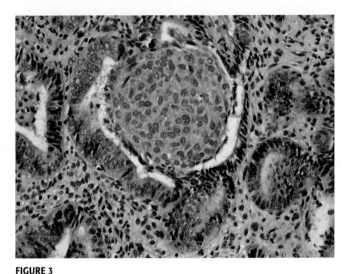

FIGURE 3

Higher magnification of a squamous morule. Note the bland cytology and collar of normal-appearing glandular epithelium.

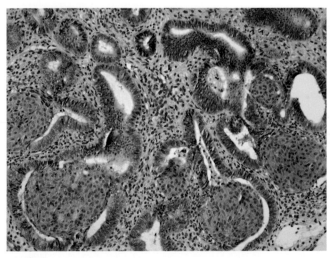

FIGURE 2

Squamous morules in the center of gland tracts. Note the mild degree of adjacent gland cell proliferation and lack of appreciable change in gland cytology relative to normal proliferative endometrium.

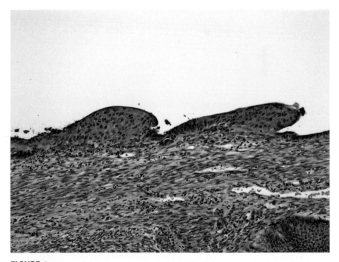

FIGURE 4

Superficial squamous metaplasia in a case of squamous morules.

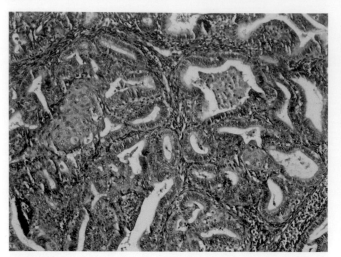

FIGURE 5

Near back-to-back glands with morular metaplasia (EIN). This form of EIN often differs somewhat from usual EIN by a lesser degree of cytologic demarcation relative to the adjacent endometrium. However, the level of gland density warrants a diagnosis of EIN.

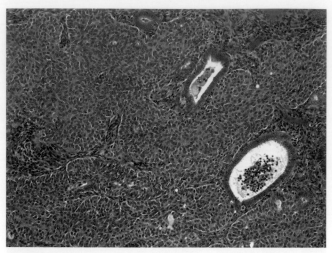

FIGURE 6

Confluent morular metaplasia. Note the absence of any visible EIN or adenocarcinoma. Nevertheless, caution is advised in managing this and additional sampling warranted.

ICHTHYOSIS UTERI

DEFINITION—Extensive, superficial endometrial squamous (nonmorular) metaplasia.

CLINICAL FEATURES

EPIDEMIOLOGY

- Ichthyosis uteri is rare. It is seen in patients with long-standing irritation of the endometrium (intrauterine device [IUD] or chronic endometritis). In postmenopausal patients care should be exercised in order to exclude concurrent adenocarcinoma.

PRESENTATION

- Patients may be asymptomatic or present with abnormal uterine bleeding.

PROGNOSIS AND TREATMENT

- Ichthyosis uteri is a benign condition; however, whenever a deceptively bland-appearing squamous epithelium is seen on the endometrial surface, an associated adenocarcinoma must be excluded. Removal of the irritant may lead to reversal. In cases clinically or histologically worrisome for carcinoma, hysterectomy may be necessary.

PATHOLOGY

HISTOLOGY

- Confluent, superficial squamous metaplasia, usually with striking differentiation and sometimes hyperkeratosis. Additional features that may be seen include large cysts, necrosis, and acute inflammation. The process may extend into the myometrium. Squamous cell carcinoma and adenocarcinoma should be searched for and excluded in every case.

IMMUNOPATHOLOGY (INCLUDING IMMUNOHISTOCHEMISTRY)

- Markers for squamous differentiation will be positive, but stains are not necessary.

MAIN DIFFERENTIAL DIAGNOSIS

- Squamous cell carcinoma of the endometrium (rare).
- Endometrial adenocarcinoma with squamous differentiation—this must always be excluded although the squamous differentiation will usually be more bizarre (but not always).
- Involvement of the endometrium by squamous cell carcinoma of the cervix—unlikely if the squamous differentiation is not atypical. Paradoxically normal-appearing squamous differentiation in the endometrium is the property of endometrial carcinomas.

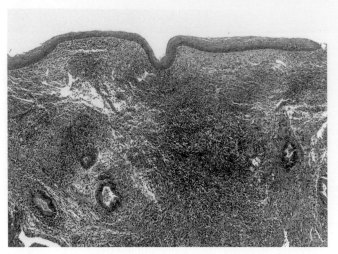

FIGURE 1

Ichthyosis uteri. Low-power view showing bland, confluent squamous metaplasia of the endometrium.

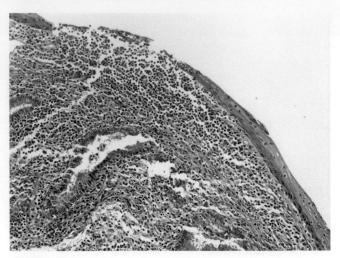

FIGURE 2

Ichthyosis uteri. Confluent squamous metaplasia of the superficial endometrium overlying endometrial glands and stroma with marked inflammation.

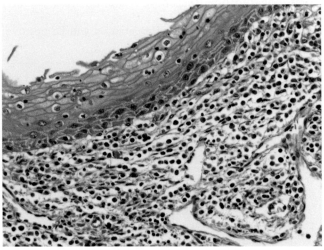

FIGURE 3

Ichthyosis uteri. Squamous metaplasia and an underlying, intense chronic inflammatory infiltrate.

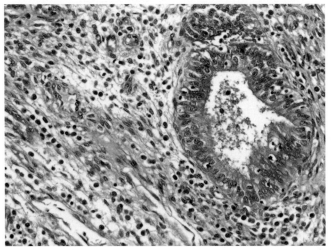

FIGURE 4

Ichthyosis uteri. An endometrial gland and stroma with marked chronic inflammation with numerous plasma cells seen in a case of ichthyosis uteri.

SQUAMOUS CARCINOMA OF THE ENDOMETRIUM

DEFINITION—An endometrial malignancy composed almost entirely of squamous carcinoma.

CLINICAL FEATURES

EPIDEMIOLOGY

- Rare, comprises less than 1% of uterine endometrial carcinomas.
- Most commonly occurs in postmenopausal women in their seventh and eighth decades.
- Usually not associated with human papillomavirus (HPV), although rare reports have linked HPV to some cases.

PRESENTATION

- Seen in endometrial curettings or biopsies of women with abnormal bleeding.

PROGNOSIS AND TREATMENT

- Prognosis is similar to other endometrial carcinomas and is comparable to the stage at the time of diagnosis.
- Managed with combined surgery, chemotherapy, and radiation as determined by stage.

PATHOLOGY

HISTOLOGY

- Classic features of squamous cell carcinoma with keratin formation and sheetlike growth.
- Papillary architecture is common.
- Differentiation may vary from well (or verrucous) to poor.
- Not infrequently, some foci exhibit deceptively bland histology, a feature not common in cervical carcinomas.

IMMUNOPATHOLOGY (INCLUDING IMMUNOHISTOCHEMISTRY)

- Positive for p53 in some reports.
- High proliferative index.

RECOMMENDED DIAGNOSIS

- Squamous cell carcinoma.

MAIN DIFFERENTIAL DIAGNOSIS

- Conventional endometrial carcinoma with squamous differentiation—these tumors usually display squamous differentiation that is rather low grade.
- Squamous cell carcinoma of the cervix—typically more moderately to poorly differentiated. p16 stains should be strong in contrast to the endometrial primary.

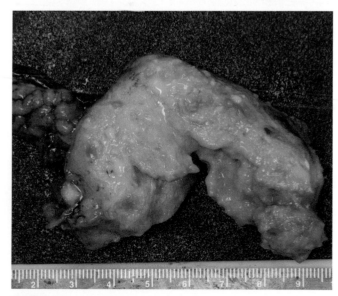

FIGURE 1

Squamous carcinoma of the endometrium. This cross section shows the endometrium and myometrium to be replaced by a necrotic tumor mass.

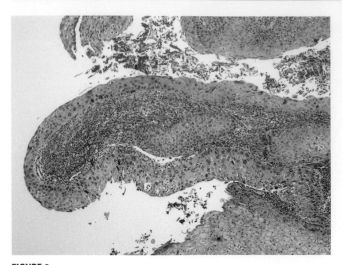

FIGURE 2

Squamous carcinoma of the endometrium with papillary architecture.

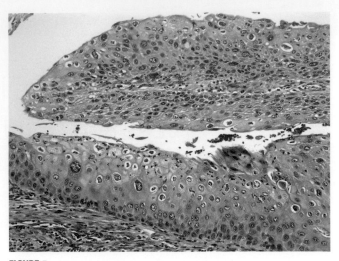

FIGURE 3

Squamous carcinoma of the endometrium. There is moderate atypia.

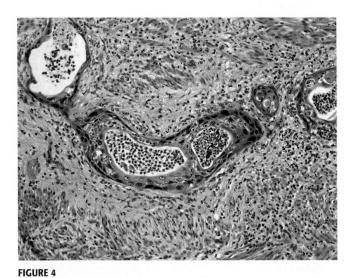

FIGURE 4

Squamous carcinoma of the endometrium infiltrating fibrous tissue.

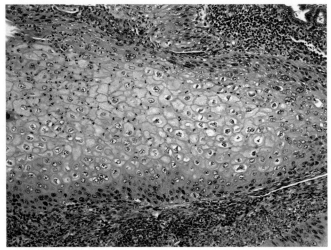

FIGURE 5

Squamous carcinoma of the endometrium. In this field the epithelial cells demonstrate pallor and minimal superficial atypia. This pale appearance to the neoplastic epithelium is more typical of endometrial versus cervical carcinomas.

TUBAL AND EOSINOPHILIC (OXYPHILIC) METAPLASIA

DEFINITION—Alteration of the epithelial cells consisting of tubular differentiation, including oxyphilic cytoplasm.

CLINICAL FEATURES

EPIDEMIOLOGY

- Tubal metaplasia is common, although clonal expansions of tubal metaplasia are less so. Eosinophilic metaplasia is an uncommon entity.
- Both tubal and eosinophilic metaplasia have been described in conjunction with endometrial intraepithelial neoplasia (EIN) and endometrial adenocarcinoma.

PRESENTATION

- Patients may be asymptomatic or present with abnormal uterine bleeding.

PROGNOSIS AND TREATMENT

- Isolated tubal or eosinophilic metaplasia limited to one or a few glands needs no additional management.
- Either tubal or eosinophilic metaplasia in a crowded expanded gland population should be managed as possible EIN.

PATHOLOGY

HISTOLOGY

- Cells composing eosinophilic metaplasia are typically large, polygonal cells with abundant oxyphilic cytoplasm, arranged in a single layer.
- The nuclei are uniform and round.

- Cells appear similar to those seen in tubal metaplasia, but without the apical cilia.

IMMUNOPATHOLOGY (INCLUDING IMMUNOHISTOCHEMISTRY)

- Noncontributory.

MAIN DIFFERENTIAL DIAGNOSIS

- Reactive-reparative changes can exhibit cytoplasmic eosinophilia and are managed similarly, depending on the complexity of gland architecture.

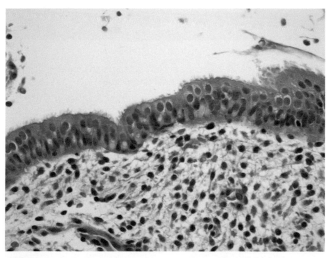

FIGURE 1

Noncomplex tubal metaplasia, typically seen on the endometrial surface epithelium.

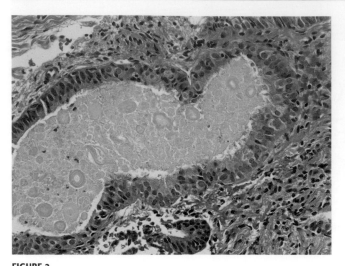

FIGURE 2

Tubal metaplasia with mild anisokaryosis, a benign feature.

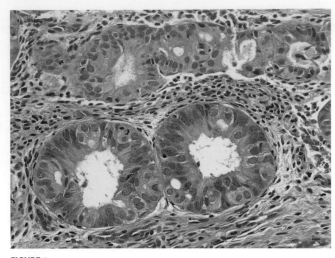

FIGURE 3

Tubal metaplasia *(center)* with mild complexity *(upper)*. This was associated with EIN.

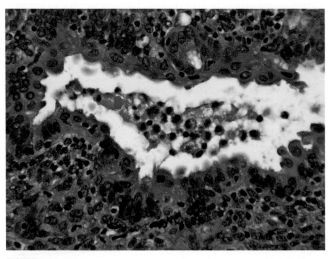

FIGURE 4

Eosinophilic metaplasia. Large, eosinophilic cells lining a normal endometrial gland. This is considered a form of tubal metaplasia.

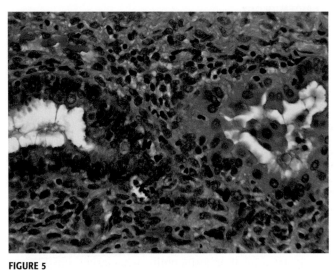

FIGURE 5

Eosinophilic metaplasia. Large, eosinophilic cells lining a normal endometrial gland. This is considered a form of tubal metaplasia.

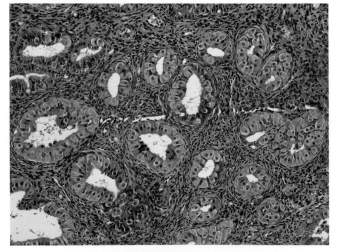

FIGURE 6

Glands showing a blend of tubal and eosinophilic metaplasia.

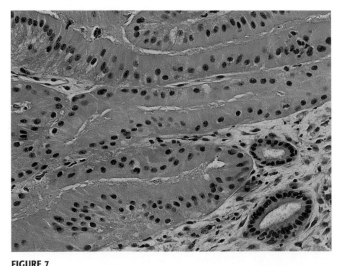

FIGURE 7

EIN with eosinophilic metaplasia. Note normal glands for reference.

MICROGLANDULAR ENDOMETRIAL ADENOCARCINOMA IN CURETTINGS

DEFINITION—A microacinar arrangement of endometrioid epithelium seen in endometrial biopsies/curettings that signifies the presence of endometrial neoplasia.

CLINICAL FEATURES

EPIDEMIOLOGY

- Most commonly occurs in postmenopausal women in their sixth and seventh decades.

PRESENTATION

- Seen in endometrial curettings or biopsies of women with abnormal bleeding.
- Not infrequently identified in relatively scant curettings.

PROGNOSIS AND TREATMENT

- A "red flag" for the presence of endometrial cancer, typically endometrioid with mucinous differentiation.

PATHOLOGY

HISTOLOGY

- Low-power examination reveals slightly irregular clusters of epithelial cells that do not exhibit the usual simple linear configuration.
- The most obvious finding is aggregated microacini with a slightly "soft" appearance relative to typical microglandular change of the cervix. However, some aggregates can be crisp appearing with vacuoles.
- Nuclei are slightly enlarged, and the mitotic index is low.
- Some neutrophils might be present.
- In their most subtle presentation they appear as small abortive acini ensconced in a linear stretch of columnar epithelium. Intervening stroma is minimal; the eosinophilic stroma seen in microglandular change is not present.
- Subcolumnar cells are inconspicuous.
- Some fine papillary architecture might be seen as well, but by itself is less specific.

IMMUNOPATHOLOGY (INCLUDING IMMUNOHISTOCHEMISTRY)

- Vimentin should be positive.
- ER and PR often positive.
- p63 will be more likely positive in microglandular change of the cervix but is not invariably negative in the endometrial lesion.

RECOMMENDED DIAGNOSIS

- Atypical endometrial glandular epithelium consistent with endometrial neoplasia.
- Well-differentiated endometrial adenocarcinoma (if sufficient).
- Comment: The curetting/biopsy specimen contains microacinar clusters of endometrial glandular epithelium. Although there is minimal cytologic atypia, this architecture is worrisome for a well-differentiated endometrial adenocarcinoma. Further tissues studies are recommended to exclude malignancy.

MAIN DIFFERENTIAL DIAGNOSIS

- Endocervical microglandular change—the lining cells are typically small and cuboidal appearing rather than taller columnar cells; reserve cells are often present; intervening stroma is distinctly cervical (if present).

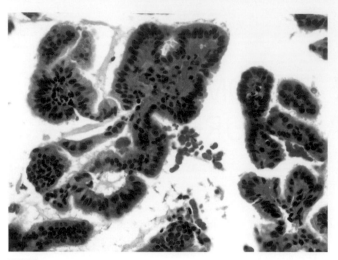

FIGURE 1

Small papillary clusters in the endometrium are relatively nonspecific but can be associated with microacinar clusters. A repeat sample would be prudent.

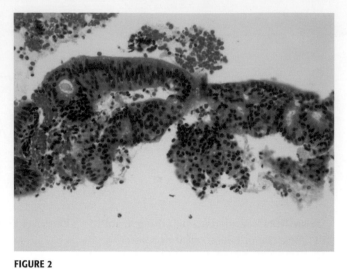

FIGURE 2

Subtle microacinar change in an endometrial biopsy. This is consistent with endometrial neoplasia (well-differentiated adenocarcinoma).

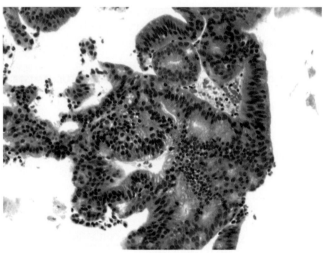

FIGURE 3

A more conspicuous cluster of microacini.

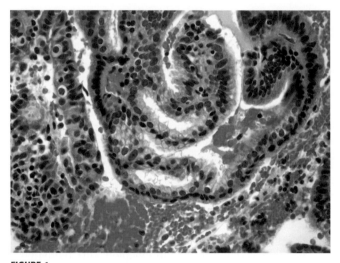

FIGURE 4

Prominent mucinous differentiation in a microacinar cluster.

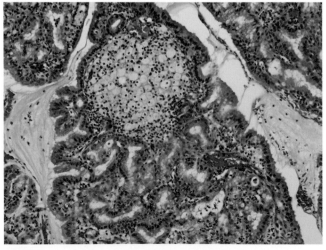

FIGURE 5

This microacinar cluster mimics endocervix. Note the foamy stromal cells.

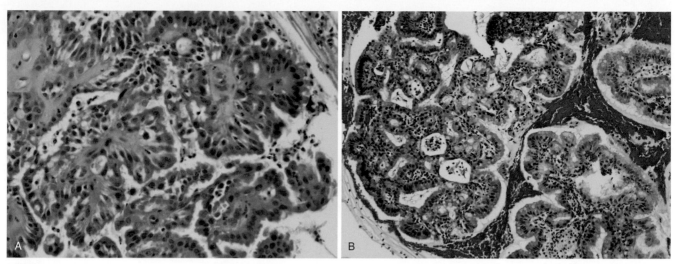

FIGURE 6

A, Microglandular change of the cervix. Note the intervening dense eosinophilic stroma, which is often seen in these cervical lesions. **B,** For comparison, microglandular adenocarcinoma.

ENDOMETRIOID ADENOCARCINOMA

DEFINITION—Adenocarcinoma of the endometrium that maintains some histologic features of normal endometrium.

CLINICAL FEATURES

EPIDEMIOLOGY

- Endometrioid endometrial carcinoma (EMCA) is the most common form of gynecologic malignancy.
- The overall lifetime incidence is between 2% and 3%.
- The majority of patients are between 55 and 65 years of age at the time of diagnosis; however, cases can occur at almost any age.
- Women with excess estrogen (whether exogenous or endogenous) are at increased risk.
- Because of the production of excess estrogens, obese women are at an increased risk.
- Patients with hereditary nonpolyposis colorectal cancer (HNPCC) (Lynch syndrome) and Cowden syndrome are at an increased risk. Approximately 4% of women with EMCA will score positive for HNPCC.
- Family history of EMCA, nulliparity, early menarche, and late menopause have all been associated with increased risk as well.
- Patients taking tamoxifen are at an increased risk of the development of endometrial intraepithelial neoplasia (EIN), which carries a 46-fold increased risk of subsequent (or concurrent) EMCA.

PRESENTATION

- Abnormal uterine bleeding or postmenopausal bleeding is the most common presenting sign.
- Increased age at the time of postmenopausal bleeding is associated with increased incidence of carcinoma. The risk of endometrial cancer may be as high as 40% 10 years out from menopause.

PROGNOSIS AND TREATMENT

- No further treatment for Stage IA, grade 1 or 2. Vaginal cuff radiation for Stage IB, grade 1 or 2, and Stage IA, grade 3. Chemotherapy +/− directed radiation for Stages III and IV. Stage IC, grade 3, and all Stage II are evolving toward chemotherapy and vaginal cuff radiation.
- Stage I, grade I or II carcinomas are associated with cure rates of ~90% or better.
- High-grade, high-stage tumors, especially undifferentiated or pleomorphic variants, have a dismal prognosis (stage III 20% to 30% 5-year survival, stage IV ~0% 5-year survival).
- Tumors exceeding 50% myometrial invasion as determined intraoperatively will usually receive lymph node dissection in the United States. However, staging is not as aggressively pursued in Europe.

PATHOLOGY

HISTOLOGY

- Tumor grade: FIGO grading is based on the percentage of nonsquamous, solid glandular component:
  - Grade 1: less than 5% solid growth
  - Grade 2: 5% to 50% solid growth
  - Grade 3: more than 50% solid growth
- Severe nuclear atypia may increase the FIGO grade by a factor of 1; however, these criteria are highly subjective and a point of controversy.
- Traditional low-grade EMCA is composed of irregular endometrioid glands with columnar cells with "cigar-shaped" nuclei, resembling the glands of proliferative endometrium. The nuclei are typically pseudostratified and have a fine, powdery chromatin with occasional small nucleoli.
- Enlarged polygonal cells with eosinophilic cytoplasm and vesicular, hyperchromatic nuclei and prominent nucleoli are signs of severe nuclear atypia.
- Numerous morphologic patterns arising in and associated with EMCA have been described:
  - Squamous differentiation is frequently found in EMCA. A wide range of squamous differentiation has been described, ranging from histologically benign squamous morules to markedly atypical

squamous epithelium indistinguishable from squamous cell carcinoma. The amount and degree of atypia of the squamous component have no effect on patient outcome.

- Mucinous differentiation is commonly identified as a minor component in many EMCA. Occasional tumors may be predominantly mucinous, prompting the diagnosis of "mucinous adenocarcinoma"; however, this has no effect on patient outcome. Morphology may range from focal columnar cell change to complete mucinous change with cribriforming or papillary growth. Cribriforming mucinous differentiation may bear a striking resemblance to microglandular hyperplasia of the cervix. Rare intestinally differentiated mucinous carcinomas have been identified. The amount and degree of atypia of the mucinous component have no effect on patient outcome.

- Secretory change, noted by scattered subnuclear or supranuclear vacuoles, can be seen in many tumors. When extensive, secretory endometrium can be ruled out by noting the enlarged glands, atypia, and loss of intervening stroma. Clear-cell carcinoma is a consideration, but the cells composing clear-cell carcinoma are typically cuboidal, lack stratification, and display marked atypia.

- Ciliated cells are common in both normal endometrium and neoplasia. Tumors composed of ciliated epithelium have been described and are termed "ciliated carcinoma."

- Villoglandular carcinoma is a term used to describe tumors composed of well-defined, slender papillae with discrete fibrovascular cores.

- Occasional tumors may display extensive eosinophilic (oxyphil) change. These tumors typically display abundant brightly eosinophilic cytoplasm and a mild degree of nuclear atypia.

- Biphasic carcinoma, composed of two distinct elements, has been reported. Commonly these tumors are composed of distinct areas of low-grade and undifferentiated carcinoma or adenocarcinoma and neuroendocrine carcinoma. Treatment and outcome are dependent on the most poorly differentiated component.

- Poorly differentiated, pleomorphic variants composed of markedly atypical cells are rare.

IMMUNOPATHOLOGY (INCLUDING IMMUNOHISTOCHEMISTRY)

- The diagnosis of EMCA is typically based on histologic findings; however, several stains may be helpful:
  - p53: Lack of diffuse, strong p53 staining is seen in most low-grade EMCAs. High-grade EMCA (FIGO grade 3) may display strong, diffuse staining similar to that seen in serous carcinoma.
  - Ki-67: Higher levels of proliferative activity are noted in more poorly differentiated cancers.
  - p63: Squamous differentiation (denoted by p63 positivity) can commonly be seen in endometrioid adenocarcinomas. Positive p63 staining may be especially helpful in identifying abortive squamous morular metaplasia.
  - Cytokeratin: Positive staining for cytokeratins can help distinguish undifferentiated carcinoma from conventional grade 3 endometrioid carcinomas.
  - CD10: Can help to identify endometrial stroma; however, care must be used as artifactual staining has been described surrounding frankly invasive glands.

MAIN DIFFERENTIAL DIAGNOSIS

- Benign endometrium (telescoping artifact).
- EIN.
- Stromal breakdown.
- Tangential sectioning.
- Microglandular hyperplasia (cervix).
- Endocervical adenocarcinoma (including in situ).
- Repair (papillary syncytial metaplasia).
- Hobnail metaplasia.
- Arias-Stella effect.
- Radiation-related changes.
- Exfoliation artifact.
- Metastasis from other sites.

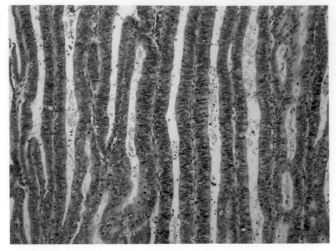

FIGURE 1

EMCA. Well-differentiated endometrial carcinoma composed exclusively of glands (FIGO grade 1).

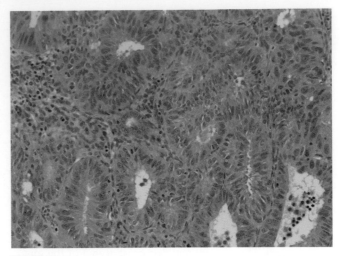

FIGURE 2

EMCA. Typical low-grade EEC morphology.

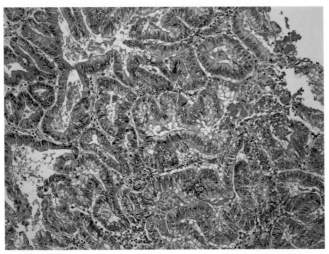

FIGURE 3

EMCA. Glands are irregular and there is minimal supporting stroma.

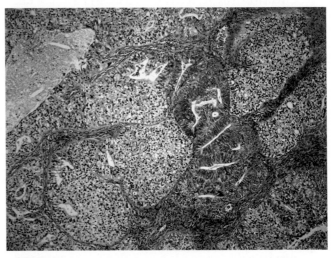

FIGURE 4

EMCA. Focal secretory change is seen here with numerous vacuoles.

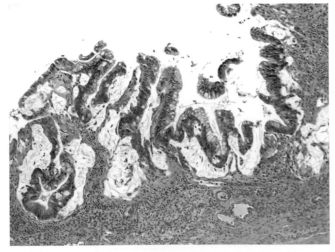

FIGURE 5

EMCA. This focus has rare intestinal differentiation.

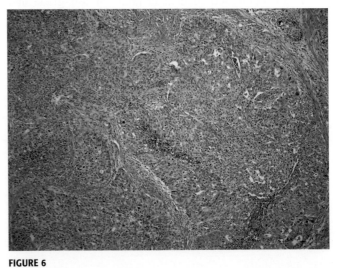

FIGURE 6

EMCA. FIGO grade 2 carcinoma based on solid growth. Note the well-differentiated component in the lower half.

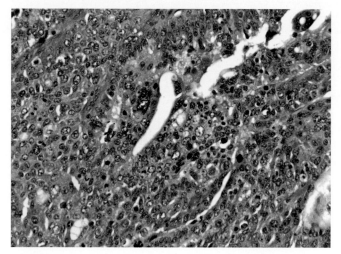

FIGURE 7

EMCA. FIGO grade 3 EEC composed almost exclusively of solid tumor growth with nuclear atypia.

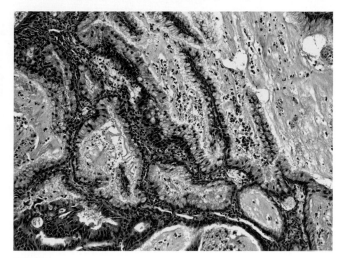

FIGURE 8

EMCA. High-grade adenocarcinoma with mucinous differentiation.

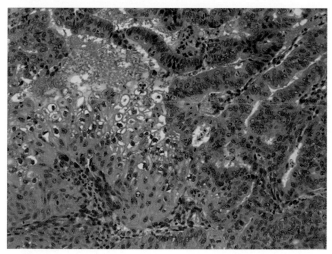

FIGURE 9

EMCA. Squamous differentiation *(lower left)*; note the presence of vacuoles and mild nuclear atypia.

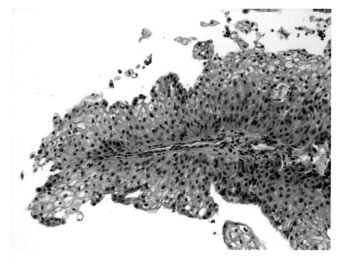

FIGURE 10

EMCA. Papillary architecture is seen here.

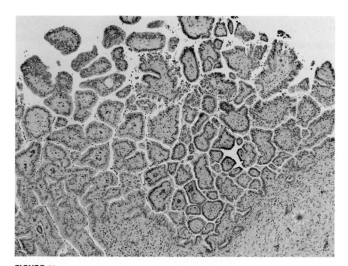

FIGURE 11

EMCA. This focus is markedly papillary; serous carcinoma must be excluded by careful histologic exam and immunostaining for p53, if deemed necessary.

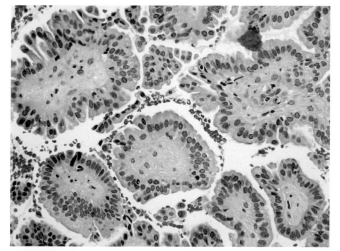

FIGURE 12

EMCA. Mucinous differentiation composed of a single layer of columnar mucinous cells simulating endocervix.

LOWER UTERINE SEGMENT ADENOCARCINOMA

DEFINITION—Adenocarcinoma arising in the lower uterine segment (LUS).

CLINICAL FEATURES

EPIDEMIOLOGY

- Uncommon variant of endometrial adenocarcinoma, accounting for from 3% to 6%.
- Associated with Lynch syndrome in up to 29% versus approximately 2% of conventional endometrial adenocarcinoma. A higher frequency of MSH2 loss has been reported by some.
- More commonly associated with higher-grade, deep myometrial invasion and less likely to have an associated endometrial intraepithelial neoplasia (atypical hyperplasia) or reproductive risk factors (such as parity and polycystic ovaries).

PRESENTATION

- Abnormal uterine bleeding or postmenopausal bleeding is the most common presenting sign.
- Imaging studies will often depict a mass in the region of the cervix, and distinction from cervical carcinoma may be difficult.

PROGNOSIS AND TREATMENT

- The prognosis is generally stage and grade dependent. Management is similar to other uterine carcinomas.
- Tumors may be more poorly differentiated and thus have a more adverse outcome.
- LUS involvement in conventional adenocarcinomas is associated with decreased survival, although in some studies this is not an independent prognostic factor.

PATHOLOGY

HISTOLOGY

- Tumor in the LUS with lesser involvement of the corpus and often extending into the endocervix.
- Higher-grade variants are common, including poorly differentiated endometrioid and serous subtypes.
- Mixed patterns with squamous, neuroendocrine carcinosarcomas have been described. Poorly differentiated, pleomorphic variants composed of markedly atypical cells have also been occasionally seen.

IMMUNOPATHOLOGY (INCLUDING IMMUNOHISTOCHEMISTRY)

- Vimentin might be helpful in confirming endometrial origin versus cervix.
- Should routinely be negative for human papillomavirus (HPV).
- p16 usually heterogeneous (as opposed to diffuse) excepting cases with serous histology.

MAIN DIFFERENTIAL DIAGNOSIS

- Cervical cancer—this can usually be excluded because although high-grade elements can be found, including squamous differentiation and neuroendocrine differentiation, these components are more haphazardly distributed in the LUS carcinomas.

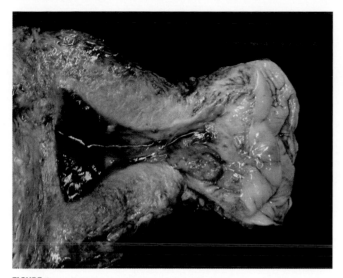

FIGURE 1

LUS carcinoma seen here as a small mass with involvement of the high endocervix.

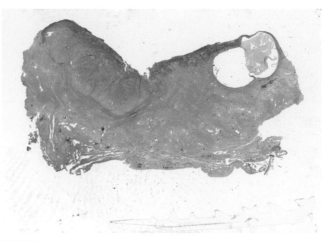

FIGURE 2

Poorly differentiated LUS carcinoma *(left)*. The endocervix is to the right.

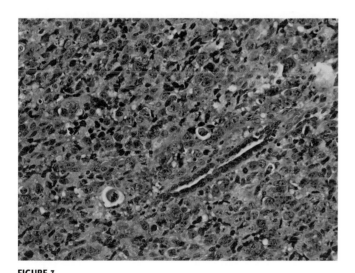

FIGURE 3

Higher magnification of the tumor in previous figure. Note the tumor is essentially undifferentiated.

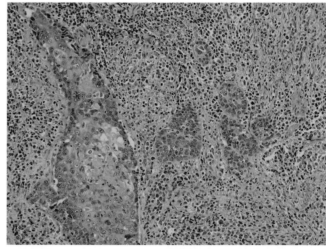

FIGURE 4

Another LUS carcinoma composed of squamous differentiation with an undifferentiated component.

LYNCH SYNDROME SCREENING

■ **Brooke E. Howitt, MD**

DEFINITION—Detecting abnormalities in immunohistochemical expression of mismatch repair proteins to identify patients at risk of harboring germline mutations in these genes (i.e., Lynch syndrome).

CLINICAL FEATURES

EPIDEMIOLOGY

- Lynch syndrome results from a germline mutation in a mismatch repair gene (MLH1, PMS2, MSH2, MSH6). The lifetime risk of colonic or endometrial cancer is from 40% to 60%.
- Approximately 60% of initial tumors in Lynch syndrome are endometrial in origin.
- Approximately 2% to 4% of endometrial carcinomas will have mismatch repair gene mutations.
- Risk of Lynch syndrome increases for women under age 50 who develop endometrial carcinomas, but can be seen at any age.
- Lifetime endometrial cancer risk of women with MLH1 or MSH2 mutations is about 40%, for PMS2 15%, and for MSH6 17% to 44%.
- Lifetime ovarian cancer risk is 6% to 8% for women with Lynch syndrome.

PRESENTATION

- Virtually any endometrial adenocarcinoma can be associated with Lynch syndrome.
- Most Lynch syndrome–associated tumors are endometrioid, but serous, poorly differentiated, and even carcinosarcoma subtypes may occur. Lower uterine segment carcinomas (up to 29%) are associated with Lynch syndrome. Lower uterine segment involvement is the only factor significantly separating Lynch syndrome–associated tumors from the general population.

PROGNOSIS AND TREATMENT

- The prognosis is generally stage and grade dependent like any endometrial cancer.

SCREENING

IMMUNOHISTOCHEMISTRY

- Sequencing of the MMR genes is the most sensitive approach and can be based on a strong family history of colon or endometrial cancer under age 60. However, the most cost-effective approach is immunohistochemical staining of all cases with triage to sequencing if staining is lost (abnormal).
- A panel of immunostains targeting the four genes (PMS2, MSH2, MSH6, MLH1) is employed.
- Loss of staining for MSH2 and/or MSH6 strongly correlates with a germline mutation. If no signal is detected, screening will then typically proceed to sequence analysis.
- Loss of staining for PMS2 and MLH1 is usually (but not always) a result of methylation of these genes. The next step is promoter methylation analysis, which if positive will generally exclude Lynch syndrome. If negative, sequencing will be offered.

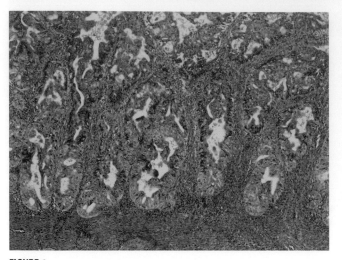

FIGURE 1

An endometrial endometrioid carcinoma.

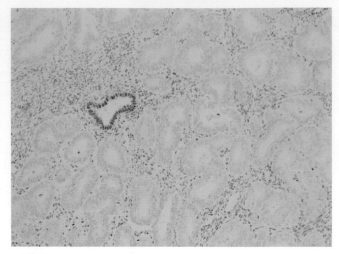

FIGURE 2

Loss of staining for MSH2.

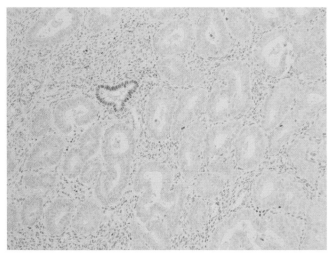

FIGURE 3

Loss of staining for MSH6.

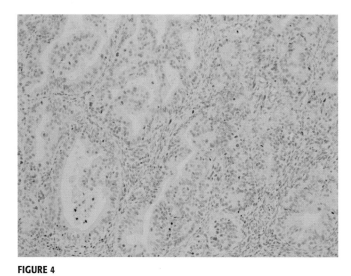

FIGURE 4

Retained staining for PMS2. MLH1 staining was also retained. This case was confirmed to be Lynch syndrome following sequencing.

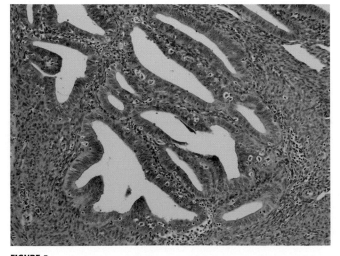

FIGURE 5

Another endometrial adenocarcinoma.

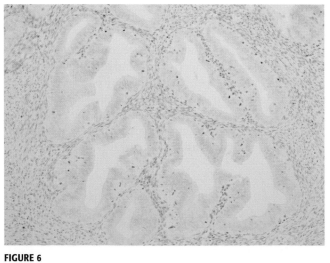

FIGURE 6

Absence of staining for PMS2.

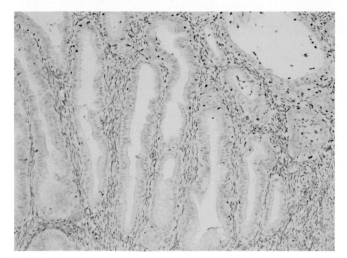

FIGURE 7

Absence of staining for MLH1.

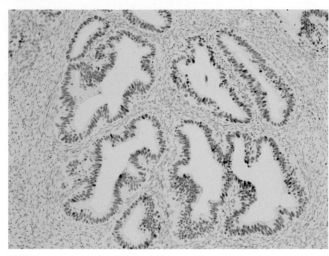

FIGURE 8

Intact staining for MSH2. Staining for MSH6 was also intact. This case was subjected to promoter methylation analysis, which was negative, a rather uncommon occurrence but one that justifies this confirmatory test. This case was subsequently confirmed to be Lynch syndrome following sequencing.

MYOINVASION IN ENDOMETRIAL ADENOCARCINOMA

DEFINITION—A diagnostic conundrum influencing management and outcome.

PRESENTATION

- Abnormal uterine bleeding or postmenopausal bleeding is the most common presenting sign.
- Increased age at the time of postmenopausal bleeding is associated with increased incidence of carcinoma. The risk of endometrial cancer may be as high as 40% 10 years out from menopause.

PROGNOSIS AND TREATMENT

- The prognosis is stage and grade dependent.
- Stage I, grade 1 carcinomas are associated with cure rates exceeding 90%.
- High-grade, high-stage tumors, especially undifferentiated or pleomorphic variants, have a dismal prognosis (stage III 20% to 30% 5-year survival, stage IV ~0% 5-year survival).
- Tumors exceeding 50% myometrial invasion will usually receive radiation therapy or lymph node dissection.

PATHOLOGY

HISTOLOGY

- Several patterns of myoinvasion have been described:
  - Infiltrating glands: The most common pattern of myoinvasion. This pattern is composed of a single gland to small clusters of glands that infiltrate the myometrium with or without a desmoplastic response.
  - Adenomyosis like: A pattern of invasion composed of large islands of malignant glands set in the myometrium. This pattern may be confused for malignant involvement of adenomyosis; however, the presence of irregular outlines and the lack of normal endometrial glands and stroma can aid in this distinction.
  - Broad front: Also known as a pushing border. Broad front invasion is composed of sheets of malignant glands that push into the myometrium. If present, adjacent normal endometrium can help to estimate the depth of invasion.
  - Microcystic elongated and fragmented glands (MELF): MELF is composed of small, fragmented clusters of eosinophilic cells set in a myxoid, desmoplastic stroma. Accompanying inflammatory cells, notably neutrophils, are typically seen. This pattern is believed to be the result of a stromal response to the infiltrating glandular pattern.
  - Adenoma malignum: A rare pattern of myoinvasion comprised of histologically unremarkable glands that infiltrate the myometrium with no surrounding tissue response.
- Issues concerning the diagnosis and staging of EEC are discussed in the following:
  - Carcinoma involving adenomyosis is a common occurrence that can be confused with adenomyosis-like tumor infiltration. Several features can help distinguish adenomyosis including the presence of normal (usually compressed) glands and stroma surrounding the malignant glands and a smooth interface between the adenomyotic nest and the surrounding endometrium. Invasion occurring at the edge of an area of adenomyosis is measured from the edge of the adenomyosis, as adenomyosis is seen as a direct extension of endometrium that can communicate with the surface.

IMMUNOPATHOLOGY (INCLUDING IMMUNOHISTOCHEMISTRY)

- CD10—can help to identify endometrial stroma; however, staining has been described surrounding invasive glands. For this reason, CD10 staining must be viewed critically.

MAIN DIFFERENTIAL DIAGNOSIS

- Myometrial invasion.

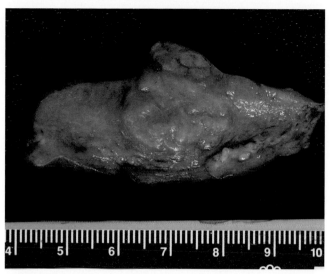

FIGURE 1

Gross image of adenocarcinoma involving adenomyosis, seen here as a nodular focus in the myometrium.

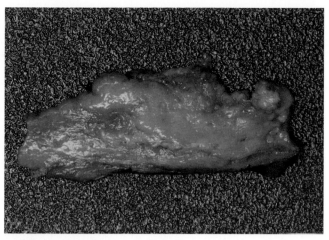

FIGURE 2

Gross image of myoinvasion. Note the less well-demarcated, yellowish thickening that is nearly transmural in this section.

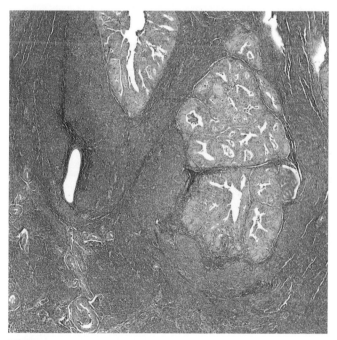

FIGURE 3

Endometrioid endometrial carcinoma involving adenomyosis. Here the stroma can be appreciated at the interface of the neoplasm and the myometrium.

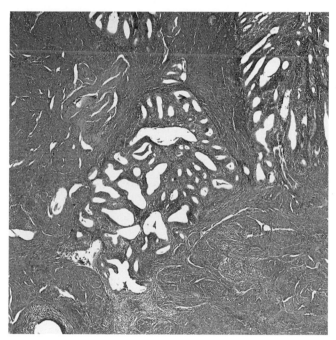

FIGURE 4

Endometrioid endometrial carcinoma involving adenomyosis. This is similar to the prior image except note the stromal reaction at the bottom, suggesting invasion developing from adenomyosis.

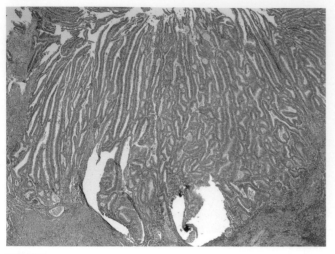

FIGURE 5

Confluent endometrioid endometrial carcinoma with a uniform epithelial stromal interface. Presumably the degree of invasion is slight.

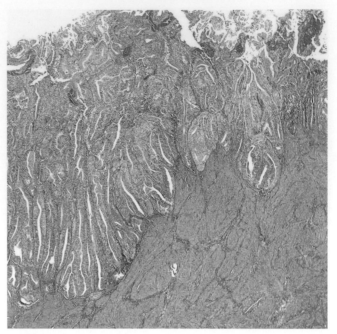

FIGURE 6

Confluent endometrioid endometrial carcinoma with a uniform epithelial stromal interface. Presumably the degree of invasion is slight.

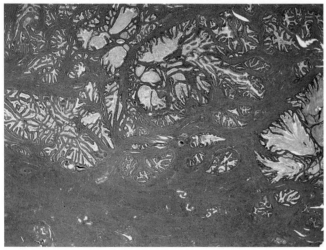

FIGURE 7

An adenomyosis-like pattern of myometrial invasion. Note the extent and downward direction of the growth pattern are characteristic of myoinvasion.

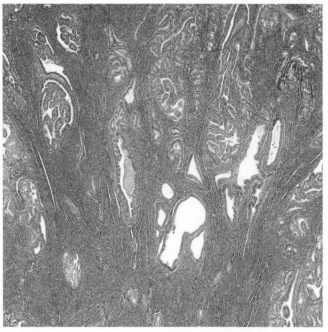

FIGURE 8

An adenomyosis-like pattern of myometrial invasion. Note the extent and downward direction of the growth pattern are characteristic of myoinvasion.

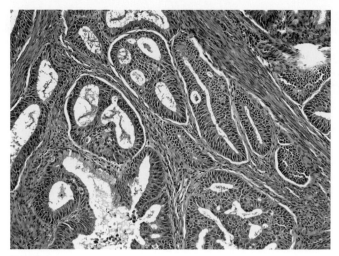

FIGURE 9

An adenomyosis-like pattern of myometrial invasion. Note the extent and downward direction of the growth pattern are characteristic of myoinvasion.

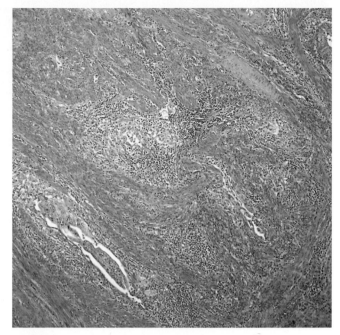

FIGURE 10

MELF-like invasion with subtle myxoid stromal changes and inconspicuous nests of epithelium. This pattern increases the risk of lymph node metastases.

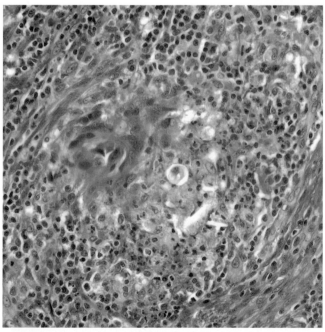

FIGURE 11

MELF-like invasion with subtle myxoid stromal changes and inconspicuous nests of epithelium. This pattern increases the risk of lymph node metastases.

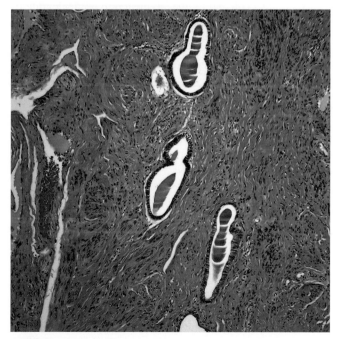

FIGURE 12

Adenoma malignum–like invasion. Uniform glands invade stroma without a desmoplastic response.

INTRAPERITONEAL KERATIN GRANULOMA

DEFINITION—Implants of keratinous material within the peritoneal cavity causing an associated granulomatous response.

CLINICAL FEATURES

EPIDEMIOLOGY

- Overall, peritoneal keratin granulomas are an uncommon finding; however, they most commonly occur in patients with gynecologic tumors.
- The most common associated tumor is endometrioid adenocarcinoma with squamous differentiation, but squamous cell carcinoma, atypical polypoid adenomyomas, and ruptured dermoid cysts have been known to cause this finding as well.

PRESENTATION

- Typically found at the time of surgery.
- If widely disseminated, it may mimic peritoneal metastasis.

PROGNOSIS AND TREATMENT

- Peritoneal keratin granulomas have not been associated with an adverse outcome, and no additional treatment is required.

PATHOLOGY

HISTOLOGY

- Microscopic examination of the small nodules reveals keratinous debris, necrotic keratinocytes (ghost cells) and surrounding foreign body giant cells, and chronic inflammatory cells.
- Variable amounts of fibrosis will be seen encasing the granulomas.

IMMUNOPATHOLOGY (INCLUDING IMMUNOHISTOCHEMISTRY)

- Noncontributory.

MAIN DIFFERENTIAL DIAGNOSIS

- Metastatic carcinoma—this will exhibit neoplastic glandular epithelium.
- Other causes of granulomatous disease (i.e., sarcoid, tuberculosis (TB), fungal infection, foreign material such as talc)—these should not exhibit keratin debris.

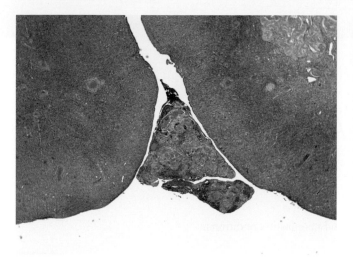

FIGURE 1

Keratin granuloma. A nodule of amorphous, eosinophilic material present on the ovarian surface.

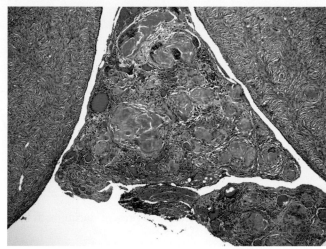

FIGURE 2

Keratin granuloma. Granulomatous inflammation and associated chronic inflammatory cells.

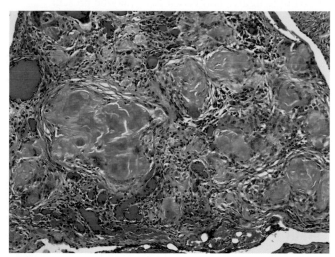

FIGURE 3

Keratin granuloma. Amorphous keratinous material and associated foreign body giant cells.

ENDOMETRIAL HISTIOCYTES AND FOAMY STROMAL MACROPHAGES

DEFINITION—Nonepithelial cells present during both benign and neoplastic conditions.

CLINICAL FEATURES

EPIDEMIOLOGY/SIGNIFICANCE

- Histiocytes are common in postmenopausal endometrial samples, often associated with surface injury or erosion. They do not confer an increased risk of malignancy.
- Foamy stromal macrophages are commonly associated with, although not specific for, well-differentiated endometrial adenocarcinomas.

PRESENTATION

- Typically found in curettings and hysterectomy specimens.
- Associated with a polyp (histiocytes) or malignancy (foamy macrophages).

PROGNOSIS AND TREATMENT

- Management is tailored to the underlying disorder.

PATHOLOGY

HISTOLOGY

Histiocytes

- Loosely cohesive aggregates of small cells with slightly irregular nuclei.

- Often admixed with fibrin or hyaline stromal changes when degenerated polyp is present.
- Cohesive sheets may mimic epithelium.
- Cytoplasmic borders are vague.
- Mitotic figures and eosinophils may be present.

Foamy macrophages

- Discrete sharply demarcated groups of foamy cells.
- May be adjacent to neoplasia (endometrial intraepithelial neoplasia [EIN] or carcinoma).

IMMUNOPATHOLOGY (INCLUDING IMMUNOHISTOCHEMISTRY)

- Keratin or macrophage markers will help in distinguishing histiocytes from epithelial cells.

MAIN DIFFERENTIAL DIAGNOSIS

- Carcinoma—macrophages can mimic carcinoma, but can be distinguished by immunohistochemical stains (cytokeratins) if needed.

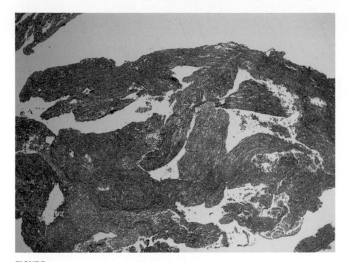

FIGURE 1

Endometrial histiocytes. A typical low-power image.

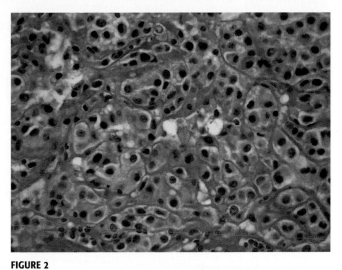

FIGURE 2

Endometrial histiocytes. At higher magnification the polyhedral cells seem to form an epithelial structure and may mimic small tumor cells. Note in particular the small nuclei with uniform chromatin.

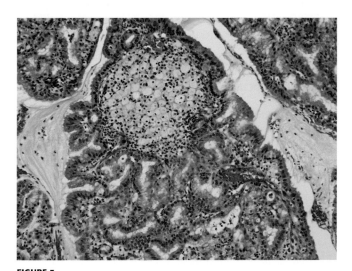

FIGURE 3

Foamy stromal macrophages. This image shows discrete clusters adjacent to endometrial neoplasms.

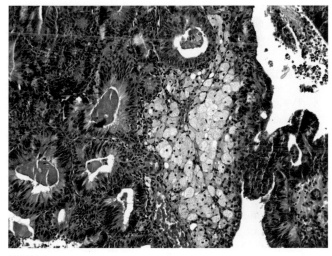

FIGURE 4

Another example of foamy stromal macrophages in a glandular neoplasm.

SEROUS CANCER PRECURSORS

DEFINITION—Epithelial proliferations with evidence of p53 mutations that do not fulfill the criteria for intramucosal carcinoma.

CLINICAL FEATURES

EPIDEMIOLOGY

- These lesions are rare and occur around menopause.
- Occasionally seen in endometrial polyps.
- Link between p53 positive epithelium with minimal atypia and cancer risk (of subsequent serous cancer) unknown.

PRESENTATION

- Typically detected in biopsies or curettings of menopausal or postmenopausal women.
- May be associated with abnormal bleeding by default.
- A subset present incidentally, in an endometrial polyp.

PROGNOSIS AND TREATMENT

- Management of a histologically normal endometrium should not include immunostaining for p53. However, positive staining for p53 might be encountered accidentally.
- So-called p53 signatures (benign appearing p53-positive mucosa) should be managed as clinically appropriate (i.e., repeat sampling if there are clinical indications such as abnormal bleeding).
- More extensive proliferations with evidence of clonal expansion but lacking marked atypia and substantially increased proliferative activity should be managed with repeat sampling and consultation as needed.

PATHOLOGY

HISTOLOGY

- p53 signatures: These are localized, histologically normal expansions of cells with a clonal p53 mutation.

They are encountered in less than 2% of endometrial polyps.
- Atypical proliferations (so-called endometrial glandular dysplasia). These are multilayered populations of cells with strong p53 (or completely absent p53) staining. Proliferative index is usually low (less than 20%).
- Both p53 signatures and endometrial glandular dysplasia can be associated with serous carcinoma including intramucosal (or intraepithelial) carcinoma.

IMMUNOPATHOLOGY (INCLUDING IMMUNOHISTOCHEMISTRY)

- Strong, diffuse (or completely null) staining for p53 should be seen in the cells. Some will have a deletion mutation and
- Ki-67 index is low.

PREFERRED DIAGNOSTIC TERMS (WHEN AN ISOLATED FINDING)

- For p53 signature: Benign endometrium with a comment that focal p53 staining is present, but there is no evidence of malignancy. Suggest repeat sampling if clinically indicated.
- For atypical proliferations that are p53 positive: Glandular atypia, possibly early serous neoplasia, with a comment that while serous endometrial intraepithelial carcinoma (EIC) is not seen, follow-up sampling is advised to exclude this possibility.

MAIN DIFFERENTIAL DIAGNOSIS

- Serous EIC—this entity will display multilayered atypia with an increased proliferative index and greater loss of polarity.

414

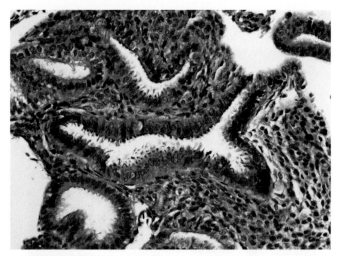

FIGURE 1

p53 signature in the endometrium discovered incidentally. Note the normal appearing mucosa. There is no current evidence that this is a risk factor for subsequent serous carcinoma.

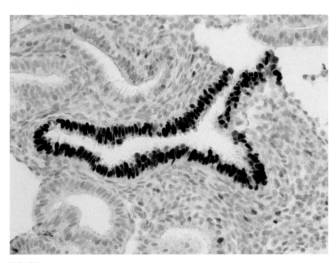

FIGURE 2

p53 immunostain of Figure 1.

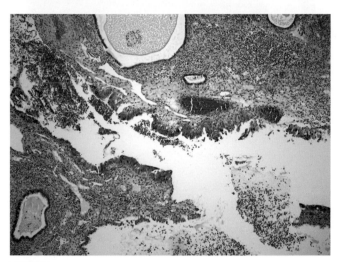

FIGURE 3

Endometrial glandular dysplasia showing multilayered epithelium with a relatively low nuclear-to-cytoplasmic (N/C) ratio.

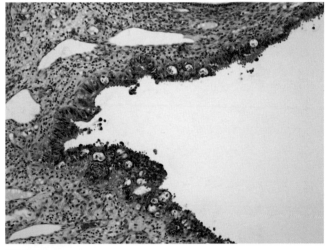

FIGURE 4

Endometrial glandular dysplasia showing multilayered epithelium with a relatively low nuclear-to-cytoplasmic (N/C) ratio.

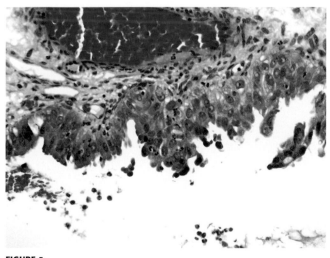

FIGURE 5

Endometrial glandular dysplasia. There is moderate atypia with some multi-layering of the epithelium.

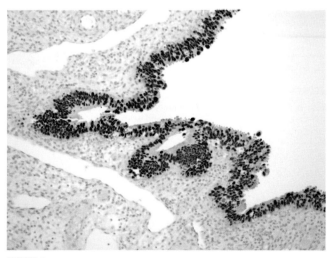

FIGURE 6

Endometrial glandular dysplasia. There is strong staining for p53.

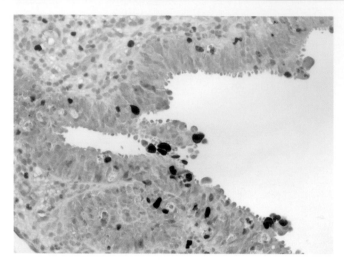

FIGURE 7

Endometrial glandular dysplasia. Note the low proliferative index.

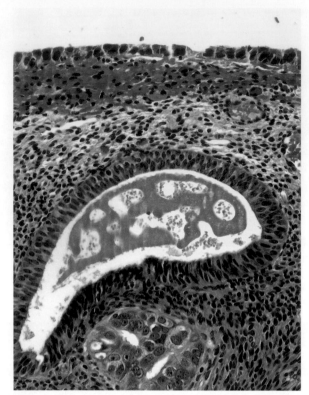

FIGURE 8

A small gland *(bottom center)* contains atypia befitting a serous EIC. Note the contrast with the surface epithelial changes, which are not diagnostic for malignancy.

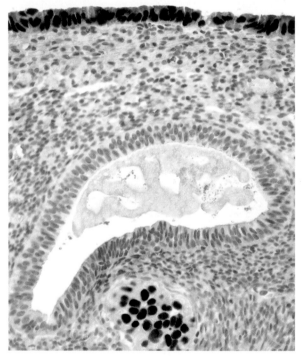

FIGURE 9

Both epithelia in Figure 8 stain strongly for p53. Note, however, that the surface epithelium is deceptively bland and would not by itself justify a diagnosis of serous EIC (see Figure 9).

SEROUS ENDOMETRIAL INTRAEPITHELIAL CARCINOMA

DEFINITION—An early, noninvasive form of serous adenocarcinoma of the endometrium.

CLINICAL FEATURES

EPIDEMIOLOGY

- Serous endometrial intraepithelial carcinoma (EIC) is a rare neoplasm.
- The vast majority of patients are postmenopausal.
- EIC is most commonly seen in a background of endometrial atrophy and associated with endometrial polyps.

PRESENTATION

- Patients may present with abnormal bloody or blood-tinged discharge.
- Patients may be asymptomatic or present with signs and symptoms of lower genital tract or abdominal spread of tumor.
- A subset present incidentally in an endometrial polyp.

PROGNOSIS AND TREATMENT

- The prognosis in serous EIC is guarded. Notably patients who are completely staged and found to have low-stage disease have a favorable prognosis with a relapse rate of approximately 5%.
- Serous EIC does display metastatic potential.
- Primary therapy includes full surgical staging.
- The value of chemotherapy in an intramucosal carcinoma without spread is controversial.

PATHOLOGY

HISTOLOGY

- Nuclear enlargement, hyperchromasia, and pleomorphism of the endometrial glandular cells are prominent.

- No increase in the gland density should be appreciated as serous EIC spreads along the surface of the endometrium and into existing gland tracts.
- Prominent exfoliation of cells may be present (mechanism of early spread).
- Increased mitotic figures with atypical forms are easily identifiable.
- A background of cystic atrophy or endometrial polyp (or both) is common.
- *A subset of these lesions are subtle.* Careful inspection of the surface epithelium may disclose an increased nuclear-to-cytoplasmic (N/C) ratio with mild nuclear enlargement only.

IMMUNOPATHOLOGY (INCLUDING IMMUNOHISTOCHEMISTRY)

- Strong, diffuse (or completely null) staining for p53 should be seen in the malignant cells. Some will have a deletion mutation and exhibit no staining.
- Increased but often quite variable proliferative index with Ki-67.

PREFERRED DIAGNOSIS (WHEN AN ISOLATED FINDING)

- Serous intramucosal (intraepithelial) carcinoma, see comment.
- Comment: This serous carcinoma is confined to the mucosa (in this specimen) without stromal invasion. Appropriate clinical management is recommended to exclude extrauterine (tubes, ovaries, peritoneal surfaces) disease.

MAIN DIFFERENTIAL DIAGNOSIS

- Surface repair; the N/C ratio is typically low, but the nuclear atypia can be striking. This paradoxical finding (atypia, low N/C ratio) is not typical of early serous carcinoma, which can show deceptively uniform nuclei.

- Papillary syncytial metaplasia can mimic serous carcinoma, but true papillary architecture is absent.
- Arias-Stella (like) effect has pronounced atypia but should have weak to patchy p53 staining.
- Metastasis (from the upper genital tract/tube) is possible in very superficial involvement, hence the necessity for full staging.
- Exfoliation artifact produces a hobnail pattern in the endometrium resulting from discohesion of the lining cells brought about by preservation artifacts. Look for a regional distribution of the changes and evidence of preservation artifact in the adjacent stroma.
- Benign (ischemic) atypia associated with polyps can show marked nuclear changes. This may mimic both serous intramucosal carcinoma and clear-cell carcinoma.
- Lower-grade precursors to serous cancer, including atypias that border on serous EIC (akin to endometrial glandular dysplasia). These can display a lower proliferative index and less atypia, suggesting that they are precursors to EIC. Their management is problematic.

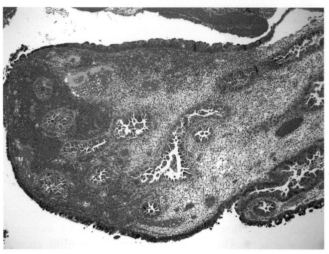

FIGURE 1

Serous EIC. At low power the process involves an endometrial polyp. The lesion conforms to existing glands but note the marked nuclear atypia.

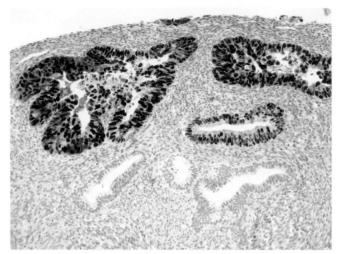

FIGURE 3

Serous EIC. p53 staining highlights the neoplastic epithelial cells with strong nuclear signal.

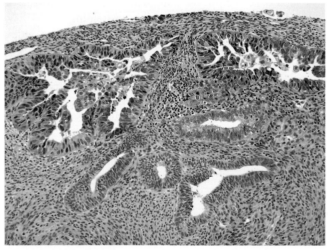

FIGURE 2

Serous EIC. Note the contrast with underlying benign glands.

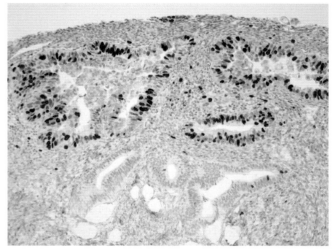

FIGURE 4

Serous EIC. A high proliferative index (MIB1) is the usual finding.

ISCHEMIC ATYPIAS OF THE ENDOMETRIUM

DEFINITION—A form of hobnail atypia associated with adjacent necrosis or hyaline degeneration signifying regional ischemia.

CLINICAL FEATURES

EPIDEMIOLOGY

- Most commonly occurs in women in their fifth to seventh decades who have endometrial polyps.

PRESENTATION

- Seen in endometrial curettings or biopsies of women with abnormal bleeding.

PROGNOSIS AND TREATMENT

- Inconsequential by itself. Management is directed to the underlying condition (e.g., polyps).

PATHOLOGY

HISTOLOGY

- The presence of endometrial polyps is common.
- Background of ischemic changes, with hemorrhage or hyaline stromal changes, either in the polyp or adjacent endometrium.

- Striking "hobnail" metaplasia.
- Often a noticeable transition from normal to hobnail changes.
- Relatively low nuclear-to-cytoplasmic (N/C) ratio and mild nuclear enlargement.

IMMUNOPATHOLOGY (INCLUDING IMMUNOHISTOCHEMISTRY)

- p53 staining is weak to heterogeneous.
- Low Ki-67 index.

RECOMMENDED DIAGNOSIS

- Reactive epithelial changes associated with infarction/ischemic change.

MAIN DIFFERENTIAL DIAGNOSIS

- Clear-cell carcinoma—nuclear enlargement and high N/C ratio with prominent nuclear enlargement.
- Serous carcinoma—high N/C ratio and high p53 and Ki-67 indices.
- Arias-Stella effect—appropriate clinical setting (pregnancy or progestin therapy) and the absence of stromal necrosis.

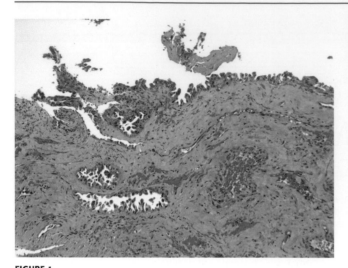

FIGURE 1

Ischemic atypia. This polyp is infarcted with prominent hobnail changes in the glands.

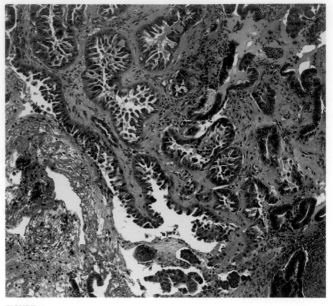

FIGURE 2

Ischemic atypia. Note the transition from nonischemic *(upper right)* to ischemic *(lower left)* zones with hyaline stromal changes.

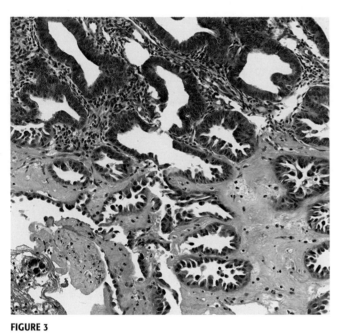

FIGURE 3

Ischemic atypia. In this field the preserved glands *(upper)* merge with the ischemic area *(lower)* with hyaline stromal changes and hobnail features.

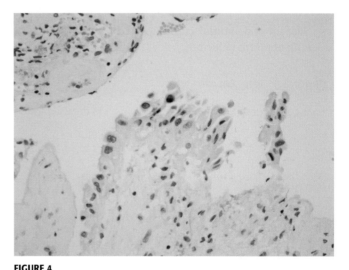

FIGURE 4

p53 staining of ischemic atypia displays heterogeneous distribution consistent with normal expression.

REACTIVE ATYPIA IN THE ENDOMETRIUM

DEFINITION—A form of atypia associated with abnormal bleeding.

CLINICAL FEATURES

EPIDEMIOLOGY

- Most commonly occurs in women in their fifth to seventh decades.

PRESENTATION

- Seen in endometrial curettings or biopsies of women with abnormal bleeding.

PROGNOSIS AND TREATMENT

- Inconsequential by itself. Management is directed to the underlying condition (e.g., polyps).

PATHOLOGY

HISTOLOGY

- The presence of endometrial polyps is common.
- Background of breakdown, with or without repair but might be seen in isolation.
- Nuclear enlargement, hyperchromasia, and in some cases multinucleation.

- Relatively low nuclear-to-cytoplasmic (N/C) ratio and mild nuclear enlargement.

IMMUNOPATHOLOGY (INCLUDING IMMUNOHISTOCHEMISTRY)

- p53 staining is weak to heterogeneous.
- Low Ki-67 index.

RECOMMENDED DIAGNOSIS

- Reactive epithelial changes associated with infarction/ischemic change.

MAIN DIFFERENTIAL DIAGNOSIS

- Clear-cell carcinoma—nuclear enlargement and high N/C ratio with prominent nuclear enlargement.
- Serous carcinoma—high N/C ratio and high p53 and Ki-67 indices. Notably many early intramucosal serous carcinomas display less variation in nuclear size, albeit a much higher N/C ratio.
- Arias-Stella effect—appropriate clinical setting (pregnancy or progestin therapy) and the absence of stromal necrosis.
- Ischemic atypia—this is probably a related entity, albeit more pronounced and described in association with infarcted endometrium or polyps.

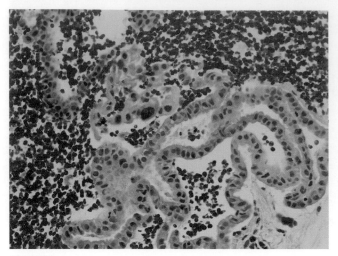

FIGURE 1

Typical reactive atypia in surface endometrium. Note the nuclear enlargement, uniform chromatin (smudged) and relatively low N/C ratio.

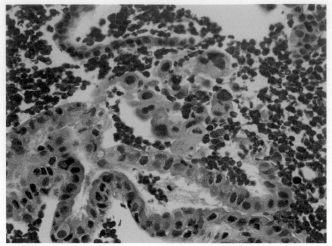

FIGURE 2

Another focus of reactive atypia *(center)* in strips of benign-appearing endometrial lining.

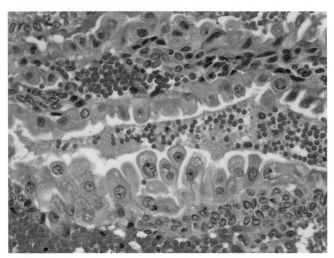

FIGURE 3

Another example of reactive atypia with breakdown. This overlaps with so-called ischemic atypia.

UTERINE SEROUS CARCINOMA

DEFINITION—High-grade adenocarcinoma arising from the endometrium and invariably associated with mutations in the p53 tumor suppressor gene.

CLINICAL FEATURES

EPIDEMIOLOGY

- Uterine serous carcinoma is relatively uncommon, comprising around 10% of endometrial primaries.
- Patients are most commonly in their seventh or eighth decade.
- Uterine serous carcinoma is not associated with obesity, diabetes, or estrogen excess.
- Precursors to serous carcinoma have been described (endometrial glandular dysplasia) and are being studied.

PRESENTATION

- Abnormal uterine bleeding, abnormal cervical cytology.

PROGNOSIS AND TREATMENT

- Serous carcinoma is automatically considered high grade and carries a worse prognosis for similarly staged endometrioid tumors.
- Tumor cell exfoliation may occur early in the course of disease and lead to pelvic or abdominal metastasis.
- Lymph node or peritoneal metastasis can be seen in over one third without myometrial invasion.
- Treatment consists of total abdominal hysterectomy with bilateral salpingo-oophorectomy and omental sampling. Some stage IA cases might be managed by observation alone but otherwise vaginal brachytherapy and platinum-based chemotherapy are frequently employed.
- Recurrence rates for stage I are approximately 15% to 20%; 5% or less for tumors confined to the endometrium with no residual disease following surgery. Three-year survival for advanced disease (Stage III or greater is 40%).

PATHOLOGY

HISTOLOGY

- Cells composing serous carcinoma are cuboidal to stratified, with marked nuclear pleomorphism, a high nuclear-to-cytoplasmic (N/C) ratio, and prominent nucleoli.
- Different patterns of growth have been described:
  1. Broad papillary projections lined by malignant cells
  2. Micropapillae, which consist of shed cells and lack fibrovascular cores
  3. Slit-forming glandular spaces.
  4. Solid growth (typically seen in more poorly differentiated/large cell serous carcinomas)
  5. Scattered angular glands with abundant fibrous stroma (so-called carcinofibroma).
  6. Microcystic growth (more common in ovarian/tubal primaries)
  7. Superficial epithelial growth, which commonly occurs in the setting of an (atrophic) endometrial polyp. These tumors may spread early and carry a poor prognosis, despite being noninvasive.

IMMUNOPATHOLOGY (INCLUDING IMMUNOHISTOCHEMISTRY)

- Serous carcinoma shows strong, diffuse positivity for p53. Occasional cases (~15%) may be completely negative for p53 (relative to the background), consistent with a p53 null mutant.
- Ki-67 is markedly increased in serous carcinoma.
- p16 (as in diffuse and intense) and IMP4 are also positive in most. Combined p16 and p53 positivity correlates strongly with serous carcinoma but does not exclude a small percentage of higher-grade endometrioid carcinomas.

MAIN DIFFERENTIAL DIAGNOSIS

- Metastatic serous carcinoma from fallopian tube or ovary—the general consensus is that most combined endometrial and tubal/ovarian carcinomas arose in the uterus; however, it may be difficult to determine primary site, since in some cases there may be multiple primary tumors. In general an invasive or large serous carcinoma in the uterus is assigned as the primary.
- Poorly differentiated endometrioid carcinoma—these tumors can be immunophenotypically identical to serous carcinoma. The distinction is primarily histological, based on lower N/C ratio, greater nuclear uniformity.

- Clear-cell carcinoma—these are relatively uncommon in the uterus. Some tumors will have features of both clear-cell and serous carcinomas. p53 immunostaining should be heterogeneous; HINF1B, Napsin A, and AMACR staining might be helpful as well.
- Undifferentiated carcinoma—these tumors typically have a very monomorphic population of undifferentiated epithelioid cells with prominent nucleoli. Some can be highly pleomorphic. In either case the necessary architectural features of serous carcinoma should be absent. In fact, many undifferentiated carcinomas will be near a small component of lower-grade endometrioid carcinoma.

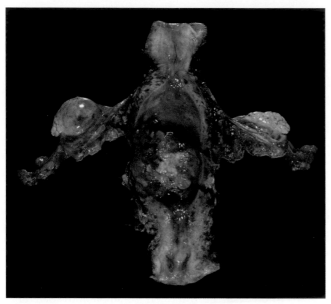

FIGURE 1

Uterine serous carcinoma. Gross photo of serous carcinoma forming a polypoid endometrial lesion.

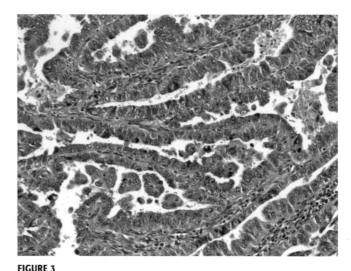

FIGURE 3

Uterine serous carcinoma. Angulated, slitlike glands with tumor cell exfoliation forming micropapillae.

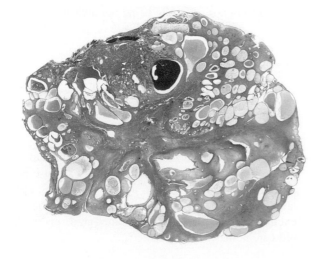

FIGURE 2

Uterine serous carcinoma. An atrophic polyp with a focus of serous carcinoma *(top half)*.

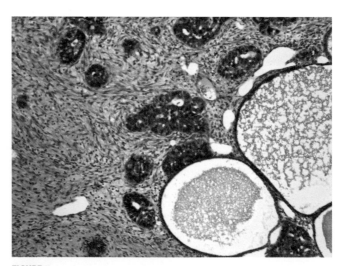

FIGURE 4

Uterine serous carcinoma. Nests of serous carcinoma with a markedly increased N/C ratio. Note the presence of cystic atrophic endometrial glands.

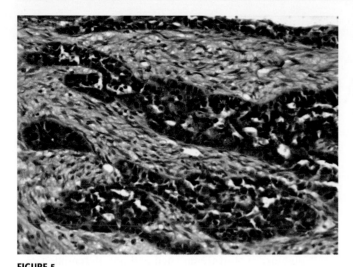

FIGURE 5

Uterine serous carcinoma. Increased N/C ratio and numerous slitlike spaces.

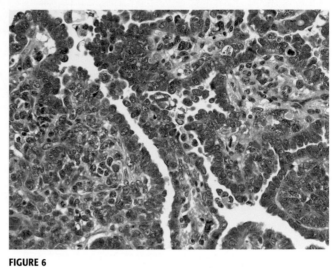

FIGURE 6

Uterine serous carcinoma. Cuboidal to low-stratified epithelium with marked nuclear pleomorphism and prominent nucleoli.

MIXED-PATTERN ADENOCARCINOMA

DEFINITION—A variant of endometrial carcinoma with two distinct differentiation patterns, usually separated, with minimal evidence of a histologic transition.

CLINICAL FEATURES

EPIDEMIOLOGY

- Relatively uncommon.
- Can occur at any age.
- Presumed to be a single original clone followed by divergence into two distinct phenotypes.

PRESENTATION

- Similar to any endometrial carcinoma.
- May be a component of a diffusely undifferentiated carcinoma or part of a biphasic carcinoma that includes a conventional endometrioid component.

PROGNOSIS AND TREATMENT

- Prognosis is poor in cases in which there is undifferentiated carcinoma or serous carcinoma as the higher-grade component. Prognosis is not affected when the second component is a lower-grade spindle cell carcinoma.
- Managed as undifferentiated carcinoma if this is the second component.

PATHOLOGY

HISTOLOGY

At least two patterns can be encountered, but any combination is possible:

- Combined endometrioid and high-grade serous carcinoma, with divergent immunophenotypes.

- Combined well-differentiated and undifferentiated carcinomas, including neuroendocrine differentiation in the latter. Neuroendocrine differentiation is common in these poorly differentiated areas but does not justify classification of the tumor as a neuroendocrine carcinoma.

IMMUNOPATHOLOGY (INCLUDING IMMUNOHISTOCHEMISTRY)

- Immunostains may be necessary to exclude carcinosarcoma.
- p53 staining will highlight the more aggressive serous component when suspected.

PREFERRED DIAGNOSIS (WHEN AN ISOLATED FINDING)

- Biphasic endometrial carcinoma with a note specifying the different components.

MAIN DIFFERENTIAL DIAGNOSIS

- Grade II endometrioid carcinoma—this diagnosis is based on amount of solid growth, but two distinct patterns are not seen.
- Carcinosarcoma—excluded when necessary by cytokeratin stains.
- Stromal sarcoma or sarcomas with sex cord–like differentiation.

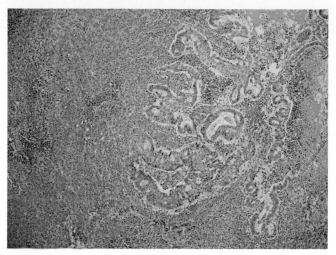

FIGURE 1

Biphasic carcinoma of the endometrium. Here a well-differentiated component on the right suddenly merges with an undifferentiated carcinoma on the left.

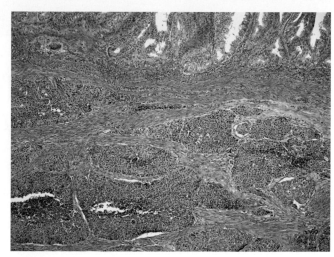

FIGURE 2

This biphasic carcinoma depicts a well-differentiated adenocarcinoma above, and a poorly differentiated carcinoma with neuroendocrine features below.

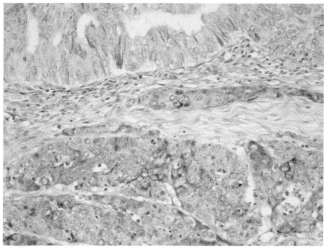

FIGURE 3

The interface of the lesion in the previous figure, with synaptophysin staining in the lower neuroendocrine component.

p53-POSITIVE ENDOMETRIOID ADENOCARCINOMA

DEFINITION—A common conundrum in endometrial cancer classification in which an endometrioid histology coexists with strong p53 staining.

CLINICAL FEATURES

EPIDEMIOLOGY

- Outcomes for serous carcinoma are distinctly less favorable relative to both low- and high-grade endometrioid carcinomas.
- Some tumors do not readily fall into either category, specifically those with both endometrioid histology and a high level of p53 expression.

PRESENTATION

- Abnormal uterine bleeding and abnormal cervical cytology.

PROGNOSIS AND TREATMENT

- High (more than 50%) expression of p53 is independently associated with a worse clinical outcome in patients with endometrioid adenocarcinomas.
- In serous carcinomas, p53 expression is not independently associated with survival.
- Cases with ambiguous results, either histologically or diagnostically (i.e., interobserver disagreement), are more likely to be p53 positive.
- p53 immunohistochemistry might provide prognostic information in cases that would otherwise be classified as endometrioid adenocarcinomas.

PATHOLOGY

HISTOLOGY

- Diagnostically ambiguous, p53-positive tumors fall into three general categories:

1. Tumors with variable histology, part of which is classically serous carcinoma. The latter exhibits the typical papillary, micropapillary, and slit-forming glandular growth with conspicuous nuclear atypia.
2. Tumors with endometrioid glandular morphology but increased (grade 2) nuclear atypia. The latter may take the form of less stratified more cuboidal cells, higher nuclear-to-cytoplasmic (N/C) ratio, and nuclear enlargement.
3. Rare tumors that are indistinguishable from endometrioid adenocarcinomas. These may not prompt suspicion but are nonetheless diffusely positive for p53.

IMMUNOPATHOLOGY (INCLUDING IMMUNOHISTOCHEMISTRY)

- p53 staining is most useful in delineating these tumors and should be found in at least 50% of the tumor cells and typically is higher.

RECOMMENDED DIAGNOSTIC TERMINOLOGY

- Endometrial adenocarcinoma, endometrioid-type grade (specify 1, 2, or 3).
- Comment: Immunostain for p53 is positive (more than 50% of cells). p53 has been independently associated with a more adverse outcome in endometrioid adenocarcinoma. Clinical correlation is advised.

MAIN DIFFERENTIAL DIAGNOSIS

- Serous carcinoma is the obvious exclusion and is done by the application of histologic criteria.

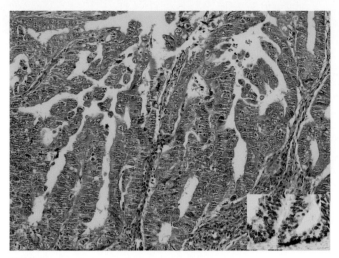

FIGURE 1

p53-Positive endometrioid adenocarcinoma. There is mild cell discohesion in an otherwise pseudostratified epithelium.

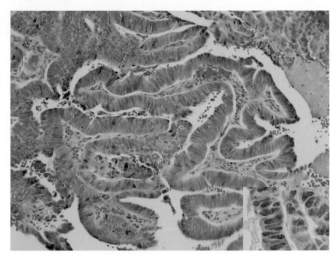

FIGURE 2

p53-Positive endometrioid adenocarcinoma. This endometrioid gland population demonstrates a higher N/C ratio.

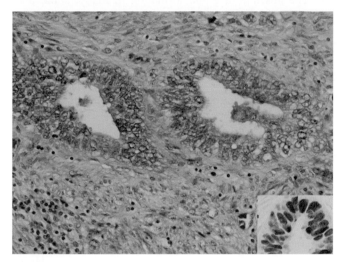

FIGURE 3

p53-Positive endometrioid adenocarcinoma. Another endometrioid glandular lesion with strong p53 staining.

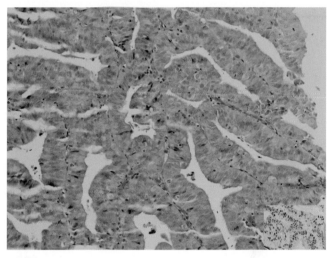

FIGURE 4

p53-Positive endometrioid adenocarcinoma. This population has moderate atypia, some loss of polarity, and some tubal-type differentiation.

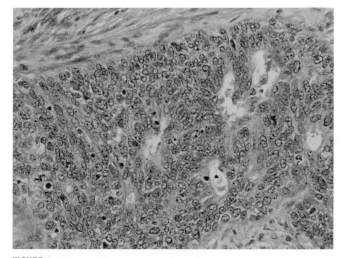

FIGURE 5

A biphasic tumor that ultimately would be classified as a serous carcinoma. The endometrioid component merges with a p53-positive serous component (see Figure 6).

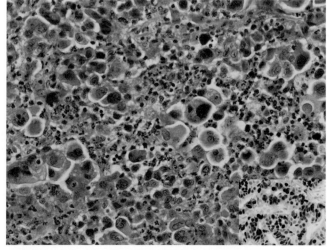

FIGURE 6

The endometrioid component (see Figure 5) merges with a p53-positive serous component *(shown here)*.

NEUROENDOCRINE DIFFERENTIATION IN ENDOMETRIAL CARCINOMA

DEFINITION—A variant of endometrioid carcinoma with neuroendocrine features.

CLINICAL FEATURES

EPIDEMIOLOGY

- A variant pattern seen in poorly differentiated carcinomas of the endometrium.
- The vast majority of patients are postmenopausal with a median age in the sixth to eighth decades.

PRESENTATION

- Typically presents as stage III or IV (75%).
- May be a component of a diffusely undifferentiated carcinoma or part of a biphasic carcinoma that includes a conventional endometrioid component.

PROGNOSIS AND TREATMENT

- Prognosis is poor. Median survival was less than 1 year.
- Empiric therapy with neuroendocrine regimens is of unclear value, and the rationale for treating such tumors as neuroendocrine carcinomas is equally uncertain. In general, focal neuroendocrine differentiation does not justify treatment as such, whereas a tumor that is diffusely positive with multiple neuroendocrine markers might justify a neuroendocrine-specific regimen.

PATHOLOGY

HISTOLOGY

- Can be both large and small cell types.
- Typically a diffuse proliferation of cells with a high nuclear-to-cytoplasmic (N/C) ratio and uniform nuclei, with variable nucleoli and stippled chromatin. Apoptosis is common. Vascular space invasion is the norm.
- The absence of gland formation in many; some may have tubular, cordlike, or sertoliform differentiation reminiscent of more well-defined neuroendocrine carcinomas.
- Geographic necrosis may be conspicuous.

IMMUNOPATHOLOGY (INCLUDING IMMUNOHISTOCHEMISTRY)

- Neuron-specific enolase is often positive but not specific. Staining with chromogranin and synaptophysin is more reliable, but extent will vary greatly from case to case. Most cases do not exhibit diffuse staining with these markers.
- p53 and p16 are usually strong.

PREFERRED DIAGNOSIS (WHEN AN ISOLATED FINDING)

High-grade (grade 3) endometrial carcinoma with neuroendocrine differentiation.

MAIN DIFFERENTIAL DIAGNOSIS

- Grade 3 endometrioid adenocarcinoma—usually a lower N/C ratio, more homogeneous distribution of chromatin, and solid growth without neuroendocrine-like architecture.
- Undifferentiated carcinoma—this distinction may be a judgment call based on immunostains.
- Lymphoma—usually easily distinguished.
- Stromal sarcoma or sarcomas with sex cord–like differentiation.
- Cervical neuroendocrine carcinoma—p16 positive but p53 weak or heterogeneous.

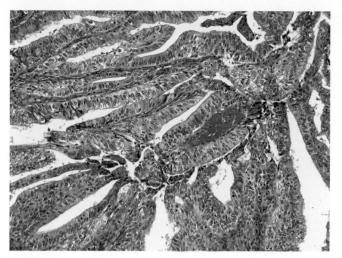

FIGURE 1

Neuroendocrine differentiation in carcinoma of the endometrium may coexist with conventional endometrioid histology as seen here.

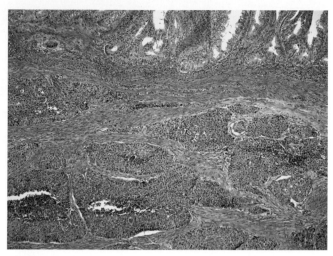

FIGURE 2

Neuroendocrine carcinoma of the endometrium. The endometrioid histology above is juxtaposed with undifferentiated carcinoma below. Note the necrosis.

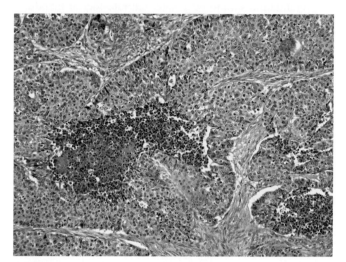

FIGURE 3

Neuroendocrine differentiation in endometrial carcinoma. Note the poorly differentiated albeit uniformly arranged cells.

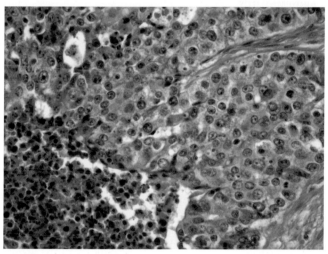

FIGURE 4

Neuroendocrine differentiation in carcinoma of the endometrium. At higher magnification the cells display uniform spacing, fine to coarse chromatin, and variable nucleoli.

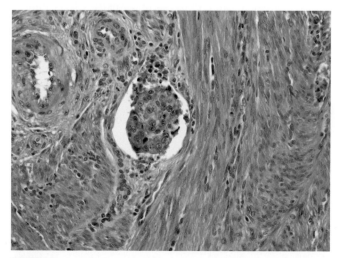

FIGURE 5

Neuroendocrine differentiation in carcinoma of the endometrium with vascular space involvement.

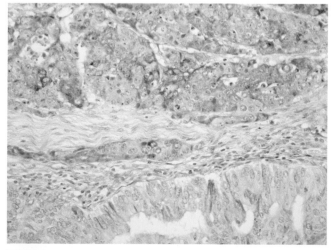

FIGURE 6

Neuroendocrine differentiation in carcinoma of the endometrium. The synaptophysin stain is positive.

UNDIFFERENTIATED CARCINOMA OF THE ENDOMETRIUM

DEFINITION—Poorly differentiated carcinomas in which a line of differentiation cannot be determined.

CLINICAL FEATURES

EPIDEMIOLOGY

- Pure undifferentiated carcinomas are rare.
- Patients may present at a wide range of ages, with a mean age of 63 years.

PRESENTATION

- Abnormal vaginal bleeding.
- Diffuse lymphadenopathy may be present at the time of diagnosis, giving the false clinical impression of a hematologic neoplasm.

PROGNOSIS AND TREATMENT

- About 79% of stage I (up to 100% if tumor is in the inner half of the myometrium) and 33% stage II survive 5 years.
- Total abdominal hysterectomy with lymph node dissection followed by adjuvant chemotherapy or radiation is typically employed.

PATHOLOGY

HISTOLOGY

- Undifferentiated carcinomas are typically composed of small- to medium-sized cells with vesicular nuclei and prominent nucleoli.
- The tumor cells may appear discohesive, mimicking lymphoma.
- Mitotic activity is markedly increased with many bizarre forms.

- Tumor-infiltrating lymphocytes may be prominent.
- Features of endometrioid (glands, squamous morules), serous, or clear cell (hyaline stroma, hobnailing) differentiation should be absent, but rare foci of glandular differentiation are not uncommon.

IMMUNOPATHOLOGY (INCLUDING IMMUNOHISTOCHEMISTRY)

- Keratin immunostaining may be focally positive (AE1/AE3, CK18).
- EMA may be focally positive.
- Markers of other lines of differentiation (CD45, MyoD1, SMA, Desmin) are negative NSE or synaptophysin are found in 10% to 30% but do not correlate with prognosis.
- ER and PR are typically negative.

MAIN DIFFERENTIAL DIAGNOSIS

- The International Federation of Gynecology and Obstetrics (FIGO) grade III endometrioid adenocarcinoma.
- Serous adenocarcinoma (solid variant)—these tumors typically demonstrate marked nuclear atypia.
- Poorly differentiated stromal sarcoma—these may be difficult to distinguish but should demonstrate a reticulin pattern of a mesenchymal tumor.
- Lymphoma—distinguished principally by immunohistochemistry.
- Neuroendocrine carcinoma—neuroendocrine differentiation (positive for chromogranin, synaptophysin, and NSE).
- Rhabdomyosarcoma—skeletal muscle differentiation.
- Leiomyosarcoma—smooth muscle differentiation.

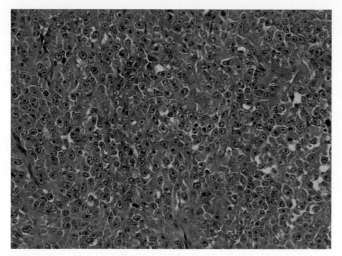

FIGURE 1

Undifferentiated carcinoma. Pleomorphic cells with prominent nucleoli.

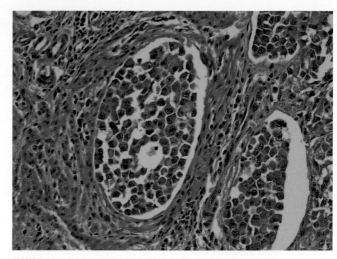

FIGURE 2

Undifferentiated carcinoma. Discohesive, plasmacytoid cells present within the lymphatics.

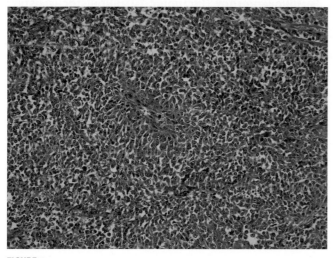

FIGURE 3

Undifferentiated carcinoma. Sheets of discohesive cells. Note the lack of architectural differentiation.

CLEAR-CELL CARCINOMA

DEFINITION—A high-grade, malignant neoplasm of the endometrium.

CLINICAL FEATURES

EPIDEMIOLOGY

- Clear-cell carcinoma of the endometrium is a rare malignancy comprising less than 1% of all endometrial cancers.

PRESENTATION

- Patients present with findings typical of endometrial carcinoma including bleeding, pain, and mass effect.
- Rarely patients may be asymptomatic.

PROGNOSIS AND TREATMENT

- Although classified as a high-grade carcinoma, 5-year progression-free and overall survival (OS) are 61% and 78%, respectively, and OS is 94% and 88% for stage I and II, respectively.
- Surgical staging is considered first-line therapy with chemotherapy and radiation as an option for high-stage cases.

PATHOLOGY

HISTOLOGY

- Large, polyhedral cells with distinct cell borders compose most tumors.
- Growth patterns range from small tubular glands to papillae to solid growth.
- In the glandular and papillary patterns these structures are lined by a single row of pleomorphic cells with distinct cell borders and varying levels of clear, vacuolated cytoplasm.

- Stromal hyalinization often accompanies the malignant epithelium and can be a helpful diagnostic clue.
- The presence of diffuse atypia and mitotic activity can help to differentiate clear-cell carcinoma from Arias-Stella effect (ASE).

IMMUNOPATHOLOGY (INCLUDING IMMUNOHISTOCHEMISTRY)

- Immunostaining for p53 typically shows an increased level of staining compared with low-grade endometrioid adenocarcinoma and a lower level of staining than serous carcinoma.
- Staining for hepatocyte nuclear factor (HNF-1beta) stains clear-cell neoplasms, but overlap can be seen in ASE and some endometrioid carcinomas.
- Napsin A is a sensitive marker (and should usually be positive) and AMACR a relatively specific marker for clear-cell carcinoma.

MAIN DIFFERENTIAL DIAGNOSIS

- Uterine serous carcinoma—typically more stratified, strongly p53 positive (or negative), and hyaline stromal changes are less conspicuous.
- ASE—can be particularly challenging in older women where the ASE is discrete (clonal-like).
- Endometrioid adenocarcinoma with secretory differentiation—less nuclear atypia with a lower nuclear-to-cytoplasmic (N/C) ratio and admixing of the vacuoles and nuclei with less hobnailing.
- Poorly differentiated endometrial carcinoma with clear-cell features—the predominant pattern is a stratified neoplastic epithelium with haphazardly arranged vacuoles. Staining for HNF1-beta may be positive but Napsin A and AMACR less so.

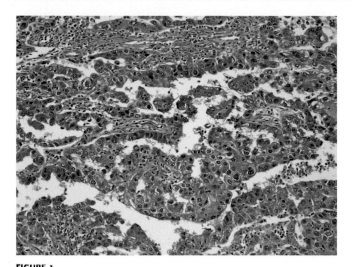

FIGURE 1

Clear-cell carcinoma. A single lining of pleomorphic epithelial cells. Note the focal cytoplasmic clearing in the middle aspect of the picture.

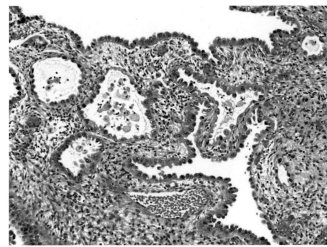

FIGURE 2

Clear-cell carcinoma. Glands with hobnail cells projecting into the lumen.

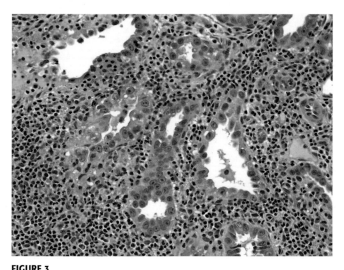

FIGURE 3

Clear-cell carcinoma. A single layer of markedly pleomorphic cells projecting into the glandular lumen.

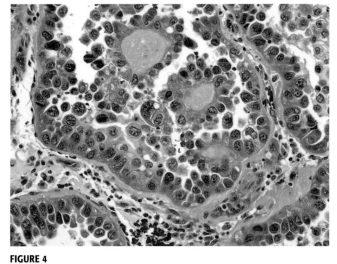

FIGURE 4

Clear-cell carcinoma. Small papillary cores with hyalinization and hobnail cells.

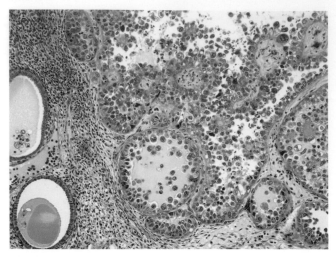

FIGURE 5

Clear-cell carcinoma. Pleomorphic, hobnail cells with focal cytoplasmic clearing. Uninvolved glands are on the left.

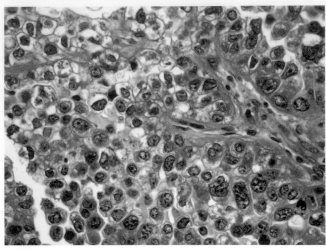

FIGURE 6

Clear-cell carcinoma. A solid sheet of pleomorphic cells with cytoplasmic clearing and distinct cell borders.

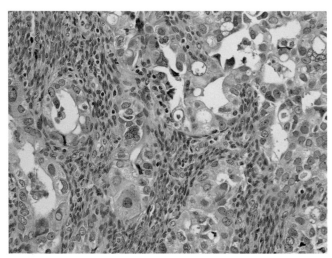

FIGURE 7

Clear-cell carcinoma. This tumor exhibits a more heterogeneous cell population.

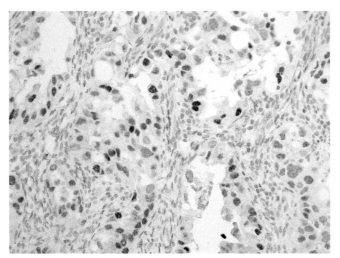

FIGURE 8

The field in Figure 7 following HNF-1beta immunostaining.

ENDOMETRIOID OR CLEAR-CELL CARCINOMA?

DEFINITION—A problematic endometrioid carcinoma with some clear-cell features.

CLINICAL FEATURES

EPIDEMIOLOGY

- Similar to other endometrioid carcinomas.

PRESENTATION

- Patients present with findings typical of endometrial carcinoma including bleeding, pain, and mass effect.
- Rarely patients may be asymptomatic.

PROGNOSIS AND TREATMENT

- Approached as an endometrioid adenocarcinoma and managed based on stage and grade.
- Surgical staging is considered first-line therapy with chemotherapy and radiation as an option for high-stage cases.

PATHOLOGY

HISTOLOGY

- There should be a recognizable endometrioid component.

- Clear cells show modest atypia and are arranged mostly in solid sheets or glands.
- In the glandular and papillary patterns, lining epithelium largely demonstrates monomorphic nuclei.
- Stromal hyalinization is absent or inconspicuous.

IMMUNOPATHOLOGY (INCLUDING IMMUNOHISTOCHEMISTRY)

- Immunostaining for p53 should be heterogeneous.
- Staining for clear-cell carcinoma markers hepatocyte nuclear factor (HINF1-β) is positive.
- Napsin-A and AMACR will be contradictory.

MAIN DIFFERENTIAL DIAGNOSIS

- Uterine serous carcinoma—greater nuclear atypia and strongly p53 positive (or negative).
- Clear-cell carcinoma—greater atypia, stromal hyalinization, and hobnailing.

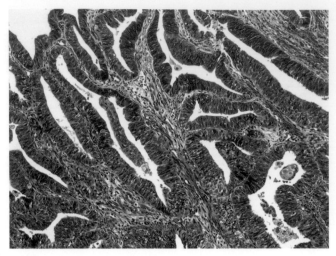

FIGURE 1

Endometrioid carcinoma with secretory clear-cell features. This focus contains typical endometrioid histology.

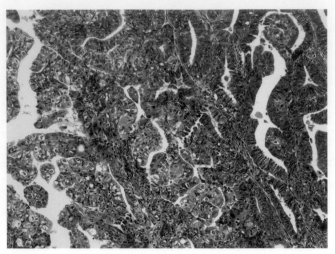

FIGURE 2

Endometrioid carcinoma with secretory clear-cell features. Transition from endometrioid to the secretory clear-cell pattern.

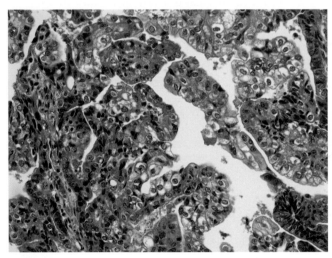

FIGURE 3

Endometrioid carcinoma with secretory clear-cell features. These areas show sheet-forming, glandlike, or ill-defined papillary architecture. Note the minimal nuclear atypia.

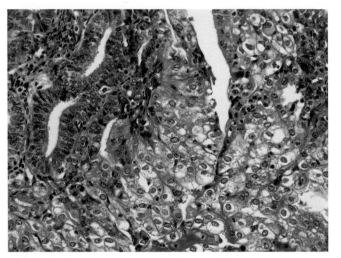

FIGURE 4

Endometrioid carcinoma with secretory clear-cell features. These areas show sheet-forming, glandlike, or ill-defined papillary architecture. Note the minimal nuclear atypia.

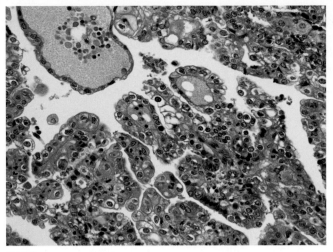

FIGURE 5

Endometrioid carcinoma with secretory clear-cell features. This one focus exhibits a few pseudopapillae. Note the absence of hyalinized stromal cores.

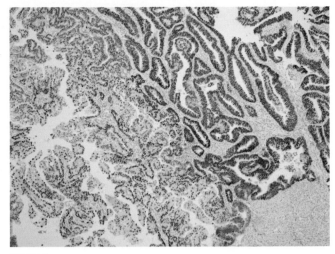

FIGURE 6

Endometrioid carcinoma with secretory clear-cell features. An HINF1 stain is positive but strongest in the endometrioid areas *(right)*, diminishing somewhat in the secretory clear-cell region *(center)*.

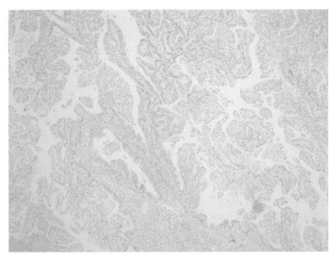

FIGURE 7

Napsin-A, a sensitive marker for clear-cell carcinoma, is negative.

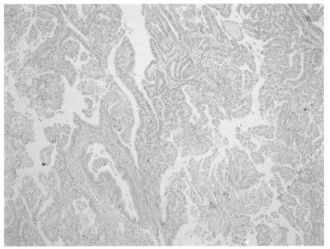

FIGURE 8

AMACR, a specific marker for clear-cell carcinoma, is also negative.

CARCINOSARCOMA

DEFINITION—A highly malignant neoplasm composed of malignant glandular and stromal elements.

CLINICAL FEATURES

EPIDEMIOLOGY

- Occurs almost exclusively in women over 60 years of age.
- An association with prior radiation has been described.
- Some studies show an increased frequency in African-American women.

PRESENTATION

- Most cases present with postmenopausal bleeding.
- Occasional cases present with the striking finding of a vaginal mass, representing prolapsed uterine tumor.

PROGNOSIS AND TREATMENT

- Carcinosarcoma carries a dismal prognosis with a 5-year survival of around 30% to 40%.
- First-line treatment consists of a total abdominal hysterectomy, bilateral salpingo-oophorectomy, lymphadenectomy, and full surgical staging.
- Most patients will receive adjuvant chemotherapy and radiation therapy.

PATHOLOGY

HISTOLOGY

- Malignant glandular and stromal elements with marked heterogeneity are present.
- The glandular component is often high grade and may display typical serous, endometrioid, or clear-cell patterns of growth. Uncommon patterns, such as neuroendocrine differentiation, primitive-appearing "secretory" changes, and bizarre squamous differentiation, should prompt a closer look for a malignant mesenchymal component.
- Poorly differentiated carcinoma with no discernible pattern of growth may be present.
- A common finding is that of solid carcinomatous growth with marked pleomorphism and necrosis.
- The sarcomatous component has typically been defined as homologous (stromal or smooth muscle) or heterologous (chondrosarcoma, rhabdomyosarcoma, osteosarcoma, or liposarcoma).
- The composition of the epithelial and stromal components is highly variable, and either may represent a focal finding.
- Poorly differentiated carcinomas with spindled areas or extensive desmoplasia may mimic carcinosarcoma, and in these cases the assessment of pattern variability coupled with immunostains for keratin may be helpful.
- Metastasis is typically composed of the malignant glandular component; however, either component of the primary tumor may be present.

IMMUNOPATHOLOGY (INCLUDING IMMUNOHISTOCHEMISTRY)

- Pan-cytokeratin staining may be helpful in identifying the carcinomatous element in a tumor with sarcomatoid differentiation or extensive desmoplasia.
- Smooth muscle markers (SMA, desmin, h-caldesmon) may be helpful in identifying the mesenchymal component of some tumors.

MAIN DIFFERENTIAL DIAGNOSIS

- Sarcomatoid or spindled variants of carcinoma—this usually appears as a spindle cell component in an otherwise well-differentiated endometrioid adenocarcinoma.
- Extensive desmoplasia mimicking sarcoma.

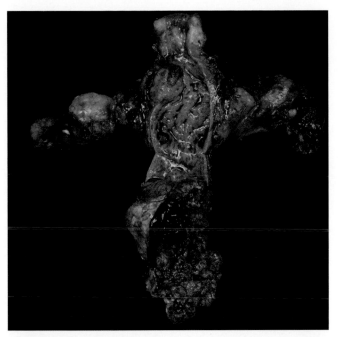

FIGURE 1

Carcinosarcoma. Gross example of carcinosarcoma presenting as a fungating, polypoid mass with associated hemorrhage.

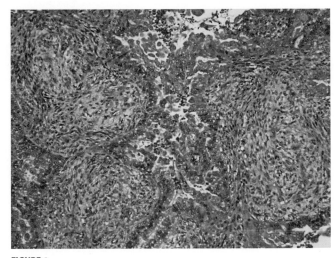

FIGURE 2

Carcinosarcoma. Typical arrangement of malignant glands and stroma. Note the faint basophilic hue to the stromal component.

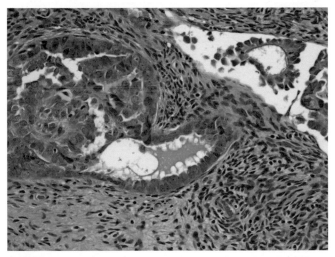

FIGURE 3

Carcinosarcoma. Malignant glandular component composed of serous adenocarcinoma.

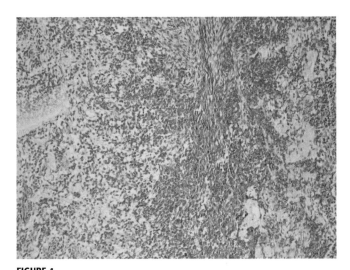

FIGURE 4

Carcinosarcoma. Primitive, high-grade carcinoma.

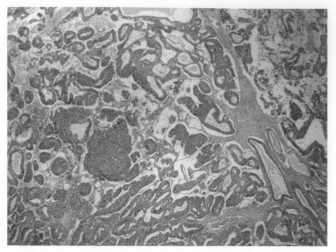

FIGURE 5

Carcinosarcoma. Endometrioid adenocarcinoma with focal solid growth (sarcomatous component is not pictured).

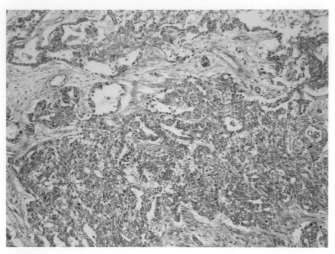

FIGURE 6

Carcinosarcoma. High-grade carcinoma with a primitive, "yolk sac–like" growth pattern.

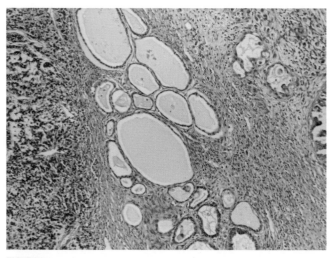

FIGURE 7

Carcinosarcoma. Atypical glands *(right)* with malignant stroma seen surrounding the glands on the right and filling the left side.

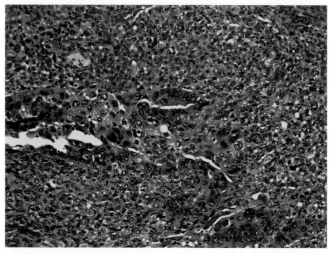

FIGURE 8

Carcinosarcoma. High-grade adenocarcinoma with marked nuclear pleomorphism and surrounding undifferentiated sarcoma.

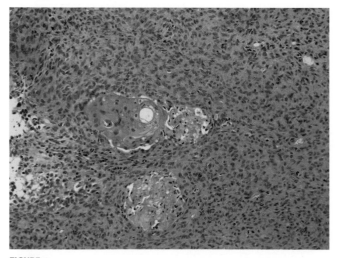

FIGURE 9

Carcinosarcoma. Sarcoma with focal glandular elements with abnormal keratinization.

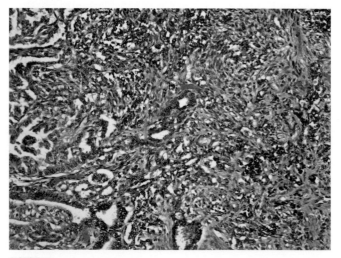

FIGURE 10

Carcinosarcoma. Malignant glands and stroma.

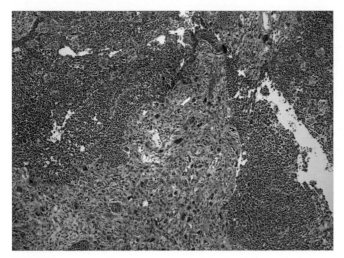

FIGURE 11

Carcinosarcoma. High-grade carcinoma with marked pleomorphism and sarcoma resembling endometrial stromal sarcoma.

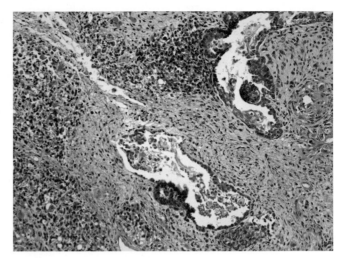

FIGURE 12

Carcinosarcoma. Malignant glands and stroma. A faint basophilic hue can be seen adjacent to one of the malignant glands.

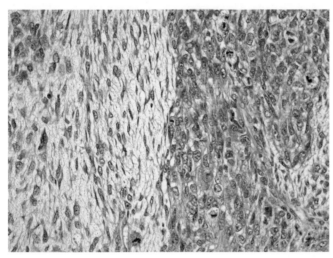

FIGURE 13

Carcinosarcoma. Sarcoma within a carcinosarcoma with a biphasic pattern of growth.

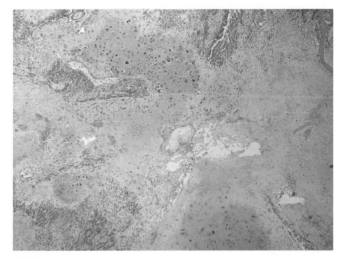

FIGURE 14

Carcinosarcoma. Heterologous cartilaginous differentiation.

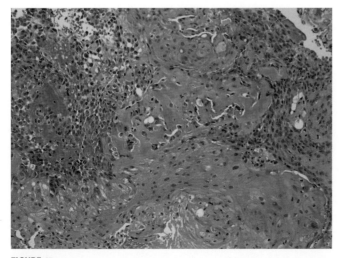

FIGURE 15

Carcinosarcoma. Heterologous osteoid formation *(center)* with adjacent keratinization.

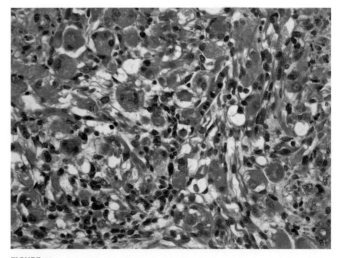

FIGURE 16

Carcinosarcoma. Malignant sarcoma with rhabdoid differentiation and marked pleomorphism.

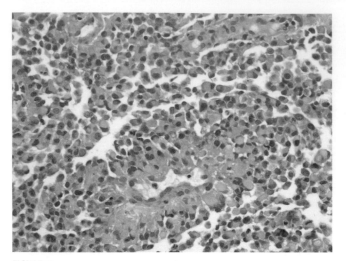

FIGURE 17

Carcinosarcoma. Rhabdoid differentiation.

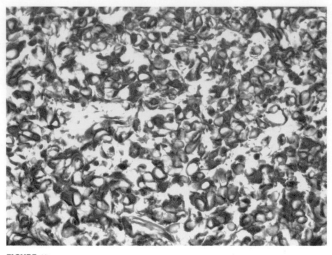

FIGURE 18

Carcinosarcoma. Rhabdoid cells staining positive for smooth muscle actin.

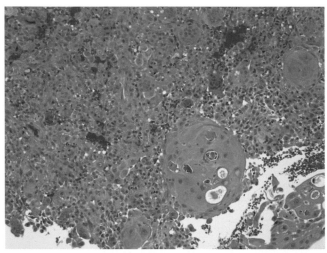

FIGURE 19

Carcinosarcoma. Syncytiotrophoblastic-like giant cells.

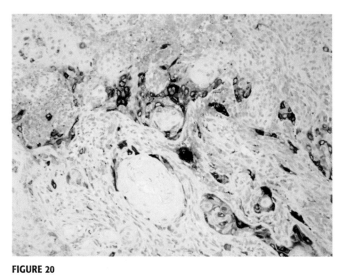

FIGURE 20

Carcinosarcoma. Syncytiotrophoblastic-like giant cells staining positive for human chorionic gonadotropin (HCG).

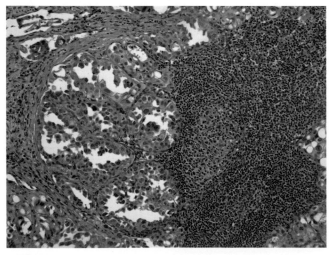

FIGURE 21

Carcinosarcoma. Lymph node metastasis composed of high-grade adenocarcinoma.

ADENOCARCINOMA WITH SPINDLE CELL FEATURES

DEFINITION—A variant of endometrial carcinoma with pseudomesenchymal or spindle cell differentiation.

CLINICAL FEATURES

EPIDEMIOLOGY

- Similar to that of conventional endometrioid adenocarcinoma.

PRESENTATION

- Detected during histologic examination.

PROGNOSIS AND TREATMENT

- Outcome parallels that of conventional adenocarcinoma and distinct from that for carcinosarcoma.
- Management is based on stage and grade, similar to adenocarcinomas.

PATHOLOGY

HISTOLOGY

- These tumors will typically (but not always) contain a component of well-differentiated adenocarcinoma, as opposed to carcinosarcomas, in which the glandular component is often poorly differentiated or demonstrates unusual patterns.
- Squamous differentiation may be present.
- A separate spindle cell component exhibits features not typical of sarcoma, including bland-appearing nuclei, an eosinophilic matrix, and eosinophilic cytoplasm.

- The spindle cells stream in an orderly fashion, often blending with the glandular or squamous component.
- The spindle cells are keratin positive.

IMMUNOPATHOLOGY (INCLUDING IMMUNOHISTOCHEMISTRY)

- Spindle cells are positive for pan-cytokeratin and negative for desmin and SMA.

MAIN DIFFERENTIAL DIAGNOSIS

- Carcinosarcoma, which has an immunohistochemically defined stromal component.

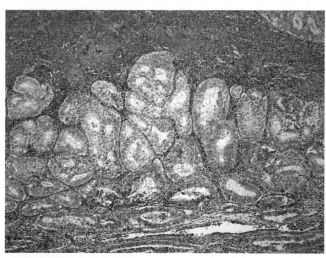

FIGURE 1

Endometrioid adenocarcinoma with spindle cell differentiation. The glandular component is distinctly bland and grade I when present.

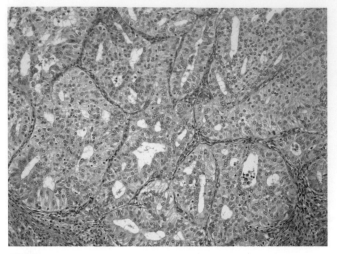

FIGURE 2

Endometrioid adenocarcinoma with spindle cell differentiation. The glandular component is distinctly bland and grade I when present.

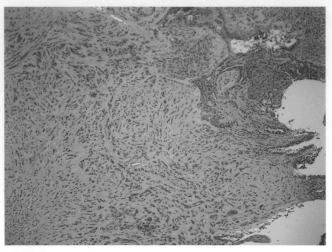

FIGURE 3

Endometrioid adenocarcinoma with spindle cell differentiation carcinosarcoma. At low magnification the spindle cell component demonstrates an orderly growth pattern, streaming into an eosinophilic matrix.

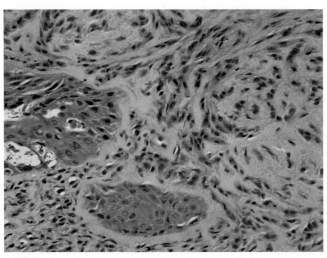

FIGURE 4

Endometrioid adenocarcinoma with spindle cell differentiation. At higher magnification the spindle cells are seen to stream from areas of squamous metaplasia.

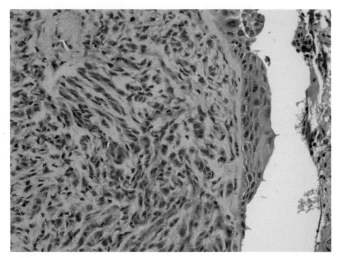

FIGURE 5

Endometrioid adenocarcinoma with spindle cell differentiation. Note the bland nuclei and conspicuous cytoplasm in the spindle cell component.

WILMS' TUMOR OF THE ENDOMETRIUM

DEFINITION—A variant of carcinosarcoma recapitulating Wilms' tumor.

CLINICAL FEATURES

EPIDEMIOLOGY

- Occurs over a wide age range from childhood to the eighth decade.
- Rare.
- Possibly arises from displaced metanephric rests.

PRESENTATION

- Abnormal bleeding.
- Pelvic mass.
- Cervical polyp.

PROGNOSIS AND TREATMENT

- Numbers are small, but many have shown a favorable outcome and no recurrence.
- Managed by hysterectomy and salpingo-oophorectomy.
- Most patients will receive adjuvant chemotherapy and radiation therapy.

PATHOLOGY

HISTOLOGY

- Classic triphasic pattern with epithelium, blastema, and stromal differentiation.

- Monotonous repetitive pattern is typical and distinguishes this tumor from a carcinosarcoma.
- Glomeruloid bodies.

IMMUNOPATHOLOGY (INCLUDING IMMUNOHISTOCHEMISTRY)

- Neuron-specific enolase, CD99, CD56, WT-1 positive.

MAIN DIFFERENTIAL DIAGNOSIS

- Carcinosarcoma—should be more heterogeneous and lack the glomeruloid bodies. Uniform primitive tubules should be less conspicuous.
- Mesonephric carcinoma—may be a mixture of both spindle and epithelial cells, but the blastema and glomeruloid bodies should not be seen.
- Primitive neuroectodermal tumor—should be negative for WT-1 and lack glomeruloid bodies.

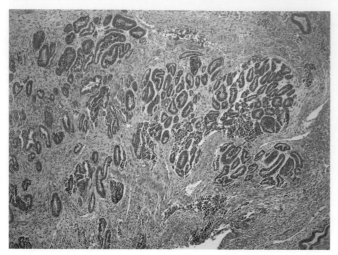

FIGURE 1

Extrarenal Wilms' tumor of the uterus. Note the uniform hyperchromatic glandlike structures.

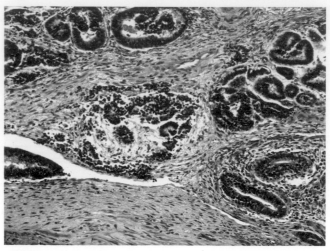

FIGURE 2

Extrarenal Wilms' tumor of the uterus. Glandlike structures are admixed with stroma.

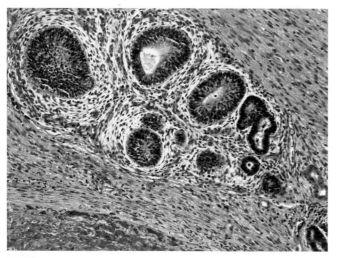

FIGURE 3

Extrarenal Wilms' tumor of the uterus. Spindled stromal envelops glands with focal eosinophilic rhabdoid cells.

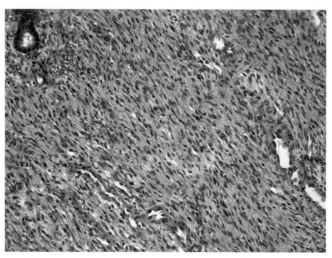

FIGURE 4

Extrarenal Wilms' tumor of the uterus. Another focus with a distinct mesenchymal appearance.

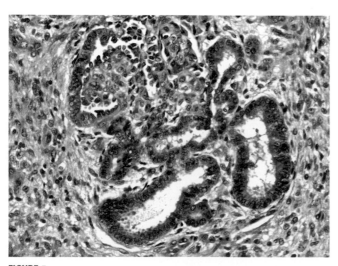

FIGURE 5

Extrarenal Wilms' tumor of the uterus. In this field there is a distinct glomeruloid structure.

ENDOMETRIAL STROMAL NODULE

DEFINITION—A benign neoplasm composed of cells resembling normal endometrial stroma.

CLINICAL FEATURES

EPIDEMIOLOGY

- Endometrial stromal nodules (ESNs) are uncommon neoplasms that occur at any age.
- Most often identified during the fifth and sixth decades of life.
- JAZF1/JJAZ1 gene fusion.

PRESENTATION

- Patients are usually asymptomatic.
- ESN may be associated with abnormal uterine bleeding or mass effect, similar to the symptoms seen with leiomyomata.

PROGNOSIS AND TREATMENT

- ESN is a benign neoplasm; the prognosis is excellent.
- A stromal neoplasm suspected on biopsy or curettage should be excised to exclude the possibility of a low-grade endometrial stromal sarcoma.
- Conservative excision is curative.

PATHOLOGY

HISTOLOGY

- Grossly ESN may be located intramurally, submucosally, or as an exophytic polypoid mass.

- The gross appearance is similar to that of a leiomyoma; however, ESNs are softer and do not bulge on cut section.
- At low power the hallmark feature of an ESN is the well-circumscribed border with adjacent myometrium.
- Foci of infiltrative fingerlike tumor projections of less than 0.3 cm are allowed in otherwise unremarkable ESN.
- At high power, ESN is composed of small spindled cells with scant cytoplasm that resemble normal proliferative-phase endometrial stroma.
- Small, uniformly sized arterioles are regularly interspersed throughout the tumor.
- Lymphatic or vascular invasion is absent.
- Scattered stromal foam cells may be present in varying amounts.
- Tumor size varies but is usually less than 10 cm (larger ESNs have been reported).

IMMUNOPATHOLOGY (INCLUDING IMMUNOHISTOCHEMISTRY)

- Positive for CD10.
- Negative or weakly positive for SMA, desmin, and h-caldesmon.

MAIN DIFFERENTIAL DIAGNOSIS

- Cellular leiomyoma—larger caliber vessels, positive for SMA, desmin, caldesmon.
- Endometrial stromal sarcoma, low grade—infiltrative borders, vascular invasion.

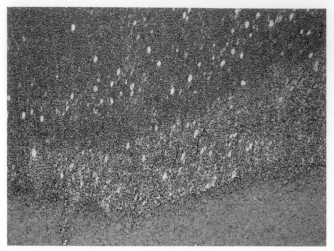

FIGURE 1

ESN. At low power the well-circumscribed border with adjacent myometrium is apparent. Note that slight irregularities are present.

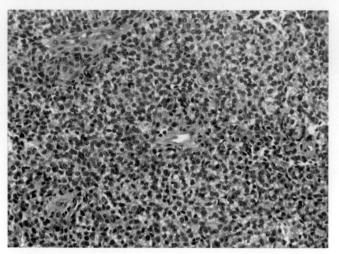

FIGURE 2

ESN. The neoplastic cells are small, with rounded nuclei and scant cytoplasm. Note the regularly spaced arterioles.

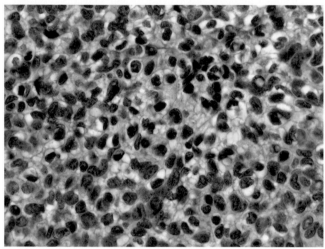

FIGURE 3

ESN. At high power the cells are small and bland.

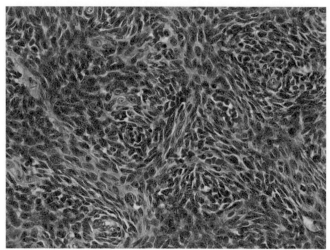

FIGURE 4

ESN. The spindled cells often whorl around the small vascular spaces.

STROMOMYOMA

DEFINITION—A low-grade stromal tumor with smooth muscle differentiation.

CLINICAL FEATURES

EPIDEMIOLOGY

- Same as endometrial stromal nodules (ESNs); are uncommon neoplasms that occur at any age.
- Most often identified during the fifth and sixth decades of life.

PRESENTATION

- Patients are usually asymptomatic.
- Stromomyoma may be associated with abnormal uterine bleeding or mass effect, similar to the symptoms seen with leiomyomata.

PROGNOSIS AND TREATMENT

- Stromomyoma is a benign neoplasm if configured like a stromal nodule. This may require hysterectomy to confirm and exclude a low-grade stromal sarcoma.
- Conservative excision, if possible, is curative, provided that the uterus is monitored for regrowth.

PATHOLOGY

HISTOLOGY

- Stromomyoma may be intramural, submucosal, or an exophytic polypoid mass.
- The gross appearance will vary from that of a leiomyoma to a softer neoplasm if predominantly stromal.
- At low magnification a stromomyoma will have a well-circumscribed border with adjacent myometrium if a nodule; careful scrutiny of borders will be important in assigning risk.
- Key features at low power include less nuclear dense areas with smooth muscle differentiation and fascicle formation intertwined with the stromal component.

- At high power, stromomyoma will display both stromal and smooth muscle differentiation.
- Lymphatic or vascular invasion is absent in nodules.
- Tumor size varies but is usually less than 10 cm (larger ESNs have been reported).

IMMUNOPATHOLOGY (INCLUDING IMMUNOHISTOCHEMISTRY)

- Positive for CD10 in stromal areas and SMA, desmin, h-caldesmon in the smooth muscle foci.

MAIN DIFFERENTIAL DIAGNOSIS

- Cellular leiomyoma—will not display a stromal phenotype, but this may require immunostains to confirm.
- Endometrial stromal sarcoma, low grade with smooth muscle differentiation—this may require excision to exclude infiltrative borders or vascular space invasion.

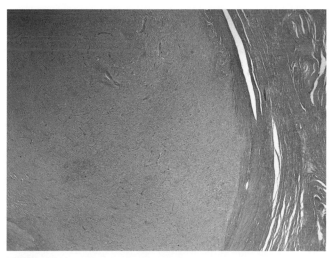

FIGURE 1

Stromomyoma. At low power there is a well-circumscribed border with adjacent myometrium.

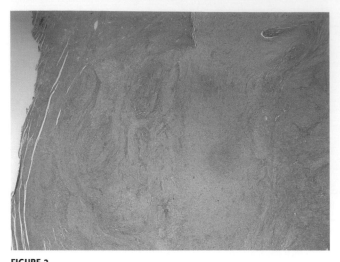

FIGURE 2

Stromomyoma. Note the admixed stromal and smooth muscle components in the center of the tumor. The periphery *(left)* is still circumscribed.

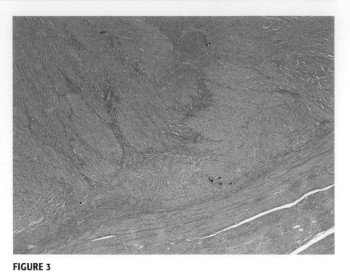

FIGURE 3

Stromomyoma. At higher power the juxtaposed stromal and smooth muscle elements can be appreciated. Again note the sharply demarcated border at the lower right, characteristic of a nodule.

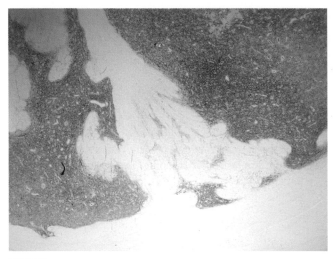

FIGURE 4

Stromomyoma. CD10 staining is strong in the stromal component.

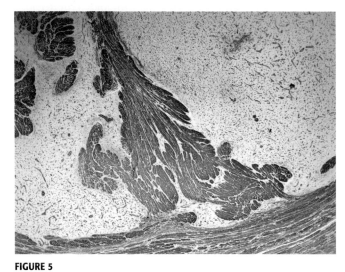

FIGURE 5

Stromomyoma. Desmin is strong in the areas of smooth muscle differentiation.

ENDOMETRIAL STROMATOSIS

DEFINITION—An endometrial polyp, composed of benign smooth muscle and glands.

CLINICAL FEATURES

EPIDEMIOLOGY

- Same as for adenomyosis, predominating in the fourth and fifth decades. However, the absence of glands is more likely to be seen postmenopause after glandular atrophy has taken place.

PRESENTATION

- In premenopausal women, dysmenorrhea, pelvic discomfort, and abnormal bleeding.
- Postmenopause may be an incidental finding.

PROGNOSIS AND TREATMENT

- None required.

PATHOLOGY

HISTOLOGY

- Stromal condensations in the endometrium.
- Stellate configuration is common.

- Somewhat vague interface between stroma and myometrium.
- Glands rare or nonexistent.

IMMUNOPATHOLOGY (INCLUDING IMMUNOHISTOCHEMISTRY)

- CD10 positive but this entity is usually easily recognized on hematoxylin and eosin (H&E) stains.

MAIN DIFFERENTIAL DIAGNOSIS

- Low-grade endometrial stromal sarcoma (ESS)—this entity will typically display a more rounded, sharply demarcated border.

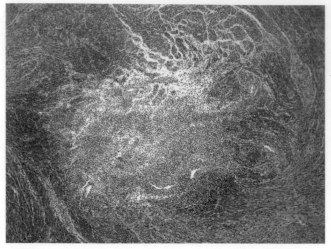

FIGURE 1

Endometrial stromatosis. Note the slightly stellate appearance relative to the surrounding myometrium and the vague stromal-myometrial interface.

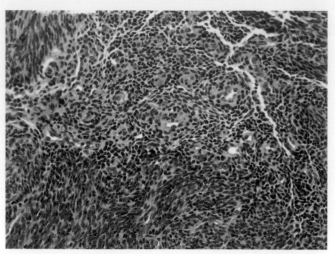

FIGURE 2

Endometrial stromatosis. At higher magnification the constituent cells are typical of benign endometrial stroma.

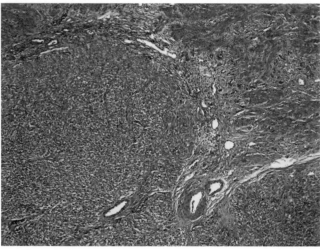

FIGURE 3

ESS. In contrast to stromatosis the neoplastic cells form a sharp interface with the surrounding myometrium.

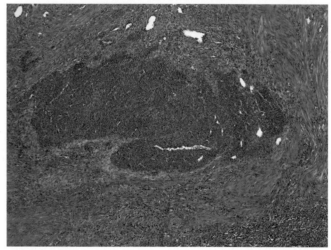

FIGURE 4

ESS. Note the rather sharp interface between tumor cells and myometrium; contrast to Figure 1.

LOW-GRADE ENDOMETRIAL STROMAL SARCOMA

DEFINITION—A malignancy composed of cells resembling proliferative-phase endometrial stroma.

CLINICAL FEATURES

EPIDEMIOLOGY

- Endometrial stromal sarcoma (ESS) is rare; it accounts for less than 0.5% of all uterine malignancies and only 10% to 15% of mesenchymal uterine malignancies.
- ESS tends to occur in younger women more than other mesenchymal uterine tumors and is typically seen in women in their 40s and 50s.
- The so-called low-grade endometrial stromal sarcomas (LGESSs) account for the majority of these tumors; high-grade and undifferentiated types are rare and are discussed separately.

PRESENTATION

- Abnormal uterine bleeding is the most common presenting symptom.
- Patients may complain of pelvic pain or pressure.
- Up to one quarter of patients are asymptomatic.
- Endometrial sampling does not usually reveal the diagnosis.

PROGNOSIS AND TREATMENT

- If confined to the uterus, LGESS has an excellent prognosis (~90% 5-year survival).
- Up to one third of patients have extrauterine spread at the time of presentation.
- Standard treatment for LGESS is hysterectomy and bilateral salpingo-oophorectomy (with or without pelvic lymphadenectomy).
- Recurrence is common and seen in up to 25% of patients with stage I disease at the time of hysterectomy.
- Distant metastases usually occur late and most commonly involve the lungs.
- Treatment for advanced or metastatic disease often includes hormonal therapy as most LGESSs are strongly progestin receptor positive.
- Undifferentiated ESSs have a poor prognosis.

PATHOLOGY

HISTOLOGY

- LGESS is characterized by a proliferation of cells that resemble nonneoplastic proliferative endometrial stroma.
- The tumor cells are spindled, with elongated round to oval nuclei and scant amounts of eosinophilic or amphophilic cytoplasm.
- At low power, LGESS is notable for its distinctive pattern of myometrial invasion, which is recognized by the characteristic "tongues" or "fingers" of tumor that dissect between the background smooth muscle bundles.
- Prominent (plugging) lymphovascular invasion is commonly noted.
- These growth and lymphovascular invasion patterns can impart a "wormlike" appearance grossly.
- At higher power, small round arterioles (analogous to the spiral arterioles) are interspersed within the tumor.
- Stromal hyalinization may occur and can be prominent.
- Divergent differentiation has been described and may consist of the following:
  1. Smooth muscle differentiation: Greater than 30% of the tumor should be composed of smooth muscle to qualify. The smooth muscle component may merge imperceptibly with the traditional ESS component, may have prominent central hyalinization in a so-called "starburst pattern," or may be present as irregular islands of differing morphology. Molecularly, these tumors are part of the ESS family of tumors and should be evaluated as such.
  2. Sex cord–like areas: Cords, tubules, and/or anastomosing trabeculae of cells resembling patterns seen in sex cord stromal tumors are present. These areas may be positive for inhibin. The presence of sex cord–like areas has no adverse prognostic implication.
  3. Endometrioid glands: Scattered endometrioid glands can be seen. Occasionally it may be difficult to

determine whether the glands are entrapped (as in adenomyosis) or truly part of the neoplastic process. The glands are most often well-formed endometrioid glands.

4. Fibrous or myxoid variants: Extensive hyalinization or myxoid change may be present, making the diagnosis of ESS challenging.

- Conventional LGESS (and variants) commonly exhibit a t(7;17) translocation involving the JAZF1 gene.

IMMUNOPATHOLOGY (INCLUDING IMMUNOHISTOCHEMISTRY)

- Traditional LGESS is usually positive for CD10 and negative for SMA and desmin.
- Occasionally LGESS will show a mixture of CD10 and smooth muscle marker (SMA, desmin) positivity reflecting combined stromal and smooth muscle differentiation.
- h-Caldesmon is more specific for true smooth muscle and may be helpful when there is increased SMA or desmin; it should be negative in ESS.
- Leiomyosarcoma may display areas of CD10 positivity.

MAIN DIFFERENTIAL DIAGNOSIS

- Endometrial stromal nodule—this distinction may not be possible on curettage specimens if sufficient fragments of myometrium are not available to assess the border of the tumor and whether myometrial invasion is present.
- Leiomyoma—cellular leiomyomas may mimic ESS and can usually be distinguished by the different vascular pattern and special stains, if needed.
- Leiomyosarcoma—typically are not confused with ESS but may mimic higher-grade stromal sarcomas. The fascicular arrangement of mesenchymal cells is helpful as is special stains for desmin, SMA, and h-caldesmon.
- Carcinosarcoma—this entity can be easily confused with ESS in small samples.

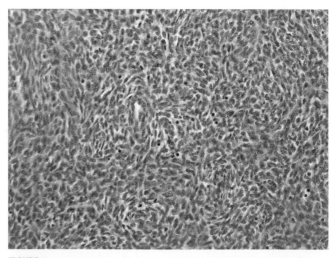

FIGURE 2

ESS. At low power the characteristic invasion pattern consisting of tongues and fingers of tumor pushing between smooth muscle bundles is apparent.

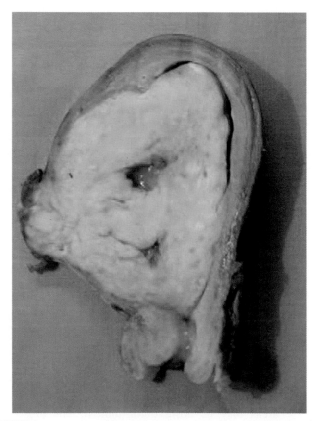

FIGURE 1

ESS. On sectioning, a somewhat irregular yellowish tumor mass distends the endometrial cavity. Note the solid appearance and the absence of any macroscopic features such as fascicle formation to suggest a smooth muscle tumor.

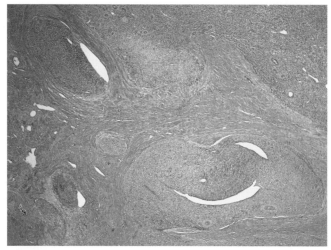

FIGURE 3

ESS. At high power LGESS is composed of small, spindled cells with elongated nuclei and scant cytoplasm. The tumor cells resemble proliferative stroma.

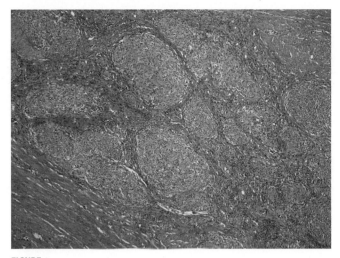

FIGURE 4

ESS. The fibrous variant of LGESS is present as multiple small nodules in this image. Note the resemblance to smooth muscle.

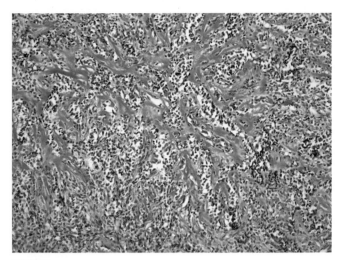

FIGURE 5

ESS. LGESS with extensive stromal hyalinization.

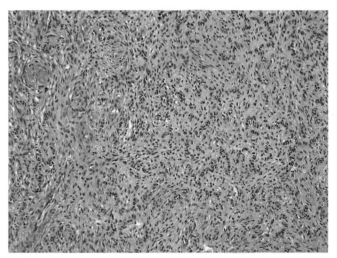

FIGURE 6

ESS. Cords of cells are prominent in this ESS with sex cord–like areas.

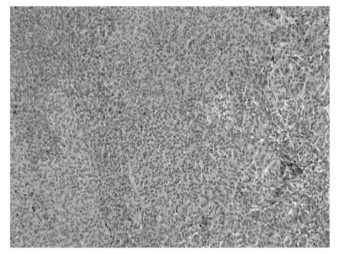

FIGURE 7

ESS. A subtle trabecular pattern *(right side of the image)* of sex cord–like growth is present in this ESS.

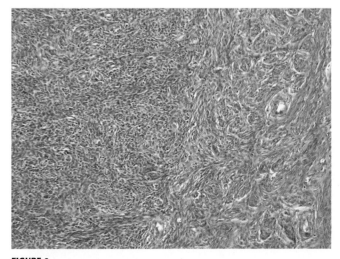

FIGURE 8

ESS. A typical appearance of LGESS *(left)* merges with an area of smooth muscle differentiation *(right)*.

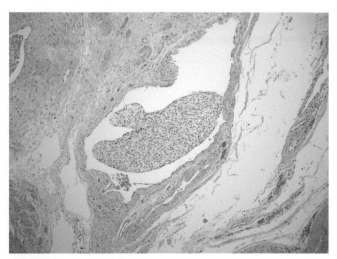

FIGURE 9

ESS. ESS commonly involves large vascular spaces in the myometrium and parametrium, as seen here.

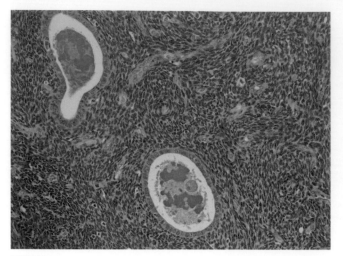

FIGURE 10

ESS. Scattered benign endometrioid glands are present in this metastatic focus.

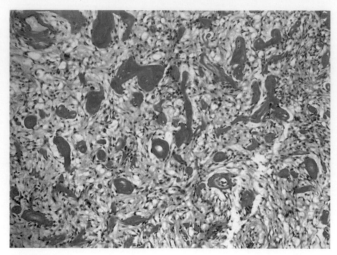

FIGURE 11

ESS. At low power this tumor is characterized by its prominent myxoid stroma rather than the more typical, densely cellular basophilic appearance of ESS. Note the presence of stromal collagen.

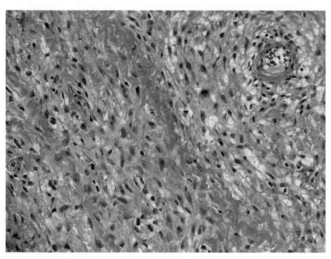

FIGURE 12

ESS. At high power this fibrous/myxoid example of ESS may be difficult to recognize. Note the round arteriole on the right.

UTERINE TUMOR RESEMBLING SEX CORD STROMAL TUMOR

DEFINITION—A benign low-grade mesenchymal tumor of the uterus.

CLINICAL FEATURES

EPIDEMIOLOGY

- Uterine tumor resembling sex cord tumor (UTRSCT) is rare; it accounts for less than 0.5% of all uterine malignancies and only 10% to 15% of mesenchymal uterine malignancies.
- Tumors are usually diagnosed in women in the fourth to sixth decades.
- These tumors in their pure form are held separate from low-grade endometrial stromal sarcomas (ESS) with sex cord—like areas. The latter have different biologic behavior.

PRESENTATION

- Abnormal uterine bleeding is the most common presenting symptom.
- Patients may complain of pelvic pain or pressure.
- Up to a quarter of patients are asymptomatic.
- Endometrial sampling does not usually reveal the diagnosis.

PROGNOSIS AND TREATMENT

- UTRSCT is typically benign with survival approaching 100% and rare (5%) recurrences, so long as there is no evidence of coexisting stromal sarcoma. In the latter the recurrence risk is high and disease-free survival poor (~25%).
- Treated by excision.

PATHOLOGY

HISTOLOGY

- UTRSCT is characterized by a repetitive pattern of cordlike or tubular growth.
- The tumor cells are bland appearing with noncomplex chromatin and round to oval features.

IMMUNOPATHOLOGY (INCLUDING IMMUNOHISTOCHEMISTRY)

- Positive for inhibin and calretinin.
- Negative for CD10.

MAIN DIFFERENTIAL DIAGNOSIS

- ESS—may have sex cord–like areas, but such lesions are heterogeneous. UTRSCT will be uniformly sex cord like throughout. The presence of CD10 would support ESS.
- Mesonephric carcinoma—these tumors are usually seen in the cervix but can present with ill defined tubules or other sex cord–like features, as well as spindled areas.

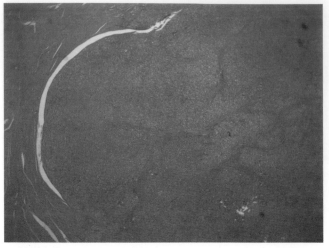

FIGURE 1

UTRSCT. The tumor is circumscribed at low magnification and resembles a stromal or smooth muscle neoplasm.

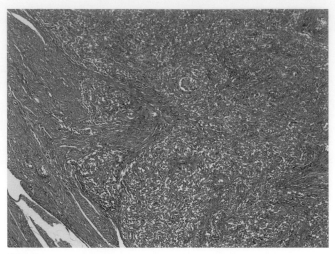

FIGURE 2

UTRSCT. At higher magnification a cordlike or ribbonlike pattern is seen, with vague acinar formation.

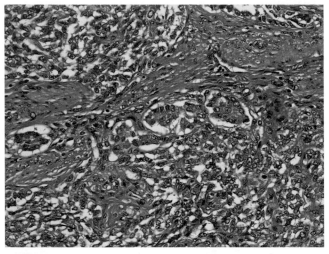

FIGURE 3

UTRSCT. At higher power a combination of some cordlike and acinar growth is seen.

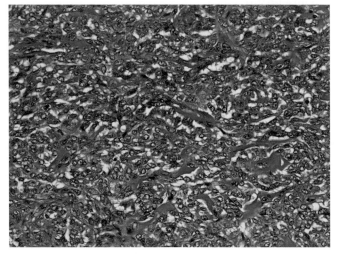

FIGURE 4

UTRSCT. This field appears vaguely ribbon like.

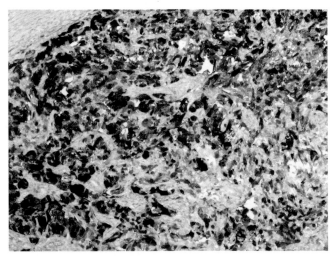

FIGURE 5

Stains for inhibin are strongly positive in UTRSCT.

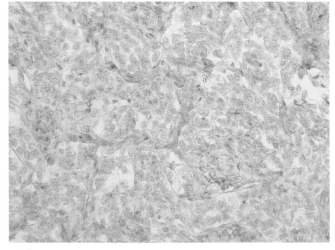

FIGURE 6

Typically UTRSCT is negative for CD10, as in this case.

HIGH-GRADE ENDOMETRIAL STROMAL SARCOMA

DEFINITION—An intermediate to high-grade stromal sarcoma with a distinct molecular genotype.

CLINICAL FEATURES

EPIDEMIOLOGY

- Overall endometrial stromal sarcoma (ESS) is rare; it accounts for less than 0.5% of all uterine malignancies and only 10% to 15% of mesenchymal uterine malignancies.
- This particular variant has a novel gene fusion between YWHAE and FAM22A/B harboring t(10 : 17)(q22;p13).
- Majority occur in the fifth and sixth decades, but can be seen at any decade in adulthood.

PRESENTATION

- Abnormal uterine bleeding is the most commonly reported presenting symptom.
- Over 80% present as stage II or higher.
- Tumors range in size, with a mean diameter of around 8 cm.

PROGNOSIS AND TREATMENT

- In contrast to low-grade ESS, which commonly presents at stage I with an 80% or higher survival, most with this tumor either die of their disease or are alive with disease in recent studies.
- Standard treatment would be total hysterectomy and bilateral salpingo-oophorectomy with surgical staging. Most patients would also receive adjuvant chemotherapy and/or radiation therapy.
- Abdominal and pulmonary recurrences are common.

PATHOLOGY

HISTOLOGY

- Tumors can be predominantly round or spindled cell or both.
- Extensive permeative growth in the myometrium.
- High mitotic index, exceeding 10/10 high-power fields.
- Invariable lymphovascular space invasion.

IMMUNOPATHOLOGY (INCLUDING IMMUNOHISTOCHEMISTRY)

- CD10 negative except in spindle cell foci, when present.
- Typically strongly positive for cyclin D1 (>75% of cells).

MAIN DIFFERENTIAL DIAGNOSIS

- Low-grade ESS—significantly lower nuclear grade, positive for CD10, and typical stromal cell phenotype.
- Leiomyosarcoma—fascicle formation, desmin and caldesmon positive.
- Undifferentiated carcinoma—uniform population with prominent nucleoli.
- Undifferentiated uterine sarcomas—CD10 negative and cyclin D1 negative (also negative for the gene fusion).

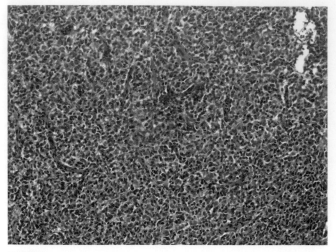

FIGURE 1

High-grade ESS. At low power the characteristic vascular pattern can be seen with a sea of round to slightly epithelioid cells lacking the more orderly elongated nuclei of lower-grade ESS.

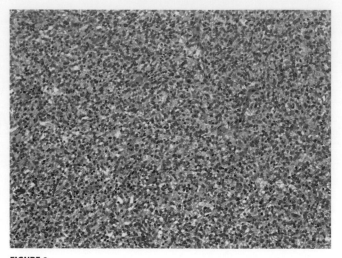

FIGURE 2

High-grade ESS.

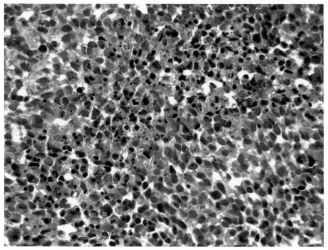

FIGURE 3

High-grade ESS. Image at higher magnification underscores the featureless arrangement of poorly differentiated stromal cells, with conspicuous mitoses, apoptosis, and focal necrosis.

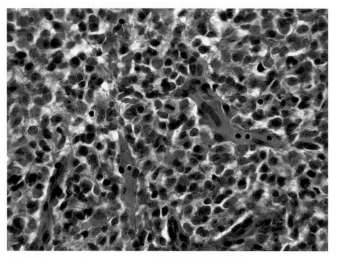

FIGURE 4

High-grade ESS. In this field a confluent array of cells with a high N/C ratio are punctuated by small vessels.

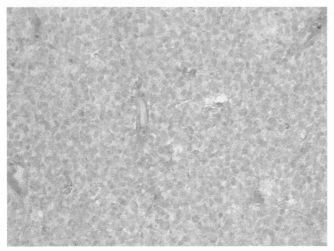

FIGURE 5

High-grade ESS. An area of predominantly round cells is CD10 negative.

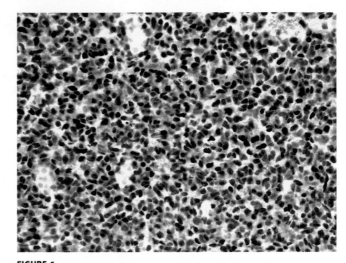

FIGURE 6

High-grade ESS. Strong staining for cyclin D1 is characteristic of these tumors, although confirmatory genetic testing (fluorescence in situ hybridization [FISH]) is needed to confirm.

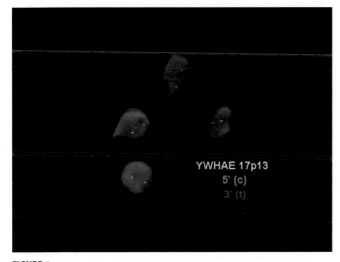

FIGURE 7

YWHAE-FAM22A/B fusion seen on FISH from tumor cells. The fusion is seen as a blend of green and red signals in each nucleus (yellow).

UNDIFFERENTIATED UTERINE SARCOMA

DEFINITION—A mesenchymal tumor of the uterus without smooth muscle or endometrial stromal differentiation.

CLINICAL FEATURES

EPIDEMIOLOGY

- Undifferentiated uterine sarcomas are rare and account for less than 0.5% of all uterine malignancies and only 10% to 15% of mesenchymal uterine malignancies.
- Mostly occur in the fifth and sixth decades, but can be seen at any decade in adulthood.

PRESENTATION

- Abnormal uterine bleeding is the most commonly reported presenting symptom.
- Over 60% present as stage III or higher.

PROGNOSIS AND TREATMENT

- Survival is poor irrespective of stage in most cases.
- Standard treatment would be total hysterectomy and bilateral salpingo-oophorectomy with surgical staging. Most patients would also receive adjuvant chemotherapy and/or radiation therapy.
- Over 60% will respond to chemotherapy, either gemcitabine/docetaxel or doxorubicin.
- Responses are usually short lived, with mean progression-free and overall survival of less than a year. Survival is improved (1-year survival of 80%) if there is no measurable disease following surgery and prior to chemotherapy.
- Residual disease and vascular invasion worsen the outcome expectations. Low-stage tumors without vascular invasion have up to an 83% 5-year survival in some studies in contrast to 17% when vascular invasion is present.
- A subset of tumors has been described with more uniform nuclear morphology and a somewhat more favorable prognosis. Authors have suggested that these tumors may be more like the traditionally designated high-grade endometrial stromal sarcoma (ESS). In retrospect at least some of these tumors are probably within the currently resurrected and genetically classified high-grade ESS group.

PATHOLOGY

HISTOLOGY

- Tumor cells are typically highly pleomorphic.
- Extensive permeative growth in the myometrium but lacking the more sinuous wormlike invasion seen in recognizable ESSs.
- High mitotic index, often exceeding 50/10 high-power fields.
- Occasionally a lower-grade component will be seen, suggesting that the tumor is a de-differentiated ESS.

IMMUNOPATHOLOGY (INCLUDING IMMUNOHISTOCHEMISTRY)

- CD10 variable and not helpful in separation from other tumors.
- Cyclin D1 should be weak or negative to exclude high-grade ESS.
- Smooth muscle markers (desmin and h-caldesmon) will be helpful in ruling out a poorly differentiated leiomyosarcoma, as will the lack of fascicle development.

MAIN DIFFERENTIAL DIAGNOSIS

- Low-grade ESS—significantly lower nuclear grade, positive for CD10, and typical stromal cell phenotype.
- Leiomyosarcoma—fascicle formation, desmin and caldesmon positive.
- Undifferentiated carcinoma—uniform population with prominent nucleoli and the absence of mesenchymal markers.
- High-grade stromal sarcoma—CD10 negative and cyclin D1 positive (also positive for the YWHAE-FAM22A/B gene fusion).

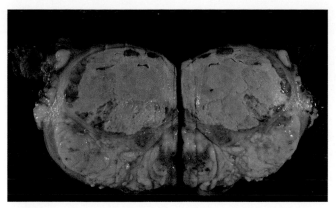

FIGURE 1

Undifferentiated uterine sarcoma. This gross photograph of the uterus shows a myometrium distended by multiple yellow nodules of necrotic tumor.

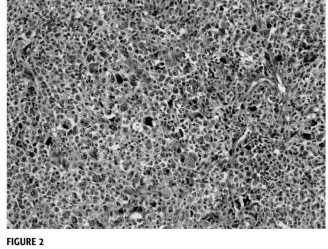

FIGURE 2

Undifferentiated uterine sarcoma. The cells lie in a featureless landscape; too pleomorphic for stromal sarcoma and without the fascicles that typify leiomyosarcoma.

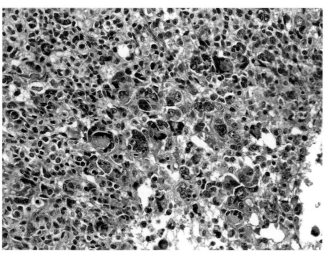

FIGURE 3

Undifferentiated uterine sarcoma. Note the tumor giant cells.

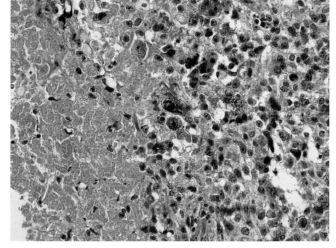

FIGURE 4

Undifferentiated uterine sarcoma showing necrosis.

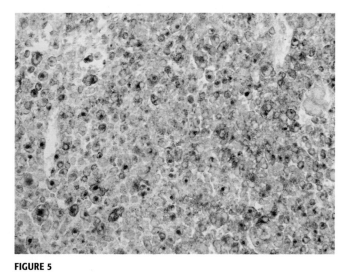

FIGURE 5

Positive staining for IFITM1 in this tumor raises the possibility of a stromal origin; however, these tumors are best approached as undifferentiated sarcomas.

ADENOSARCOMA OF THE ENDOMETRIUM

■ **Brooke E. Howitt, MD**

DEFINITION—A low-grade stromal malignancy of the uterus with preservation of the normal resident endometrial epithelium.

CLINICAL FEATURES

EPIDEMIOLOGY

- Most cases occur in postmenopausal women in their 60s, but a wide age range has been reported (teenagers to centenarians).
- Tamoxifen therapy for breast cancer, as well as prolonged hyperestroginism (either exogenous or endogenous), has been linked to endometrial malignancy, including adenosarcoma.

PRESENTATION

- Presenting symptoms are nonspecific and may include vaginal bleeding, pelvic mass, and tissue protruding through the cervical os.
- Recurrent endometrial polyps may be in the patient's medical history.

PROGNOSIS AND TREATMENT

- Hysterectomy with surgical staging is the treatment of choice.
- Oophorectomy is usually recommended, but the necessity of this procedure is not clear, particularly in the setting of noninvasive tumors.
- Prognosis is better than that of other uterine mesenchymal malignancies, but up to one third of patients will experience a recurrence.

PATHOLOGY

HISTOLOGY

- Grossly, the tumor is bulky, and the soft exophytic mass fills the endometrial cavity.
- The histology is characterized by a biphasic tumor composed of malignant stroma and benign endometrial glands.
- At low power the endometrial glands may be dilated, have a leaflike (phyllodes-like) architectural pattern, or may be present as slitlike spaces.
- Also notable at low power is stromal condensation (cuffing) around the glandular elements.
- At higher power the epithelial elements are benign and may appear cuboidal, endometrial, or even metaplastic (such as tubal or mucinous).
- The stromal element is most often homologous, with a fibrous or endometrial stromal appearance.
- Less commonly, heterologous elements such as rhabdomyosarcoma are identified.
- Nuclear atypia in the stromal component is variable and ranges from mild to marked.
- Mitotic activity is present in the stromal element and must be greater than 2/10 high-power field.
- Stromal overgrowth at the time of initial resection is thought to indicate poor prognosis and higher risk of recurrence.

Immunopathology (Including Immunohistochemistry)

- Epithelial elements: keratin positive.
- Stromal/mesenchymal elements: CD10 or CD34 may be positive.
- Epithelial and stromal elements: variable ER and PR expression.

Main Differential Diagnosis

- Endometrial stromal sarcoma—this tumor does not have the organized epithelial component, but in a small sample the distinction may be difficult.
- Uterine adenofibroma—this diagnosis is becoming obsolete as the existence of adenofibromas is called into question. "Borderline" adenosarcomas are typically classified as atypical endometrial polyps and, in contrast to adenosarcomas, should lack stromal atypia in the form of high cellularity, increased mitoses, and nuclear pleomorphism with overlap.
- Carcinosarcoma—look for neoplastic epithelium. However, there are carcinosarcomas that are distinctly "adenosarcoma like."

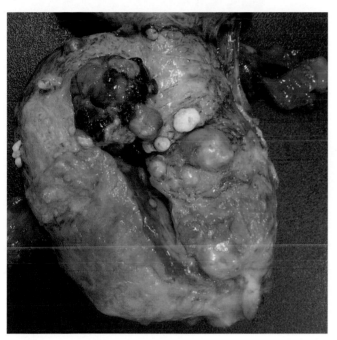

FIGURE 1

Adenosarcoma of the uterus presenting as an irregular, partially gelatinous, and hemorrhagic polypoid mass confined to the lumen in the opened uterus. Several intramural leiomyomata can be seen for comparison in the sectioned myometrium.

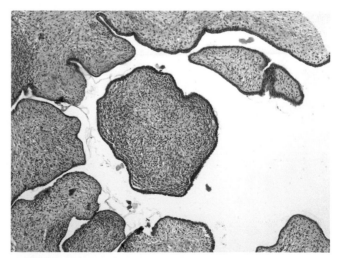

FIGURE 3

Adenosarcoma. Low-power view of cellular, stromal cuffing surrounding "leaf-like" glandular spaces.

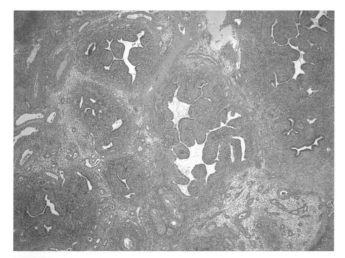

FIGURE 2

Adenosarcoma. Low-power view of cellular, stromal cuffing surrounding "leaf-like" glandular spaces.

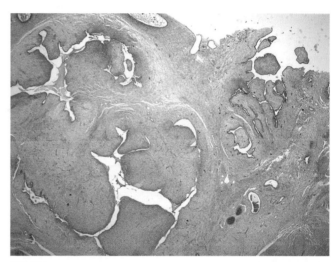

FIGURE 4

Adenosarcoma. Leaflike architecture with hypercellular stroma. Note that it may not be highly cellular, but there is a clear increase in stromal density under the surface epithelium. Note the benign glandular epithelium.

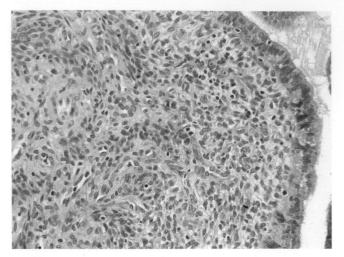

FIGURE 5

Adenosarcoma. Variably dense but consistently atypical subepithelial stromal cells with mitoses.

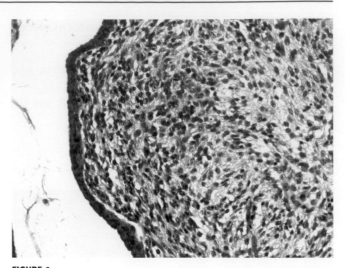

FIGURE 6

Adenosarcoma. In this focus the subepithelial cells are particularly hyperchromatic.

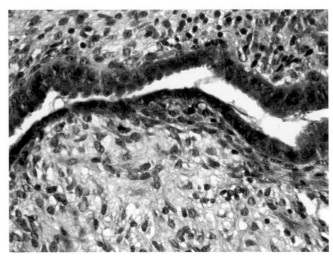

FIGURE 7

Adenosarcoma. Another focus with subepithelial stromal condensation.

ATYPICAL ENDOMETRIAL POLYP

■ **Brooke E. Howitt, MD**

DEFINITION—An endometrial polyp with features suggestive, but not diagnostic, of an müllerian adenosarcoma.

CLINICAL FEATURES

EPIDEMIOLOGY

- Wide age range.
- Typically fourth to sixth decades.

PRESENTATION

- Abnormal vaginal bleeding.
- Can be asymptomatic, with a polyp identified on ultrasound or during exam.

PROGNOSIS AND TREATMENT

- Atypical polyps are presumably benign and so have an excellent prognosis.
- Excision of the polyp or mass is required for diagnosis and is also the treatment of choice; additional therapy is not warranted, but monitoring of the endometrium for regrowth is advised.

PATHOLOGY

HISTOLOGY

- Adenosarcoma-like endometrial polyps display some architectural resemblance to low-grade adenosarcoma.
- The most common feature is the presence of irregularly shaped glands with occasional cleftlike, branching spaces that are reminiscent of phyllodes tumor of the breast.

- These irregular glands are best appreciated at low power.
- High-power examination reveals a notable lack of significant cytologic atypia.
- Mitotic activity is often very low, but may be elevated when the stromal cells are morphologically similar to proliferative-type endometrial stroma.
- Periglandular stromal condensation (cuffing) may be present but is typically ill-defined and not a prominent feature.
- Typically the atypical or unusual histologic features are seen in only a portion of the polyp.

IMMUNOPATHOLOGY (INCLUDING IMMUNOHISTOCHEMISTRY)

- Noncontributory.

MAIN DIFFERENTIAL DIAGNOSIS

- Endometrial polyp—typical polyps present no problem given the lack of stromal hypercellularity.
- Low-grade endometrial adenosarcoma—these should have conspicuous nuclear atypia in the periglandular stroma, coupled with mitotic activity.
- Adenomyoma—the key to this diagnosis is the presence of smooth muscle fascicles between the irregularly shaped glands.
- Atypical polypoid adenomyoma—this is a tumor with both smooth muscle differentiation and an atypical glandular proliferation with squamous metaplasia.

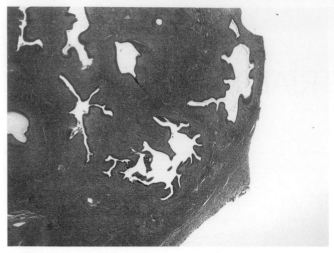

FIGURE 1

Atypical endometrial polyps. Low-power examination shows various degrees of branching or phyllodiform architecture.

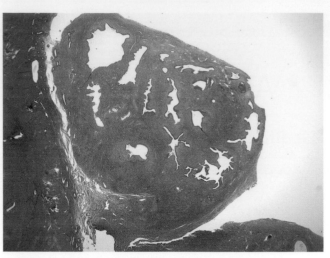

FIGURE 2

Atypical endometrial polyps. Low-power examination shows various degrees of branching or phyllodiform architecture.

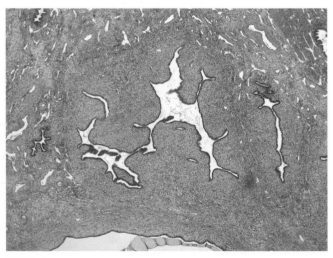

FIGURE 3

Atypical endometrial polyps. Low-power examination shows various degrees of branching or phyllodiform architecture but a lack of prominent periglandular cuffing.

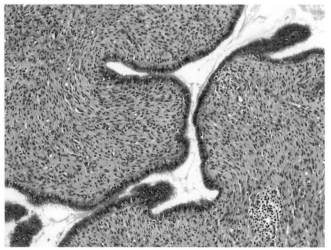

FIGURE 4

Atypical endometrial polyps. At higher magnification the stromal cells are uniform, and there is minimal nuclear enlargement or crowding.

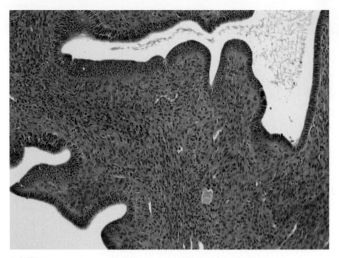

FIGURE 5

Atypical endometrial polyps. At higher magnification the stromal cells are uniform, and there is minimal nuclear enlargement or crowding.

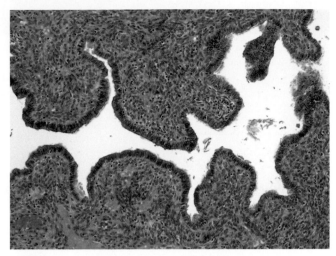

FIGURE 6

Atypical endometrial polyps. At higher magnification the stromal cells are uniform, and there is minimal nuclear enlargement or crowding.

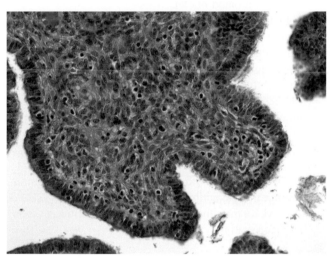

FIGURE 7

Atypical endometrial polyps. Higher magnification confirms a lack of stromal cell atypia.

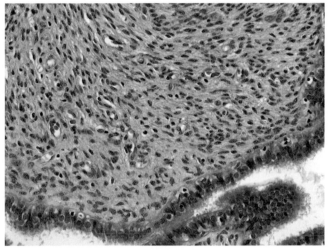

FIGURE 8

Atypical endometrial polyps. Higher magnification confirms a lack of stromal cell atypia.

ADENOMATOID TUMOR

DEFINITION—A benign tumor composed of smooth muscle and mesothelium that is most common in the outer myometrium and fallopian tube.

CLINICAL FEATURES

EPIDEMIOLOGY

- Uncommon but not rare.
- Reproductive-age to perimenopausal women.

PRESENTATION

- Most often incidental and less than 2 cm in size.
- May be associated with symptomatic leiomyomata.

PROGNOSIS AND TREATMENT

- Prognosis is excellent; this is a benign tumor.
- Excision is adequate treatment.

PATHOLOGY

HISTOLOGY

- On gross examination, tumors are rubbery and white to gray, and lack prominent bulging on cut section.
- The border with myometrium is less defined than that seen with leiomyomata.
- At low power, fascicles of brightly eosinophilic smooth muscle cells with bland, elongated nuclei are apparent.
- The mesothelial component is interspersed between bundles of smooth muscle and can vary from inconspicuous to prominent.

- Mesothelial cells are usually arranged in small glandlike spaces with frequent "chaining," although other patterns have been described, including sheets and densely glandular appearing proliferation.
- Mesothelial cells are epithelioid and cuboidal to squamoid, with bland nuclei.
- Signet-ring–like cells and pseudolipoblasts are almost always seen.
- An infiltrative growth pattern, with tumor cells involving adjacent myometrium, is not uncommon; extension beyond the uterus is rare.
- Marked nuclear atypia, tumor necrosis, and atypical mitotic figures are absent.

IMMUNOPATHOLOGY (INCLUDING IMMUNOHISTOCHEMISTRY)

- Positive for smooth muscle components: desmin, smooth muscle actin, and CD34.
- Positive for mesothelial components: calretinin (nuclear) and pankeratins.

MAIN DIFFERENTIAL DIAGNOSIS

- Lipoleiomyoma—the key here is to pay close attention to the spaces and whether they are adipose tissue or mesothelial lined.
- Carcinomas, particularly signet-ring cell tumors—the mesothelial-lined spaces may be less conspicuous, and the mesothelial cells may take on a "signet ring" appearance, which can be misleading.

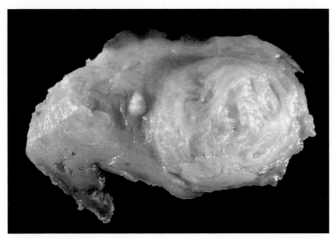

FIGURE 1

Adenomatoid tumor. This myometrial tumor resembles a leiomyoma. If the mesothelial lined spaces are prominent, the lesion may take on a spongy consistency.

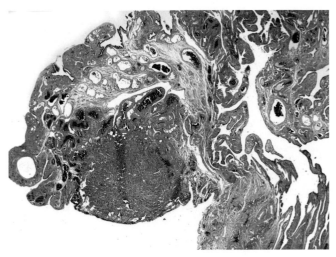

FIGURE 2

Adenomatoid tumor. A small tubal tumor within the fimbria.

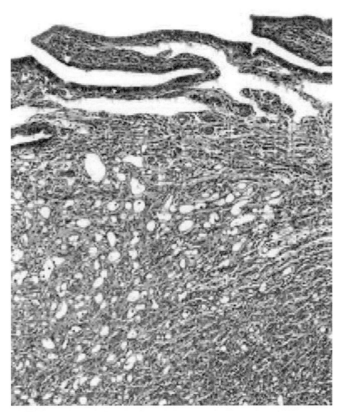

FIGURE 3

Adenomatoid tumor. This is a common appearance at low magnification, with numerous small spaces creating a honeycomb pattern.

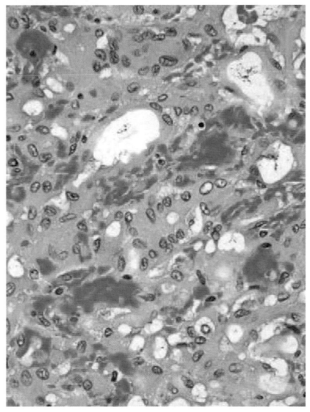

FIGURE 4

Adenomatoid tumor. In this variant the mesothelial cells are plump and glandlike, and may be confused with malignancy.

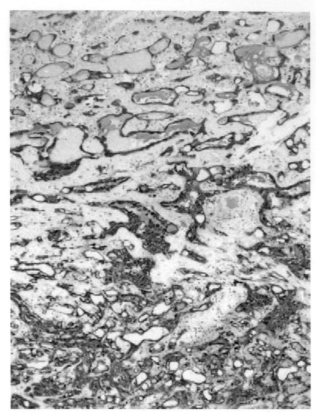

FIGURE 5

Calretinin staining is strong in these lesions and will distinguish them from adenocarcinomas.

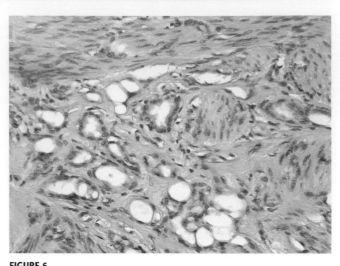

FIGURE 6

At high magnification note the variably sized spaces. When small, they may mimic signet-ring tumor cells.

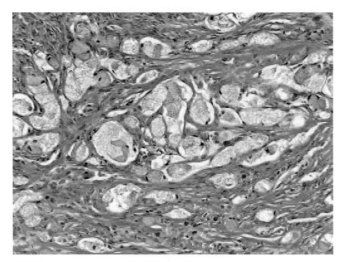

FIGURE 7

A signet-ring cell adenocarcinoma for comparison.

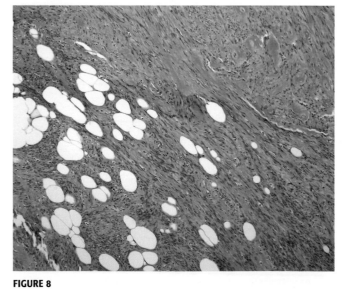

FIGURE 8

A lipoleiomyoma may mimic an adenomatoid tumor, both on gross exam and at low-power magnification.

LIPOLEIOMYOMA

DEFINITION—A benign tumor of the uterus composed of both smooth muscle and adipose cells.

CLINICAL FEATURES

EPIDEMIOLOGY

- Rare.
- Postmenopausal women.
- t(12;14) a common chromosomal rearrangement similar to other leiomyomas.

PRESENTATION

- Abnormal vaginal bleeding.
- Pelvic pressure or pain.

PROGNOSIS AND TREATMENT

- Excellent; these are benign tumors.

PATHOLOGY

HISTOLOGY

- Grossly a yellow (even bright yellow) appearance may be noted.

- Histologically these tumors are characterized by an admixture of smooth muscle cells and adipose cells.
- The bland, brightly eosinophilic smooth muscle cells are arranged in the usual bundles and fascicles of a leiomyoma.
- Adipocytes are interspersed within the bundles of smooth muscle singly and in groups.
- Rarely the adipocytic component may constitute the majority of tumor cells.

IMMUNOPATHOLOGY (INCLUDING IMMUNOHISTOCHEMISTRY)

- Noncontributory. However, HMGI-C is aberrantly expressed in this tumor.
- Cytogenetic and molecular data suggest that these tumors represent a distinct variant and are not simply a degenerative phenomenon, as was traditionally presumed.

MAIN DIFFERENTIAL DIAGNOSIS

- Lipoma (when adipocytes predominate).

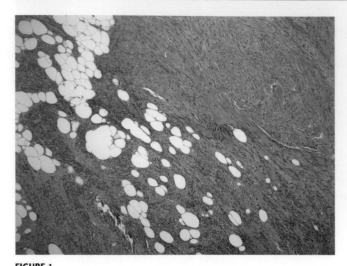

FIGURE 1

Lipoleiomyoma. Fascicles of smooth muscle with interspersed mature adipose tissue.

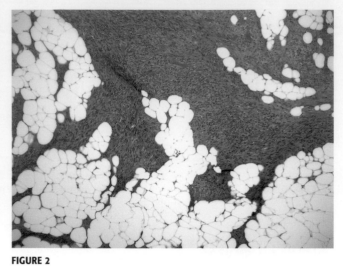

FIGURE 2

Lipoleiomyoma. Fascicles of smooth muscle with interspersed mature adipose tissue.

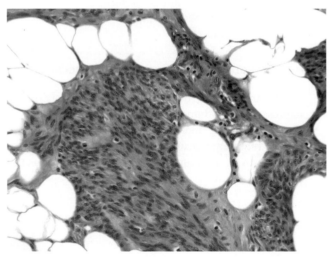

FIGURE 3

Lipoleiomyoma. Fat cells with spindled smooth muscle cells.

CELLULAR LEIOMYOMA

DEFINITION

- A smooth muscle tumor with conspicuous increased cellularity.

CLINICAL FEATURES

EPIDEMIOLOGY

- The same as for usual leiomyoma.

PRESENTATION

- The same as for usual leiomyoma.
- On gross exam these tumors tend to be softer and "fleshier" than usual leiomyomas, with a slightly more gray or pink color.

PROGNOSIS AND TREATMENT

- Generally excellent; these are benign tumors. However, the cellular leiomyoma phenotype with loss of 1p has been described in some reports as behaving more aggressively.

PATHOLOGY

HISTOLOGY

- At low power, cellular leiomyomas are notable for increased cellularity.
- The degree of increased cellularity required for a designation of "cellular leiomyoma" is debatable, and strict criteria are not available, although there is a suggestion that these more cellular tumors have a distinct molecular signature.
- The tumor cells themselves are bland, with minimal amounts of eosinophilic cytoplasm, and are arranged (at least focally) in the usual fascicles and bundles of leiomyomata.

- Highly cellular leiomyomas, in particular, may have an irregular border with surrounding myometrium, which can be mistaken for the infiltrative borders of more worrisome lesions.
- Interspersed large thick-walled blood vessels are present.
- Characteristic cleftlike spaces between the tumor and surrounding myometrium.
- Nuclear atypia and tumor necrosis are absent.
- Cellular leiomyomas are often also mitotically active (see Mitotically Active Leiomyoma).

IMMUNOPATHOLOGY (INCLUDING IMMUNOHISTOCHEMISTRY)

- Positive for desmin (strong positive) and h-caldesmon.
- Negative for CD10 (in most cases).
- Overall the use of immunohistochemistry to distinguish cellular leiomyoma from endometrial stromal sarcoma is not advisable as the profiles share significant overlap.

MAIN DIFFERENTIAL DIAGNOSIS

- Leiomyosarcoma—the keys to a diagnosis of leiomyosarcoma are atypia, increased mitotic activity, and tumor necrosis. Cellular leiomyomas exhibit increased nuclear density and may exhibit an increase in mitotic index but should contain neither atypia nor necrosis.
- Low-grade endometrial stromal sarcoma—careful scrutiny of a cellular leiomyoma will reveal the fasciculated pattern of a smooth muscle tumor. Moreover, the fine vascular pattern of an endometrial stromal tumor should not be present and thick-walled blood vessels should be seen. In difficult cases, smooth muscle (desmin, h-caldesmon, increased) and stromal (CD10, decreased relative to endometrial stromal sarcoma) staining should make the distinction.

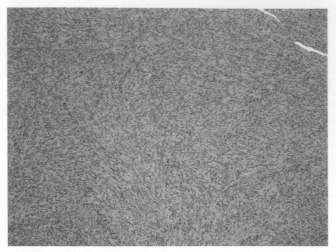

FIGURE 1

Cellular leiomyoma. Increased cellularity and nuclear density evident at low power.

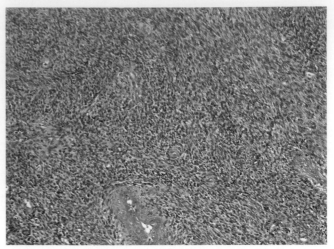

FIGURE 2

Cellular leiomyoma. A highly cellular variant, with numerous overlapping nuclei.

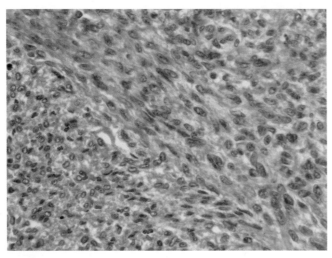

FIGURE 3

Cellular leiomyoma. High-power view displaying bland smooth muscle cells with cigar-shaped nuclei.

HYDROPIC LEIOMYOMA

DEFINITION—Uterine smooth muscle tumor with prominent degenerative changes.

CLINICAL FEATURES

EPIDEMIOLOGY

- Same as for leiomyoma.
- Degenerative change within leiomyomata is extremely common.

PRESENTATION

- Same as for leiomyoma.
- Some believe that a component of the pain associated with leiomyomata is due to degeneration.

PROGNOSIS AND TREATMENT

- Excellent; these are benign tumors.

PATHOLOGY

HISTOLOGY

- The gross appearance of degenerative change is variable; in some instances it may appear as a round, white area in the center of a leiomyoma.
- In other cases the mass may be diffusely yellow and gelatinous, or extensively calcified.
- Occasionally the tumoral mass may be extensively replaced by cystic structures filled with serous fluid.
- Hemorrhage may also be seen, resulting in a pink or even red appearance (carneous).

- Histologically the areas of necrosis have a characteristic interface (transition zone) between viable and nonviable tissues.
- The interface is composed of fibroblasts, viable and nonviable smooth muscle cells, and inflammation, similar to granulation tissue.
- The interface or transition zone should be relatively uniform (although not easily demarcated) around the area of necrosis, and at least several cells thick.
- Within the necrotic tissue, cells should not have prominent or well-defined cell outlines (ghost cells).
- Other patterns of degeneration are characterized by prominent edema and accumulation of fluid ("hydropic" change).
- The hydropic areas generally lack cellular debris within the areas of fluid accumulation.
- In any pattern of degeneration the border with background myometrium should be sharp; infiltration of the surrounding smooth muscle should not be present.

IMMUNOPATHOLOGY (INCLUDING IMMUNOHISTOCHEMISTRY)

- Positive for smooth muscle actin and desmin.

MAIN DIFFERENTIAL DIAGNOSIS

- Myxoid leiomyosarcoma. Look for increased mitotic activity, atypia, necrosis, and infiltration of the adjacent myometrium.

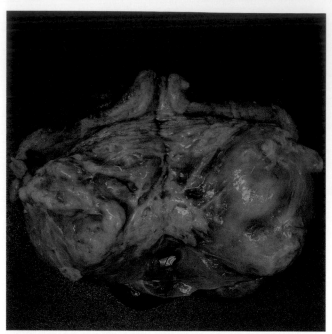

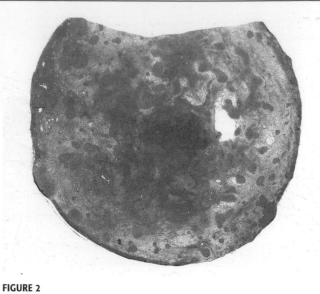

FIGURE 2
Hydropic leiomyoma. Low-power view showing alternating areas of hyper-cellularity and hypocellularity within a well-circumscribed mass.

FIGURE 1
Hydropic leiomyoma. Gross specimen with cystic degeneration.

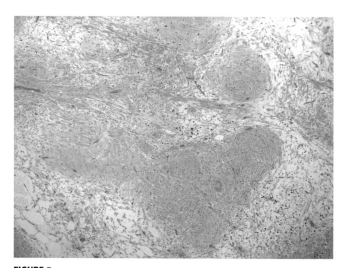

FIGURE 3
Hydropic leiomyoma. Bundles of bland smooth muscle with areas of edema.

MITOTICALLY ACTIVE LEIOMYOMA

DEFINITION—A morphologic variant of uterine leiomyoma.

CLINICAL FEATURES

EPIDEMIOLOGY

- Mitotic activity within normal and leiomyomatous smooth muscle cells is a well-established phenomenon.
- Exogenous progesterones increase the observed mitotic rate in leiomyomata.

PRESENTATION

- Same as for usual leiomyoma.

PROGNOSIS AND TREATMENT

- Excellent; these are benign tumors.

PATHOLOGY

HISTOLOGY

- Overall these tumors are histologically identical to other leiomyomata and are composed of fascicles and bundles of smooth muscle cells with brightly eosinophilic cytoplasm and bland, blunt-ended nuclei.
- Significant mitotic activity is present (up to 15/10 high-power fields), but atypical mitotic figures should not be present.
- Mitotic activity should always be assessed in the most mitotically active area, and at least 30 high-power fields should be examined.
- Mitotically active tumors are often cellular or highly cellular; it is critical to ensure that nuclear atypia and tumor necrosis are absent in these lesions.

IMMUNOPATHOLOGY (INCLUDING IMMUNOHISTOCHEMISTRY)

- The proliferation marker Ki-67 may be useful in some cases to exclude overinterpretation of pyknotic nuclei as mitotic figures.

MAIN DIFFERENTIAL DIAGNOSIS

- Smooth muscle tumor of uncertain malignant potential—these will be considered when there is atypia and moderately increased mitotic activity (5 to 10 mitoses per 10 HPF).
- Leiomyosarcoma—atypia and mitoses exceeding 10 per 10 HPF or the presence of tumor necrosis.

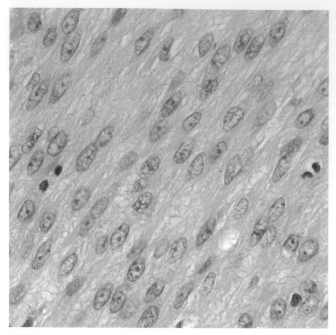

FIGURE 1

Mitotically active leiomyoma. A typical leiomyoma with two mitotic figures (anaphase).

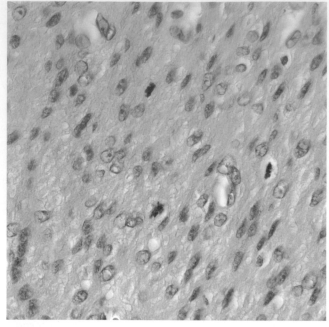

FIGURE 2

Mitotically active leiomyoma. Three mitotic figures admixed with bland smooth muscle cells.

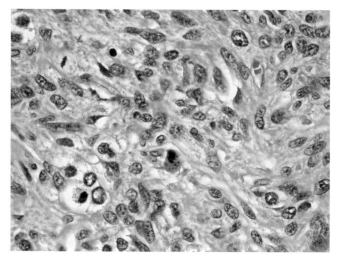

FIGURE 3

Mitotically active leiomyoma. An atypical leiomyoma with one mitotic figure (*upper left,* metaphase) and one pseudomitosis noted by its bright pink, well-defined cytoplasm *(center).*

ATYPICAL LEIOMYOMA (LEIOMYOMA WITH BIZARRE NUCLEI)

DEFINITION—A benign smooth muscle tumor with prominent nuclear atypia.

CLINICAL FEATURES

EPIDEMIOLOGY

- Uncommon.
- Identified in the same patient population as typical leiomyomata.

PRESENTATION

- The same as for usual leiomyoma.

PROGNOSIS AND TREATMENT

- Complete excision is recommended, with periodic monitoring if only a myomectomy has been performed.
- Rarely, recurrent atypical leiomyomata and association with leiomyosarcoma have been reported.
- Risk of recurrence or malignant behavior is very low (under 5%).

PATHOLOGY

HISTOLOGY

- This diagnosis is restricted to tumors that exhibit atypia discernible at low power.

- The striking atypia is appreciated at low power and often brings to mind the possibility of leiomyosarcoma.
- Nuclear atypia may consist of enlargement, hyperchromasia, multinucleated cells or multilobated nuclei, prominent nucleoli, or any combination of them.
- Cytoplasmic atypia may also be demonstrated and may consist of abundant eosinophilic cytoplasm, with or without cytoplasmic whorling.
- Tumor "giant" cells may be seen.
- The markedly atypical cells may be very focal or may be diffusely present throughout the tumor.
- By definition, geographic tumor necrosis and increased mitotic activity (>10/10 high-power fields) are absent.

IMMUNOPATHOLOGY (INCLUDING IMMUNOHISTOCHEMISTRY)

- Positive for p53, desmin, and smooth muscle actin.
- A Ki-67 proliferation index is low.

MAIN DIFFERENTIAL DIAGNOSIS

- Smooth muscle tumor of uncertain malignant potential (STUMP)—this might be considered if mitoses approach 10/10 HPF or if infiltrative borders are present.
- Leiomyosarcoma—considered if there is tumor necrosis.

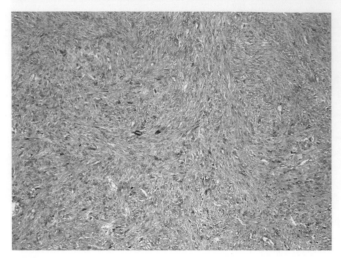

FIGURE 1

Atypical leiomyoma. Atypical nuclear features evident at low magnification.

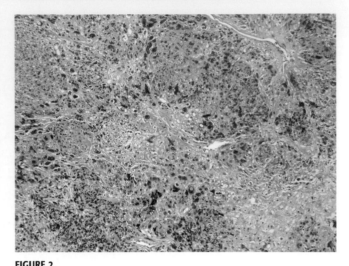

FIGURE 2

Atypical leiomyoma. 10× view (definition of low power according to the Bell criteria) of diffuse nuclear atypia.

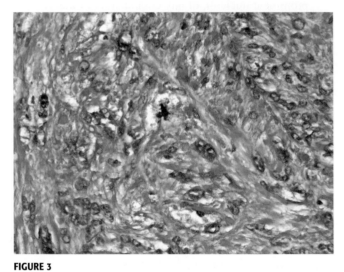

FIGURE 3

Atypical leiomyoma. Pseudomitosis within an atypical leiomyoma. Note the vacuolization and the eosinophilic, cytoplasmic clumping.

LEIOMYOMATOSIS

DEFINITION—Uterine smooth muscle tumor composed of multiple repetitive fascicles of smooth muscle diffusely involving the myometrium without a definable border.

CLINICAL FEATURES

EPIDEMIOLOGY

- Same as for leiomyoma, but extremely rare.

PRESENTATION

- Same as for leiomyoma, dysmenorrhea, bleeding, pelvic pressure, discomfort, and infertility.
- Uterus is diffusely enlarged due to the absence of a discrete intramural nodule.

PROGNOSIS AND TREATMENT

- Excellent; these are benign tumors, but hysterectomy is the only effective approach given the diffuse nature of the process.

PATHOLOGY

GROSS AND MICROSCOPIC

- The gross appearance is that of a diffusely expanded myometrium with confluent variably defined nodules of variable size, ranging from a few millimeters to several centimeters.
- Isolated infarcts may be seen.
- On microscopy the nodules may blend but overall display the histology of typical leiomyomas.

IMMUNOPATHOLOGY (INCLUDING IMMUNOHISTOCHEMISTRY)

- Not usually necessary; positive for smooth muscle markers.

MAIN DIFFERENTIAL DIAGNOSIS

- Leiomyosarcoma—this may be considered on gross exam given the unexpected diffuse appearance and presence of infarcts; however, this can be readily excluded on histologic examination.
- Hydropic leiomyoma—this entity will display small confluent nodules similar to leiomyomatosis, but this process is within a discrete mass.

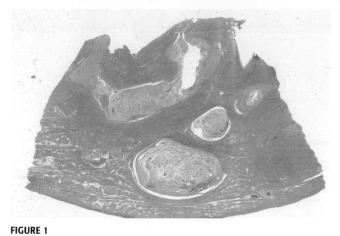

FIGURE 1

Intravenous leiomyomatosis. Note the multiple distended vascular spaces with tumor.

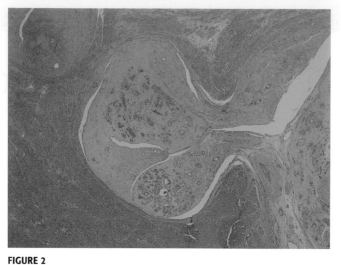

FIGURE 2

Intravenous leiomyomatosis. Tumor permeates vascular spaces. Note the prominent collagenized appearance with small vessels in the tumor.

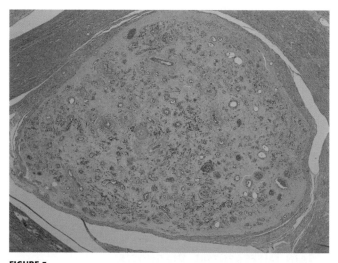

FIGURE 3

Intravenous leiomyomatosis. Here the multiple small vessels are prominent, some with thick walls.

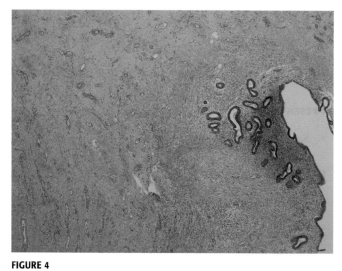

FIGURE 4

In this case of intravenous leiomyomatosis the tumor is closely associated with adenomyosis.

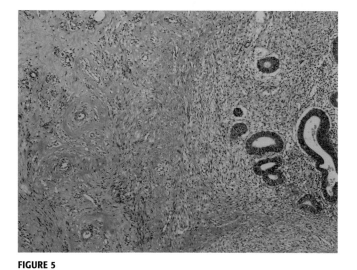

FIGURE 5

Higher magnification illustrates the relationship of the smooth muscle and endometrial tissue in a case of intravenous leiomyomatosis with an adenomyotic focus.

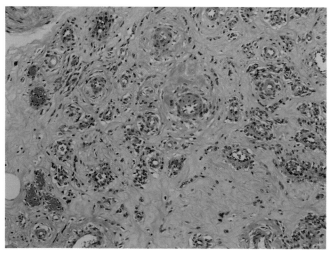

FIGURE 6

Higher magnification of small vessels and capillaries.

MORCELLATION-RELATED DISSEMINATION OF SMOOTH MUSCLE NEOPLASIA

■ **Bradley J. Quade, MD, PhD**

DEFINITION—A specific syndrome caused by the iatrogenic dissemination of a morcellated smooth muscle tumor, which is distinct from spontaneous disseminated peritoneal leiomyomatosis.

CLINICAL FEATURES

EPIDEMIOLOGY

- Power morcellation has been a commonly used technique for removing intraabdominal smooth muscle tumors and may disseminate both normal and tumor tissues in the peritoneal cavity.
- Unexpected leiomyosarcoma occurs in approximately 1 to 2 per 1000 routine hysterectomies for presumed benign leiomyomata.
- Malignancies can be detected in as high as 1:350 morcellation procedures for presumed symptomatic leiomyomata.

PRESENTATION

- Recurrent neoplasms following morcellation are typically seen as multiple tumor nodules or plaques on peritoneal surfaces.
- In comparison to the typical case of sporadic disseminated peritoneal leiomyomatosis, morcellation-associated cases tend to have fewer and larger peritoneal or omental tumors.

PROGNOSIS AND TREATMENT

- Morcellation is associated with a higher frequency of abdominal-pelvic recurrence relative to conventional hysterectomy, for both benign and malignant soft tissue tumors.
- Morcellation is associated with a significantly shorter median recurrence-free survival (10 vs. 40 months for conventional hysterectomy) in cases of leiomyosarcoma.

PATHOLOGY

HISTOLOGY

- Implantation of normal endometrium and other mesenchymal tumors also have been observed.
- The characteristic histologic features of benign and malignant smooth muscle tumors will be seen.
- However, given the random nature of the fragmentation at the time of morcellation, the deposits may be irregular.
- Evaluation of the interface between tumor and normal tissues may be limited, as is the assessment of tumor size.
- A high proliferative rate or infiltration into adjacent normal tissues at site(s) of dissemination may herald an aggressive clinical course.

IMMUNOPATHOLOGY (INCLUDING IMMUNOHISTOCHEMISTRY)

- Usually noncontributory unless the histology of the tumor is unclear.

MAIN DIFFERENTIAL DIAGNOSIS

- Disseminated peritoneal leiomyomatosis—may have a similar distribution, but without a history of power morcellation, and sporadic disseminated peritoneal leiomyomatosis typically presents with higher numbers of smaller tumorlets.

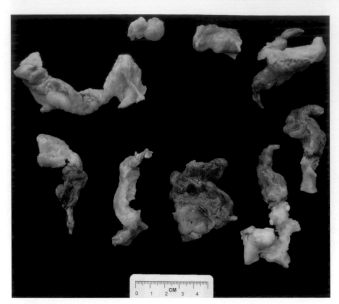

FIGURE 1

Typical morcellation specimen with irregular fragments of smooth muscle tumor.

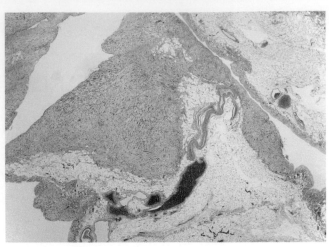

FIGURE 2

Recurrent leiomyosarcoma post morcellation. Note the irregular size and shape of the tumor on histology, corresponding to a variable clinical presentation.

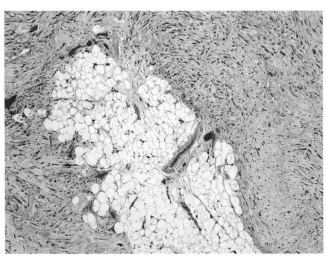

FIGURE 3

Recurrent leiomyosarcoma post morcellation. At higher magnification obvious infiltration of adipose tissue can be appreciated.

DISSEMINATED PERITONEAL LEIOMYOMATOSIS

■ **Bradley J. Quade, MD, PhD**

DEFINITION—An uncommon disorder marked by the presence of multiple smooth muscle tumors that are scattered throughout the peritoneum and omentum.

CLINICAL FEATURES

EPIDEMIOLOGY

- Disseminated peritoneal leiomyomatosis (DPL) is a rare disorder.
- It is most commonly seen in reproductive-age women; however, cases have been identified after menopause.

PRESENTATION

- Patients may be asymptomatic or may present with symptoms of mass effect.

PROGNOSIS AND TREATMENT

- Overall, DPL has a benign (and sometimes protracted) clinical course.
- Surgical intervention may be warranted in severe or symptomatic cases.
- Several reports suggest that aggressive surgical intervention may be detrimental as it can be associated with increased morbidity.

PATHOLOGY

HISTOLOGY

- The tumorlets of DPL may range from 1 to 2.5 cm and may be limited to a few nodules or present as hundreds of nodules.

- Histologically each nodule should represent a discreet leiomyoma.
- The leiomyomas should not display any atypia, significant mitotic activity, or necrosis, in keeping with their uterine counterparts.
- Malignant transformation has been known to occur and is marked by the same features that are diagnostic of leiomyosarcoma in the uterus. The presence of necrosis, atypia, and increased mitotic activity should be readily apparent.

IMMUNOPATHOLOGY (INCLUDING IMMUNOHISTOCHEMISTRY)

- The individual tumorlets will stain positive for SMA and desmin, analogous to their uterine counterparts.

MAIN DIFFERENTIAL DIAGNOSIS

- Metastatic leiomyosarcoma.
- Metastatic carcinoma (clinically and grossly).
- Seeding of the abdominal cavity following morcellation procedures.

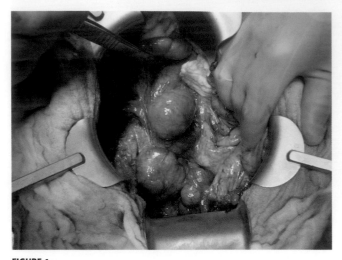

FIGURE 1

DPL. Numerous smooth muscle tumors can be seen growing within the abdominal cavity.

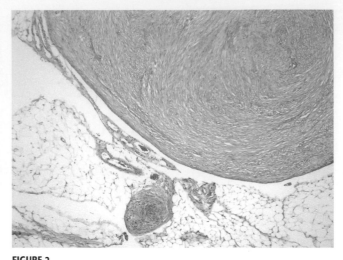

FIGURE 2

DPL. Two leiomyomas within the omentum.

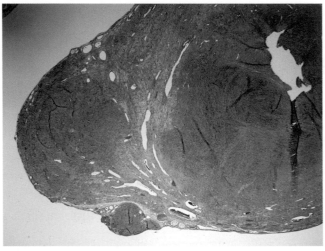

FIGURE 3

DPL. Low-power view of three discrete leiomyomas within the abdominal cavity.

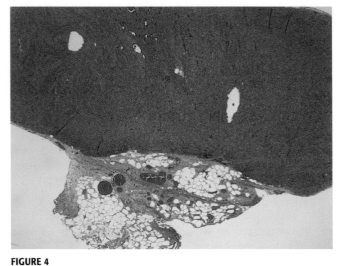

FIGURE 4

DPL. Mesentery with a cellular leiomyoma.

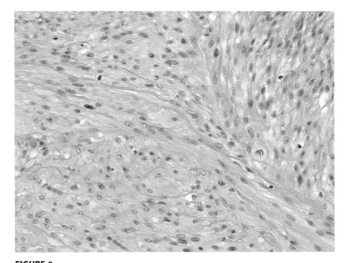

FIGURE 5

DPL. Malignant transformation may occur. Note the increased mitotic activity and subtle nuclear pleomorphism.

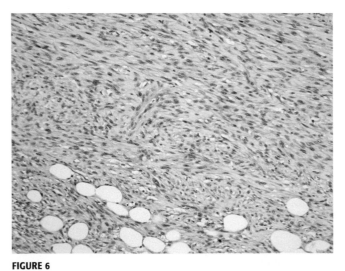

FIGURE 6

DPL. The tumor pictured in Figure 5, infiltrating omental fat.

PATHOLOGY FOLLOWING UTERINE ARTERY EMBOLIZATION

■ **Bradley J. Quade, MD, PhD**

DEFINITION—Changes in the myometrium following an embolization procedure for a presumed leiomyoma using synthetic material.

CLINICAL FEATURES

EPIDEMIOLOGY

- Uterine embolization procedures are performed about 25,000 times per year in the United States.

PRESENTATION

- The procedure is performed by introducing a catheter into the uterine artery and injecting synthetic material (often polyvinyl alcohol or tris-acryl gelatin microspheres).
- Continued growth or postprocedure pain may result in subsequent hysterectomy and examination of these embolized tumors by pathologists.

PROGNOSIS AND TREATMENT

- In rare cases leiomyosarcomas have been embolized, resulting in slightly delayed diagnosis and treatment.

PATHOLOGY

HISTOLOGY

- On gross examination, ischemic necrosis with or without calcification is present, usually as circumscribed soft yellow change of the myometrial mass.

- Spheres of foreign material can be seen grossly, filling and distending vessels within and adjacent to the ischemic tumor mass.
- At low power, homogenous acellular bluish-purple to pink material is apparent within vascular spaces and sometimes associated with foreign body giant cell reaction around the microsphere.
- Bland ischemic necrosis is often prominent; mitotic activity may be present, particularly immediately adjacent to the zone of necrosis.
- Ischemic necrosis is characterized by pink necrotic debris without prominent cell borders (ghost cells) and with a transition zone (similar to granulation tissue) from viable to nonviable areas.
- Tumor necrosis, atypical mitotic figures, and significant mitotic activity are not present.

IMMUNOPATHOLOGY (INCLUDING IMMUNOHISTOCHEMISTRY)

- Positive for smooth muscle actin and desmin.

MAIN DIFFERENTIAL DIAGNOSIS

- Leiomyosarcoma, if ischemic necrosis is misclassified as tumor necrosis.

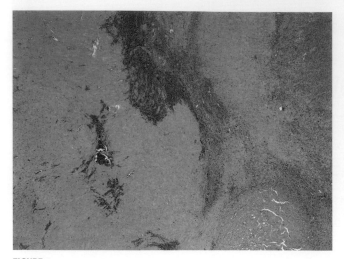

FIGURE 1

Leiomyoma embolization artifact. An abrupt transition to ischemic necrosis with hemorrhage.

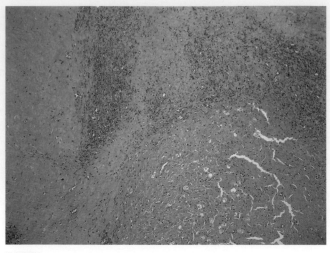

FIGURE 2

Leiomyoma embolization artifact. Ischemic necrosis.

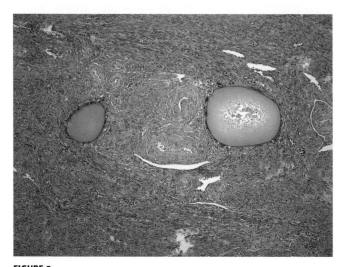

FIGURE 3

Leiomyoma embolization artifact. Blue to pink embolization material is seen within the vascular spaces in the adjacent myometrium.

HEREDITARY LEIOMYOMATOSIS AND RENAL CELL CARCINOMA SYNDROME

PITFALL

DEFINITION—A unique variant of uterine smooth muscle tumor associated with a genetically transmitted increased risk of renal cell carcinoma (RCC) (loss of heterozygosity [LOH] at 1q43).

CLINICAL FEATURES

EPIDEMIOLOGY

- The underlying defect is a germ-line heterozygous loss of function mutation in the fumarate hydratase gene with LOH at 1q43. Cases can be both germ-line and sporadic.
- Patients typically (77%) present with leiomyomas, often at a young age.
- The associated RCC is aggressive and often presents at a late stage.

PRESENTATION

- Typically younger age of onset and with multiple leiomyomata up to 8 cm.

PROGNOSIS AND TREATMENT

- The leiomyoma carries no risk to the patient other than signifying an increased risk of RCC.
- Identification of subjects at risk for RCC may reduce mortality by earlier detection.

PATHOLOGY

HISTOLOGY

- Three characteristic low-power features include increased cellularity, multinucleation, and increased atypia.

- The hallmark feature is a large orangeophilic nucleolus with a perinuclear halo.
- Modest (up to 3 per 10 HPF) increase in mitotic index.
- Features of sarcoma (high mitotic index, tumor necrosis) are not present.

IMMUNOPATHOLOGY (INCLUDING IMMUNOHISTOCHEMISTRY)

- Same as any conventional leiomyoma.

MAIN DIFFERENTIAL DIAGNOSIS

- Cellular leiomyoma—the prominent nucleolar features exclude this tumor.
- Leiomyosarcoma—contains both necrosis and high mitotic index as well as prominent atypia.

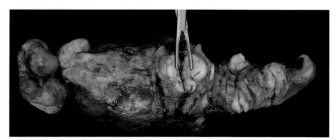

FIGURE 1

Suspected hereditary leiomyomatosis and renal cell carcinoma (HLRCC). Multiple leiomyomata in the uterus of a young woman whose tumor contained the characteristic histologic features associated with fumarate hydratase deficiency.

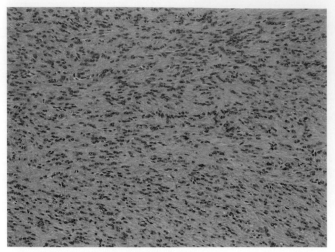

FIGURE 2

Leiomyoma in a case of documented HLRCC. Note the modest increase in cellularity. Some nuclear variation is visible at this power.

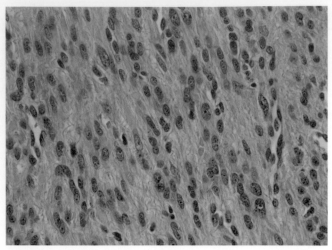

FIGURE 3

Leiomyoma in a documented case of HLRCC. The atypia is more conspicuous at this magnification.

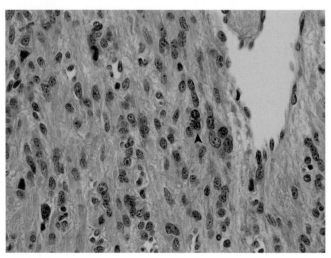

FIGURE 4

HLRCC. Nuclear overlap suggesting multinucleation *(arrow)*.

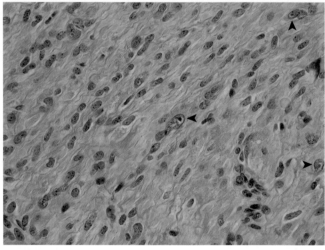

FIGURE 5

HLRCC. This field contains several prominent orangeophilic nuclei *(arrows)*.

LEIOMYOSARCOMA

DEFINITION—A malignant tumor of smooth muscle originating in the myometrium.

CLINICAL FEATURES

EPIDEMIOLOGY

- Rare (estimated incidence of 0.64 per 100,000 women).
- Account for 1% of all uterine malignancies and more than 25% of uterine mesenchymal malignancies.
- Mostly occurs in postmenopausal women.

PRESENTATION

- Most cases of leiomyosarcoma are discovered following a procedure for symptomatic leiomyoma.
- Less often, postmenopausal patients present with a rapidly enlarging uterine mass.

PROGNOSIS AND TREATMENT

- The mainstay of primary treatment includes hysterectomy and resection of extrauterine disease. Adjuvant chemotherapy is of unclear benefit at this time.
- Aggressive behavior, with frequent aggressive local growth, recurrence, and distant metastases (lung, liver).
- The 5-year survival rate has been reported between 15% and 25%.
- A new disease pattern is being encountered following morcellation for what was assumed to be a benign leiomyoma. Morcellation can result in dissemination of the tumor within the peritoneal cavity with an anticipated poor outcome.

PATHOLOGY

HISTOLOGY

- Grossly, leiomyosarcomas are often seen as a solitary or dominant mass (usually at least 10 cm) with grossly evident infiltration of the myometrium, and a soft, tan cut surface (fish flesh).
- On cut section the tumor does not bulge and often has a gray or variegated appearance.

- The three basic histologic components of leiomyosarcoma are atypia, increased numbers of mitoses, and tumor necrosis (not ischemic necrosis). Tumor cell necrosis is abrupt, with irregular borders and abundant "ghost nuclei" present within the zone of necrosis. As opposed to ischemic necrosis, a reactive rim of myofibroblasts is not present (although this distinction is sometimes difficult).
- If all three features are present, the diagnosis is straightforward, but this is often not the case.
- In the presence of true, multifocal, tumor necrosis, a high mitotic rate and nuclear atypia are not required.
- Evaluation of tumor necrosis is both the most critical and the most controversial aspect of smooth muscle neoplasms.
- If tumor necrosis is absent, then marked diffuse nuclear atypia and a mitotic rate greater than 10/10 high-power fields must be present.
- Mitotic activity should be assessed in more than one area; usually at least three sets of 10 high-power fields should be counted (be sure to exclude pyknotic cells).
- Atypical mitotic figures (multipolar mitoses, lagging chromosomes, and extreme aneuploidy) are often seen.
- Nuclear atypia is usually identifiable at low power and is characterized by any nuclear enlargement and irregularity, hyperchromasia, clumped chromatin, prominent nucleoli, and multilobation, often in combination.
- Other helpful features include increased cellularity or marked hypercellularity and infiltration into the surrounding myometrium.

IMMUNOPATHOLOGY (INCLUDING IMMUNOHISTOCHEMISTRY)

- Positive for desmin and smooth muscle actin.
- Negative for S100.

MAIN DIFFERENTIAL DIAGNOSIS

- Smooth muscle tumor of uncertain malignant potential (see chapter on STUMP).
- Endometrial stromal sarcoma (on small samples). See chapter on ESS.

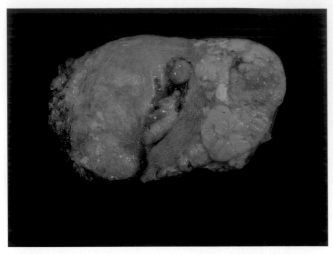

FIGURE 1

Leiomyosarcoma. Gross image of an irregular tumor with a tan-brown, fleshy cut surface. Note how the tumor does not bulge as seen in a typical leiomyoma.

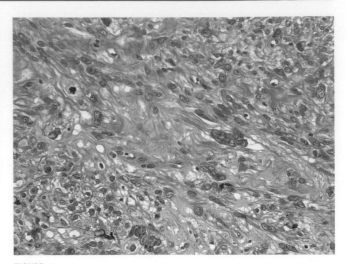

FIGURE 2

Leiomyosarcoma. Nuclear atypia.

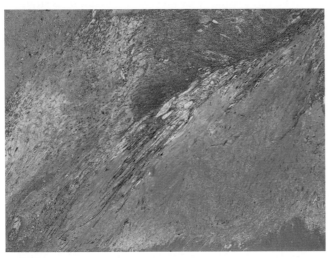

FIGURE 3

Leiomyosarcoma. Low-power view of an area of geographic necrosis. Note the abrupt transition between viable and necrotic areas.

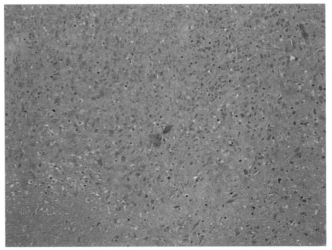

FIGURE 4

Leiomyosarcoma. Tumor cell (ghost cells) within an area of coagulative tumor necrosis.

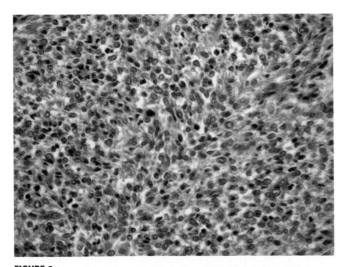

FIGURE 5

Leiomyosarcoma. A cellular area with nuclear atypia and numerous mitotic figures.

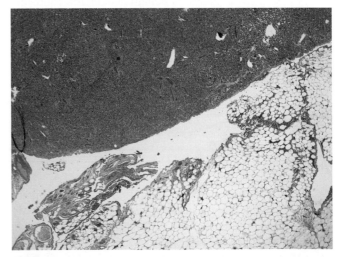

FIGURE 6

Leiomyosarcoma. A nodule of leiomyosarcoma, metastatic to the omentum.

MYXOID LEIOMYOSARCOMA

DEFINITION—An aggressive histologic variant of uterine leiomyosarcoma.

CLINICAL FEATURES

EPIDEMIOLOGY

- Rare, even among uterine leiomyosarcomas.

PRESENTATION

- Similar to usual leiomyosarcoma.

PROGNOSIS AND TREATMENT

- Prognosis is poor, and overall survival seems to be lower than in usual leiomyosarcoma.

PATHOLOGY

HISTOLOGY

- The gross appearance is usually characterized by a large mass with a soft, gelatinous cut surface.
- At low power these tumors often appear relatively hypocellular due to the accumulation of blue intracellular myxoid material.

- Criteria for a diagnosis of malignancy in myxoid smooth muscle lesions (leiomyosarcoma) include at least one of the following features:
- Mitoses greater than 2/10 high-power fields.
  - Significant cytologic atypia (e.g., nuclear irregularity and hyperchromasia).
  - True tumor cell necrosis.
  - Destructive infiltration into the surrounding myometrium.
- The presence of vascular involvement may be helpful, but it is not diagnostic of malignancy and must be distinguished from myxoid intravascular leiomyomatosis.

IMMUNOPATHOLOGY (INCLUDING IMMUNOHISTOCHEMISTRY)

- Noncontributory.

MAIN DIFFERENTIAL DIAGNOSIS

- Other, less aggressive, myxoid smooth muscle neoplasms of the uterus.

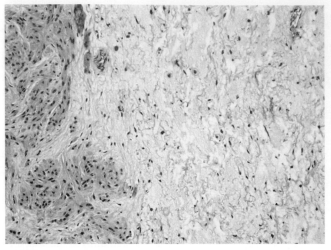

FIGURE 1

Myxoid leiomyosarcoma. A myxoid neoplasm is seen adjacent to bundles of smooth muscle.

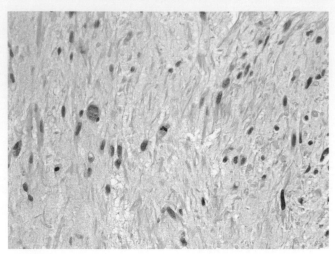

FIGURE 2

Myxoid leiomyosarcoma. A mitotic figure. Note the cigar-shaped smooth muscle cells that are present within the myxoid stroma.

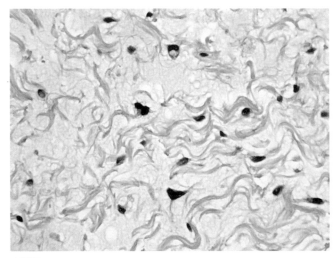

FIGURE 3

Myxoid leiomyosarcoma. Nuclear pleomorphism may be present but is usually mild.

EPITHELIOID LEIOMYOSARCOMA

DEFINITION—A distinctive histopathologic variant of uterine leiomyosarcoma.

CLINICAL FEATURES

EPIDEMIOLOGY

- Rare.

PRESENTATION

- Similar to usual leiomyosarcoma with nonspecific symptoms including vaginal bleeding, pelvic pressure, and pain.

PROGNOSIS AND TREATMENT

- This variant appears to have a lower overall survival than usual leiomyosarcoma.

PATHOLOGY

HISTOLOGY

- The defining feature of this variant is the presence of nonspindled, round, epithelioid cells.

- The cells have abundant brightly eosinophilic cytoplasm and often appear slightly discohesive.
- Criteria for a diagnosis of leiomyosarcoma are slightly altered if an epithelioid phenotype is present: either true tumor necrosis *or* mitotic count greater than 5/10 high-power fields is sufficient.
- Nuclear atypia, vascular invasion, and large tumor size are also indicative of aggressive behavior but are not sufficient for diagnosis.
- The epithelioid component may be focal or diffuse.

IMMUNOPATHOLOGY (INCLUDING IMMUNOHISTOCHEMISTRY)

- Less positivity for desmin and smooth muscle actin compared with usual leiomyosarcoma.
- Cytokeratin stains will be negative.

MAIN DIFFERENTIAL DIAGNOSIS

- Epithelioid smooth muscle tumor of uncertain malignant potential.
- Undifferentiated carcinoma. Smooth muscle markers will be negative.

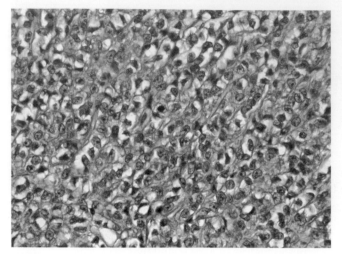

FIGURE 1

Epithelioid leiomyosarcoma. Smooth muscle cells with abundant clear cytoplasm arranged in cords.

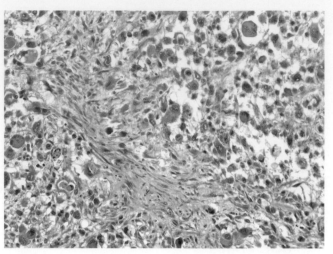

FIGURE 2

Epithelioid leiomyosarcoma. Epithelioid cells with abundant, eosinophilic cytoplasm and distinct cell borders. These cells can appear similar to those seen in poorly differentiated carcinoma.

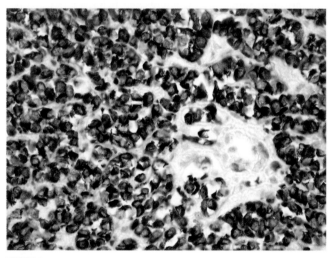

FIGURE 3

Epithelioid leiomyosarcoma. Immunohistochemical stain for desmin showing strong cytoplasmic positivity.

PEComa

DEFINITION—A tumor composed of a morphologically and immunohistochemically distinct cell type with features of smooth muscle and melanocytic differentiation.

CLINICAL FEATURES

EPIDEMIOLOGY

- Very rare; a somewhat controversial diagnosis at this site (uterus).
- Cases have been reported in a wide age range (40s to 80s).

PRESENTATION

- Presumably similar to leiomyomata, although the number of reported cases is very small.

PROGNOSIS AND TREATMENT

- Prognosis is difficult to estimate due to the small number of cases, although some histologic features are associated with aggressive behavior.
- Hysterectomy is the treatment of choice.

PATHOLOGY

HISTOLOGY

- The overriding histologic feature that should prompt the pathologist to consider this diagnosis is the presence of epithelioid cytomorphology.
- In particular the epithelioid cells tend to have abundant clear to eosinophilic (and sometimes granular) cytoplasm with a centrally placed nucleus.

- In some areas these cells can be seen in a distinctly perivascular distribution and located just under the endothelial layer.
- A commonly identified invasive growth pattern is similar to that seen in an endometrial stromal sarcoma, with fingers and tongues of tumor cells permeating the myometrium.
- Important histologic features that apparently portend a worse prognosis include large size (greater than 5 cm), an infiltrative growth pattern, high nuclear grade, the presence of true tumor necrosis, and identifiable mitotic activity (>1/50 high-power fields).
- As this entity is controversial in the uterus, strict application of histologic and immunophenotypic criteria should be used before rendering this diagnosis.

IMMUNOPATHOLOGY (INCLUDING IMMUNOHISTOCHEMISTRY)

- Positive for muscle markers: desmin, smooth muscle actin, and calponin.
- Positive for melanocytic markers: HMB45, Melan-A, and MiTF.

MAIN DIFFERENTIAL DIAGNOSIS

- Epithelioid leiomyoma.
- Epithelioid leiomyosarcoma.
- Endometrial stromal sarcoma with focal clear-cell features. All of these entities are best excluded by the absence of melanocytic markers.

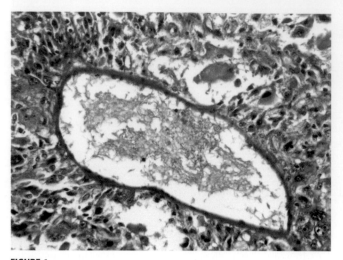

FIGURE 1

Uterine PEComa. Cells can be seen in a perivascular distribution, directly under the endothelial surface.

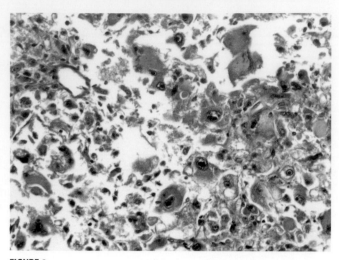

FIGURE 2

Uterine PEComa. Epithelioid cells with atypical nuclei and clear cytoplasm.

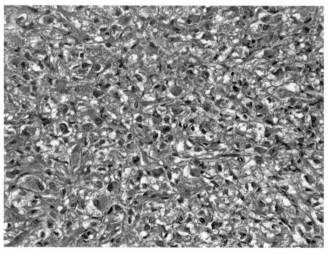

FIGURE 3

Uterine PEComa. Alternatively eosinophilic cells may predominate.

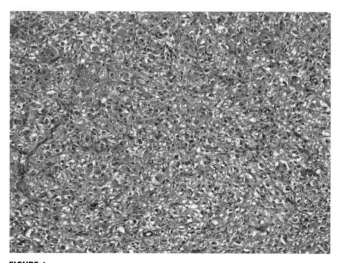

FIGURE 4

Uterine PEComa. In some cases a vague, nested pattern may be present.

REPRODUCTIVE TRACT LYMPHOMA

■ **Emily E.K. Meserve, MD, MPH**

DEFINITION—A malignant lymphoid process involving the reproductive tract.

CLINICAL FEATURES

EPIDEMIOLOGY

- Reproductive tract lymphoma is exceedingly rare but about two thirds will be primary tumors.
- In about one third of cases the tumor will be a manifestation of a systemic lymphoma.

PRESENTATION

- Patients may present with abnormal uterine bleeding. About two thirds involve the adnexae, followed by the uterus and cervix.

PROGNOSIS AND TREATMENT

- Uterine or adnexal involvement by lymphoma typically represents advanced stage disease and has a dismal prognosis.
- Chemotherapy specific to the type of lymphoma present is the treatment of choice.

PATHOLOGY

HISTOLOGY

- An infiltrate of monomorphic lymphocytes is invariably present.
- Loss of normal architecture and glands (effacement) may occur.
- In small biopsy specimens of the endometrium the fragments may resemble those seen in submucosal leiomyomas (aglandular functionalis); however, the stroma will appear hypercellular.
- The most common cell types are diffuse large B-cell lymphoma, follicular lymphoma, and Burkitt lymphoma.

IMMUNOPATHOLOGY (INCLUDING IMMUNOHISTOCHEMISTRY)

- Immunostains for lymphoid differentiation (CD45) and B and T cell markers are helpful for the classification of lymphoid neoplasms.

MAIN DIFFERENTIAL DIAGNOSIS

- Marked chronic inflammation (cervicitis, endometritis, salpingitis)—there will be a mixed infiltrate.

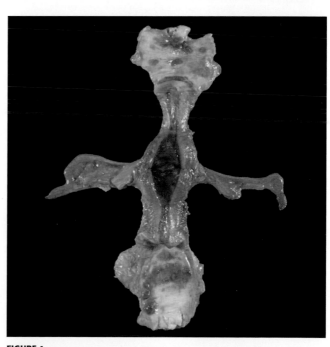

FIGURE 1

Vaginal lymphoma, seen as multiple small submucosal nodules *(top)*.

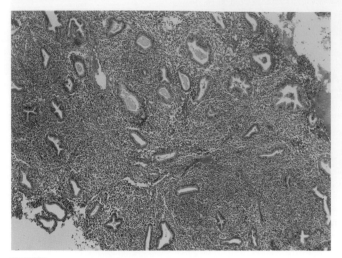

FIGURE 2

Diffuse large B cell lymphoma of the endometrium.

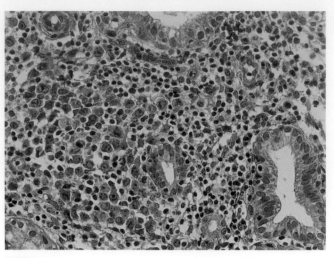

FIGURE 3

Diffuse large B cell lymphoma of the endometrium.

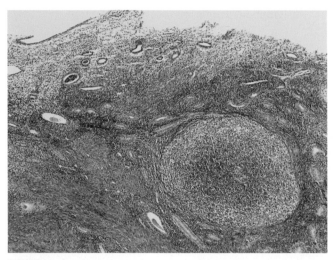

FIGURE 4

Non-Hodgkin's lymphoma involving the endometrium.

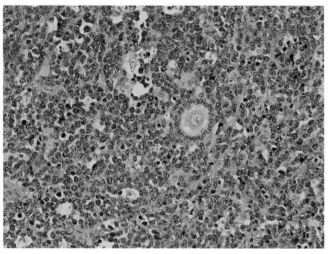

FIGURE 5

Burkitt lymphoma of the ovary. Note the residual oocyte *(center)*.

Fallopian Tube

ADRENAL REST

DEFINITION—A developmental rest of adrenal tissue in the adnexal soft tissue.

CLINICAL FEATURES

EPIDEMIOLOGY

- Can be seen at all ages and in up to one fourth of fallopian tubes examined. Presumably adrenal rests are misplaced deposits of adrenal tissue.

PRESENTATION

- This is an incidental finding seen in surgical specimens. The most common location is the paratubal or paraovarian soft tissue.

PROGNOSIS AND TREATMENT

- None.

PATHOLOGY

HISTOLOGY

- The appearance is identical to adrenal tissue, consisting of polyhedral cortical cells. Some smaller cells similar to those seen on the surface may also be present. The cells are within a well-defined delicate vascular network. The rest is composed of cortex only; no medullary cells are present.

IMMUNOPATHOLOGY (INCLUDING IMMUNOHISTOCHEMISTRY)

- Noncontributory, although will be negative for inhibin or calretinin (excluding hilar cells).

MAIN DIFFERENTIAL DIAGNOSIS

- Macrophages or histiocytes—typically will manifest with finely granular cytoplasm and pigment deposition.
- Hilar cells—typically found in the ovarian hilus, but might be seen in the adnexae where they will mimic adrenal rest. Will be inhibin or calretinin positive.

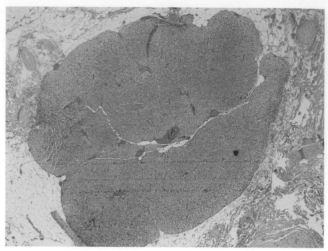

FIGURE 1

Low magnification of an adrenal rest, seen as a lobular, well-circumscribed mass.

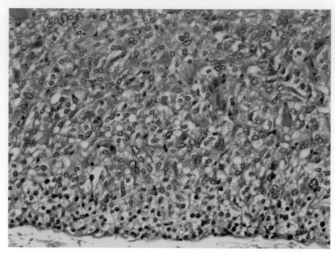

FIGURE 2

Adrenal rest at higher magnification; note the smaller cells at the periphery, similar to those seen in the peripheral cortex of the normal adrenal gland.

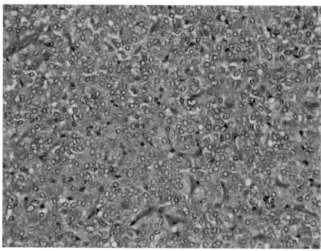

FIGURE 3

Uniform cortical cells with open nuclei. Note the regular vascular network.

PSEUDOXANTHOMATOUS SALPINGIOSIS

DEFINITION—Accumulation of histiocytic cells within the fallopian tube in association with pelvic endometriosis.

CLINICAL FEATURES

EPIDEMIOLOGY

- Pseudoxanthomatous salpingiosis is an uncommon entity that may be found in association with endometriosis.

PRESENTATION

- Usually found incidentally at the time of histologic examination of the fallopian tube. Patients may present with clinical symptoms or signs of endometriosis and/or endometrioma formation.

PROGNOSIS AND TREATMENT

- Pseudoxanthomatous salpingiosis is benign, and treatment of the underlying cause (endometriosis) may be necessary for symptomatic relief. There is an increased risk for infertility and ectopic pregnancy in patients with this process.

PATHOLOGY

HISTOLOGY

- Histiocytes with foamy cytoplasm can be seen within the tubal plica. Evidence of hemorrhage may be seen within the histiocytes and the stroma. A conspicuous lack of other acute and chronic inflammatory cells should be present (hence the alternate name salpingiosis).

IMMUNOPATHOLOGY (INCLUDING IMMUNOHISTOCHEMISTRY)

- Noncontributory.

MAIN DIFFERENTIAL DIAGNOSIS

- Xanthogranulomatous salpingitis—this entity has considerable inflammation and fibroblast proliferation.
- Chronic salpingitis—may overlap with xanthogranulomatous salpingitis.

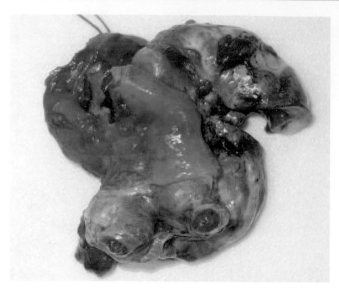

FIGURE 1

Sectioned tubes *(near bottom of picture)* display a golden-brown appearance to the endosalpinx.

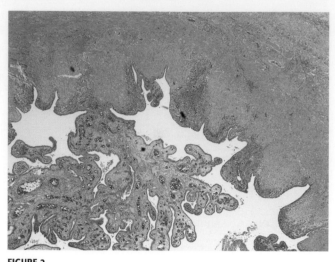

FIGURE 2

Low magnification of tubal lumen shows blunt plica with increased stromal cellularity.

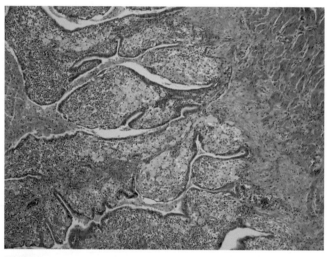

FIGURE 3

Low magnification of mucosa showing prominent macrophages and xanthoma cells.

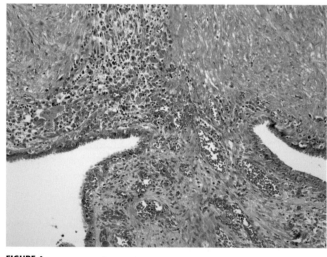

FIGURE 4

A plica with old hemorrhage but few inflammatory cells.

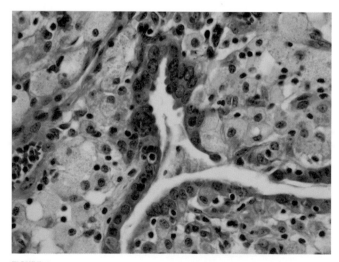

FIGURE 5

Higher magnification shows xanthoma cells in the lamina propria.

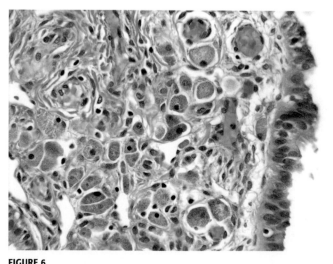

FIGURE 6

These macrophages are heavily pigmented.

XANTHOGRANULOMATOUS SALPINGITIS

DEFINITION—An admixture of inflammatory cells and histiocytes within the fallopian tube.

CLINICAL FEATURES

EPIDEMIOLOGY

- Xanthogranulomatous salpingitis is an uncommon entity. It is most commonly seen in association with pelvic inflammatory disease, extensive endometriosis, and intrauterine contraceptive devices. Infection with one of a variety of coliform bacteria likely plays a role in some cases. Rare cases have been associated with contrast agents.

PRESENTATION

- Patients present with signs and symptoms of pelvic inflammatory disease including pelvic pain, abnormal bleeding, and fever. The presence of xanthogranulomatous salpingitis is typically identified at the time of histologic examination of the tube in these cases.

PROGNOSIS AND TREATMENT

- Xanthogranulomatous salpingitis is benign; however, treatment of the underlying cause is required (antibiotics and surgery).

PATHOLOGY

HISTOLOGY

- Xanthogranulomatous salpingitis displays a prominent acute and chronic inflammatory infiltrate with admixed foamy histiocytes. The presence of the acute and chronic inflammatory infiltrate differentiates this from pseudoxanthomatous salpingitis.

IMMUNOPATHOLOGY (INCLUDING IMMUNOHISTOCHEMISTRY)

- Noncontributory.

MAIN DIFFERENTIAL DIAGNOSIS

- Pseudoxanthomatous salpingitis—typically characterized by xanthoma cells and pigment in the lamina propria with preservation of architecture, but without the prominent inflammatory component.
- Granulomatous salpingitis—well-developed granulomas are present.

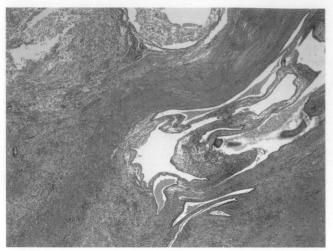

FIGURE 1

Xanthogranulomatous salpingitis. At low magnification the tubal architecture is distorted by the prominent inflammatory process.

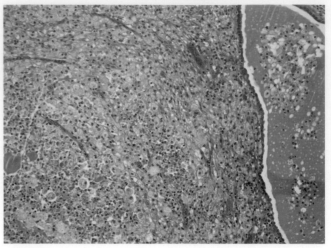

FIGURE 2

Xanthogranulomatous salpingitis. A prominent inflammatory infiltrate with foamy histiocytes. This distinguishes this entity from pseudoxanthomatous salpingitis, which typically does not cause marked distortion of plical architecture.

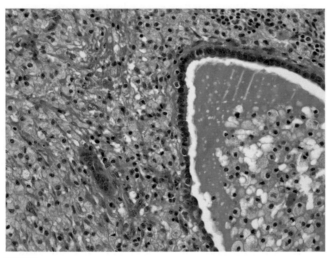

FIGURE 3

High magnification shows numerous foamy histiocytes.

FOLLICULAR SALPINGITIS

DEFINITION—The chronic phase of pelvic inflammatory disease.

CLINICAL FEATURES

EPIDEMIOLOGY

- Follicular salpingitis is the chronic phase of pelvic inflammatory disease, which is common in the United States (as well as the remainder of the world). The majority of cases happen in young adults and are related to sexual activity. The majority of the remaining cases are secondary to instrumentation or intrauterine device use.

PRESENTATION

- Patients may be asymptomatic, and the follicular salpingitis may be discovered after it has resolved (as hydrosalpinx or chronic follicular salpingitis).

PROGNOSIS AND TREATMENT

- As a result of scarring after resolution, fertility may be greatly diminished or lost. With repeated bouts of salpingitis the risk of infertility climbs over 50%. There is a greatly increased risk of ectopic (tubal) pregnancy following cases of pelvic inflammatory disease. About one half of ectopic pregnancies are related to chronic salpingitis and the presence of pre-existing inflammation increases the risk of ectopic to greater than 7 fold that of the general population. Antibiotic therapy with multiagent drugs is the typical first-line treatment choice; however, severe or refractory cases (including tubo-ovarian abscess formation) may require surgery.

PATHOLOGY

HISTOLOGY

- During the chronic phase of pelvic inflammatory disease (follicular salpingitis), the inflammatory infiltrate within the tubal lamina propria is comprised of lymphocytes and plasma cells. As the lesion progresses, the plica becomes scarred and fused and the inflammatory infiltrate decreases. In resolved lesions the inflammatory infiltrate is sparse and the lamina propria is fibrotic; eventual hydrosalpinx (tubal dilation) may occur.

Diagnostic terminology—Chronic follicular salpingitis (e.g., with or without hydrosalpinx, adhesions).

IMMUNOPATHOLOGY (INCLUDING IMMUNOHISTOCHEMISTRY)

- Noncontributory.

MAIN DIFFERENTIAL DIAGNOSIS

- Acute salpingitis—typically will exhibit intraluminal acute inflammatory exudate and neutrophils.
- Salpingitis isthmica nodosum—this entity is not associated with inflammation, and the "follicles" are separated by the smooth muscle of the tubal wall.

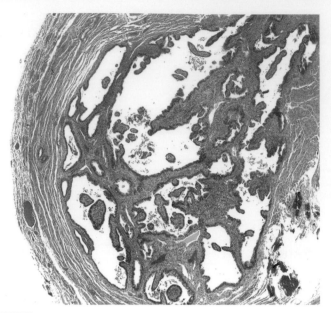

FIGURE 1

Chronic follicular salpingitis. Note the prominent fusion of the plicae imparting a follicle-like appearance.

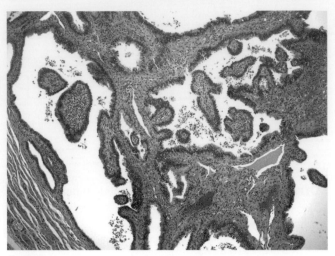

FIGURE 2

Chronic follicular salpingitis. Entrapment of epithelium within adhered plicae is characteristic of this disorder and cannot be produced by tangential sectioning.

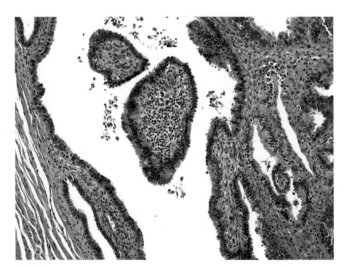

FIGURE 3

Chronic follicular salpingitis. There is virtually always a lymphoid infiltrate with plasma cells.

SALPINGITIS ISTHMICA NODOSUM

DEFINITION—A proliferation of smooth muscle with accompanying epithelium in the fallopian tube, analogous to adenomyosis/adenomyoma seen within the uterus.

CLINICAL FEATURES

EPIDEMIOLOGY

- Salpingitis isthmica nodosum (SIN) is a relatively common phenomenon seen in up to 11% of thoroughly examined fallopian tubes.

PRESENTATION

- SIN can be grossly identified as a beadlike nodule within the tube, usually in the more proximal aspects. The patient may present clinically with infertility or ectopic pregnancy, both of which are heavily associated with SIN.

PROGNOSIS AND TREATMENT

- SIN is benign. Because of the proximal location within the tube, surgical repair is rarely considered. If the patient elects to have in vitro fertilization (IVF), the tubes may be removed to lower the risk of tubal pregnancy.

PATHOLOGY

HISTOLOGY

- A nodule is typically present within the fallopian tube. Within this nodule there is a proliferation of smooth muscle with multiple, discrete tubal lumina. Inflammation is typically sparse, and reactive fibrosis, as seen in follicular salpingitis, is absent.

IMMUNOPATHOLOGY (INCLUDING IMMUNOHISTOCHEMISTRY)

- Noncontributory.

MAIN DIFFERENTIAL DIAGNOSIS

- Follicular salpingitis—this is characterized by fusion of the plica, which will be suspended in the lumen and not ensconced in the wall of the tube, as seen in SIN.
- Sectioning of the fallopian tube in the cornu—this may be difficult to distinguish from SIN, but some endometrial stroma should be seen.

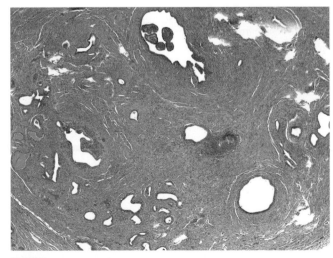

FIGURE 1

SIN. Giving the impression of tubal "adenomyosis," the epithelium is arranged in glandlike structures spaced between smooth muscle of the tubal wall.

GRANULOMATOUS SALPINGITIS

DEFINITION—Granulomatous inflammation of the fallopian tube.

CLINICAL FEATURES

EPIDEMIOLOGY

- Granulomatous salpingitis is uncommon. The granulomatous inflammation may be secondary to infectious causes (*Mycobacterium tuberculosis*, actinomyces, and parasitic infections) or noninfectious causes (sarcoid, Crohn's disease, or foreign-body giant cell reaction).

PRESENTATION

- Patients may be asymptomatic or may present with symptoms of the underlying condition responsible for the inflammation.

PROGNOSIS AND TREATMENT

- Granulomatous salpingitis in isolation is a benign process; however, the underlying cause should be sought out and treated.

PATHOLOGY

HISTOLOGY

- Granuloma formation is the hallmark of granulomatous salpingitis. The accompanying giant cells are frequently large, with abundant eosinophilic cytoplasm and numerous nuclei. Variable amounts of acute and chronic inflammation may be present. In cases secondary to foreign material, polarizable debris may be identified.

DIAGNOSTIC TERMINOLOGY

- Granulomatous salpingitis. Note: Granulomatous salpingitis is not specific. Infectious etiology (e.g., tuberculosis [TB]) or other inflammatory etiologies should be excluded as clinically appropriate.

IMMUNOPATHOLOGY (INCLUDING IMMUNOHISTOCHEMISTRY)

- In cases of infectious granulomatous salpingitis special stains for fungus (Grocott's methenamine silver [GMS]) and mycobacterium (acid-fast stains) may be helpful in identifying organisms; however, molecular methods, such as polymerase chain reaction (PCR) in the case of TB, are more sensitive.

MAIN DIFFERENTIAL DIAGNOSIS

- Crohn's disease, sarcoid, other nontuberculous infections, and foreign material can all produce granulomas and should be excluded, as appropriate to the clinical setting.

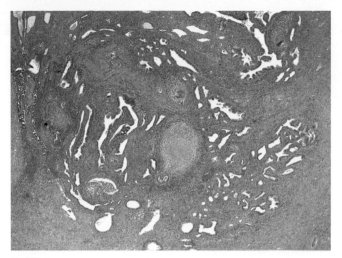

FIGURE 1

Granulomatous salpingitis. At low power note the prominent follicular salpingitis pattern with fused plicae.

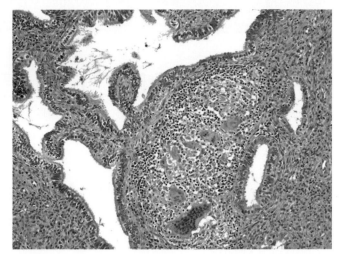

FIGURE 2

Granulomatous salpingitis. At higher magnification a granuloma is seen in the center just beneath the epithelium.

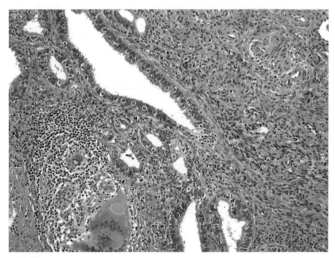

FIGURE 3

Granulomatous salpingitis. At higher magnification a granuloma with prominent giant cells is seen.

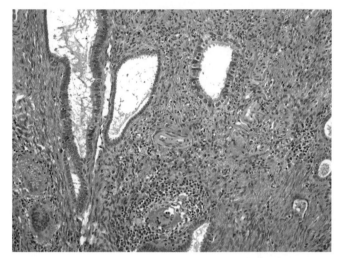

FIGURE 4

Granulomatous salpingitis. There is a variable lymphoplasmacytic infiltrate.

TORSION OF THE TUBE AND OVARY

DEFINITION—Mechanical interruption of the adnexal arterial and/or venous blood flow by mechanical factors.

CLINICAL FEATURES

EPIDEMIOLOGY

- Rare (reported in as few as 1 in every 1.5 million women), can occur at any age but usually in reproductive-age women.
- Most commonly seen with pregnancy, hydrosalpinx, ovarian cysts, tubal ligation, and benign tumors.
- Uncommonly associated with malignancies.
- Caused by rotation on the vascular pedicle. Fallopian tube and ovary can torse together or individually via rotation of the mesosalpinx and mesovarium, respectively.

PRESENTATION

- Abdominal pain, nausea, and vomiting.
- Fever can occur if the torsion results in tissue necrosis.
- Ultrasound and Doppler evidence of a uniformly expanded ovary with decreased blood flow.

PROGNOSIS AND TREATMENT

- Immediate management entails untwisting the adnexa.
- Recurrence rates are high with mechanical relief alone, and fixation of the ovary (oophoropexy) is often required.
- Salpingo-oophorectomy may be required if the torsion has resulted in extensive loss of tissue viability.

PATHOLOGY

HISTOLOGY

- Early on, torsion manifests as marked vascular congestion followed by early hemorrhagic necrosis in the form of interstitial hemorrhage.
- Prolonged torsion leads to devitalized tissue and variable inflammatory response.

IMMUNOPATHOLOGY (INCLUDING IMMUNOHISTOCHEMISTRY)

- Noncontributory.

MAIN DIFFERENTIAL DIAGNOSIS

- Massive ovarian edema—this is not characterized by hemorrhagic necrosis.
- Excluding malignancy—this diagnostic dilemma occurs when there is an obvious tumor that has undergone necrosis due to torsion. In such instances the pathologist must carefully examine the devitalized tissue for clues that might indicate malignancy, focusing on the most well-preserved portion of the tumor and taking into account cell density, uniformity, or lack of in nuclear size and overall architecture.

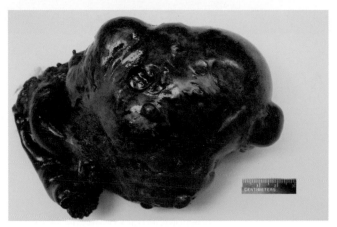

FIGURE 1

Adnexal torsion. In this case the tube and ovary are a single ischemic and hemorrhagic mass.

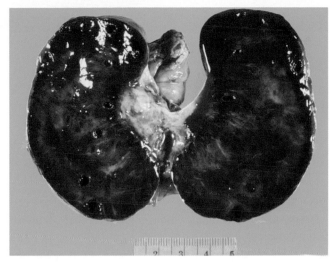

FIGURE 2

Ovarian torsion. The ovary is diffusely hemorrhagic and uniformly expanded.

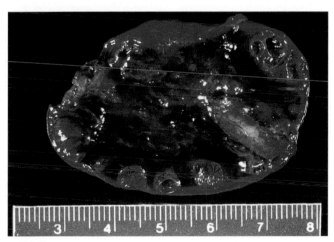

FIGURE 3

Ovarian torsion during pregnancy. The follicles are pushed to the periphery by the interstitial hemorrhage.

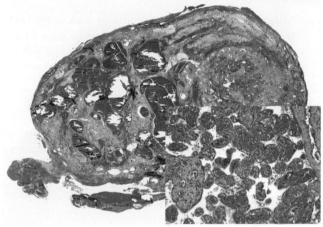

FIGURE 4

Low-power photomicrograph of a torsed fallopian tube. The lumen is designated by the dotted circle, with marked congestion of adnexal vessels on the left. The inset shows interstitial hemorrhage in the plicae.

TUBAL ARIAS-STELLA EFFECT

DEFINITION—Hormonally induced changes that occur within the epithelium of the gynecologic tract (typically secondary to pregnancy).

CLINICAL FEATURES

EPIDEMIOLOGY

- Arias-Stella effect is most commonly seen in the background of pregnancy; however, it can be seen in any case of hormonal alteration (whether exogenous or endogenous).

PRESENTATION

- Arias-Stella effect is typically an incidental finding on microscopic examination of the fallopian tube removed for other reasons.

PROGNOSIS AND TREATMENT

- Arias-Stella effect associated with pregnancy or exogenous hormone effect is benign, and no further treatment is warranted.

PATHOLOGY

HISTOLOGY

- Arias-Stella effect of the fallopian tube is similar to that seen elsewhere in the gynecologic tract. It can be discrete or more generalized as a form of hypersecretory change. Variable cellular and nuclear enlargement may be seen. The affected cells typically have abundant eosinophilic cytoplasm. Despite the large nuclei and cells, the nuclear-to-cytoplasmic (NC) ratio will usually remain low (as opposed to a high NC ratio as seen in serous tubal intraepithelial neoplasia). Mitotic activity should be absent; however, very rare mitoses have been described in association with Arias-Stella effect in other sites.

IMMUNOPATHOLOGY (INCLUDING IMMUNOHISTOCHEMISTRY)

This is a good example of where immunostaining can be helpful in excluding a serous tubal intraepithelial carcinoma (STIC), although the suspicion would be very low in a central section of a tube from a reproductive-age woman. Arias-Stella effect is negative (i.e., weakly staining) for p53. This is a key piece of confirming evidence. Arias-Stella effect should also have a low proliferative index (under 50%) by Ki-67 immunohistochemistry.

MAIN DIFFERENTIAL DIAGNOSIS

- Serous tubal intraepithelial neoplasia: This is vanishingly rare in the fallopian tubes of women who are pregnant. It can be excluded by the aforesaid approach.

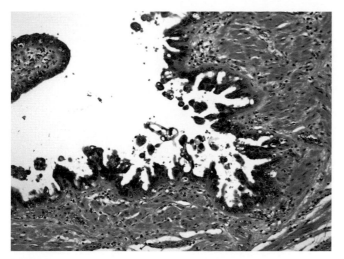

FIGURE 1

Arias-Stella effect in the fallopian tube. Note the exfoliative nature of the process at low magnification.

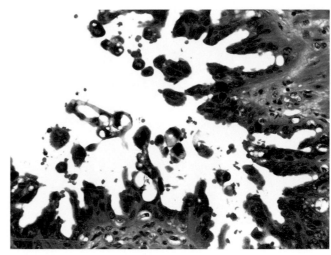

FIGURE 2

Arias-Stella effect in the fallopian tube. At higher power the vacuolated cells and enlarged nuclei are present

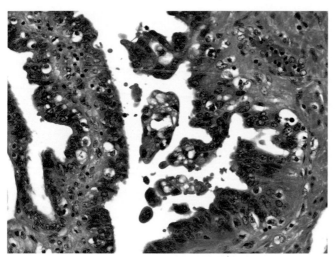

FIGURE 3

Arias-Stella effect. Another field showing mild nuclear enlargement.

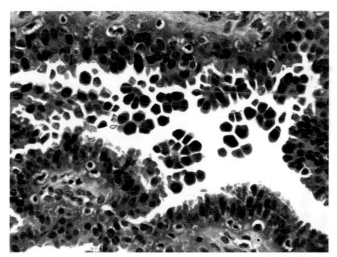

FIGURE 4

Hypersecretory changes in the fallopian tube of a pregnant woman.

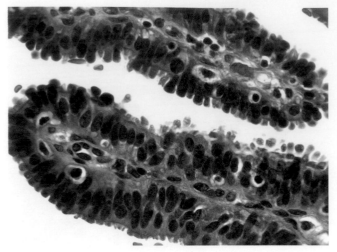

FIGURE 5

Hypersecretory change at higher power. Note the prominent admixture of ciliated and secretory type cells, many with extruded nuclei at the luminal border.

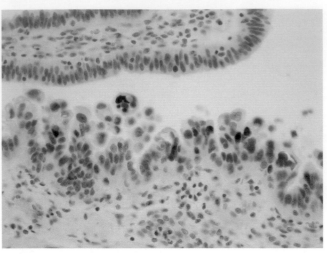

FIGURE 6

Arias-Stella effect stained for p53, showing scattered weak to moderate staining.

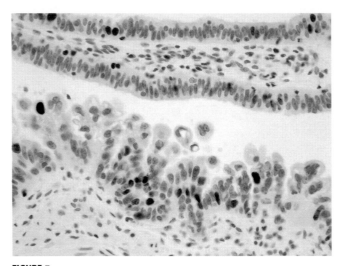

FIGURE 7

Arias-Stella effect, showing a low MIB1 index.

ADENOFIBROMA

DEFINITION—A benign neoplasm of the distal tube.

CLINICAL FEATURES

EPIDEMIOLOGY

- Adenofibromas are thought to be relatively common entities within the fallopian tube and are found predominantly within the fimbriated end of the tube.

PRESENTATION

- Tubal adenofibromas are typically found incidentally at the time of histologic examination for other causes. There are essentially two forms. One is a conspicuous lesion seen on gross exam, and the other is a microscopic lesion that cannot be seen with the naked eye.

PROGNOSIS AND TREATMENT

- The prognosis of these tumors is uneventful when not complicated by any other form of neoplasia. Adenofibromas themselves are benign and carry no risk of subsequent malignancy. Occasional malignancies are found in association with an adenofibroma, the best examples being ovarian adenocarcinomas.

PATHOLOGY

HISTOLOGY

- The fimbriated end of the fallopian tube may show focal stromal proliferations that are not mass forming and are associated with minor changes in the overlying benign epithelium, and these foci may be a millimeter or less in dimension. These are synonymous with microscopic or "early" adenofibromas. Larger lesions have a more well-developed glandular component and are macroscopically visible.

IMMUNOPATHOLOGY (INCLUDING IMMUNOHISTOCHEMISTRY)

- The stromal compartment within an adenofibroma typically marks positive for CD10 and inhibin (as their ovarian counterparts do).

MAIN DIFFERENTIAL DIAGNOSIS

- Paratubal cystadenoma—This arises within a paratubal cyst.
- Leiomyoma (stromal compartment only)—A discrete lesion with smooth muscle differentiation.

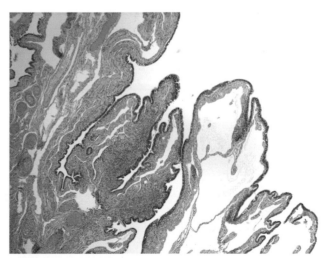

FIGURE 1

Microscopic adenofibroma with stromal condensation and minimal change in the overlying epithelium.

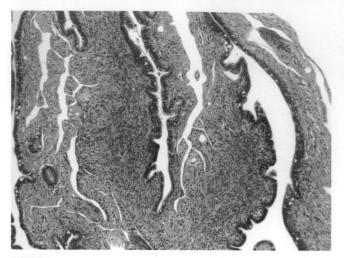

FIGURE 2

At higher magnification the stroma abuts the epithelium.

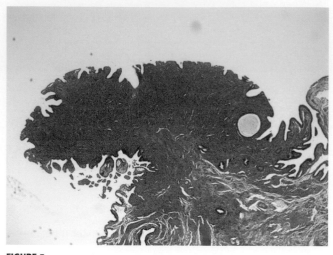

FIGURE 3

A larger adenofibroma with slight papillary change in the overlying epithelium.

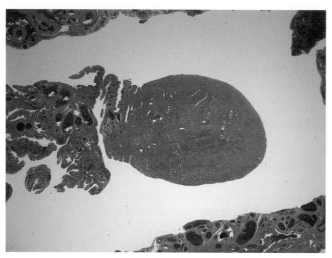

FIGURE 4

This fimbrial adenofibroma has a predominance of fibrous stroma.

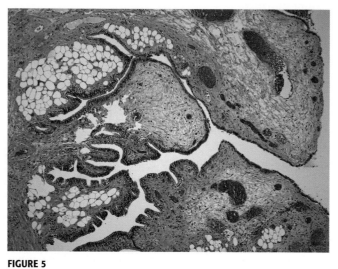

FIGURE 5

This adenofibroma contains adipose tissue.

BENIGN EPITHELIAL HYPERPLASIA (SECRETORY CELL OUTGROWTHS)

DEFINITION—Benign, self-limited clonal proliferations of tubal secretory-type cells with variable ciliation.

CLINICAL FEATURES

EPIDEMIOLOGY AND PATHOGENESIS

- Secretory cell outgrowths (SCOUTs) are common proliferations seen most commonly in the sixth and seventh decades of life but may be found earlier.
- They are increased somewhat in fallopian tubes of women with borderline or malignant serous tumors. However, whether they have a direct relationship to serous neoplasia is unknown.
- SCOUTs are presumably an outgrowth from a specialized progenitor cell in the fallopian tube.

PRESENTATION

- SCOUTs are encountered as an incidental finding during the pathologic examination of the fallopian tubes.

PROGNOSIS AND TREATMENT

- SCOUTs require no treatment and pose no risk to the patient. They are an incidental finding.

PATHOLOGY

HISTOLOGY

- There are two types of SCOUTs, and this is for descriptive (not diagnostic) purposes.
- Type 1 SCOUTs closely resemble normal mucosa and may be predominantly secretory or have conspicuous cilia.

- Type 2 SCOUTs are expansions of pseudostratified epithelial cells that can be more easily distinguished from the surrounding epithelium and may be "endometrioid," resembling endometrial lining.
- Occasionally SCOUTs may appear mildly papillary and call to mind a papillary neoplasm. However, the papillae are usually rather bland appearing.

IMMUNOPATHOLOGY (INCLUDING IMMUNOHISTOCHEMISTRY)

- Most but not all SCOUTs are PAX2 negative.
- Type 1 SCOUTs are also ALDH1 negative.
- Type 2 SCOUTs are ALDH1 positive and, interestingly, β-catenin positive (nuclear and cytoplasmic).

RECOMMENDED DIAGNOSTIC TERMINOLOGY

- If prominent, a diagnosis of benign epithelial hyperplasia is appropriate.

MAIN DIFFERENTIAL DIAGNOSIS

- p53 signatures may be similar but are p53 positive (or completely negative in some instances) and are more likely to be seen in the distal tube.
- Localized intraepithelial endometrioid carcinomas are rare but should be distinguished by the greater degree of atypia.

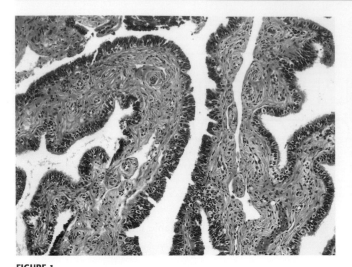

FIGURE 1

A subtle type 1 SCOUT that would not be appreciated by inspection of a hematoxylin and eosin (H&E) slide alone.

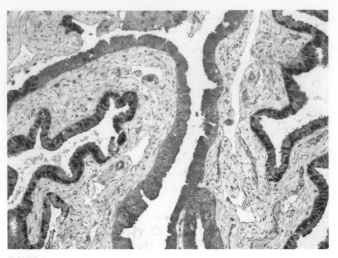

FIGURE 2

Note the discrete loss of PAX2, which highlights the epithelium.

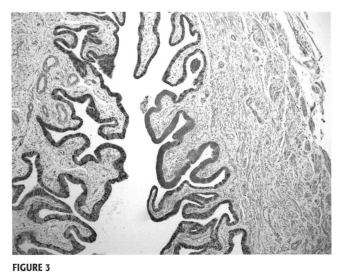

FIGURE 3

A low-power microphotograph of a PAX2-stained fallopian tube reveals a focus of slightly more pseudostratified epithelium (Type 2 SCOUT).

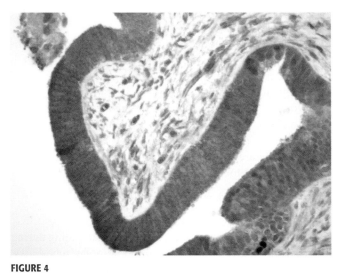

FIGURE 4

At higher magnification, note the lack of epithelial atypia despite the slight increase in thickness reminiscent of endometrioid differentiation.

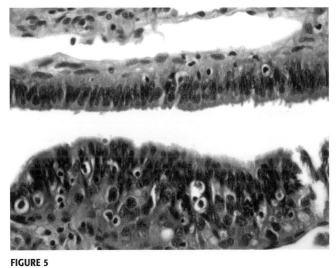

FIGURE 5

A SCOUT *(lower)* with multilayered mixed secretory and ciliated differentiation.

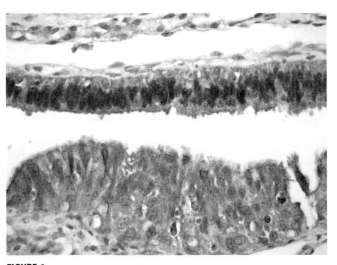

FIGURE 6

Loss of PAX2 staining highlights the same focus.

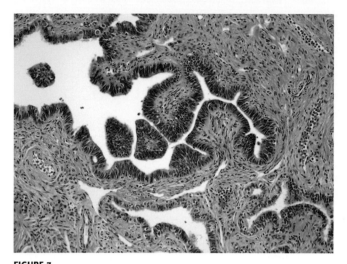

FIGURE 7

H&E-stained section shows a central focus with slight architectural complexity.

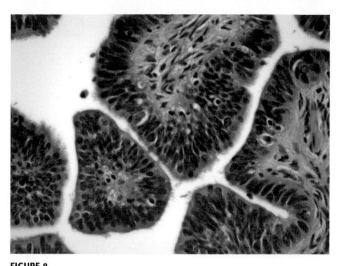

FIGURE 8

At higher power this focus takes on an appearance resembling endometrial epithelium (Type 2 SCOUT).

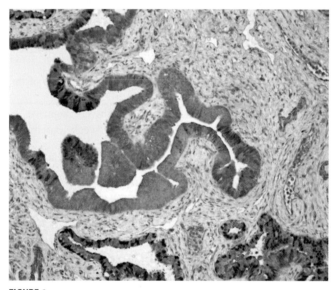

FIGURE 9

There is an absence of PAX2 staining.

p53 SIGNATURES

DEFINITION—A limited clonal expansion of secretory cells associated with mutations in p53 exhibiting minimal or atypia. Seen as perhaps the very first step in serous carcinogenesis in the tube; often termed a "latent precursor" to pelvic serous carcinoma.

CLINICAL FEATURES

EPIDEMIOLOGY

- p53 signatures exhibit features consistent with very early or latent serous cancer precursors. They are common (up to 70%) in thoroughly sectioned fallopian tubes of older women, predominate in the fimbria, exhibit evidence of DNA damage response, and are more frequently found in association with cancer. However, they are benign and their high frequency indicates that this entity, like many precursors, confers no risk to the patient.

PRESENTATION

- p53 signatures are almost always an incidental finding at the time of examination of the fallopian tube that has been removed routinely or during a risk reduction procedure for an inherited BRCA1 or BRCA2 mutation.

PROGNOSIS AND TREATMENT

- p53 signatures require no further treatment. Although they theoretically may have a low risk of developing into a malignancy, the circumstances of their discovery (in tubes that have been removed) indicate that they are clinically insignificant.

PATHOLOGY

HISTOLOGY

- The features are of a secretory cell expansion with mild atypia including
  - A continuous row of nonciliated cells
  - Variable nuclear enlargement
  - Nuclear molding (may be present)
  - Mild disturbances in nuclear orientation with preserved cell-to-cell cohesion

  - Ciliated cells, usually toward the luminal surface
- Large numbers of p53 signatures may be encountered in cases of Li-Fraumeni syndrome due to the greater likelihood of loss of p53 function (with a secondary mutation or loss of heterozygosity [LOH]).

IMMUNOPATHOLOGY (INCLUDING IMMUNOHISTOCHEMISTRY)

- p53 stains are typically strongly and diffusely positive, highlighting the cells.
  - MIB1 stains typically highlight less than 20% of the cells.
  - PAX2 stains are usually but not always negative.
  - Cyclin E and p16ink4 are usually weak, patchy, or negative.

RECOMMENDED DIAGNOSTIC TERMINOLOGY

- No diagnosis is required.
- If the changes are found in a risk-reducing specimen and found incidentally, the diagnosis of benign epithelial changes is permissible with the comment that the p53 stain is positive but there is no evidence of atypia or malignancy.

MAIN DIFFERENTIAL DIAGNOSIS

- Moderate or secretory cell atypia will exhibit greater degree of atypia, usually involve a larger surface area and demonstrate an increased proliferative index (low-grade serous tubal intraepithelial neoplasia or serous tubal intraepithelial lesion).
- High-grade serous tubal intraepithelial neoplasia (or serous tubal intraepithelial carcinoma) contains the above in addition to loss of polarity and epithelial cell disorganization.
- Li-Fraumeni syndrome. In this condition a germ-line mutation in p53 renders the tube prone to multiple p53 signatures. However, atypia is usually minimal.

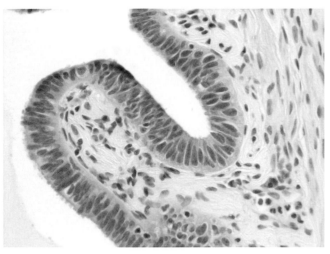

FIGURE 1

p53 signature. This entity is often limited to a portion of a tubal plica. Note the minimal nuclear enlargement and preservation of polarity. This would attract little notice in a routine specimen.

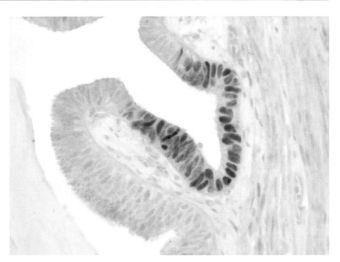

FIGURE 2

Strong nuclear staining for p53 highlights the cells.

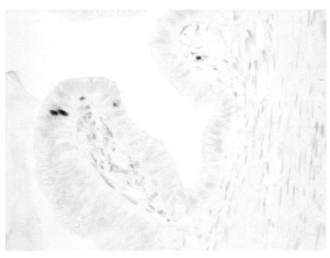

FIGURE 3

MIB1 staining typically highlights less than 20% of the cells in these mild secretory cell atypias.

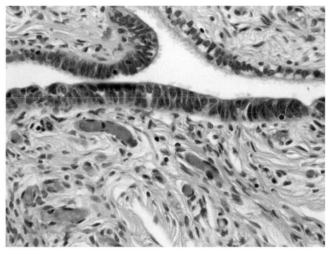

FIGURE 4

Another mild atypia (p53 signature). Note the presence of ciliated cells.

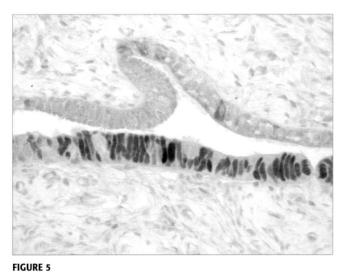

FIGURE 5

p53 staining spares the ciliated cells.

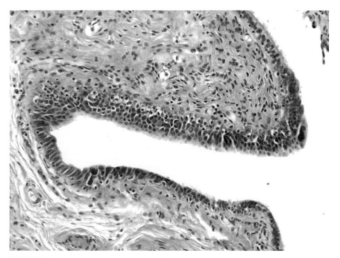

FIGURE 6

A p53 signature with greater anisokaryosis. The tangential staining lends an appearance of epithelial disorganization.

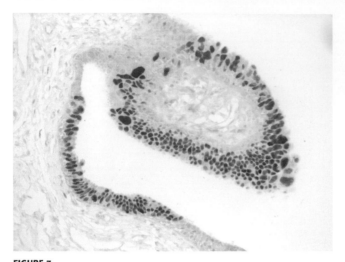

FIGURE 7

p53 staining is strong in most cells. Note the prominent nuclear enlargement in some. This by itself is not uncommon in milder forms of atypia.

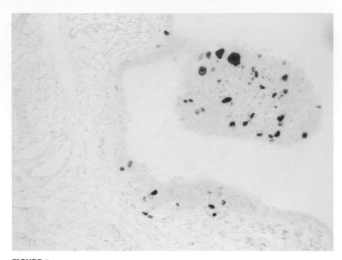

FIGURE 8

The MIB1 index is low.

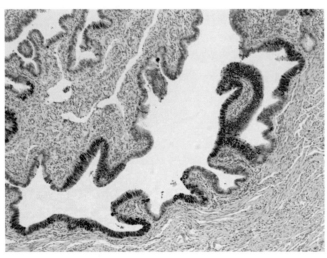

FIGURE 9

Li-Fraumeni syndrome. This p53-stained tube exhibits multiple p53 signatures. However, note that there is little atypia.

LOW-GRADE SEROUS TUBAL INTRAEPITHELIAL NEOPLASIA (SEROUS TUBAL INTRAEPITHELIAL LESION)

DEFINITION—A serous intraepithelial neoplasm of uncertain risk that does not fulfill the criteria for serous tubal intraepithelial carcinoma (STIC).

CLINICAL FEATURES

EPIDEMIOLOGY

- Low-grade serous tubal intraepithelial neoplasia (STIN) is synonymous with a proliferation produced when there are both a mutation and an inactivation of p53 and is similar to STIC.
- Like STICs, STINs are uncommon, found in less than 1 : 500 routine salpingectomies. It is found in less than 10% of tubes removed during risk reduction salpingo-oophorectomy (RRSO) for inherited BRCA1 or BRCA2 mutations, the percentages fluctuating as a function of patient age. It is discovered more commonly (just how commonly we do not know) in fallopian tubes of women with high-grade pelvic serous carcinoma. It can be associated with, and presumably preceded by, a benign non-atypical clonal expansion of secretory cells with p53 mutations (p53 signatures).

PRESENTATION

- Low-grade STINs are discovered on histologic exam of the tubes, either in RRSOs or tubes removed during surgery for advanced serous carcinoma. The former are usually asymptomatic, and the latter present with the usual signs and symptoms of advanced disease. Low-grade STINs are uncommon in the asymptomatic woman without an inherited BRCA1 or BRCA2 mutation.

PROGNOSIS AND TREATMENT

- Low-grade STINs are removed during surgery and when found in the setting of pelvic serous cancer may imply a relationship of the tumor to the tube, particularly if the STIN is in continuity with the cancer. This would imply that the STIN was a direct precursor to invasive carcinoma if not an actual intraepithelial carcinoma.
- When found in an RRSO, low-grade STINs do not require further surgery, although thorough examination is required to exclude STIC.
- The need to test for BRCA1 or BRCA2 germ-line mutations is unclear when low-grade STINs are found incidentally. If they are particularly worrisome in appearance, testing should be considered.

PATHOLOGY

HISTOLOGY

- Low-grade STIN is diagnosed using histologic criteria, but it is helpful to take advantage of ancillary tests to clarify the diagnosis. The most helpful histologic criteria include the following:
  - Cilia: Some cilia (and occasionally abundant) may be found in low-grade STINs (they are much less likely in STICs).
  - Pseudostratified epithelial growth with minimal loss of epithelial polarity.

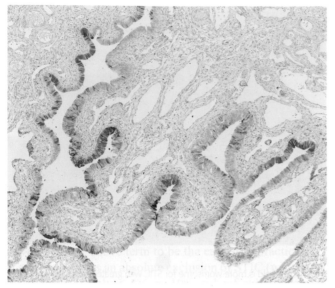

FIGURE 6

Staining for p16 is heterogeneous, more in keeping with nonmalignant epithelium, but not excluding STIC.

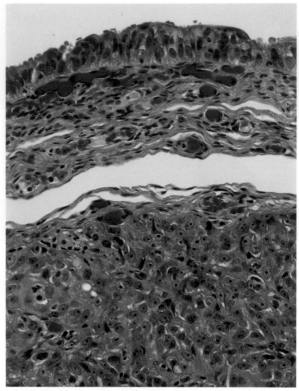

FIGURE 7

A low-grade STIN overlying an invasive carcinoma in the tube.

PAPILLARY HYPERPLASIA

DEFINITION—An increase in thickness of the epithelial layer, occasionally forming papillary tufts within the tubal lumen.

CLINICAL FEATURES

EPIDEMIOLOGY

- Papillary hyperplasia is an uncommon entity, and no associations have been made regarding incidence or predisposing factors. They have some resemblance to borderline serous tumors and have been proposed as a potential precursor to these tumors. However, they are not associated with most borderline tumors.

PRESENTATION

- May be discovered incidentally at the time of examination of the tube for other reasons.

PROGNOSIS AND TREATMENT

- Papillary hyperplasia is benign, and no further treatment is warranted.

PATHOLOGY

HISTOLOGY

- The histologic appearance can vary, likely due to different etiologies. Some are associated with tubal inflammation, in which case the lining cells closely resemble the adjacent tube with pseudostratified ciliated and secretory cells. The underlying stroma may form papillary fronds that project into the tubal lumen. These papillomas are differentiated from normal plica in that they are more architecturally complex compared with the background tube. Of note, cases of acute salpingitis may be accompanied by a florid epithelial hyperplasia that is benign. Other papillary lesions may more closely resemble mesothelium, with a cuboidal appearance.

IMMUNOPATHOLOGY (INCLUDING IMMUNOHISTOCHEMISTRY)

- Calretinin stains will be negative or focally positive.

MAIN DIFFERENTIAL DIAGNOSIS

- Normal fallopian tube—tube has a plicate rather than papillary architecture.
- Papillary adenofibromas of the fallopian tube—these are associated with a prominent dense stroma that is often immunopositive for inhibin and calretinin, similar to ovarian stroma.
- Borderline serous tumors of the tube—these may overlap with this entity but typically form cystic masses rather than single intraluminal foci.
- Salpingoliths—psammomatous calcification can be encountered in the tube, associated with some alterations in tubal architecture. They are often seen in association with regionally located borderline tumors of the ovary or peritoneum.
- Serous tubal intraepithelial carcinoma—marked atypia and p53 positive (or null [from a deletion mutation]).

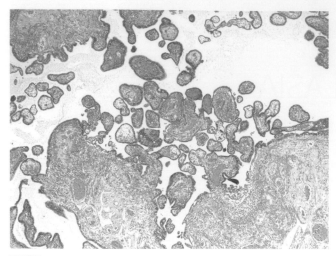

FIGURE 1

Papillary hyperplasia associated with inflammation. Note the small diameter papillae in contrast to larger tubal plicae.

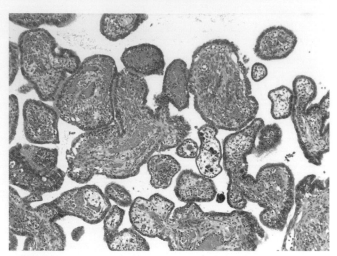

FIGURE 2

Papillary hyperplasia of the tube. Occasional calcification is present *(center).*

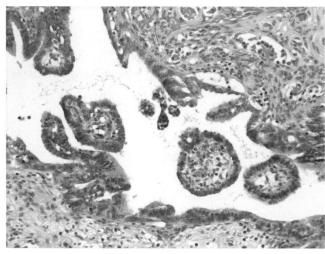

FIGURE 3

Papillary hyperplasia of the tube. Note the small, free-floating papillae.

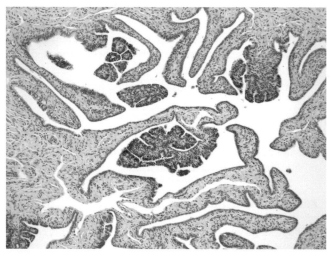

FIGURE 4

Papillary hyperplasia, present as multiple small outgrowths of ciliated and secretory cells.

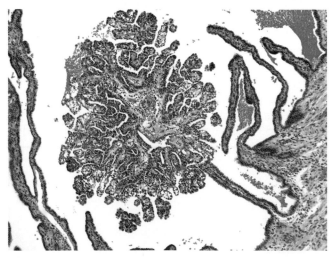

FIGURE 5

Papillary hyperplasia (a.k.a. papilloma). Note the appearance resembling a small borderline serous tumor of the tube.

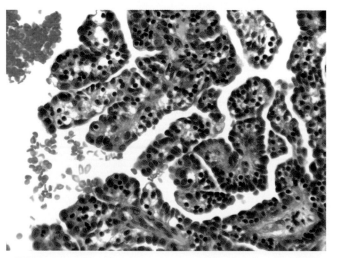

FIGURE 6

Papillary hyperplasia. At higher magnification the lining is composed of non-descript cuboidal cells.

HIGH-GRADE SEROUS TUBAL INTRAEPITHELIAL NEOPLASIA (SEROUS TUBAL INTRAEPITHELIAL CARCINOMA)

DEFINITION—Intramucosal (noninvasive) serous carcinoma. Undisputable origin of pelvic serous cancer when found in isolation or with early invasion. A plausible candidate of origin when found in association with advanced disease.

CLINICAL FEATURES

EPIDEMIOLOGY

- Serous tubal intraepithelial carcinoma (STIC) is rare, found in less than 1:1000 routine salpingectomies. It is found in from 1% to 12% of tubes removed during risk reduction salpingo-oophorectomy (RRSO) for inherited BRCA1 or BRCA2 mutations, the percentages increase with increasing patient age. It is discovered in up to 50% of fallopian tubes of women with high-grade pelvic serous carcinoma. It can be associated with, and presumably preceded by, a benign clonal expansion of secretory cells with p53 mutations (p53 signatures). Depending on the study, up to 30% of women with a carcinoma arising in the fallopian tube (with STIC) harbor a BRCA1 or BRCA2 mutation.

PRESENTATION

- STICs are discovered on histologic exam of the tubes, either in RRSOs or tubes removed during surgery for advanced serous carcinoma. The former are usually asymptomatic and the latter present with the usual signs and symptoms of advanced disease. STIC is very uncommon in the asymptomatic woman without an inherited BRCA1 or BRCA2 mutation. Discovery of STIC is maximized using a protocol that thoroughly examines the distal fallopian tube (SEE-FIM protocol).

PROGNOSIS AND TREATMENT

- STICs are removed during surgery and when found in the setting of pelvic serous cancer are important as indicators of a tubal primary. When found in an RRSO they may or may not prompt further surgery (such as omentectomy or hysterectomy) to exclude residual disease. When found incidentally in nonmalignant circumstances, testing for BRCA1 or BRCA2 should be seriously considered to determine if other family members are at risk. If there is no evidence of immediate spread and pelvic washings are negative, the risk of subsequent pelvic serous cancer is low (under 10%) and in most institutions will not result in chemotherapy. Patients must be counseled that there is always some recurrence risk in a patient with a germ-line BRCA1/2 mutation.

PATHOLOGY

HISTOLOGY

- STIC is diagnosed using histologic criteria, but it is helpful to take advantage of ancillary tests to clarify the diagnosis. The most helpful histologic criteria include the following:
  - Absence of cilia: The cell involved is a secretory cell.
  - An (slightly) irregular growth pattern with variable epithelial thickness, sometimes subtle.
  - Loss of normal nuclear orientation, imparting an appearance of abnormal polarity.
  - In extreme examples, horizontal fracture lines with exfoliation.
  - High nuclear-to-cytoplasmic (N/C) ratio.
- Features that may be present but are not specific are as follows:
  - Multilayered epithelium, which can be seen with any admixture of ciliated and secretory cells.

541

- Nuclear molding, which often occurs focally in the tubal lining.
- Nuclear enlargement (anisokaryosis), which is common in ciliated epithelium.
- Review by a second pathologist is encouraged if there is a difference of opinion.

PREFERRED DIAGNOSTIC TERM

STIC (or intramucosal serous carcinoma), with the mention that up to 10% of these lesions will recur.

IMMUNOPATHOLOGY (INCLUDING IMMUNOHISTOCHEMISTRY)

- The neoplastic cells are usually strongly and diffusely positive for p53 but will be conspicuously negative if the antigenic target sequence is deleted.
- Stains for p16ink4, cyclin E, EZH2, and stathmin are often positive; however, EZH2 and stathmin are *not specific and can be seen in benign epithelial hyperplasias* as can loss of PAX2 and ALDH1.
- The MIB1 index (Ki-67) is usually over 50% in parts of the lesion; however, STICs with low proliferative index can occur.
- A marker of polarity (p-ERM) typically shows loss of normal surface staining, highlighting irregular serrated luminal borders often with single cell membranous staining.
- Generic markers of tubal epithelium, PAX8, WT1, and CK7 will be positive.
- Use of p53 and Ki-67 is encouraged to support the diagnosis in difficult cases, but in such cases the ultimate verdict is *based on the degree of histologic certainty that the epithelium is malignant.*

MAIN DIFFERENTIAL DIAGNOSIS

- Benign epithelial hyperplasia (secretory cell outgrowths [SCOUTs])—these may exhibit multilayering but usually include ciliated cells. Polarity is preserved.

- Reactive epithelial changes, including Arias-Stella effect—these can be striking but have normal p53 expression and a low proliferative index. Moreover, they are typically found in younger women in the setting of inflammation or pregnancy.
- p53 signatures—these are typically small and unimpressive histologically, and exhibit low proliferative index. However, they may be associated with higher proliferation indices overlapping with lower-grade tubal intraepithelial neoplasms (e.g., serous tubal intraepithelial lesion [STIL], tubal intraepithelial lesions in transition [TILTs]).
- Lower-grade tubal intraepithelial neoplasms (a.k.a. tubal intraepithelial lesions or TILTs) share features of both p53 signatures and STICs and may signify the beginning of a transition from benign to malignant. Key distinguishing features are a casual appearance of benign pseudostratified epithelium with preserved polarity and a proliferative index under 25%.

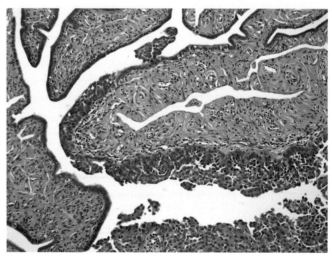

FIGURE 1

A classic STIC with multilayered epithelium and loss of polarity with horizontal fracture lines in the epithelium and exfoliation.

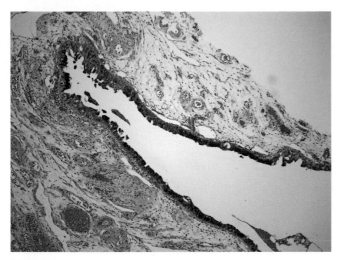

FIGURE 2

This STIC shows disorganized multilayered growth in the upper left, trailing off toward the lower right with a thinner epithelium that still displays a loss of normal cell orientation.

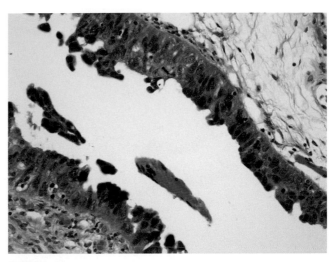

FIGURE 3

Higher power view of the STIC depicted in Figure 2.

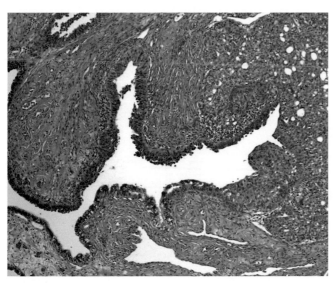

FIGURE 4

STIC *(center left)* merging with invasive serous carcinoma *(right)*.

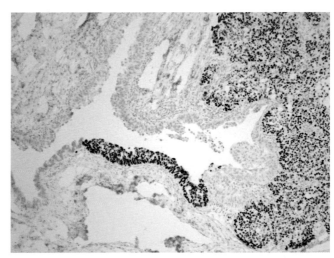

FIGURE 5

Strong p53 staining highlights part of the STIC and the cancer. The remainder of the STIC is negative, consistent with deletion of the gene encoding the protein recognized by the antibody.

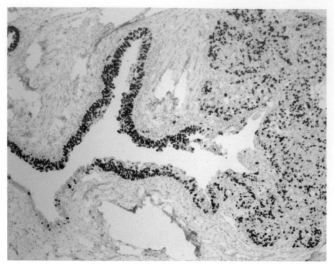

FIGURE 6

Note the strong MIB1 staining throughout both the STIC and invasive cancer. This can be highly variable from lesion to lesion, with occasional STICs having a low proliferative index.

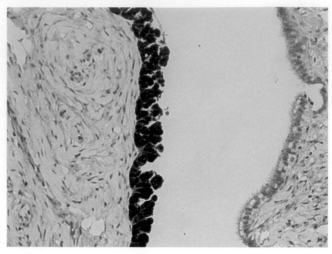

FIGURE 7

An STIC *(left)* highlighted by strong p53 staining. Note that p53 staining alone is not sufficient for a diagnosis of malignancy (also present in premalignant atypias and p53 signatures).

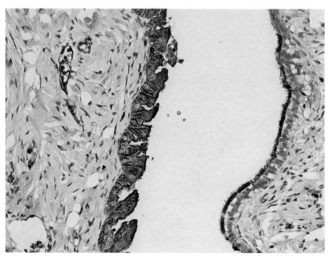

FIGURE 8

Staining for p-ERM, a marker of cell polarity, is abnormal in the STIC, tracing its irregular contour and highlighting the cell borders. Note the strictly luminal distribution in the normal epithelium *(right)*.

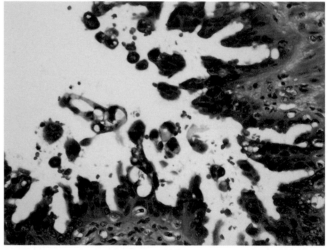

FIGURE 9

Arias-Stella reaction in a tube from a postpartum woman. This can be confused with STIC but lacks proliferative activity and will show normal p53 staining.

THE RISK REDUCING SALPINGO-OOPHORECTOMY

DEFINITION—A procedure designed to remove the tubes and ovaries prior to the development of malignancy in women at high risk for ovarian cancer (BRCA1/2 germ-line mutations).

CLINICAL FEATURES

EPIDEMIOLOGY

- Heterozygous germ-line mutations in BRCA1 or BRCA2 occur in approximately 1 in 400 women in the general population and 1 in 40 women of Ashkenazi Jewish descent.
- Lifetime risk of a pelvic fimbrial ovarian cancer is estimated at 40% and 10% for BRCA1 and BRCA2 mutation carriers respectively, without surgical intervention.
- The vast majority of carcinomas are variants of high-grade serous carcinoma including "SET" (solid, endometrioid-like and transitional) patterns.

PRESENTATION

- All fallopian tubes and ovaries should be submitted for pathologic evaluation and completely sectioned. The sectioning and extensively examining the fimbria (SEE-FIM) protocol, which provides for extensive and thin sectioning of the distal one third of the tube, will maximize detection of small neoplasms.
- In about 95% of risk reduction salpingo-oophorectomies (RRSOs) no abnormality will be found. Virtually all RRSOs in asymptomatic women are grossly unremarkable.
- If a small cancer is present in the fimbria, it may be detected as a small 1 to 2 mm nodule on palpation.
- In some cases, examination of the peritoneal fluid will disclose malignant cells.

PROGNOSIS AND TREATMENT

- RRSO will reduce the risk of cancer by approximately 80% to 90%. Residual risk of developing malignancy following RRSO is estimated at approximately 1% to 5%, depending on the study.
- Most institutions do not treat women with intraepithelial carcinoma alone. From 1% to 10% will be followed by a pelvic serous cancer.
- Importantly, recurrences following risk reduction surgery will often not be detected for several (2 to 5) years.
- If either invasion or local spread is found at RRSO, treatment with combination chemotherapy will usually be instituted, and up to 50% will recur over the next 5 years. Short- to intermediate-term survival is high (>80%); 10-year survival approximately 25% to 35%.

PATHOLOGY

HISTOLOGY

- In 5% to 10% of RRSOs an early carcinoma is detected and will be classified as a tubal primary in about 80% (see chapters on tubal intraepithelial neoplasia). Virtually all carcinomas will be found in the distal one third of the fallopian tube, including the fimbria, infundibulum, and nearby tubal segment.
- A range of tubal abnormalities will be encountered. Most are high-grade intraepithelial neoplasia (serous tubal intraepithelial carcinoma [STIC]). Others will consist of atypias that fall short of STIC and are variously classified as low-grade tubal intraepithelial neoplasia, tubal intraepithelial lesion, or moderate atypias. Occasionally, *endometrioid* intraepithelial carcinomas can be seen.
- If STIC is suspected, the following should be searched for:
  - Absence of cilia: The cell involved is a secretory cell.
  - A slightly irregular growth pattern with variable epithelial thickness, sometimes subtle.
  - Loss of normal nuclear orientation, imparting an appearance of abnormal polarity.
  - In extreme examples, horizontal fracture lines with exfoliation.
  - High nuclear-to-cytoplasmic (N/C) ratio.
- Features that are not particularly helpful are:
  - Multilayered epithelium, which can be seen with any admixture of ciliated and secretory cells.

- Nuclear molding, which often occurs focally in the tubal lining.
- Nuclear enlargement (anisokaryosis), which is common in ciliated epithelium.
- In difficult cases, staining for p53 and Ki-67 may be helpful, but the diagnosis is ultimately based on histologic features. Review by a second pathologist is encouraged if there is a difference of opinion.

PREFERRED DIAGNOSTIC TERMINOLOGY

- Terminology for high- and low-grade tubal intraepithelial neoplasia is sufficient (see respective chapters).
- If STIC alone is found, the risk of recurrence (1% to 10%) should be specified.
- If STIC and/or invasive carcinoma or spread are documented, this should be specified as it increases the recurrence risk to up to nearly 50%.
- If the specimen is entirely normal histologically or contains a lower-grade atypia, no diagnosis is necessary other than benign epithelial changes. However, a note should be added that even in the absence of a neoplasm there is still a small (1% to 5%) risk of a subsequent pelvic cancer, which is greater than the general population.
- Terms such as tubal dysplasia and p53 signature should not be used, or if they are, should be qualified with a carefully written explanation to distinguish them from higher-risk (STIC) lesions.

IMMUNOPATHOLOGY (INCLUDING IMMUNOHISTOCHEMISTRY)

- Use of p53 and Ki-67 is encouraged to support the diagnosis in difficult cases, but in such cases the ultimate verdict is *based on the degree of certainty that the epithelium is malignant.*

MAIN DIFFERENTIAL DIAGNOSIS

- These are detailed in the appropriate chapters on tubal intraepithelial neoplasia.

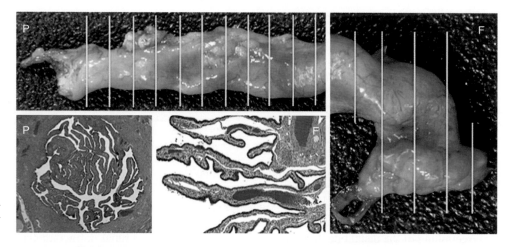

FIGURE 1

The SEE-FIM sectioning protocol specifies complete tubal sectioning and multiple sections of the fimbria..

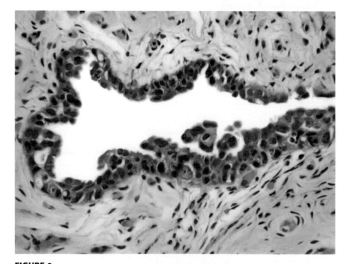

FIGURE 2

A typical STIC found in an RRSO.

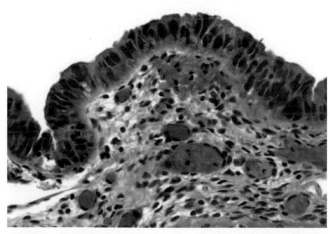

FIGURE 3

A low-grade tubal intraepithelial neoplasm with lesser atypia (serous tubal intraepithelial lesion [STIL] or tubal intraepithelial lesion in transition [TILT]).

SALPINGOLITHS

DEFINITION—Psammous calcifications in the lumen and plica of the fallopian tube.

CLINICAL FEATURES

EPIDEMIOLOGY

- Uncommon.
- Approximately one half are associated with low-grade serous tumors of the ovary (borderline or low-grade malignancies).

PRESENTATION

- Discovered incidentally at the time of examination of the tube for other reasons.
- When found in association with low-grade serous tumors, they are usually at higher stage perhaps because salpingoliths signify a form of spread from the primary tumor.

PROGNOSIS AND TREATMENT

- Depends entirely on the associated epithelial lesion.
- Incidentally discovered salpingoliths require immediate workup, but periodic follow-up is prudent given the association with low-grade serous tumors.

PATHOLOGY

HISTOLOGY

- Numerous concentric calcifications are situated in the plical stroma.

- Calcifications may be bare or surrounded by scant cytoplasm.
- Location in the lamina propria suggests lymphatic spread from the primary tumor.

IMMUNOPATHOLOGY (INCLUDING IMMUNOHISTOCHEMISTRY)

- Noncontributory.

MAIN DIFFERENTIAL DIAGNOSIS

- The main issue is whether the salpingoliths are incidental or associated with a benign or malignant tumor. This is resolved usually by analysis of the remainder of the adnexa.
- Primary borderline or malignant serous tumor originating in or involving the tube. This is confirmed if there is a proliferating neoplastic epithelium associated with psammous calcifications.

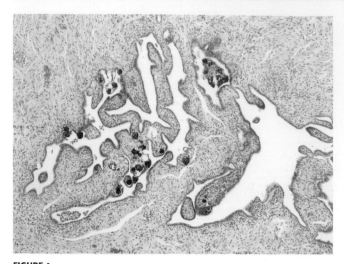

FIGURE 1

Salpingoliths at low magnification. Note the predominance in the lamina propria.

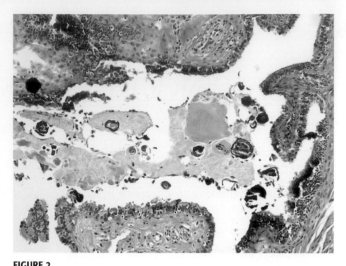

FIGURE 2

Salpingoliths. In some areas they may present as intraluminal calcifications.

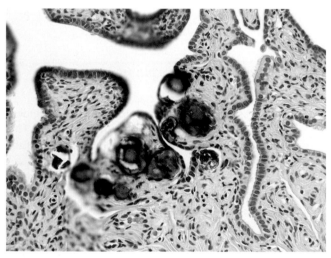

FIGURE 3

Salpingoliths at higher magnification. Note the distinctive location in the stroma. This raises the intriguing question of whether they were transported by lymphatics versus directly incorporated from the lumen.

ADENOCARCINOMA OF THE FALLOPIAN TUBE

DEFINITION—Adenocarcinoma arising in the tubal mucosa.

CLINICAL FEATURES

EPIDEMIOLOGY

- Historically a small fraction (5% or less) of pelvic serous carcinomas relative to the ovary; however, with the attention being paid to the distal tube (using the section and extensively examine the fimbriated end [SEE-FIM] protocol) as a source of many high-grade serous carcinomas, the incidence is presumed to be much higher.
- Linked to chronic tubal inflammation.
- Up to 30% have been reported to be associated with BRCA1 or BRCA2 germ-line mutations.

PRESENTATION

Two major presentations are as follows:

- A bulky, sausage-shaped tube filled with tumor. This is presumed to occur when the distal fallopian tube is closed by peritubal or tubal-ovarian adhesions.
- A microscopic intramucosal carcinoma (serous tubal intraepithelial carcinoma [STIC]) that (presumably) spreads by direct exfoliation onto the pelvic surfaces.

PROGNOSIS AND TREATMENT

- Generally seen as synonymous with high-grade serous carcinoma of the ovary or pelvis in terms of outcome, which is dependent on stage at presentation.
- Stage I tumors confined by fimbrial adhesions have a much better prognosis.

PATHOLOGY

HISTOLOGY

- Classic criteria for diagnosis as a tubal carcinoma include (1) intramucosal carcinoma; (2) absence of a coexisting endometrial carcinoma of same histology; and (3) minimal parenchymal involvement of the ovaries, with primarily surface involvement. Each of these has a caveat. First, not all intramucosal carcinomas can necessarily be assumed to be sites of origin in the absence of a lesser precursor condition (such as a low-grade serous tubal intraepithelial neoplasia [STIN]/ serous tubal intraepithelial lesion [STIL]). Coexisting tubal and endometrial carcinomas can be concurrent primary tumors in some instances. There is no evidence that a cystic tumor in the ovary is necessarily more likely to be a primary ovarian tumor than a surface implant given recent data indicating that ovulating mice are highly prone to cystic metastases from pelvic carcinomas (via entry of repairing ovulation sites).
- Most tumors are high-grade müllerian carcinomas including those with classic high-grade serous carcinoma and solid, endometrioid-like, and transitional (SET) patterns. Occasional endometrioid lesions in the tube have been described but primary low-grade endometrioid carcinomas of the tube are uncommon and many likely come from endometriosis.

IMMUNOPATHOLOGY (INCLUDING IMMUNOHISTOCHEMISTRY)

- The neoplastic cells are usually strongly and diffusely positive for p53 but will be conspicuously negative if the antigenic target sequence is deleted.

- Generic markers of tubal epithelium, PAX8, WT1, and CK7 will be positive.

MAIN DIFFERENTIAL DIAGNOSIS

- Metastatic carcinomas of the gastrointestinal and pancreaticobiliary tracts—these are usually mucin producing.

- Metastatic carcinomas from the uterus and/or ovary—determining origin may be difficult, but at present a dominant ovarian mass in the absence of a tubal STIC may favor an ovarian origin. Endometrial carcinomas that invade the myometrium are generally held to be primary in the setting of a coexisting STIC or carcinoma.
- Female adnexal tumor of wolffian origin—may mimic a low-grade endometrioid adenocarcinoma. These are typically inhibin and calretinin positive.

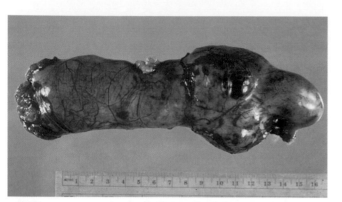

FIGURE 1

Typical sausage-shaped tube filled with a seemingly confined serous carcinoma.

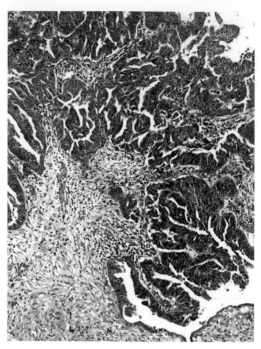

FIGURE 3

Exophytic high-grade serous carcinoma.

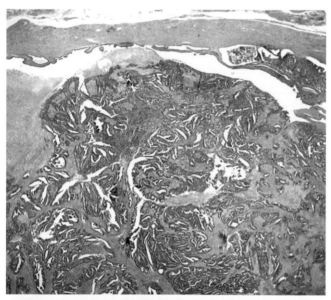

FIGURE 2

Low-power magnification of a fallopian tube distended by carcinoma. This is not specific for a tubal origin by itself.

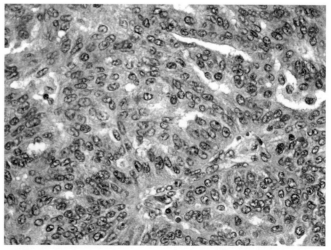

FIGURE 4

Endometrioid differentiation in a high-grade müllerian carcinoma (SET type).

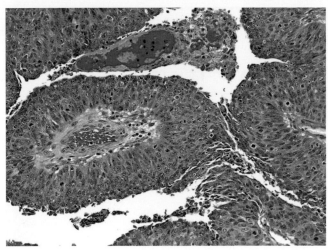

FIGURE 5

Transitional pattern in a high-grade müllerian carcinoma of the tube (SET type).

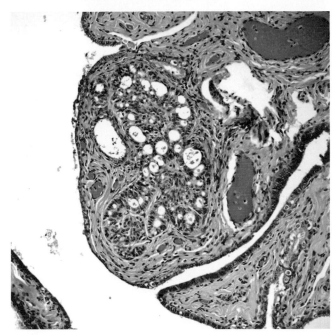

FIGURE 6

Small focus of endometrioid atypia involving a plica. This was the only abnormality in this patient, indicating that lower-grade endometrioid differentiation can occur in the fallopian tube and possibly give rise to endometrioid carcinomas. However, these are quite rare.

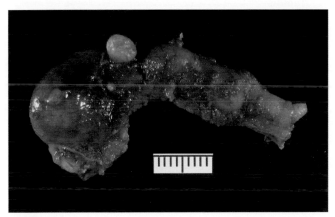

FIGURE 7

Small endometrioid carcinoma in the distal tube in a patient with endometrial adenocarcinoma. This would be designated as a metastasis in most cases.

ENDOSALPINGEAL IMPLANTS FROM REMOTE TUMORS

DEFINITION—Intraepithelial neoplasms of presumed nontubal origin.

CLINICAL FEATURES

EPIDEMIOLOGY

- Uncommon but a function of the thoroughness to which the tube is examined.
- Can be seen with both gynecologic and nongynecologic tumors.
- Mucosal involvement will be seen in about one third of cases where the tube is involved.
- Colon and breast are the most common sites of origin.

PRESENTATION

- Discovered incidentally during tubal examination.
- Clinical features related to the nature of the tumor of origin.

PROGNOSIS AND TREATMENT

- Depends on the biologic behavior of the original tumor.

PATHOLOGY

HISTOLOGY

- Tumor cells are in the mucosa, lending the appearance of an "intraepithelial" neoplasm.

- Degree of atypias varies depending on the nature of the tumor.
- Bland-appearing mucinous epithelium is seen in cases with either gynecologic or intestinal (appendiceal) tumors.
- The absence of a clear precursor condition, although with bland lesions this may be impossible to exclude.

IMMUNOPATHOLOGY (INCLUDING IMMUNOHISTOCHEMISTRY)

- PAX8 and WT1 may be helpful in differentiating gastrointestinal and other sites from a primary lesion of the fallopian tube, but both may be negative in mucinous lesions even if from the female genital tract.

MAIN DIFFERENTIAL DIAGNOSIS

- Primary tubal intraepithelial carcinoma with mucinous differentiation—diagnosis of exclusion (must rule out concomitant gastrointestinal including appendiceal primary).
- Mucinous metaplasia of fallopian tube epithelium—again this is a diagnosis of exclusion.

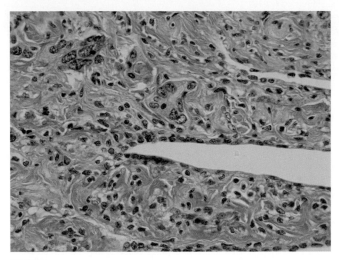

FIGURE 1

Metastatic colonic carcinoma present in lymphatics beneath a normal tubal mucosa.

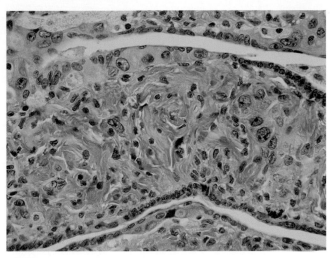

FIGURE 2

Here the tumor cells have migrated onto the mucosa, displacing normal epithelial cells. In this case there is no question that the tumor is from another site, but this illustrates the potential for intraepithelial spread in such tumors.

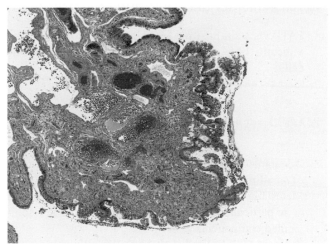

FIGURE 3

Tumor implant on the fimbrial mucosa from a low-grade mucinous tumor of the appendix.

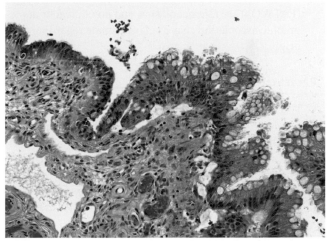

FIGURE 4

At higher magnification the metastatic epithelium is virtually indistinguishable from what would be expected if this were a mucinous metaplasia.

FEMALE ADNEXAL TUMOR OF WOLFFIAN ORIGIN

DEFINITION—A low-grade neoplasm that is thought to arise in the mesonephric remnants of the broad ligament.

CLINICAL FEATURES

EPIDEMIOLOGY

- Female adnexal tumors of (probable) wolffian origin (FATWOs) are rare neoplasms, and no clinical or demographic associations have yet been made regarding their origin.

PRESENTATION

- FATWOs usually present as unilateral, expansile tumors arising in the broad ligament but may be seen less commonly in the fallopian tube, ovary, and adjacent peritoneal region. The patient may describe mass effect symptoms if the tumor is large enough or may be completely asymptomatic.
- FATWOs present as solid or solid and cystic masses.

PROGNOSIS AND TREATMENT

- FATWOs are considered low-grade malignancies, and after conservative surgical excision, the patient can be closely followed. About 20% have an adverse outcome and concern is raised when there is capsular invasion, necrosis, and increased mitotic counts.

PATHOLOGY

HISTOLOGY

- Histologically, FATWOs closely resemble mesonephric tumors of the cervix. Histologic patterns include solid to spindled with variable amounts of retiform tubule formation. In solid tumors, irregular cleftlike spaces may form. Nuclear grade is low and necrosis should be rare or absent.

IMMUNOPATHOLOGY (INCLUDING IMMUNOHISTOCHEMISTRY)

- FATWOs stain positive for calretinin, cytokeratin, and vimentin. EMA and CEA are negative in the neoplastic cells.

MAIN DIFFERENTIAL DIAGNOSIS

- Adenomatoid tumor—this tumor has a regular pattern of small mesothelial lined acini.
  Metastatic adenocarcinoma—endometrioid carcinomas in particular may mimic this when they have a spindled component.
  Sarcoma (solid/spindled variant)—calretinin and cytokeratin stains should exclude this entity.
- Sex cord stromal tumors may mimic this neoplasm; however, Sertoli-Leydig cell tumors are not seen in the broad ligament. Granulosa cell tumors can be and the distinction is based on histology and the cytologic features (nuclear grooves) when present.

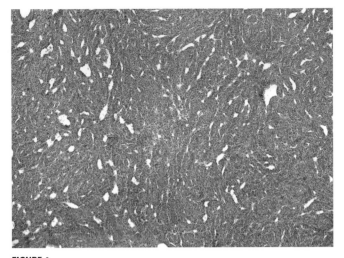

FIGURE 1

FATWO. Note the monomorphic population of cells with ill-defined spaces.

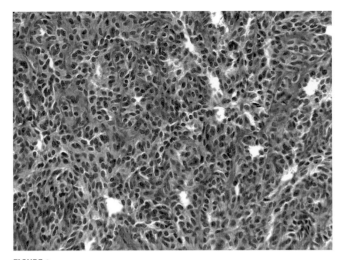

FIGURE 2

At higher magnification the nuclei are uniform and slightly fusiform with minimal coarsening of the chromatin

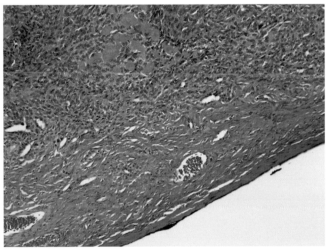

FIGURE 3

The border of the tumor and benign stroma.

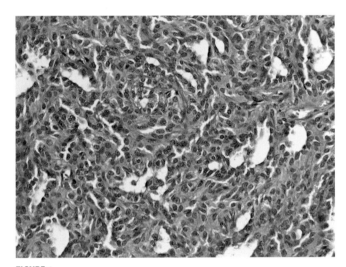

FIGURE 4

At high magnification the glands form a small slitlike space.

TANGENTIALLY SECTIONED OVARIAN FOLLICLE

PITFALL

DEFINITION—A benign sectioning artifact that can be mistaken for neoplasia.

CLINICAL FEATURES

EPIDEMIOLOGY

- Reproductive-age women.

PRESENTATION

- Found incidentally on examination of the ovaries.

PROGNOSIS AND TREATMENT

- Not neoplastic and of no clinical import unless misdiagnosed as neoplasia.

PATHOLOGY

HISTOLOGY

- Tangentially sectioned follicles will display theca cells only in a somewhat discrete microscopic nodule.

- Theca cells are enlarged and fusiform.
- Mitotic figures are common but normal appearing.

IMMUNOPATHOLOGY (INCLUDING IMMUNOHISTOCHEMISTRY)

- Noncontributory but are inhibin positive.

MAIN DIFFERENTIAL DIAGNOSIS

- Microscopic thecoma-fibroma. These will appear more discrete.
- Metastatic carcinomas. These can be distinguished by cytokeratin stains if needed. In general, serial sections will likely reveal the follicle for what it is.

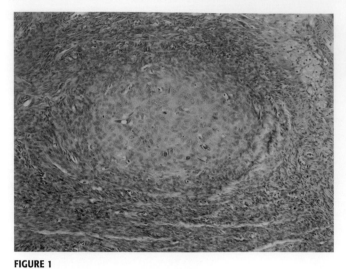

FIGURE 1

Tangentially sectioned follicle. Note the pale appearance of the theca externa.

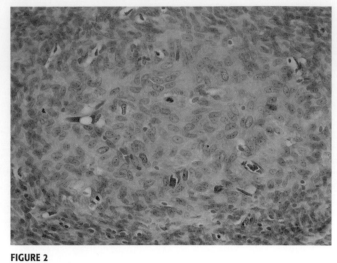

FIGURE 2

Tangentially sectioned follicle. At higher magnification the theca externa cells exhibit ovoid nuclei and open chromatin.

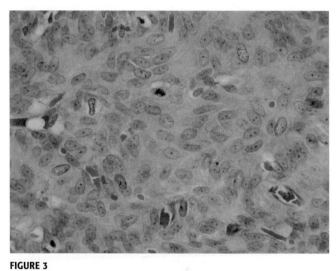

FIGURE 3

Tangentially sectioned follicle. At higher magnification the theca externa cells exhibit ovoid nuclei and open chromatin.

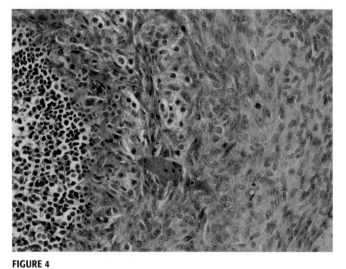

FIGURE 4

Follicles in which orientation permits distinction of the different layers. Note the theca externa on the right and the mitotic activity.

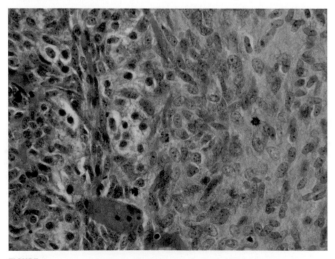

FIGURE 5

Higher magnification delineating the theca interna *(right)* and externa *(left)* of a follicle.

THE OVARY IN PREGNANCY

DEFINITION—A constellation of findings in the ovary during gestation.

CLINICAL FEATURES

EPIDEMIOLOGY

- Related to the pregnancy state.
- Linked to the effects of gonadotropins on the ovarian cortex.
- Can be particularly pronounced during multiple-gestation pregnancies and hydatidiform moles.

PRESENTATIONS

- Corpus luteum of pregnancy.
- Theca-lutein hyperplasia of pregnancy (TLHP): Presents with variable enlargement of ovaries during pregnancy, typically bilateral.
- Hyperreactio luteinalis: Bilateral multicystic ovaries.
- Solitary luteinized cyst (discussed separately).

PROGNOSIS AND TREATMENT

- Excellent; these are incidental benign lesions.

PATHOLOGY

HISTOLOGY

- Corpus luteum of pregnancy: A distinct cerebriform contour, hyaline droplets, and vacuoles.
- TLHP: Varies from focal to extensive. Thecal cells are expanded and merge with luteinized stromal cells to form small nodules (sometimes called pregnancy luteoma). Variable and less-pronounced luteinization of the granulosa cells.
- Hyperreactio luteinalis: A variant of TLHP in which there are in addition numerous follicle cysts giving rise to a multicystic ovary.

IMMUNOPATHOLOGY (INCLUDING IMMUNOHISTOCHEMISTRY)

- Not usually necessary.

MAIN DIFFERENTIAL DIAGNOSIS

- Steroid-producing tumors—these are single unilateral uninodular solid tumors. Here the distinction between a luteoma and a "pregnancy luteoma" becomes blurred. Pregnancy is believed by some to be synonymous with TLHP. However, if the tumor is single, solid, and unilateral, the term steroid cell tumor is more apt.

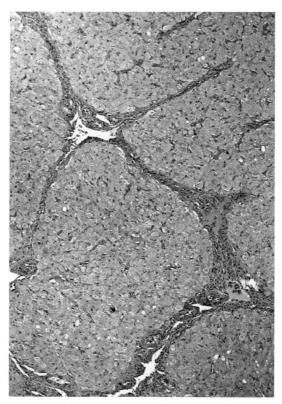

FIGURE 1

Corpus luteum of pregnancy. Low-power image with cerebriform contour.

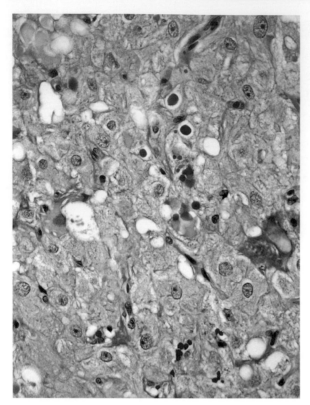

FIGURE 2

Corpus luteum of pregnancy. At higher power the characteristic vacuoles and hyaline droplets are seen.

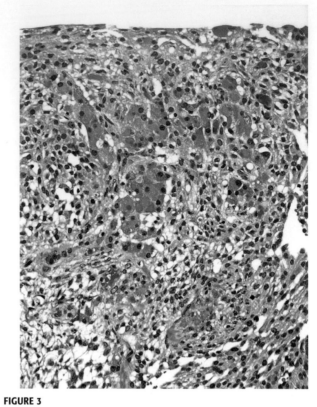

FIGURE 3

TLHP. Prominent coalescing thecal and stromal luteinized cells.

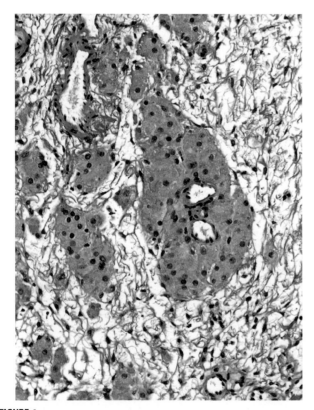

FIGURE 4

TLHP. Plump luteinized stromal cells.

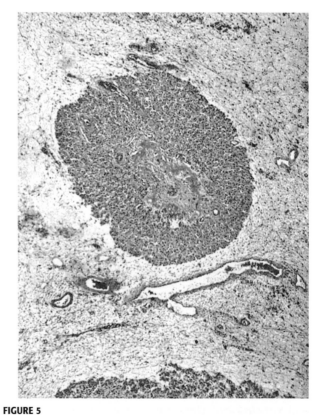

FIGURE 5

Nodular TLHP, characterized by microscopic nodular aggregates of hyperplastic thecal cells.

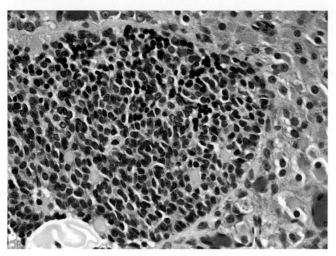

FIGURE 6

Granulosa cell proliferation in the ovary during pregnancy.

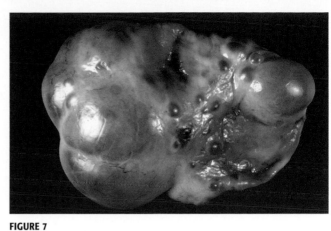

FIGURE 7

Hyperreactio luteinalis. The characteristic features are bilateral expansion of the ovaries by multiple cysts.

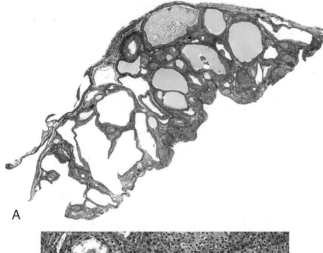

A

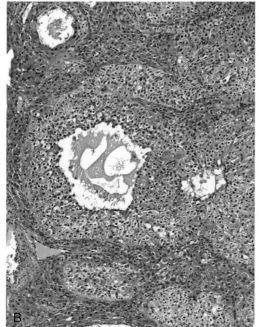

B

FIGURE 8

Hyperreactio luteinalis. **A,** Low-power microphotograph depicts multiple cystic follicles. **B,** The follicles are lined by luteinized cells.

SOLITARY LUTEINIZED FOLLICLE CYST

DEFINITION—Benign incidental ovarian cyst most often noted in pregnant women.

CLINICAL FEATURES

EPIDEMIOLOGY

- Uncommon to rare.
- Most often noted in pregnant or recently postpartum women.
- Can also be seen in nonpregnant, usually reproductive-age, women.

PRESENTATION

- May be found on imaging or the patient may present with pelvic discomfort.
- Hormonal derangement has not been reported in association with these cysts.
- Most are incidentally noted at the time of cesarean section or ultrasound examination of the ovaries/pelvis.

PROGNOSIS AND TREATMENT

- Excellent; these are incidental benign lesions.

PATHOLOGY

HISTOLOGY

- Gross examination is characterized by a thin-walled cyst filled with watery fluid.

- Median size of these cysts is 2.5 cm.
- At low power the cyst is lined by several layers of eosinophilic luteinized cells.
- At high power both a granulosa and theca cell layer can usually be appreciated.
- Occasional cells with nuclear atypia can be appreciated and are sometimes dramatic, but the overall nuclear-to-cytoplasmic (N/C) ratio remains very low.
- Mitotic activity is typically absent but rare studies have reported seeing some mitotic activity.

IMMUNOPATHOLOGY (INCLUDING IMMUNOHISTOCHEMISTRY)

- Not usually needed, although inhibin and calretinin might be helpful in excluding an epithelial lesion. Reticulin stains will highlight the individual cells.

MAIN DIFFERENTIAL DIAGNOSIS

- Cystic ovarian epithelial tumor.
- Follicle cyst.

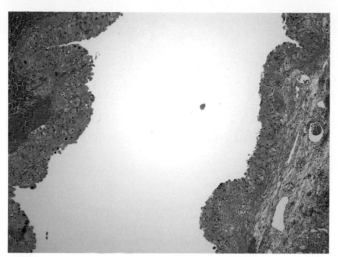

FIGURE 1

Solitary luteinized follicle cyst. At low power the cyst lining is seen, and it is composed of cells with abundant eosinophilic cytoplasm.

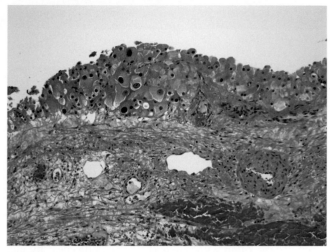

FIGURE 2

Solitary luteinized follicle cyst. In this example, at high power, cells with marked nuclear atypia are seen. Note the preserved, low N/C ratio and the absence of mitotic activity.

POLYCYSTIC OVARIAN SYNDROME

■ **Emily E.K. Meserve, MD, MPH**

DEFINITION—An apparent congenital disorder characterized by ovulatory dysfunction and biochemical evidence of androgen excess, often with polycystic ovaries detected by ultrasound.

CLINICAL FEATURES

EPIDEMIOLOGY

- First described by Stein and Leventhal.
- Can be seen in generations of families, suggesting an autosomal mode of inheritance in such cases.
- However, no single gene has been consistently linked to this disorder.
- Underlying defect is hyperandrogenism associated with ovulatory dysfunction, follicular arrest, and oligomenorrhea.
- Most common endocrinopathy in reproductive-age women, affecting from 2% to 20% of this group and up to 3.5% of women worldwide.

PRESENTATION

- Criteria for the clinical diagnosis include a variation on the following: (1) oligo-ovulation or anovulation manifested as oligomenorrhea or amenorrhea, (2) clinical or biochemical evidence of androgen excess, and (3) polycystic ovaries as defined by ultrasound (Rotterdam criteria). However, 20% of otherwise normal reproductive-age women have polycystic ovaries and up to 25% of women with signs of polycystic ovarian syndrome (PCOS) will have normal-appearing ovaries.
- Gross examination of the ovaries generally demonstrates increased ovarian size/volume and number of follicles. Often the cystic follicles appear blue through the semitranslucent overlying ovarian cortex.
- Women with PCOS often have normal or only mildly elevated serum luteinizing hormone (LH) and/or follicle stimulating hormone (FSH) levels. Importantly, however, the serum LH is often increased relative to the FSH resulting in an elevated LH:FSH ratio, especially during the follicular phase of the menstrual cycle, which is sufficient to disrupt ovulation.

PROGNOSIS AND TREATMENT

- The most common therapy used to induce ovulation is clomiphene, which has a success rate in achieving pregnancy of over 80%.
- Other manifestations are managed by weight loss, reducing hyperinsulinemia, and suppressing endometrial hyperplasia (oral contraceptives).

PATHOLOGY

HISTOLOGY

- Histologic examination demonstrates increased thickness of cortical and subcortical stroma, thickened and collagenized tunica, increased number of developing and atretic follicles, and multiple cystic follicles (1 to 2 mm) with theca-lutein hyperplasia. A normal number of primordial follicles will be present. A subset of patients show stromal hyperplasia and/or hyperthecosis. Often there is a relative paucity of evidence of recent ovulation including few corpora lutea. These findings are all in keeping with the spectrum of changes seen in long-term exposure to excess androgen, such as in female to male transsexual ovaries.

IMMUNOPATHOLOGY (INCLUDING IMMUNOHISTOCHEMISTRY)

- Noncontributory.

MAIN DIFFERENTIAL DIAGNOSIS

- Granulation tissue.
- Recurrent adenocarcinoma (in clinically appropriate setting).

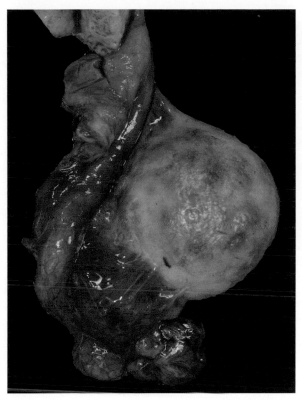

FIGURE 1

Gross examination of ovaries from a patient with PCOS, showing bluish cysts under the cortex.

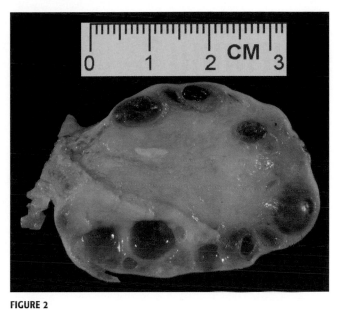

FIGURE 2

Section of ovaries demonstrating features of PCOS; note the increased number of subcortical cystic follicles.

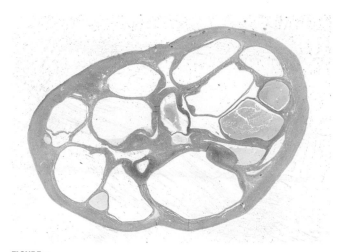

FIGURE 3

Whole mount section of PCOS ovary with cystic follicles.

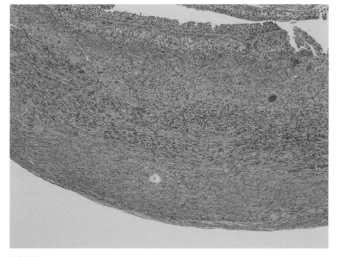

FIGURE 4

Thickened, collagenized, superficial cortex seen in PCOS.

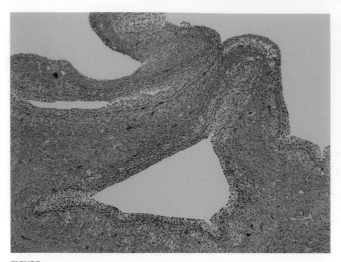

FIGURE 5

Multiple luteinized cystic follicles seen in PCOS.

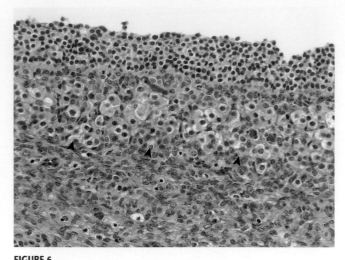

FIGURE 6

Higher magnification of cystic follicle in PCOS with expanded and luteinized theca cell layer *(arrows)*.

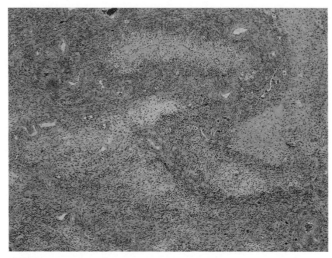

FIGURE 7

Multiple atretic follicles are common in PCOS.

CORTICAL STROMAL HYPERPLASIA AND HYPERTHECOSIS

DEFINITION—An expansion of the ovarian cortex and medulla by a benign proliferation of ovarian cortical stromal cells and associated luteinized cells. Cortical stromal hyperplasia (CSH) is a mild form seen at menopause; stromal hyperthecosis is a more pronounced variant associated with symptoms comparable to polycystic ovarian syndrome.

CLINICAL FEATURES

EPIDEMIOLOGY

- Seen in perimenopausal or postmenopausal women.
- May less commonly be seen as part of the clinical spectrum of polycystic ovarian syndrome (PCOS).

PRESENTATION

- Imaging studies will reveal a diffuse symmetric enlargment of the ovaries.
- The most common symptomatic presentation is of hyperestrogenic sequelae including abnormal uterine bleeding, occasionally with endometrial intraepithelial neoplasia (EIN) or endometrial adenocarcinoma. CSH is considered to confer an increased risk for endometrial carcinoma; however, it can be found in at least one third of ovaries at menopause.
- Rarely, virilizing symptoms attributable to excess androgen production are present when there is more pronounced stromal cell luteinization (hyperthecosis). Insulin resistance is also a manifestation.

PROGNOSIS AND TREATMENT

- Cortical stromal hyperplasia with mild stromal luteinization is usually an incidental finding requiring no further treatment.
- Hyperthecosis accompanied by excess androgen effects is managed by oophorectomy or GnRH-agonist therapy. In premenopausal women management is similar to that for PCOS.

PATHOLOGY

HISTOLOGY

- The findings should always be bilateral and symmetrical.
- Grossly, the ovaries appear slightly larger than would be expected for the patient's age, and on cut section the medulla and cortex appear expanded by a nodular, light brown to tan tissue.
- At low power the histologic appearance is strikingly different than an atrophic ovary, which would be expected in most cases (based on patient age).
- The atrophic ovarian cortex is not appreciated, and instead a diffuse to nodular proliferation of ovarian cortical stromal cells is apparent at low power.
- The cortical stromal cells are spindled, with elongated oval nuclei and scant lightly eosinophilic cytoplasm, with minimal amounts of intercellular collagen.
- Mitoses are infrequent.
- The "hyperthecosis" component is named for the small clusters, nests, and single luteinized cells that are associated with the spindled stromal cells.
- The luteinized cells are large, with relatively abundant clear to eosinophilic cytoplasm and centrally placed nuclei with prominent nucleoli.

IMMUNOPATHOLOGY (INCLUDING IMMUNOHISTOCHEMISTRY)

- Noncontributory.

MAIN DIFFERENTIAL DIAGNOSIS

- Stromal hyperthecosis and/or stromal hyperplasia alone—isolated stromal hyperthecosis has been described as a separate entity and is the extreme form of this disorder and quite rare. Similarly stromal expansion without luteinized stromal cells can occur but it is unusual to not find occasional luteinized stromal cells.
- Hilus cell hyperplasia—this is limited to the hilar region.
- Fibroma-thecoma—this will present as a discrete mass. In some cases, stromal hyperthecosis will be more fibrous in appearance, and the distinction from fibroma-thecoma is essentially one of distribution.
- Stromal luteoma— this is a homogeneous lesion with a monomorphic population of cells with abundant cytoplasm, rather than the admixture of spindled stromal cells and luteinized cells.

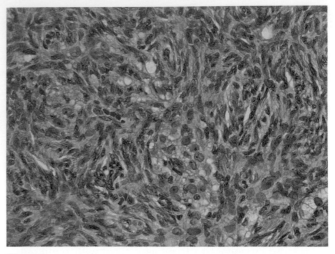

FIGURE 3

Stromal hyperplasia and hyperthecosis. At high power, single cells and small nests of luteinized cells are easily appreciated within the nodules of spindled stromal cells. The luteinized cells are epithelioid, with large round nuclei, prominent nucleoli, and eosinophilic cytoplasm.

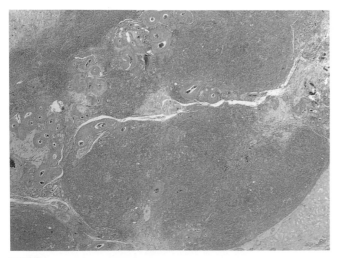

FIGURE 1

Stromal hyperplasia with luteinized stromal cells. Gross appearance. The ovary is larger than would be expected for a postmenopausal woman. The ovarian medulla and cortex appear expanded by vaguely nodular tan to brown tissue.

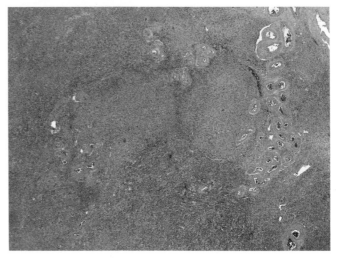

FIGURE 4

Stromal hyperplasia and hyperthecosis. In some cases the proliferation of luteinized cells is more exuberant and can have a nodular appearance at low power (center). The eosinophilic areas in the center are composed of luteinized cells.

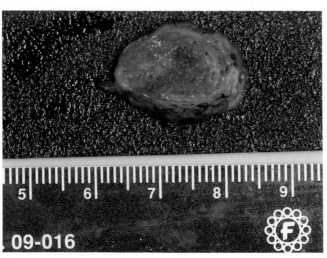

FIGURE 2

Stromal hyperplasia and hyperthecosis. A nodular proliferation of stromal cells within the medulla is apparent at low power.

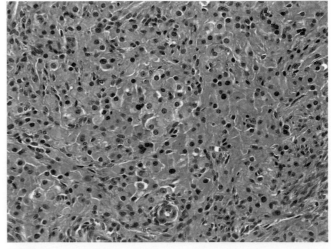

FIGURE 5

Stromal hyperplasia and hyperthecosis. At high magnification the nodules of luteinized cells are identical to those seen singly and in small nests.

ENDOMETRIOMA WITH MUCINOUS METAPLASIA

DEFINITION—Endometriotic epithelium with focal noncomplex mucinous differentiation.

CLINICAL FEATURES

PATHOGENESIS

- Occurs in endometriotic cysts. Probably a very early neoplastic change akin to other lesions associated with endometriomas, such as müllerian mucinous cystadenomas, adenofibromas, and well-differentiated endometrioid adenocarcinomas.

PRESENTATION

- An incidental finding in endometriotic cysts.

PROGNOSIS AND TREATMENT

- The prognosis is excellent, and outcome is uneventful as this process, when not complex or mass forming, is not associated with neoplasia.
- No treatment is required, but the endometrioma should be *liberally sampled* to exclude any more advanced process.

PATHOLOGY

HISTOLOGY

- A bland mucinous epithelial lining without gland formation. Mild epithelial complexity is not uncommon.

IMMUNOPATHOLOGY (INCLUDING IMMUNOHISTOCHEMISTRY)

- Noncontributory.

MAIN DIFFERENTIAL DIAGNOSIS

- Müllerian (sero) mucinous cystadenomas form larger cysts with more prominent architecture and with mucinous and often tubal differentiation. The tumors do not contain endometrial stroma in direct continuity with the mucinous proliferation, although endometrial stroma may be found in the adjacent cyst wall.

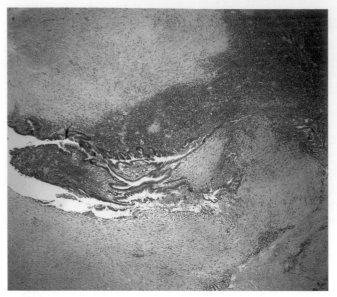

FIGURE 1

Endometrioma with mucinous differentiation. A low-power photomicrograph of a cyst wall with prominent endometrial stroma, the middle and right of the picture.

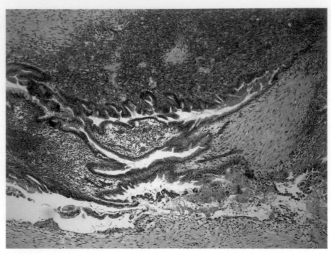

FIGURE 2

Endometrioma with mucinous differentiation. At higher magnification the stroma can be seen to abut the overlying mucinous metaplasia.

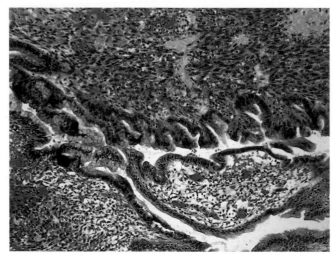

FIGURE 3

Endometrioma with mucinous differentiation. Note the lack of complex epithelial growth.

ENDOMETRIOMA WITH ATYPIA

DEFINITION—Endometriotic epithelium with noncomplex architecture and nuclear atypia.

CLINICAL FEATURES

PATHOGENESIS

- Occurs in endometriotic cysts. Possibly a very early neoplastic change akin to other lesions associated with endometriomas, such as müllerian mucinous cystadenomas, adenofibromas, and well-differentiated endometrioid adenocarcinomas. Can be associated with mutations in ARID1A.

PRESENTATION

- An incidental finding in endometriotic cysts.

PROGNOSIS AND TREATMENT

- The prognosis is excellent and outcome uneventful as this process, when not complex or mass forming, is not associated with neoplasia.
- No treatment is required, but the endometrioma should be *liberally sampled* to exclude any more advanced process.

PATHOLOGY

HISTOLOGY

- The hallmark is nuclear enlargement and hyperchromasia. The nuclear/cytoplasmic ratio remains relatively low.

IMMUNOPATHOLOGY (INCLUDING IMMUNOHISTOCHEMISTRY)

- Noncontributory.

MAIN DIFFERENTIAL DIAGNOSIS

- Arias-Stella effect in endometriotic cysts—these could be associated with pregnancy.
- Clear-cell carcinoma—the cells in this entity would harbor a higher nuclear/cytoplasmic ratio and often would be associated with adenofibromas.

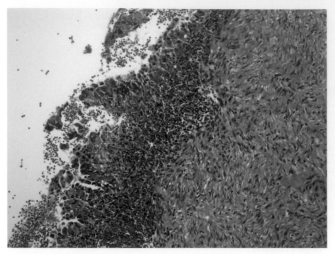

FIGURE 1

Endometrioma with epithelial atypia. A low-power photomicrograph of a cyst wall with prominent endometrial stroma *(the middle and right of the picture)*.

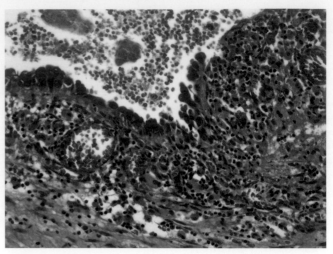

FIGURE 2

Endometrioma with atypia. At higher magnification the stroma can be seen to abut the overlying atypical epithelium.

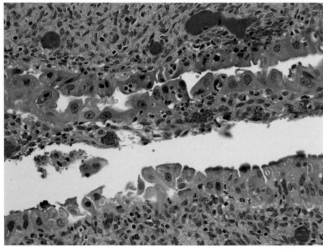

FIGURE 3

Endometrioma with atypia. Note the relatively low nuclear/cytoplasmic ratio.

DECIDUALIZED ENDOMETRIOMA

PITFALL

DEFINITION—A variant of endometrioma that may be confused with malignancy on ultrasound.

CLINICAL FEATURES

EPIDEMIOLOGY

- Relatively common.
- Seen during pregnancy.

PRESENTATION

- May be a prior history of endometriosis.
- Ovarian enlargement or cyst during pregnancy.
- The presence of mural nodules, usually but not always smoothly lobulated.
- May be interpreted on imaging studies as *potentially malignant*.

PROGNOSIS AND TREATMENT

- Because these lesions are occasionally interpreted on ultrasound as possibly malignant, they may inspire greater anxiety on the part of the physician and patient.
- Once the diagnosis of endometrioma is made, the risk or likelihood of concomitant malignancy is low in young patients.
- Outcome is uneventful, but rare cases in pregnancy can rupture (with rare deaths) and require surgery to control hemorrhage.

PATHOLOGY

HISTOLOGY

- Grossly, decidualized endometriotic cysts are notable for their thickened surface, often with a cobblestone appearance due to the prominent decidual changes.

- The range in size is broad, and the cyst diameter can be anywhere from a few millimeters to many centimeters, with a cyst wall that varies in thickness.
- At low magnification the cyst wall is lined by a prominent decidualized endometrium.
- Endometrial glands may be inconspicuous.

IMMUNOPATHOLOGY (INCLUDING IMMUNOHISTOCHEMISTRY)

- Noncontributory.

MAIN DIFFERENTIAL DIAGNOSIS

- Corpus luteum of pregnancy—these are lined by luteinized granulosa cells with a classic lobulated appearance.
- Xanthomatous pseudotumor—this variant of endometriosis is lined by foamy macrophages that might be confused with the decidualized endometrium lining endometriosis.

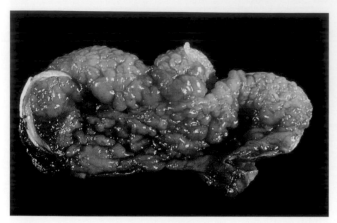

FIGURE 1

Decidualized endometrioma. Gross image. Note the thickened lining of decidualized endometrium with a vague cobblestone appearance.

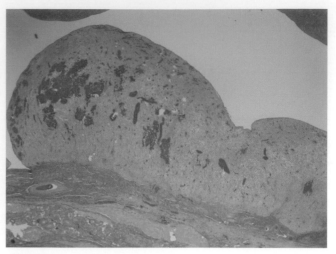

FIGURE 2

Decidualized endometrioma. At low magnification the decidualized stromal cells are most conspicuous.

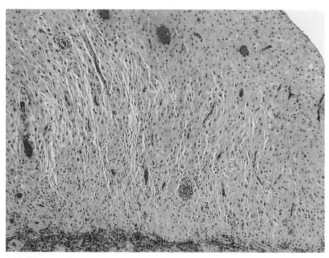

FIGURE 3

At higher magnification the polyhedral decidualized cells are uniformly arranged.

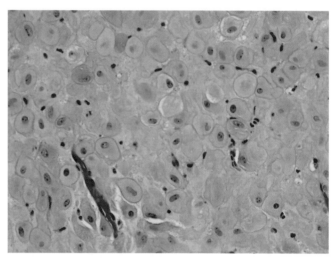

FIGURE 4

The decidualized stroma forms a characteristic pavement of non-overlapping cells.

SEROUS CYSTADENOMAS AND CYSTADENOFIBROMAS

DEFINITION—A benign epithelial or epithelial stromal tumor with a serous (ciliated) epithelial component.

CLINICAL FEATURES

EPIDEMIOLOGY

- Common; among the most frequently encountered of the benign epithelial tumors.
- Can be seen at any age, most commonly in postmenopausal women.
- Average age at presentation is in the mid-50s.
- May be associated with endometriosis.

PRESENTATION

- Ovarian mass ranging from cystic (cystadenoma) to cystic and solid (adenofibroma) or both (cystadenofibroma).
- Frequently bilateral.

PROGNOSIS AND TREATMENT

- Outcomes should be uneventful.
- Occasionally adenofibromas will have foci of adenocarcinoma, but such cases have an excellent prognosis.
- Surgical excision is adequate treatment.

PATHOLOGY

HISTOLOGY

- Cystadenomas are typically encysted without surface involvement.
- (Cyst) adenofibromas can involve the surface and occasionally may be associated with benign regional implants.
- Tumors may be confined to the ovary or adjacent (paraovarian) region. Sometimes they may be associated with fimbrial adenofibromas, which are morphologically identical.

- On histologic examination the fibromatous component consists of small bland spindled cells with short nuclei arranged in fascicles and storiform patterns, similar to a fibroma.
- The cystic spaces are irregularly shaped and are uniformly present throughout the stroma.
- The spaces are lined by benign epithelial cells resembling salpingeal epithelium.
- The epithelial cells are columnar to cuboidal and often pseudostratified.
- Nuclear atypia is not present in the glandular or stromal components.
- Endometrial-type stroma is not present, but some of these tumors may merge histologically with endometrioid adenofibromas or mucinous tumors.
- Psammomatous calcifications may be noted, particularly in the stromal component.
- Varying degrees of ischemic-type necrosis and stromal calcification may be seen.

IMMUNOPATHOLOGY (INCLUDING IMMUNOHISTOCHEMISTRY)

- Noncontributory.

MAIN DIFFERENTIAL DIAGNOSIS

- Borderline serous tumor—there should be complex epithelial architecture.
- Extensive cortical inclusion cysts—this distinction is based on degree and how discrete the changes are.
- Paratubal cysts—these have an identical lining but possess a cyst wall with loose connective rather than densely fibrotic tissue. Smooth muscle should be focally evident.
- Hydrosalpinx—the presence of plicae and a well-developed wall of smooth muscle.

577

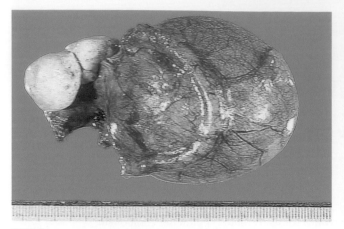

FIGURE 1

Paratubal cystadenofibroma, seen here as a unilocular cyst.

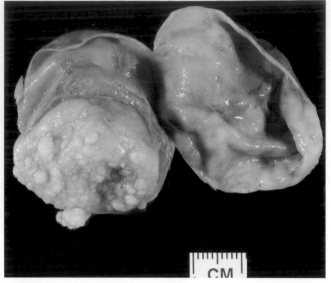

FIGURE 2

Serous cystadenoma. Note the mildly irregular cyst lining.

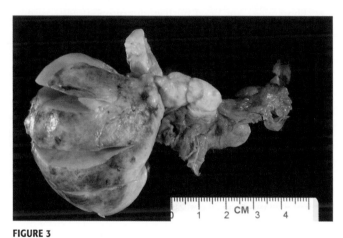

FIGURE 3

Adenofibroma of the ovary. This tumor resembles a fibroma due to the predominance of stroma.

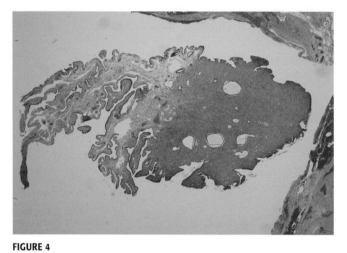

FIGURE 4

Serous adenofibroma of the tubal fimbria. These are sometimes associated with ovarian tumors of the same histology.

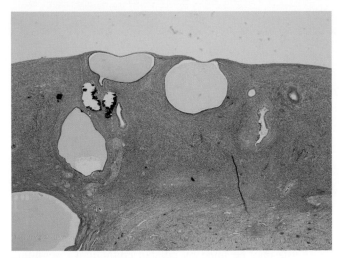

FIGURE 5

Ovarian cortical inclusion cysts are sometimes prominent and may suggest an incipient cystadenofibroma. The distinction from a cyst (adenofibroma) is based on the discrete nature of the latter.

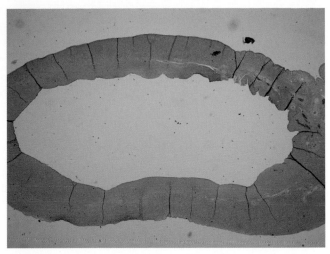

FIGURE 6

Serous cystadenoma. Note in particular the dense fibrous wall, which distinguishes this from a hydrosalpinx or paratubal müllerian cyst.

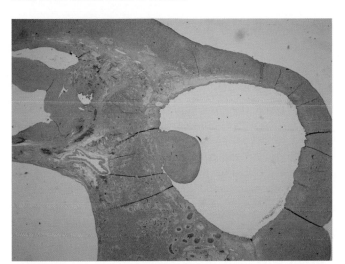

FIGURE 7

A serous cystadenofibroma. Note the nodular excrescence and abundance of stroma.

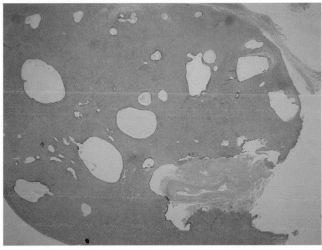

FIGURE 8

Serous adenofibroma, with a well-organized fibrous nodule punctuated by small epithelial-lined cysts.

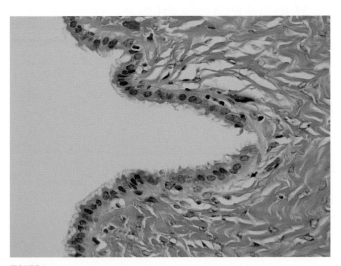

FIGURE 9

The lining of these benign serous tumors is typically uncomplicated with conspicuous cilia.

CORTICAL INCLUSION CYSTS

DEFINITION—Ovarian cortical inclusion cysts (CICs) lined by either mesothelium (ovarian surface epithelium [OSE]) or müllerian epithelium.

CLINICAL FEATURES

EPIDEMIOLOGY

- Very common.
- Found in the majority of ovaries in postmenopausal women.
- Associated with increasing age.
- Most plausible origin is entrapped tubal epithelium or shed cells from the fimbria. Another proposed mechanism is transdifferentiation of OSE.

PRESENTATION

- Usually an incidental finding.
- Occasionally a very large inclusion cyst will be removed as a cystectomy.

PROGNOSIS AND TREATMENT

- These cysts are incidental benign findings.
- CICs are postulated to give rise to epithelial tumors of the ovary, the most likely being mucinous and low-grade serous tumors.

PATHOLOGY

HISTOLOGY

- The cyst lining may be flat to cuboidal with minimal cytoplasm.

- Cysts may be lined by ciliated epithelium resembling the fallopian tube.
- Nuclear atypia is generally absent.
- Mitoses are not seen.

IMMUNOPATHOLOGY (INCLUDING IMMUNOHISTOCHEMISTRY)

- Noncontributory for diagnostic purposes. However, there is considerable interest in whether the epithelium is derived from the tube or the mesothelial covering of the ovary. The immunophenotype is typically müllerian (PAX8 positive) but occasional examples can be found where there is co-expression of both mesothelial (Calretinin) and müllerian (PAX8) markers, which prompts some speculation that the OSE is unique and capable of both mesothelial and müllerian differentiation (or transdifferentiation).

MAIN DIFFERENTIAL DIAGNOSIS

- Cystic follicle—these can be lined by very thin layers of residual theca cells and be misclassified as CICs. Alternatively cystic follicles or ovulation sites can be populated with OSE/endosalpingiosis.
- Unilocular serous cystadenoma: This is an arbitrary distinction, but the diagnosis of cystadenoma will be considered when the cyst exceeds 1 cm and is associated with a fibrous wall.

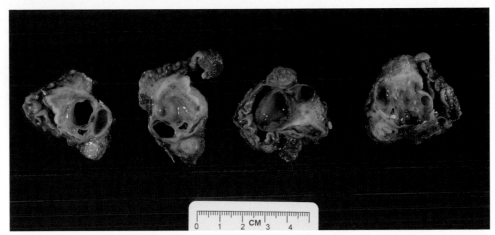

FIGURE 1

CICs associated with a corpus luteum *(center)*.

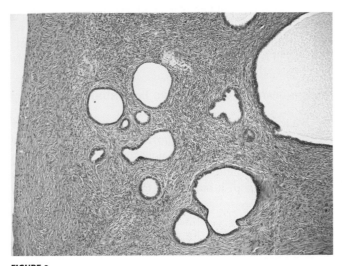

FIGURE 2

CICs. This low-power image shows several cysts within the ovarian cortex.

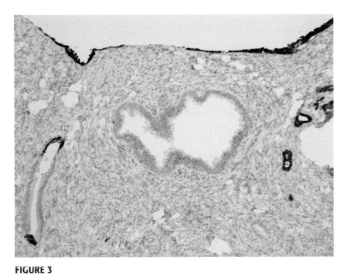

FIGURE 3

CICs stained with calretinin. Note the OSE stains positive while the cysts do not, typical of müllerian CICs.

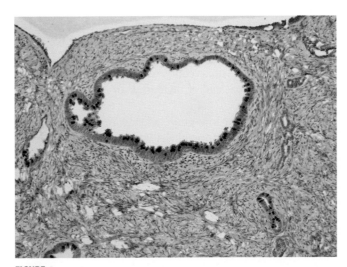

FIGURE 4

A serial section of (of Figure 3) stained with FOXJ1, a marker of ciliated cells. Note the müllerian CICs stain positive in contrast to the OSE.

ENDOSALPINGIOSIS

DEFINITION—The presence of epithelium resembling fallopian tube epithelium outside the fallopian tube.

CLINICAL FEATURES

EPIDEMIOLOGY

- Endosalpingiosis has been noted in up to 7% of reproductive-age women.
- It can be found in association with other pelvic pathologic processes including endometriosis, infection (pelvic inflammatory disease), neoplasm, and tubal processes, such as hydrosalpinx.

PRESENTATION

- Occasionally patients may present with pelvic pain; however, the majority of cases are asymptomatic and may be found incidentally at the time of surgery. May be seen in pelvic or aortic lymph nodes removed during a staging procedure.

PROGNOSIS AND TREATMENT

- Some authors have pointed out a possible association between endosalpingiosis and low-grade serous tumors; however, this has not been proven.
- Currently no further treatment is warranted.

PATHOLOGY

HISTOLOGY

- Endosalpingiosis is commonly a microscopic finding; however, mass lesions have been described.

- Typically the lesions are glandular or tubular structures lined by cuboidal epithelium with variable amounts of cilia.
- The glands should be bland with no increase in mitoses (opposed to low-grade serous carcinoma), and no surrounding desmoplasia or endometrial-like stroma should be appreciated.

IMMUNOPATHOLOGY (INCLUDING IMMUNOHISTOCHEMISTRY)

- Noncontributory for diagnostic purposes, although the distinction of endosalpingiosis from mesothelium may be of interest in studies. Endosalpingiosis should stain for PAX8, a müllerian epithelial marker, and for FOXJ1, tubulin, and p73, markers of ciliated epithelial cells.

MAIN DIFFERENTIAL DIAGNOSIS

- Implants of low-grade serous carcinoma or a serous borderline tumor—these entities should manifest with more complex/papillary architecture and will be associated with desmoplasia (both) or evidence of tissue replacement by tumor (carcinomas). Endosalpingiosis typically manifests with more uniform glandlike structures and conspicuous ciliation.
- Endometriosis—this entity is associated with endometrial stroma and/or evidence of old hemorrhage (hemosiderin).
- Metastasis from low-grade adenocarcinoma—this can occur when endosalpingiosis involves lymph nodes.

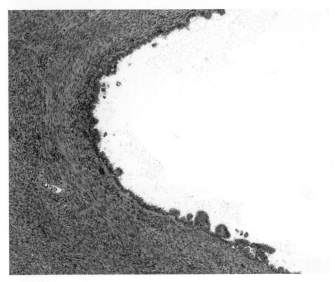

FIGURE 1

Endosalpingiosis. This focus in the ovarian cortex exhibits small papillary like structures.

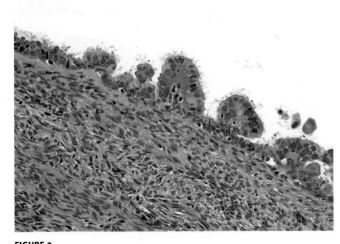

FIGURE 2

Endosalpingiosis. At higher magnification the papillary structures seen in Figure 1 exhibit an eosinophilic cytoplasm and cilia.

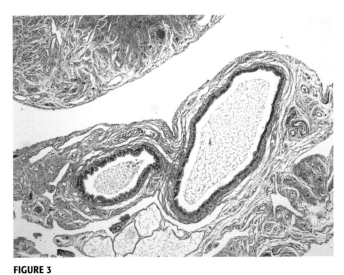

FIGURE 3

Endosalpingiosis. This focus in the mesosalpinx depicts uniform glandlike structures surrounded by loose stroma.

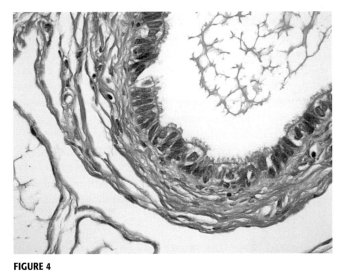

FIGURE 4

Note the conspicuous cilia lining this focus of endosalpingiosis (seen in Figure 3).

MALAKOPLAKIA

DEFINITION—A granulomatous disease of uncertain etiology characterized by histiocytic infiltrates (von Hansemann cells) with calcified inclusions (Michaelis-Gutmann bodies).

CLINICAL FEATURES

EPIDEMIOLOGY

- Most often associated with the urinary tract with a female preponderance (4 : 1). There is no relationship to gender in other sites.
- Wide age range, but the typical patient is older, with an overall mean age of 50 years.
- Invariably associated with some underlying chronic disorder, including organ transplantation, allergic conditions, chemotherapy, acquired immunodeficiency syndrome (AIDS), malignancy, chronic inflammatory or infectious conditions, and malnutrition.
- The cause is obscure, but theories include an underlying infection with an abnormal immune response that could include the inability of macrophages to digest and eliminate bacteria because of lysosomal defect, leading to the inclusions seen in the cells.

PRESENTATION

- Typically found incidentally in the context of an underlying disorder. In the gynecologic tract, abnormal bleeding is the most common.
- When seen grossly the lesions are soft tan to yellow nodules, plaques, or bands.

PROGNOSIS AND TREATMENT

- Depends on the underlying disorder, which includes a range of diseases (see earlier).
- Antibiotic therapy has been shown to be effective.

PATHOLOGY

HISTOLOGY

- The appearance will vary depending on the age of the lesions, ranging from predominantly inflammatory early on, to the development of the prominent histiocytic infiltrate with Michaelis-Gutmann bodies, and terminating in fibrosis.
- Michaelis-Gutmann bodies are diagnostic but not always present depending on the age of the lesion. These are discrete targetoid structures in which dot-forming, calcified debris is present in the cytoplasm of the macrophages.

IMMUNOPATHOLOGY (INCLUDING IMMUNOHISTOCHEMISTRY)

- Numerous CD68 positive histiocytes.
- Gram stains may be positive for gram-negative bacteria.

MAIN DIFFERENTIAL DIAGNOSIS

- Other granulomatous diseases, including tuberculosis and sarcoid.

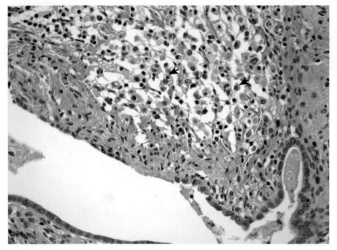

FIGURE 1

Malakoplakia in the gynecologic tract associated with chronic diverticulitis. In this image of the tubal mucosa there is a prominent macrophage response with a few targetoid Michaelis-Gutmann bodies *(arrows)*.

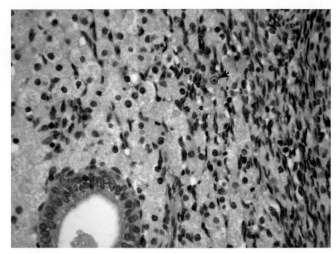

FIGURE 2

Malakoplakia in the gynecologic tract associated with chronic diverticulitis. This microscopic field in the endometrium exhibits a classic targetoid Michaelis-Gutmann body *(arrow)*.

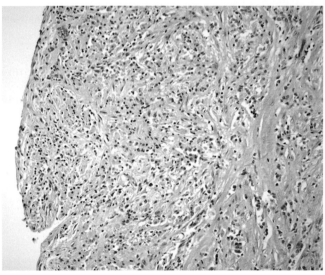

FIGURE 3

Malakoplakia in an inflammatory pseudocyst of the ovary from the same patient. Note that this lesion is more developed with some fibroblastic response.

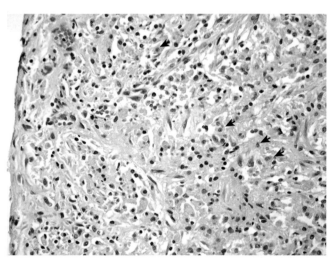

FIGURE 4

At higher magnification a few Michaelis-Gutmann bodies can be appreciated *(arrows)*.

HIGH-GRADE SEROUS CARCINOMA, CLASSIC TYPE

■ **Brooke E. Howitt, MD**

DEFINITION—A pelvic serous carcinoma with papillary architecture and high nuclear grade.

CLINICAL FEATURES

EPIDEMIOLOGY

- Approximately 15% associated with *BRCA1* or *BRCA2* germline mutation.
- Predominant in the sixth and seventh decades of life.
- Approximately 1% of women will develop this malignancy in their lifetime.
- Associated with nulliparity and talc exposure.
- Approximately 40% to 50% associated with a detectable tubal intraepithelial carcinoma in the distal fallopian tube.

PRESENTATION

- Pelvic discomfort, bloating, and frequent urination.
- Pelvic mass on physical exam or on ultrasound.

PROGNOSIS AND TREATMENT

- Forty percent 5-year survival.
- Managed with surgical debulking and chemotherapy with platinum-based agents and taxol.

PATHOLOGY

HISTOLOGY

- Papillary or micropapillary architecture.
- High nuclear grade.

- Patterns of spread are frequently infiltrative.
- Tumor is often associated with psammomatous calcifications.

IMMUNOPATHOLOGY (INCLUDING IMMUNOHISTOCHEMISTRY)

- Immunostains for p16, WT1, and PAX8 are typically positive.
- p53 is typically strongly and diffusely positive (>75% of tumor cells), or may be entirely negative (consistent with null phenotype).

MAIN DIFFERENTIAL DIAGNOSIS

- SET pattern of serous carcinoma—this pattern is frequently admixed with classic morphology.
- Low-grade serous carcinoma—less nuclear atypia with uniformity; p53 is *wild-type*.
- High-grade endometrioid adenocarcinoma—columnar tumor cells lacking exfoliative growth; squamous differentiation indicates endometrioid-type carcinoma. May also overexpress p53.
- Other metastatic carcinomas—should be considered in a limited biopsy specimen; use of immunohistochemistry (PAX8, WT-1) to confirm the diagnosis.

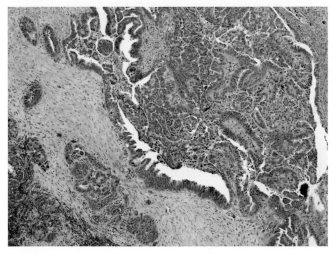

FIGURE 1

High-grade serous carcinoma, classic type. Note the poorly formed glands, papillary architecture, and dark blue appearance due to the high nuclear-to-cytoplasmic ratio.

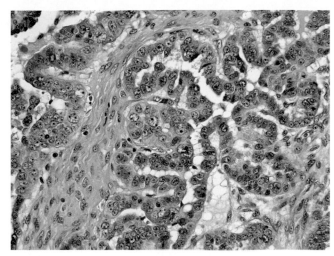

FIGURE 2

High-grade serous carcinoma, classic type. Here there is a semblance of gland architecture, but note the lining cells are largely single layer and cuboidal.

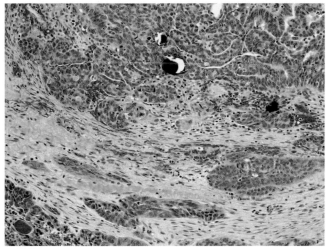

FIGURE 3

High-grade serous carcinoma, classic type. Scattered psammomatous calcifications are seen here. A dense fibrotic response is also characteristic.

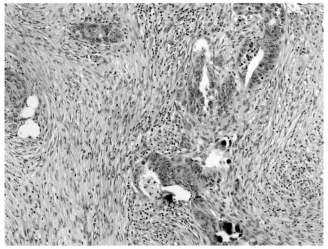

FIGURE 4

High-grade serous carcinoma, classic type. Typical area of invasion with a strong desmoplastic response and poorly formed glandular architecture.

HIGH-GRADE SEROUS CARCINOMA WITH "SET" PATTERNS

■ **Brooke E. Howitt, MD**

DEFINITION—A distinctive constellation of patterns (solid, endometrioid-like, and transitional [SET]). Defined (arbitrarily) as greater than 50% of the tumor.

CLINICAL FEATURES

EPIDEMIOLOGY

- Frequently associated with *BRCA1* or *BRCA2* germline mutation (approximately 50%).
- This pattern is seen less frequently (about 25%) in sporadic serous carcinomas, and may be associated with somatic mutations in *BRCA1* or *BRCA2*.
- Younger mean age than classic serous carcinomas.
- Lower frequency of associated serous tubal intraepithelial carcinoma than classic serous carcinoma.

PRESENTATION

- Similar to most serous carcinomas, but may present at a younger age.
- Somewhat less frequently detected incidentally or in risk-reducing salpingo-oophorectomies relative to classic serous carcinoma.

PROGNOSIS AND TREATMENT

- Based on preliminary data, these tumors trend toward a more favorable response to chemotherapy and short- to intermediate-term outcome.
- Managed like other high-grade serous carcinomas.

PATHOLOGY

HISTOLOGY

- Three patterns, including solid, endometrioid like, and transitional.

- Lower frequency of papillary architecture and micropapillary architecture.
- Patterns of spread are often less infiltrative.
- Tumor-infiltrating lymphocytes also seen.
- Necrosis ("comedo-type") is frequently present and may be extensive.
- May be associated with a serous tubal intraepithelial carcinoma, but less commonly than classic serous carcinoma.

IMMUNOPATHOLOGY (INCLUDING IMMUNOHISTOCHEMISTRY)

- Usually noncontributory. Immunostains for p53, p16, WT1, PAX8, etc. are typically strongly positive, similar to classic serous carcinoma.

MAIN DIFFERENTIAL DIAGNOSIS

- Classic serous carcinoma—this pattern may be present to some degree as well.
- High-grade and solid endometrioid adenocarcinoma—less prominent nucleoli; lacks other areas of classic serous carcinoma. Squamous differentiation indicates endometrioid pattern of adenocarcinoma.

588

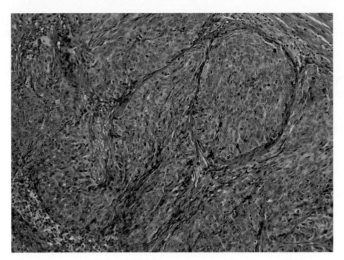

FIGURE 1

High-grade serous carcinoma, SET type. This field depicts a predominantly *solid* pattern with elongated nuclei in a nested background.

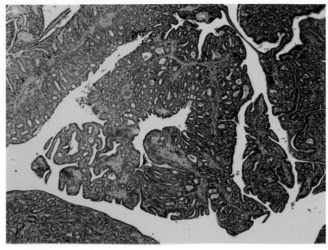

FIGURE 2

High-grade serous carcinoma, SET type. Low-power microphotograph showing gland architecture that closely mimics endometrioid carcinoma.

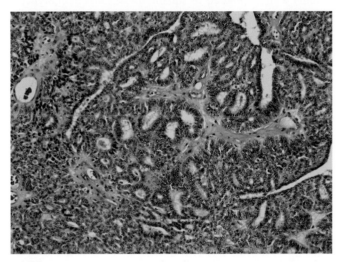

FIGURE 3

High-grade serous carcinoma, SET type. Higher-power microphotograph showing some multilayering with elongated nuclei, similar to endometrioid adenocarcinoma.

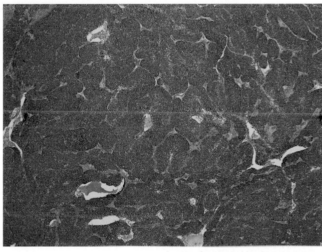

FIGURE 4

High-grade serous carcinoma, SET type. Low- and higher-power images of a tumor with transitional features.

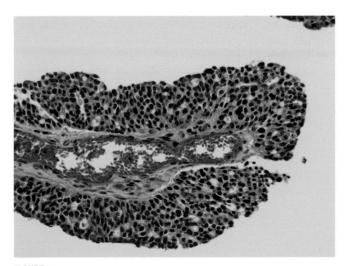

FIGURE 5

High-grade serous carcinoma, SET type. Low- and higher-power images of a tumor with transitional features.

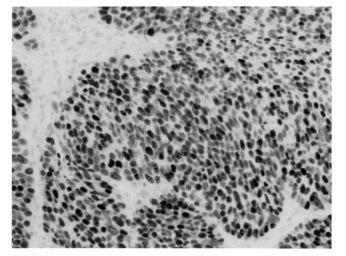

FIGURE 6

High-grade serous carcinoma, SET type. These tumors invariably contain p53 mutations, similar to classic serous carcinomas.

LOW-GRADE ENDOMETRIOID ADENOCARCINOMA WITH SQUAMOTRANSITIONAL OR SPINDLE FEATURES

DEFINITION—A distinct variant of low-grade endometrioid carcinoma with a spindled or squamotransitional phenotype.

CLINICAL FEATURES

EPIDEMIOLOGY

- Similar to other low-grade endometrioid adenocarcinomas.
- Associated with endometriosis of the ovary.

PRESENTATION

- Abdominal mass and ovarian enlargement.

PROGNOSIS AND TREATMENT

- As any low-grade endometrioid adenocarcinoma.

PATHOLOGY

HISTOLOGY

- Three intersecting patterns can be seen, including conventional endometrioid adenocarcinoma, a whirled spindled cell pattern that may appear almost morule like, and a more papillary pattern with fusiform cells giving the illusion of transitional differentiation.
- Uniform nuclear morphology and low proliferative index.
- Expansile growth pattern.

IMMUNOPATHOLOGY (INCLUDING IMMUNOHISTOCHEMISTRY)

- May be helpful. Inhibin will be negative as will be CK20. Immunostains for p53, p16, WT1, PAX8, and CK7 will be heterogeneous.

MAIN DIFFERENTIAL DIAGNOSIS

- Higher-grade carcinoma with transitional differentiation: greater nuclear atypia, higher nuclear-to-cytoplasmic (N/C) ratio with more nuclear pleomorphism, and p53 positive (or completely absent).
- Variants of granulosa cell or Sertoli cell tumors—inhibin positive.
- Proliferative Brenner tumor—these will not have background endometrioid differentiation and typically demonstrate a more delicate papillary rather than nested histology.

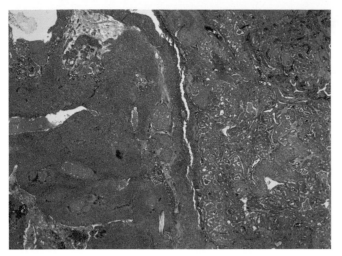

FIGURE 1

Low-grade endometrioid adenocarcinoma of the ovary with transitional features. The more conventional glandular pattern on the right merges with a transitional pattern on the left.

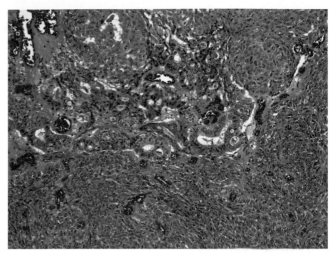

FIGURE 2

Low-grade endometrioid adenocarcinoma of the ovary with transitional features. In this field some glandular differentiation is seen centrally, with vague morule-like histology above and more spindle cell growth below.

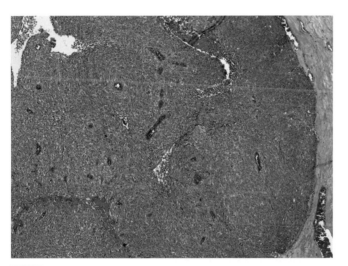

FIGURE 3

A field showing transitional growth alone. Note that the papillary architecture gives way to a more nested growth pattern.

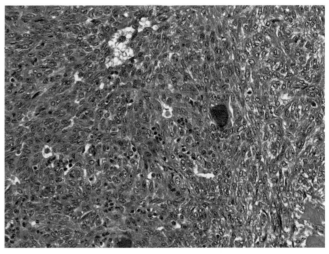

FIGURE 4

An area of solid growth. Note the uniform nuclear features.

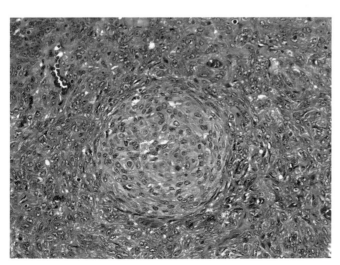

FIGURE 5

In this field a morule-like focus is seen *(center)*.

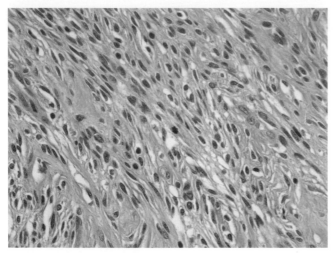

FIGURE 5

Ovarian adenosarcoma. This field shows moderate atypia with mitotic activity.

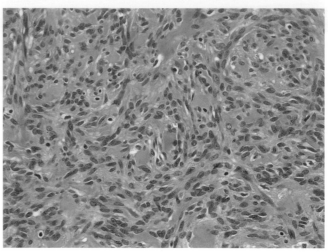

FIGURE 6

Ovarian adenosarcoma. This field resembles smooth muscle differentiation. Such stromal heterogeneity is common in these tumors and may necessitate careful examination to identify the diagnostic areas.

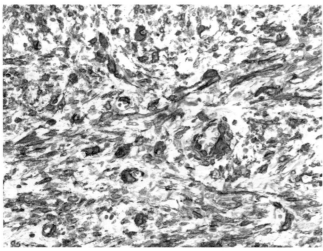

FIGURE 7

A stain for smooth muscle actin is strongly positive, underscoring the unreliability of such stains for excluding other tumors with smooth muscle differentiation.

SEROUS BORDERLINE TUMOR (SBT)

DEFINITION—A proliferative serous tumor of the ovary conferring a small (less than 5%) risk of adverse outcome.

CLINICAL FEATURES

EPIDEMIOLOGY

- The most common epithelial tumor of the ovary. Predominates in the fourth to sixth decades of life, but can be seen at virtually any age.
- These tumors can be associated with endometriosis but more often are seen as part of a continuum merging with müllerian ovarian cortical inclusions.
- There is no known relationship to BRCA, a familial syndrome or p53 mutations.

PRESENTATION

- Usually as a large, multicystic mass with papillary growth, either lining the cyst lumens or on the surface. From one third to one half will be bilateral. Peritoneal implants occur in some cases.

PROGNOSIS AND TREATMENT

- Prognosis is excellent in the absence of frank stromal invasion or invasive implants on the peritoneum (which would define a well-differentiated serous carcinoma).

PATHOLOGY

HISTOLOGY

- Cardinal features include a low-power appearance of multiple papillary structures with a mild to moderate degree of epithelial complexity. The lining epithelium typically contains ciliated cells, but this appearance can merge with both endometrioid and mucinous differentiation, the latter often termed "seromucinous" differentiation.
- Fibrosis with entrapment of epithelium, either in the cyst wall or ovarian surface, is not uncommon.

- Confluent epithelial growth, either in the form of micro-acinar or micropapillary architecture, can be seen. In the absence of invasive implants, these findings do not significantly alter prognosis.
- Microinvasion, defined as small papillary clusters of eosinophilic tumor cells in spaces totaling less than 5 mm in diameter, is found in up to 10% of SBTs. It may be associated with a greater risk of invasive implants, but in their absence confers no appreciable increase in the risk of adverse outcome over SBTs.
- Lymph node metastases can also be seen with serous borderline tumors (SBTs) but does not independently alter the prognosis in the absence of an infiltrative pattern that would suggest low-grade serous carcinoma.
- Tumors in pregnant patients may show exuberant epithelial proliferation and microinvasion.

IMMUNOPATHOLOGY (INCLUDING IMMUNOHISTOCHEMISTRY)

- Usually noncontributory. PAX8 (positive) and calretinin (negative) immunostains might aid in sorting out rare cases that resemble well-differentiated mesothelioma.
- In cases with exuberant growth or moderate nuclear atypia, wild-type p53 staining can help to rule out high-grade serous carcinoma.

MAIN DIFFERENTIAL DIAGNOSIS

- Rare mesotheliomas can overlap with SBT and may be difficult to distinguish based on immunophenotype.
- Well-differentiated serous carcinomas—look for stromal invasion or extensive confluent or micropapillary growth.
- Rare high-grade serous carcinomas might mimic SBT at low magnification due to well-developed papillae with a thin epithelial covering. Higher power inspection will confirm the high nuclear grade.

597

LOW-GRADE INVASIVE SEROUS CARCINOMA OF THE OVARY

DEFINITION—An invasive low-grade serous carcinoma.

CLINICAL FEATURES

EPIDEMIOLOGY

- The less common serous carcinoma. Predominates in the fourth to sixth decades of life, but can be seen at virtually any age.
- Can arise in a serous borderline tumor (SBT) or SBT with complex architecture (intraepithelial carcinoma).
- Associated with mutations in regulators of the MAPK pathway (KRAS, BRAF, ERBB2) in about two thirds of tumors.

PRESENTATION

- One third to one half are bilateral. Often associated with an SBT.
- Large unilocular or multilocular cystic mass.
- May respond to withdrawal of estrogen replacement. There have been responses to tamoxifen and aromatase inhibitors. MEK inhibitors are being investigated as well.

PROGNOSIS AND TREATMENT

- Prognosis is a function of stage. Tumors involving peritoneal surfaces have a poor prognosis with less than 50% 5-year survival.
- Typically responds poorly to conventional chemotherapy but regimens targeting the MAPK pathway have shown responses in some patients.

PATHOLOGY

HISTOLOGY

- Low-grade serous carcinomas are often associated with areas that merge morphologically with SBTs.

- Combine the features of both extensive papillary architecture (often with many psammoma bodies) and evidence of stromal invasion. The latter may consist of infiltrating glandlike structures or, more commonly, multiple papillae projecting into a space or embedded in a fibrous stroma that may also contain glands, cysts, irregular islands of tumor cells, or cribriform glands.
- Often the invasive papillae are suspended in space. Nuclei are uniform, round, or oval with evenly distributed chromatin, with or without a prominent nucleolus.
- Cilia are usually not conspicuous, but ciliated differentiation (tubulin, FOXJ1) can be found.
- Peritoneal invasion by low-grade serous carcinoma is an extension of the spectrum of invasive implants, but the abundance of metastatic deposits and its nuclear morphology are more in keeping with a frankly malignant process. This can take the form of numerous nests of invasive tumor, more loosely arranged clusters of papillae, the latter of which might be delicate and might mimic a noninvasive implant.
- A rare variant, psammocarcinoma, is seen on the peritoneal surfaces and, despite the predominance of psammomatous calcifications, destructively infiltrates the adjacent tissues.

IMMUNOPATHOLOGY (INCLUDING IMMUNOHISTOCHEMISTRY)

- Usually noncontributory. PAX8 and calretinin immunostains might aid in sorting out rare cases that resemble well-differentiated mesothelioma. However, we have seen hybrid tumors that share both immunophenotypes.

MAIN DIFFERENTIAL DIAGNOSIS

- Pseudoinvasion in areas of SBT.
- SBT with complex architecture (no invasion).
- Microinvasion in an SBT (less than 10 square mm).
- Well-differentiated mesothelioma (most will be PAX8 negative/calretinin positive).

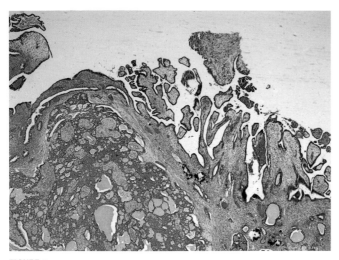

FIGURE 1

Low-grade serous carcinoma. Note the blunt, nonbranching surface papillae. This paradoxically low architectural complexity is commonly seen with low-grade serous carcinomas. Note also the confluent growth in the stroma, an expansile/replacement pattern of invasion.

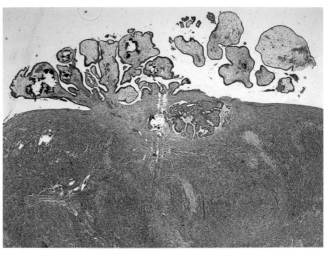

FIGURE 2

A metastasis to a contralateral ovary again demonstrates a low architectural surface complexity with subsurface invasion.

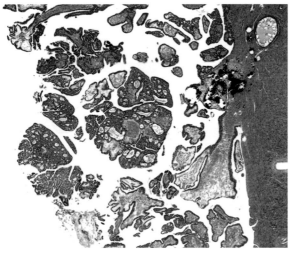

FIGURE 3

Cortical invasion by a low-grade serous carcinoma with expansile and infiltrative growth and retraction artifact.

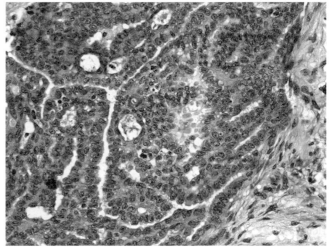

FIGURE 4

High-power image of low-grade serous carcinoma, papillary and solid patterns. There is mild atypia with inconspicuous cilia.

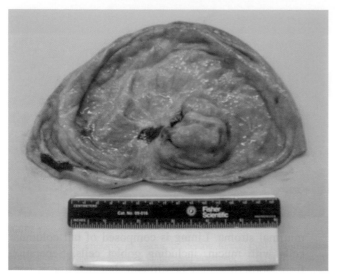

FIGURE 1

Mucinous carcinoma of the ovary arising in a borderline tumor. This tumor is a single cyst with a central tumor nodule.

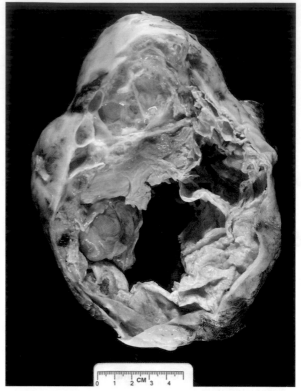

FIGURE 2

Mucinous carcinoma. This is more typical, with multiple cysts and focal solid growth.

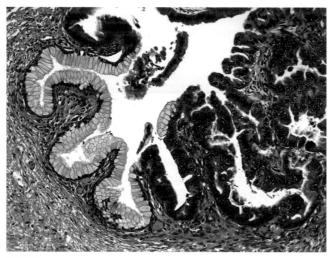

FIGURE 3

Junction of benign and malignant mucinous epithelium, not uncommon in these tumors.

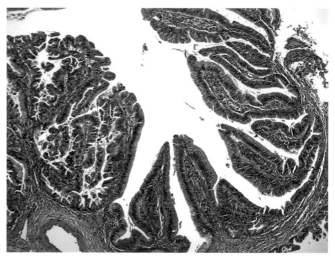

FIGURE 4

Mucinous carcinoma. In this medium-power magnification there is expansile growth with intracystic exophytic growth. This pattern portends a favorable outcome.

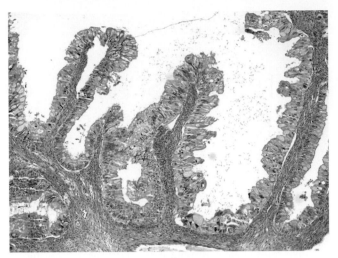

FIGURE 5

A somewhat more subtle variant of malignant epithelium, again with an expansile growth pattern and papillary architecture.

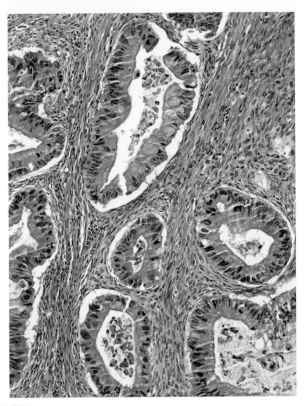

FIGURE 6

Malignant glands in stroma with retraction artifact.

MUCINOUS TUMORS WITH MURAL NODULES

DEFINITION—Mucinous tumors containing nodular foci in the cyst wall of altered mesenchymal and/or epithelial differentiation.

CLINICAL FEATURES

EPIDEMIOLOGY

- Extremely uncommon; tendency toward women in the fifth and sixth decades.
- Associated with both borderline and malignant mucinous tumors.
- Etiology is unclear; however, one recent paper noted different codon 12 k-ras mutations in a mucinous tumor and its mural nodule, suggesting that both may have originated in a mucinous precursor cell followed by clonal divergence.

PRESENTATION

- Typically found incidentally in a mucinous tumor.
- Generally uniform to variegated, yellow, pink, or red in appearance.
- Hemorrhage and necrosis may be present.
- Mural nodules may be single or multiple and range from less than 1 cm up to 30 cm.

PROGNOSIS AND TREATMENT

- Benign mural nodules will have an uneventful outcome.
- Outcome of malignant nodules varies but in general is poor. Risk of tumor-related death in patients with either anaplastic carcinomatous or sarcomatous nodules exceeds 50%. In small series of patients with stage IA tumors, 5-year disease-free survival has been as high as 100%.

PATHOLOGY

HISTOLOGY

- Three categories of benign nodules have been described. (1) Pleomorphic and epulis-like type, with osteoclast-like multinucleated giant cells, extravasated red blood cells (RBCs), and pleomorphic spindled cells similar to aneurysmal bone cysts. (2) Pure spindle cell population with no or few giant cells. (3) Multinucleated cells with ground-glass cytoplasm and thin fibrous bands. A resemblance to sarcoma (i.e., sarcoma like) is noted, but these nodules are sharply circumscribed and do not invade vessels.
- Malignant nodules include the following: (1) Anaplastic carcinoma with pleomorphic cells with markedly enlarged nuclei with prominent nucleoli and abundant eosinophilic cytoplasm, the latter sometimes imparting a rhabdoid appearance. Both epithelioid and spindle cells may be present and will stain with cytokeratin antibodies. (2) Sarcomatous and carcinosarcomatous mural nodules are even rarer, and fibrosarcomas, rhabdomyosarcomas, and pleomorphic undifferentiated sarcomas have been reported.

IMMUNOPATHOLOGY (INCLUDING IMMUNOHISTOCHEMISTRY)

- Cytokeratins will stain both spindle and epithelial components.

MAIN DIFFERENTIAL DIAGNOSIS

- Benign and malignant can be confused with each other.

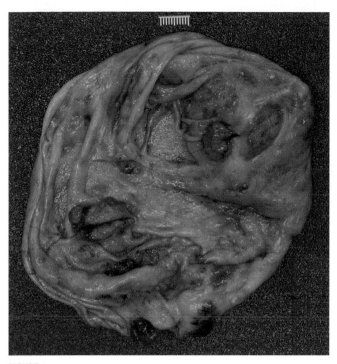

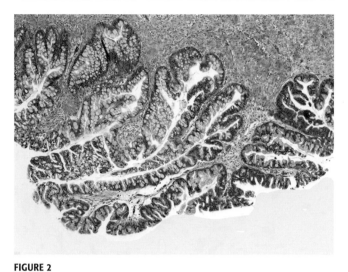

FIGURE 2

The tumor appears as a well-differentiated mucinous carcinoma without stromal invasion.

FIGURE 1

Low-grade mucinous tumor with mural nodules. Note several raised lesions in the wall of this tumor.

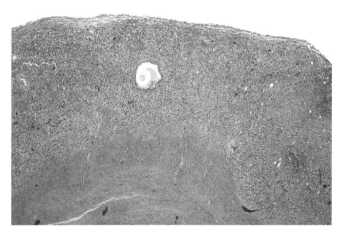

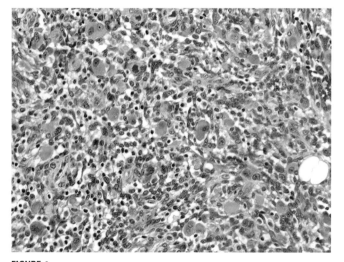

FIGURE 3

Mural nodule from above tumor, seen as a plaquelike lesion on the cyst wall.

FIGURE 4

At higher magnification there is an epithelioid population with scattered eosinophilic cells.

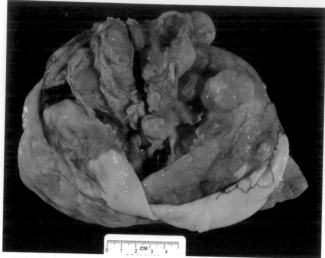

FIGURE 1

Gross pathology of a mucinous borderline tumor with soft fleshy excrescences that contain small cysts filled with mucin.

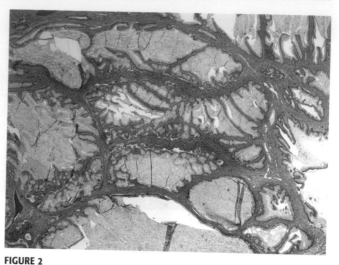

FIGURE 2

Mucinous borderline tumor. At low magnification there are abundant contiguous cysts with mild epithelial complexity.

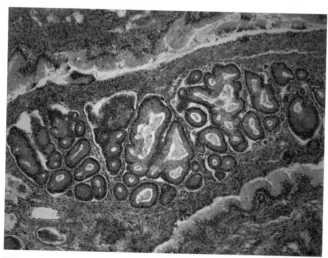

FIGURE 3

Mucinous borderline tumor. This field displays minimal atypia.

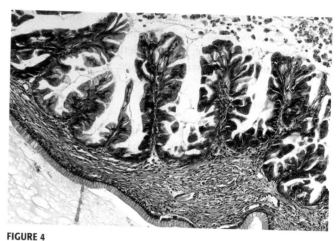

FIGURE 4

Mucinous borderline tumor. At higher magnification there are uniform papillae with mild epithelial complexity, modest atypia, and thin stromal cores.

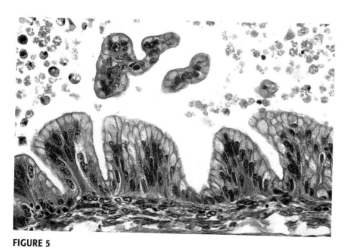

FIGURE 5

Mucinous borderline tumor. Intestinal-type differentiation is present, with mucin-producing epithelium and modest atypia.

MUCINOUS BORDERLINE TUMOR WITH INTRAEPITHELIAL CARCINOMA

DEFINITION—Marked intramucosal atypia in a borderline mucinous tumor of the ovary.

CLINICAL FEATURES

EPIDEMIOLOGY

- The second most common epithelial tumor of the ovary and 12% to 15% of ovarian tumors. Approximately 10% of mucinous tumors are borderline. The average age is in the sixth decade, but borderline tumors can be encountered over a wide age range.

PRESENTATION

- Usually as a large, multicystic mass. The solid component should be principally fibrous, but mucin-producing epithelium can produce both soft and fibrous areas.

PROGNOSIS AND TREATMENT

- Prognosis is excellent if the atypia is confined to the surface and is not accompanied by frank stromal invasion. No further therapy is warranted but thorough sampling of the tumor is indicated to exclude invasion. Undersampling of a more ominous component may explain the small risk of recurrence, approximately 5%. There is minimal risk of bilaterality, but this can rarely be seen in primary tumors.

PATHOLOGY

HISTOLOGY

- Features of a borderline tumor will virtually always be present, but rarely an intraepithelial carcinoma will emerge from a benign-appearing epithelium.

- The epithelial cell nuclei appear cytologically malignant (significant nuclear enlargement, nuclear hyperchromasia, often prominent nucleoli), but there is no obvious stromal invasion.
- In most cases there is prominent stratification of the malignant-appearing cells with stroma-free papillae or a cribriform pattern of growth.

IMMUNOPATHOLOGY (INCLUDING IMMUNOHISTOCHEMISTRY)

- Positive for CK7 and variable for CK20, PAX8, and CDX2.

MAIN DIFFERENTIAL DIAGNOSIS

- Well-differentiated metastatic mucin-producing adenocarcinomas of the appendix and pancreaticobiliary tree—usually smaller, multinodular, involving the ovarian surface, and including pseudomyxoma.
- Metastatic colonic carcinoma can present with a similar level of atypia within large cysts. However, confluent neoplastic glands are usually seen as well.

PROLIFERATIVE (BORDERLINE) ENDOMETRIOID ADENOFIBROMA

DEFINITION—Noninvasive epithelial and stromal tumors with an atypical endometrioid epithelial component.

CLINICAL FEATURES

EPIDEMIOLOGY

- Uncommon but not exceedingly rare; less than 200 reported cases but most pathologists will encounter at some point in their practice.
- Similar to other endometrioid tumors, patients are typically at the end of their reproductive period or postmenopausal.
- The average age at diagnosis is in the mid-50s.
- At least one fourth of cases are associated with endometriosis.

PRESENTATION

- Ovarian mass, usually unilateral.

PROGNOSIS AND TREATMENT

- Excellent; recurrences are exceedingly rare when the tumor is not accompanied by a frank carcinoma.
- Two cases of potential peritoneal implants at the time of initial surgery have been reported, but autochronus endometriosis could not be excluded.
- Surgical excision is adequate therapy.

PATHOLOGY

HISTOLOGY

- Gross examination is characterized by a solid and cystic mass with variable amounts of hemorrhage.
- The low-power histologic examination reveals a fibrous stroma with variable numbers of proliferative endometrioid glands scattered about.

- The epithelial cells are stratified and proliferative, with nuclear atypia that can be either mild or marked.
- The glandular architecture is variable and ranges from purely glandular (frequently with squamous morule formation), to papillary, to a combination of both.
- The glandular type of proliferation can be adenofibromatous or may consist of numerous closely packed endometrioid glands.
- The papillary growth patterns are usually villous, lack extensive branching, and project into the cystic spaces of the tumor.
- If the epithelial changes are limited to nuclear atypia, then the tumor is often referred to as a "proliferative endometrioid tumor with atypia;" if the epithelial component resembles a low-grade endometrioid carcinoma, then the tumor is often referred to as a "borderline endometrioid tumor." These distinctions have unclear clinical significance.
- By definition, stromal invasion, typified by a desmoplastic stromal response, is absent.
- In some cases there is a robust proliferation of endometrioid epithelium without intervening stroma; if this area exceeds 5 mm, some would call this microinvasion; however, recurrences have not been reported in these tumors.
- Our definition of microinvasion is limited to those tumors with one or more invasive foci, defined as irregularly shaped invasive-appearing glands with a desmoplastic stromal response, smaller than 10 mm^2.
- Tumors with a clearly invasive pattern, or those with such a degree of confluent growth that the pathologist judges it to be invasive, should be termed as such.

IMMUNOPATHOLOGY (INCLUDING IMMUNOHISTOCHEMISTRY)

- Noncontributory.

MAIN DIFFERENTIAL DIAGNOSIS

- Low-grade endometrioid carcinoma—this diagnosis is made when there is a loss of gland integrity or confluent epithelial growth.

- Endometriosis with atypia—this is defined as epithelial atypia and may be confused (or associated) with early clear-cell carcinoma. It is not characterized by glandular expansion.

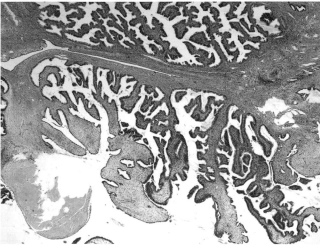

FIGURE 1

Borderline endometrioid adenofibroma. At low power note the presence of innumerable papillary growths into a cystic space.

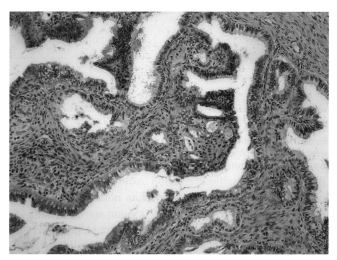

FIGURE 3

Borderline endometrioid adenofibroma. Note the focus of cribriform growth in the center of the image.

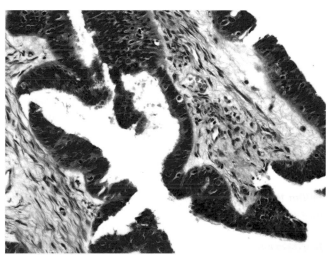

FIGURE 2

Borderline endometrioid adenofibroma. At high power note the stratified epithelium, which resembles endometrial endometrioid adenocarcinoma. There is mild nuclear atypia.

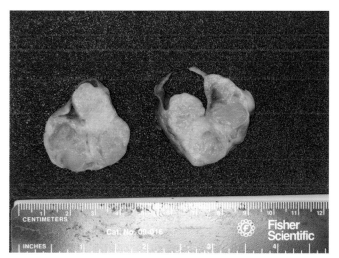

FIGURE 4

Borderline endometrioid adenofibroma with endometrioid adenocarcinoma. The borderline component is present at the top of the specimen, near the cystic structure. The nodules of carcinoma are present at the lower portion and are distinguished by their more gelatinous or fleshy appearance.

MAIN DIFFERENTIAL DIAGNOSIS

- Borderline or low-grade malignant endometrioid tumors—the two may merge in some cases.

- Borderline serous tumors—some serous tumors can appear quite "secretory." The presence of clear-cut mucinous differentiation segregates the mucinous, or if admixed with tubal differentiation, seromucinous tumors from the pure serous borderline tumors.

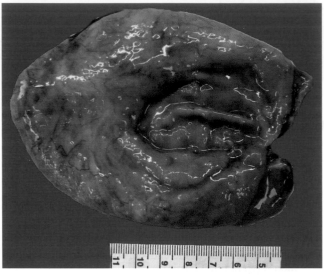

FIGURE 1

Mucinous cystic tumor, müllerian (endocervical) type in a unilocular cyst, presumably arising from an endometrioma.

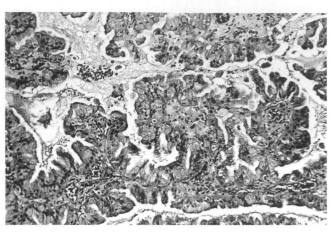

FIGURE 3

Endocervical-like mucinous borderline tumor. The papillae are lined by benign-appearing mucinous cells that resemble those of the endocervix.

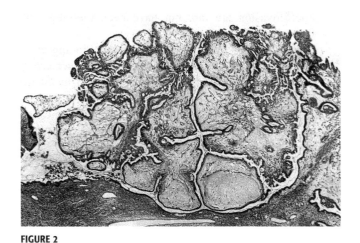

FIGURE 2

Endocervical-like mucinous borderline tumor. The low-power appearance mimics a serous borderline tumor with bulbous papillae.

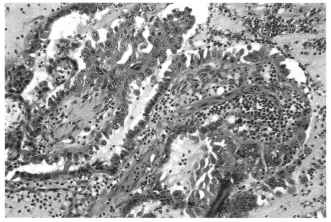

FIGURE 4

Endocervical-like mucinous borderline tumor. In this focus highly stratified eosinophilic cells line the papillae. There are numerous leukocytes in the papillae and in the mucin.

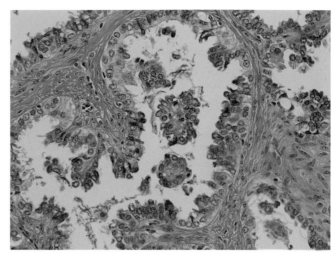

FIGURE 5

Seromucinous borderline tumor showing a mixture of phenotypes.

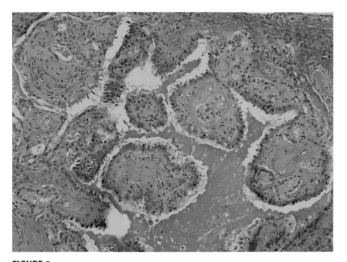

FIGURE 6

Seromucinous borderline tumor showing focal prominent ciliated differentiation.

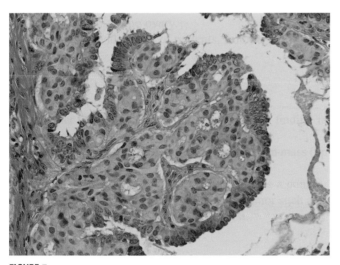

FIGURE 7

Seromucinous borderline tumor showing eosinophilic cells with mucin reminiscent of both endocervical and tubal differentiation.

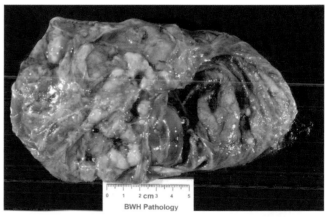

FIGURE 8

Malignant mucinous carcinoma arising in an endometrioma.

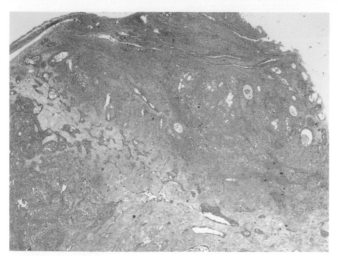

FIGURE 1

Malignant Brenner tumor. Low-power image shows a solid and focally cystic neoplasm with areas of ovarian and hyaline stroma.

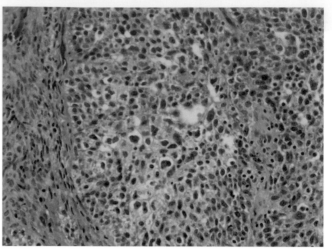

FIGURE 2

Malignant Brenner tumor. Marked atypia with pleomorphic hyperchromatic nuclei.

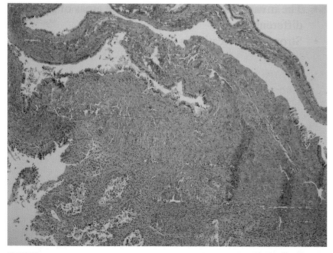

FIGURE 3

Malignant Brenner tumor. Foci of invasive carcinoma *(lower half of the image)* adjacent to a focus of benign Brenner tumor with mucinous features *(top half of the image).*

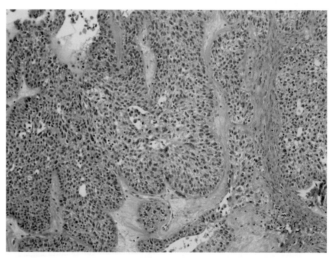

FIGURE 4

Malignant Brenner tumor. Invasive appearing nests of carcinoma with severe atypia.

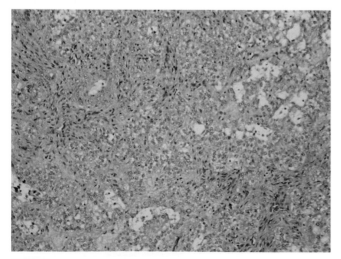

FIGURE 5

Malignant Brenner tumor. Frankly invasive nests of epithelial cells, which have a vaguely transitional morphology.

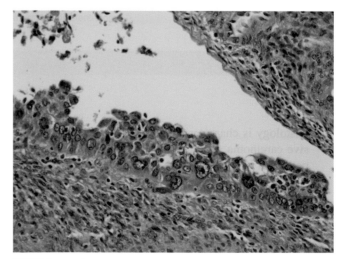

FIGURE 6

Malignant Brenner tumor. A flat focus of markedly atypical cells.

CLEAR-CELL CARCINOMA

DEFINITION—A malignant, endometriosis-associated epithelial tumor.

CLINICAL FEATURES

EPIDEMIOLOGY

- Uncommon.
- Distinct gene expression profile.
- Present in postmenopausal women with a mean age in the 50s.

PRESENTATION

- Unilateral ovarian mass in more than 95% of patients.
- Rare cases are associated with a paraneoplastic syndrome consisting of hypercalcemia. This is the most common ovarian cancer to present with thromboembolic disease.
- Frequently arise in the setting of endometriosis and/or an adenofibroma.

PROGNOSIS AND TREATMENT

- At least 40% of patients present with stage I disease (confined to the ovary).
- Data conflict on whether clear-cell carcinoma has a worse prognosis than other ovarian epithelial-stromal tumors with early stage tumors. However, with more advanced disease, clear-cell cancers are very resistant to conventional chemotherapy. Mammalian target of rapamycin (MTOR) inhibitors are being evaluated as treatment for these tumors.
- In some studies, tumors contained within a cyst have the better prognosis than those associated with adenofibromatous masses.

PATHOLOGY

HISTOLOGY

- On gross examination these tumors are often both cystic and solid; the solid component is soft and tan/brown.

- In early-stage tumors, endometriosis can often be identified nearby.
- On microscopic examination the characteristic feature of this tumor is the abundant clear cytoplasm.
- The cells may be growing in sheets, arranged in a tubuloglandular pattern, in papillae, or as a mixture of multiple patterns.
- Cells are not pseudostratified and are usually only one to two cell layers thick in any given area.
- The tumor cells have abundant cytoplasm, which is most often clear (due to glycogen accumulation) but may be eosinophilic or even granular.
- The cells often have a "hobnail" appearance, most evident when they are lining cystic spaces or the surface of papillae.
- The nuclei may be only mildly atypical or may exhibit marked pleomorphism.
- The papillary cores are characteristically hyalinized.
- In rare cases mucin-producing cells can be seen, and sometimes lymphocytes and plasma cells are prominent.

IMMUNOPATHOLOGY (INCLUDING IMMUNOHISTOCHEMISTRY)

- Broad-spectrum keratins and cytokeratin 7 are positive.
- ER, PR, and Her2-neu are variably present.
- WT1 and p53 are usually negative or patchy.
- HINF1-β is a new marker that is relatively sensitive for ovarian clear-cell carcinoma. Napsin A and AMACR are less sensitive but more specific.

MAIN DIFFERENTIAL DIAGNOSIS

- Serous carcinoma—strongly p53 positive.
- Endometrioid carcinoma with clear-cell change—this differential is more commonly encountered in the uterus. Look for classic features of clear-cell carcinoma, including staining with Napsin A and AMACR.
- Dysgerminoma—different age group, lack of glandular architecture, positive for OCT3/4.
- Metastatic renal cell carcinoma—consider if the tumor is bilateral. May be CD10 positive, CK7 negative.

OVARIAN ADENOCARCINOMA WITH YOLK SAC DIFFERENTIATION

■ **Brooke E. Howitt, MD**

PITFALL

DEFINITION—A rare tumor variant with classic carcinoma and yolk sac differentiation.

CLINICAL FEATURES

EPIDEMIOLOGY

- Extremely rare, limited to isolated reports or small case series.
- Broad age range but most are postmenopausal, averaging in the early 50s.

PRESENTATION

- The majority present with an abdominal mass at high stage (III or greater).
- Alpha-fetoprotein may be elevated.
- Large tumor mass, averaging 17 cm in one report.

PROGNOSIS AND TREATMENT

- Managed with standard chemotherapy with generally poor results.
- Behaves as any poorly differentiated epithelial tumor; most survive less than 2 years. Regimens targeting germ cell tumors (BEP) are often too toxic for elderly women with these tumors.
- Reported longer-term survival seen only in patients with stage IA disease.
- Prognosis parallels other tumors with germ cell differentiation occurring in older women.

PATHOLOGY

HISTOLOGY

- Non–germ-cell component can include endometrioid or clear-cell carcinoma and carcinosarcoma.
- Coexisting benign endometrioid lesions reported in some, including the contralateral ovary.
- Admixture of germ cell and epithelial elements, although the two are distinct from one another.

IMMUNOPATHOLOGY (INCLUDING IMMUNOHISTOCHEMISTRY)

- Strong AFP and SAL4 immunopositivity in the yolk sac tumor (YST) component.
- Adenocarcinoma is positive for ER/PR (if endometrioid).

MAIN DIFFERENTIAL DIAGNOSIS

- YST with endometrioid differentiation—younger age, not associated with an endometrioid precursor, positive for YST markers, responds to appropriate chemotherapy.

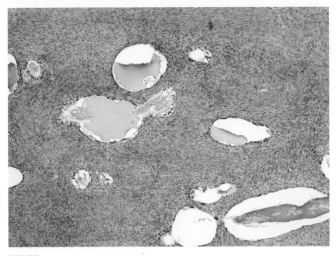

FIGURE 1

Borderline clear-cell adenofibroma in a case of mixed clear-cell carcinoma and YST of the ovary.

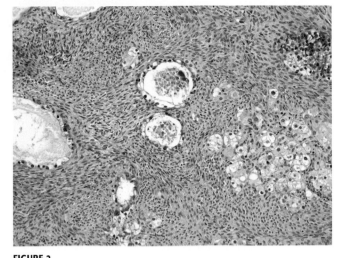

FIGURE 2

Junction of the clear-cell adenofibroma with frank clear-cell carcinoma on the right.

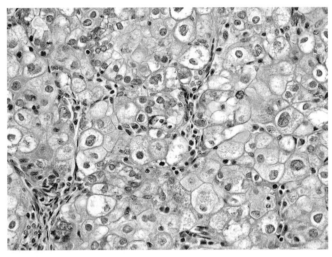

FIGURE 3

Solid growth of classic clear-cell carcinoma.

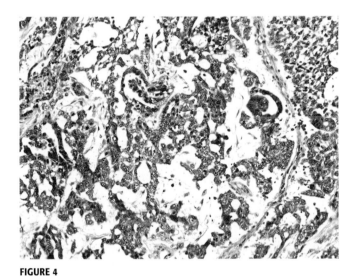

FIGURE 4

Medium magnification of the YST component with a complex but somewhat "regularly irregular" alveolar-glandular pattern.

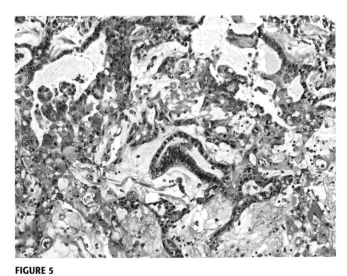

FIGURE 5

Higher magnification of the YST component with foci of glandlike differentiation. Note the numerous eosinophilic hyaline droplets.

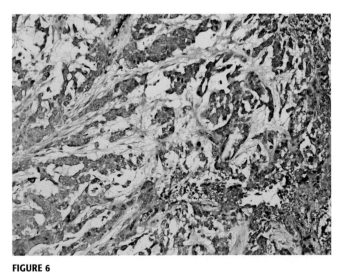

FIGURE 6

The YST component is strongly AFP positive.

BORDERLINE CLEAR-CELL ADENOFIBROMA

DEFINITION—An early form of clear-cell neoplasia with malignant cytology and the absence of invasion.

CLINICAL FEATURES

EPIDEMIOLOGY

- Clear-cell tumors of this type typically present as adenofibromas that can arise *de novo* or from within endometriotic cysts. Uncommon tumors comprising less than 1% of epithelial tumors.

PRESENTATION

- Usually as a large, unilateral multicystic mass. The cysts can give a honeycomb appearance within a fibrous stroma.

PROGNOSIS AND TREATMENT

- Prognosis is excellent in the absence of frank stromal invasion. The significance of microinvasion is unclear, but there is no evidence at present to suggest more than a minimal risk of recurrence.

PATHOLOGY

HISTOLOGY

- A cardinal feature is a low-power appearance of multiple, round, variably sized cysts within a fibrous stroma in a honeycomb pattern. The low-power image is often unimpressive because the cells lining the cysts are flattened.
- At higher magnification, enlarged, hyperchromatic nuclei, often with prominent nucleoli, should be visible to justify the diagnosis of a borderline clear-cell tumor.
- Clusters of smaller atypical glands with confluent architecture justify the diagnosis of microinvasion. This term is applied to invasive focus of less than 10 mm^2.

IMMUNOPATHOLOGY (INCLUDING IMMUNOHISTOCHEMISTRY)

- Noncontributory.

MAIN DIFFERENTIAL DIAGNOSIS

- Clear-cell adenofibroma—this is a subjective interpretation inasmuch as it will be based on whether there is sufficient atypia to justify a diagnosis of borderline tumor. Many feel that pure benign clear-cell adenofibromas do not really exist.
- Multiloculated simple or mesothelial cyst—this misclassification is a possibility. PAX8 staining should be sufficient to confirm a clear-cell tumor.

Meta

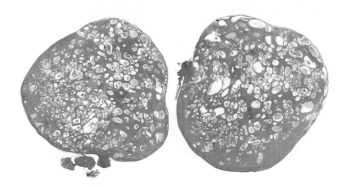

FIGURE 1

Low magnification of a borderline clear-cell adenofibroma. Note the honey-comb distribution of epithelial-lined cysts.

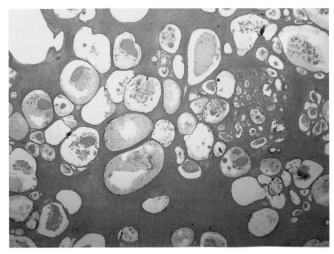

FIGURE 2

Borderline clear-cell adenofibroma. Note the focus of microinvasion at center right.

FIGUR

Meta:
necro

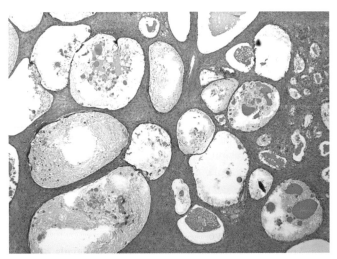

FIGURE 3

Borderline clear-cell adenofibroma. The focus of microinvasion is on the right.

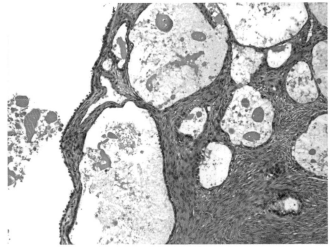

FIGURE 4

Borderline clear-cell adenofibroma. Note the nuclear enlargement in the lining cells.

FIGUR

Metast
surfac

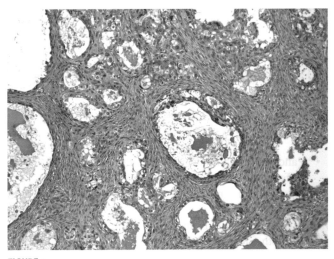

FIGURE 5

Borderline clear-cell adenofibroma. Higher magnification of the focus of microinvasion.

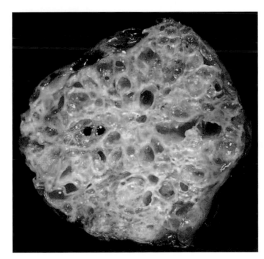

FIGURE 6

Classic honeycomb appearance of a multicystic borderline clear-cell adenofibroma.

PSEUDOMYXOMA PERITONEI

DEFINITION—A clinical term for increased mucin present within the abdominal cavity, typically associated with a low-grade mucinous tumor of the appendix or gastrointestinal tract.

CLINICAL FEATURES

EPIDEMIOLOGY

- Pseudomyxoma is frequently associated with appendiceal neoplasms; however, occasional cases occur in the absence of a detectable appendiceal tumor.
- Occasionally a large bowel, pancreatic, or coexisting ovarian mass may be present.

PRESENTATION

- Patients with pseudomyxoma typically present with increased abdominal girth; however, this is not a universal finding.

PROGNOSIS AND TREATMENT

- The prognosis is guarded. In patients with pseudomyxoma and a tumor of either appendiceal or ovarian origin the clinical course is protracted and may result in death.
- The higher the level of tumor burden and the higher the stage are associated with an adverse outcome.
- The currently recommended treatment is surgical excision of the tumor and drainage of the mucin with close clinical follow-up.

PATHOLOGY

HISTOLOGY

- The mucin itself is comprised of acellular to highly cellular mucin.

- Two general histologic groups have been described by Ronnett et al including "adenomucinosis" in which the glandular cells appear benign and "mucinous adenocarcinoma" in which the glandular cells appear malignant. A hybrid of the two has also been described with an outcome similar to the malignant form. However, adenomucinosis may also recur and prove fatal, albeit over a more protracted course.
- The primary tumor is typically appendiceal and may show distension of the appendix with mucin.
- Ovarian involvement may be unilateral or bilateral with cyst formation and pseudomyxoma ovarii.

IMMUNOPATHOLOGY (INCLUDING IMMUNOHISTOCHEMISTRY)

- Immunohistochemistry with CK7, CK20, and CDX2 may be helpful in identifying the primary site; however, there is overlap in gastrointestinal (GI), pancreatic, and ovarian tumors that may lead to confusion.
- Appendiceal tumors may show variable levels of CK7 and CK20 expression and can be uninformative in a large number of cases.
- CDX2 staining may be patchy in ovarian and appendiceal tumors as opposed to strong staining seen in most colon tumors.

MAIN DIFFERENTIAL DIAGNOSIS

All of the following may be associated with pseudomyxoma peritonei and therefore should be ruled out:
- Pancreatic mucinous tumors
- Appendiceal mucinous tumors
- Ovarian mucinous tumors
- Tubular gut mucinous tumors

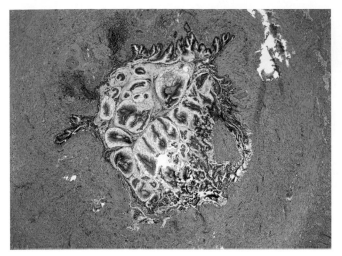

FIGURE 1

Pseudomyxoma peritonei. An appendix with luminal obliteration by a low-grade appendiceal mucinous neoplasm.

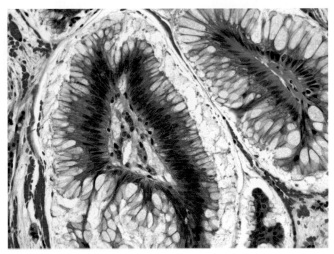

FIGURE 2

Pseudomyxoma peritonei. Low-grade appendiceal mucinous neoplasm with bland cytology.

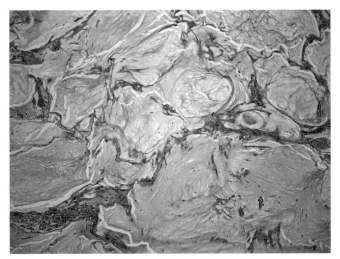

FIGURE 3

Pseudomyxoma peritonei. Pools of acellular mucin.

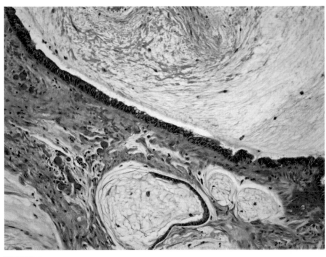

FIGURE 4

Pseudomyxoma peritonei. A peritoneal implant of epithelium from a low-grade appendiceal mucinous neoplasm.

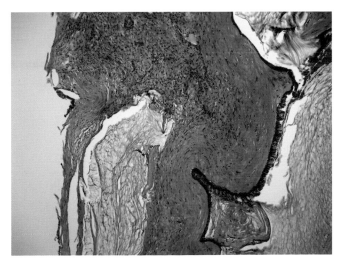

FIGURE 5

Pseudomyxoma peritonei. Ovarian involvement of a low-grade appendiceal mucinous neoplasm. The ovarian implants may closely represent a mucinous cystadenoma or borderline tumor.

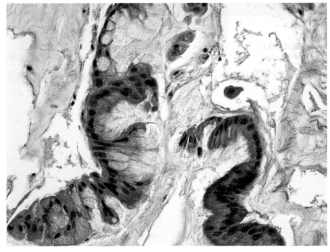

FIGURE 6

Pseudomyxoma peritonei. Strips of epithelium may be present in the mucin. Low-grade mucinous epithelium is present in this example.

FETIFORM TERATOMA

■ **Odise Cenaj, MD, PhD** ■ **Jelena Mirkovic, MD, PhD**

DEFINITION—A teratoma recapitulating human form.

CLINICAL FEATURES

EPIDEMIOLOGY

- Exceedingly rare, reproductive-age group.

PRESENTATION

- Ovarian mass.
- These tumors exhibit extremities, head and trunk, including phallus.

PROGNOSIS AND TREATMENT

- The prognosis is excellent. These tumors are not malignant.

PATHOLOGY

HISTOLOGY

- When differentiation is extreme, tissues are oriented along both the anterior-posterior, dorsal-ventral, and left-right axes.

- Virtually any germ cell layer can be found in the appropriate region including brain, eye, viscera phallus, endocrine, and blood vessels.

IMMUNOPATHOLOGY (INCLUDING IMMUNOHISTOCHEMISTRY)

- Noncontributory.

MAIN DIFFERENTIAL DIAGNOSIS

- Fetus in fetu—this is a monozygotic twin that becomes incorporated into the abdomen of the fetus. It would not be confused with a fetiform teratoma.
- Ectopic pregnancy—a fully formed embryo with an umbilical cord present.

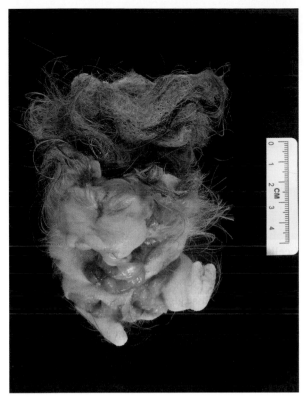

FIGURE 1

Fetiform teratoma. Note the vague resemblance to a fetus.

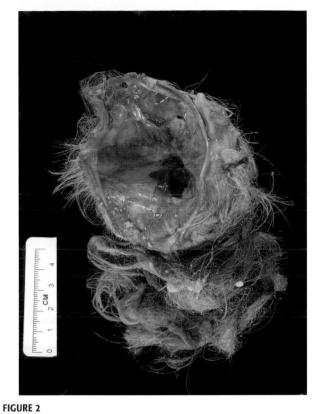

FIGURE 2

Fetiform teratoma. The "head" is opened to reveal a semblance of a cranial vault with some brain tissue.

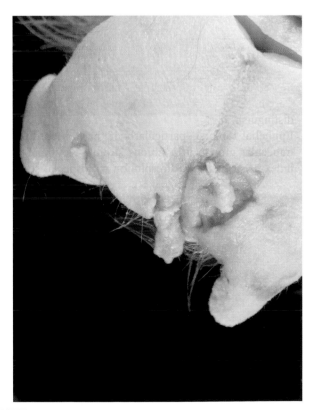

FIGURE 3

Fetiform teratoma. The lower torso exhibits limblike structures and a central phallic appendage.

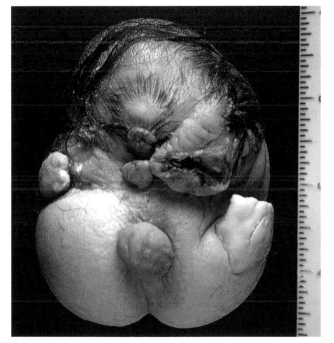

FIGURE 4

Another example of a fetiform teratoma.

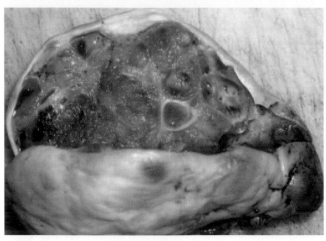

FIGURE 1

Malignant struma ovarii. A large mass-forming tumor distends the ovarian capsule. *(Courtesy Dr. Michael Roh.)*

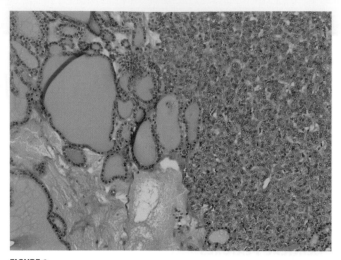

FIGURE 2

Interface of benign *(left)* and malignant (follicular variant of papillary carcinoma) *(right)*.

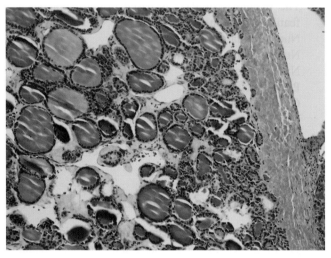

FIGURE 3

Benign strumal component at higher magnification.

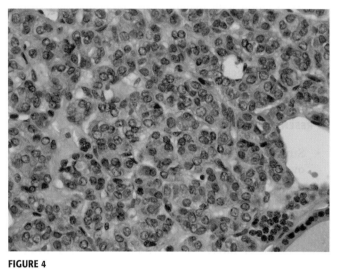

FIGURE 4

Malignant strumal component. There is nuclear enlargement, some nuclear contour irregularities, and nuclear clearing.

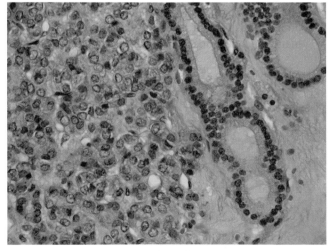

FIGURE 5

Benign thyroid follicles *(right)* are contrasted with carcinoma *(left)*.

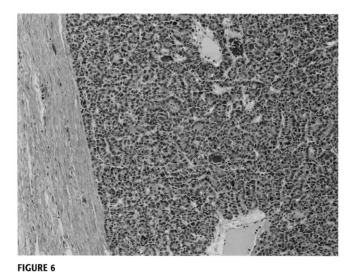

FIGURE 6

A more difficult nodule of thyroid tissue in a struma ovarii that is not conclusive for malignant struma.

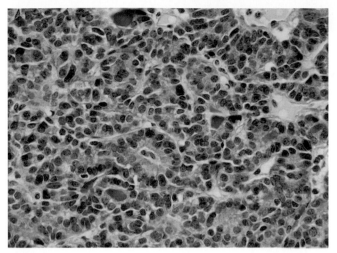

FIGURE 7

Higher power view of the focus in Figure 6 showing less pronounced nuclear abnormalities.

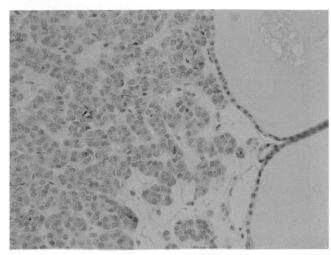

FIGURE 8

Immunostains may be helpful but are still under study. In this case (depicted in Figures 4 and 5) the malignant component stains for Galectin in contrast to the adjacent benign tissue on the right.

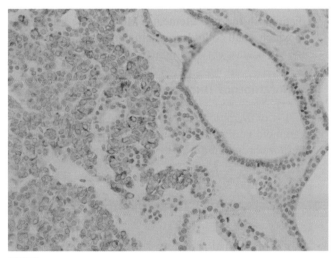

FIGURE 9

A stain for CK19 is diffusely positive.

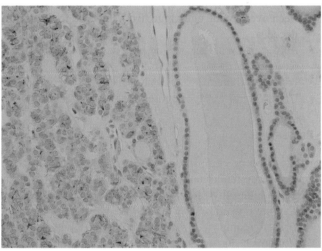

FIGURE 10

Staining for HBME-1 is also positive. Figures 8 to 10 show the "best case scenario" for immunostaining but the pathologist must use caution in their interpretation from case to case.

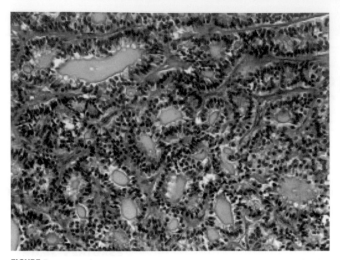

FIGURE 5

A focus of mixed differentiation in a strumal carcinoid.

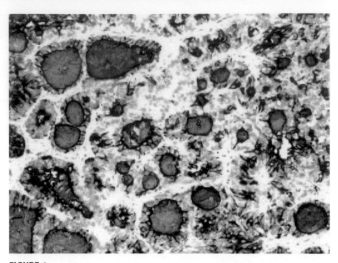

FIGURE 6

Mixed differentiation following staining for thyroglobulin.

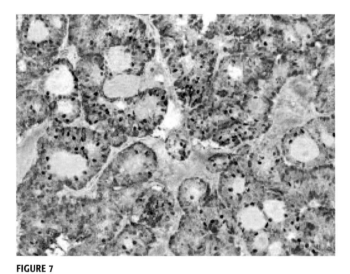

FIGURE 7

Mixed differentiation following double staining for TTF-1 (nuclear) and chromogranin (cytoplasm). This illustrates the common cell of origin for these tumors and the immunophenotypic overlap in these tumors.

METASTATIC CARCINOID

DEFINITION—Metastatic carcinoid, usually from the gastrointestinal tract.

CLINICAL FEATURES

EPIDEMIOLOGY

- The majority of metastatic carcinoids are of distal ileal origin.
- Have a wide age range, but most will be postmenopausal.

PRESENTATION

- Bilateral in up to 90%.
- Urinary uptake of hydroxyindoleacetic acid (HIAA) is increased in 90%.
- Hepatic and peritoneal involvement common.
- Solid tan to yellow tumor masses, often multinodular.

PROGNOSIS AND TREATMENT

- Despite the metastatic nature of this disease, some reports note a 5-year survival exceeding 80% due to favorable response to therapy and the generally low level of malignancy. We have seen occasional patients survive for decades after resection of their ovarian tumor.

PATHOLOGY

HISTOLOGY

- The most common pattern is an insular pattern.
- Formation of acini is common, with salt and pepper chromatin.
- Small cordlike patterns or linear arrays of tumor cells are not uncommon.
- Mucin production may also be seen, including gastrointestinal differentiation.
- Multifocal distribution, with frequent involvement of both ovaries.

IMMUNOPATHOLOGY (INCLUDING IMMUNOHISTOCHEMISTRY)

- Synaptophysin and chromogranin stains should be positive.
- CDX2 stains often positive but not specific for metastatic carcinoid.

MAIN DIFFERENTIAL DIAGNOSIS

- Sex cord–stromal neoplasms—inhibin positive.
- Struma or strumal carcinoid—TTF-1 and neuroendocrine stains will distinguish.
- Epithelial tumors—particularly if there is cordlike or trabecular growth in a fibrous stroma. Key here is an index of suspicion and resolution with special stains. Glandlike patterns will closely resemble endometrioid and other epithelial tumors.

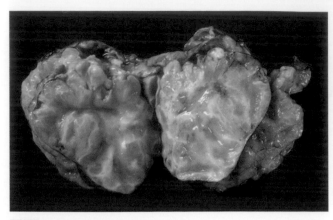

FIGURE 1

Metastatic carcinoid from the small bowel displays a brown-tan appearance.

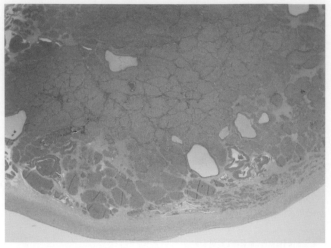

FIGURE 2

Metastatic carcinoid. Multiple confluent islands of tumor in the ovarian cortex.

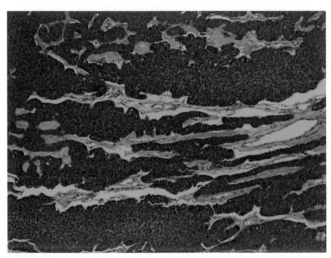

FIGURE 3

Metastatic insular carcinoid showing large cohesive sheets of tumor cells.

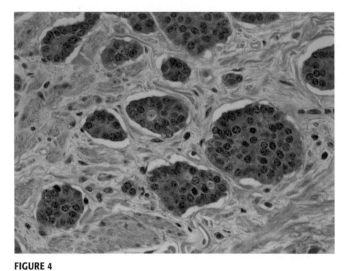

FIGURE 4

Metastatic insular carcinoid showing a range of patterns from predominantly solid nests to glandlike pattern. Key here are the nuclear features, which can be deceptive depending on fixation.

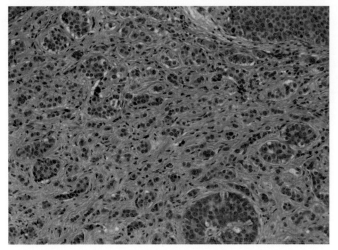

FIGURE 5

Metastatic insular carcinoid showing a range of patterns from predominantly solid nests to glandlike pattern. Key here are the nuclear features, which can be deceptive depending on fixation.

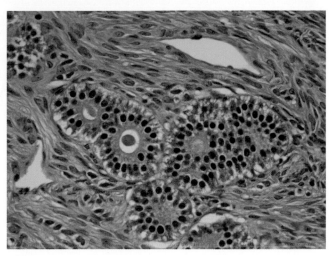

FIGURE 6

Metastatic insular carcinoid showing a range of patterns from predominantly solid nests to glandlike pattern. Key here are the nuclear features, which can be deceptive depending on fixation.

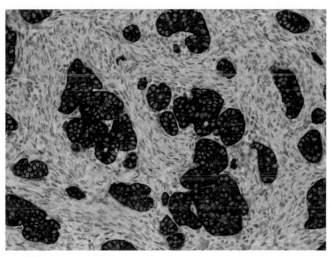

FIGURE 7

Synaptophysin staining of a metastatic carcinoma.

MALIGNANCY ARISING IN TERATOMAS

DEFINITION—A malignant tumor of somatic tissues arising from an element of mature teratoma.

CLINICAL FEATURES

EPIDEMIOLOGY

- Rare, occurring in 1% of mature cystic teratomas.
- Approximately 90% are epithelial, 80% of which are squamous carcinomas.
- Mean age is approximately 20 years older than that of benign teratomas.

PRESENTATION

- Usually discovered incidentally following removal of the teratoma (pelvic mass).
- More commonly associated with tumors of 10 cm or greater in diameter.

PROGNOSIS AND TREATMENT

- One half are advanced stage (II or greater at diagnosis).
- The prognosis varies with tumor type and stage.
- Squamous carcinomas have the worst prognosis, influenced by stage, tumor size, and older age.
- Ten-year survival is 60% for stage I and less than 25% for more advanced stages.
- Carcinoids, malignant struma, and primitive neuroectodermal tumor (PNET) are discussed separately.

PATHOLOGY

HISTOLOGY

- Most of these tumors are well-differentiated squamous carcinomas, befitting tumors of a non–human papillomavirus (HPV) pathogenesis.

IMMUNOPATHOLOGY (INCLUDING IMMUNOHISTOCHEMISTRY)

- Noncontributory, although p16 should be negative or weakly positive in contrast to metastatic squamous carcinomas of the cervix.

MAIN DIFFERENTIAL DIAGNOSIS

- Metastatic squamous carcinoma from other sites—this can usually be excluded by the presence of other teratomatous elements. Rarely we have seen metastatic squamous carcinomas from the cervix in the region of the ovary. The latter should be excluded with a p16 immunostain (positive) and appropriate history.

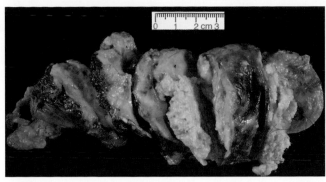

FIGURE 1

Squamous carcinoma arising in a teratoma. Note the presence of hair, coupled with a solid necrotic carcinoma.

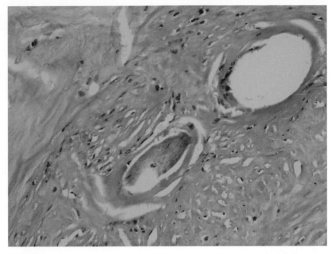

FIGURE 2

Squamous carcinoma arising in a teratoma. A portion of the normal parenchyma with hair shafts is histologic confirmation of a teratoma.

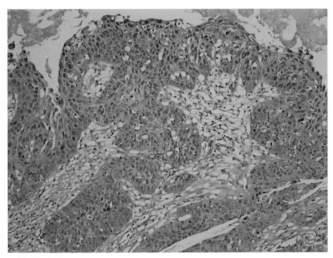

FIGURE 3

Squamous carcinoma lining a cyst.

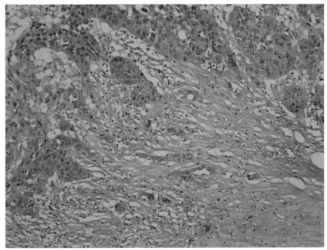

FIGURE 4

Invasive carcinoma penetrating the cyst wall.

DYSGERMINOMA

DEFINITION—A malignant, primitive germ cell tumor of the ovary that is the counterpart to testicular seminoma.

CLINICAL FEATURES

EPIDEMIOLOGY

- Rare; represents only 1% of all ovarian germ cell tumors but is the most common malignant germ cell tumor.
- Most cases arise in women in their teens or twenties with a mean age of 19 years.
- The most common malignant germ cell tumor identified in young persons.

PRESENTATION

- Rapidly growing ovarian mass with 10% to 20% showing macroscopic or microscopic involvement of the contralateral ovary.
- Elevated serum lactate dehydrogenase in at least 95% of patients.
- Incidental finding in patients with gonadal dysgenesis (rare).

PROGNOSIS AND TREATMENT

- More than half of all cases are still confined to the ovary at the time of diagnosis; metastasis to the contralateral ovary is common and can be microscopic.
- Most recurrences occur in the first 2 years after initial diagnosis.
- Metastatic spread is to lymph nodes (iliac, mediastinal, supraclavicular) and later to solid organs (liver, lungs, bone).
- With treatment, survival is over 95%.
- For tumors limited to one ovary, patients are followed with the expectation of almost 100% salvage with chemotherapy for those that relapse.
- These tumors are highly sensitive to radiation, but chemotherapy has almost completely replaced radiation therapy in their management. Some authors still recommend BEP but others feel carboplatin, with or without etoposide, is sufficient.

PATHOLOGY

HISTOLOGY

- Gross examination of the ovary is notable for a firm, solid mass that may be gray or tan-pink with or without hemorrhage and necrosis; true cystic structures should not be seen.
- The low-power appearance is characterized by large tumor cells arranged in nests or cords; occasional cases have cells arranged in thin, nearly single cell cords.
- The tumor cells have large, round to oval, vesicular nuclei with eosinophilic nucleoli and abundant pale to eosinophilic cytoplasm; cytoplasmic borders are often prominent.
- There is a moderate degree of variability in nuclear size; occasional giant cells or syncytiotrophoblastic cells may be seen, and this finding alone is not sufficient to warrant a diagnosis of mixed germ cell tumor.
- A delicate loose stroma is most commonly present; but in some cases, the stroma may be hyalinized or luteinized.
- Infiltrating inflammatory cells are variably present and usually consist of T-cells; in some cases even germinal center formation is present.
- A careful search for other germ cell elements should be undertaken, especially for yolk sac tumor.

IMMUNOPATHOLOGY (INCLUDING IMMUNOHISTOCHEMISTRY)

- Positive for PLAP (membranous), CD117, OCT-4, LDH (usually), and desmin.
- Negative for CD30, EMA, and AFP.
- Variable for keratins (usually weak) and HCG (usually only in syncytiotrophoblasts, but rarely in the cytoplasm of dysgerminoma).

MAIN DIFFERENTIAL DIAGNOSIS

- Mixed germ cell tumor; teratoma, yolk sac tumor, embryonal carcinoma, and choriocarcinoma.

- Clear-cell carcinoma. Usually forms discrete acinar or papillary structures while dysgerminoma may show a nested pattern; positive for epithelial markers; usually (but not necessarily) older age group.
- Granulosa cell tumor. These lack the nuclear characteristics; inhibin positive.

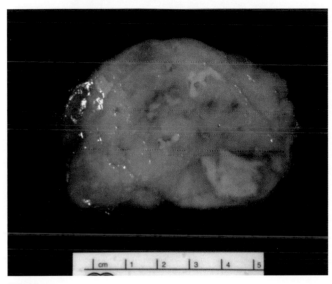

FIGURE 1

Dysgerminoma. Gross photograph demonstrating a tan, fleshy surface with foci of necrosis. Hemorrhage is also common.

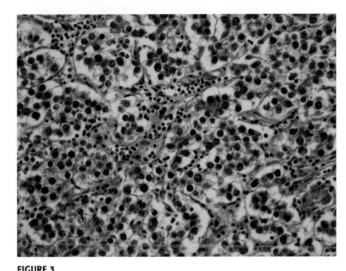

FIGURE 3

Dysgerminoma. At medium power this example is composed of small- to medium-sized nests of cells surrounded by delicate fibrovascular stroma.

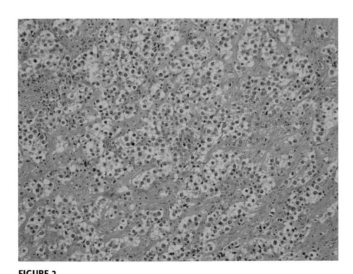

FIGURE 2

Dysgerminoma. At low power this tumor is composed of large cords of round, epithelioid neoplastic cells.

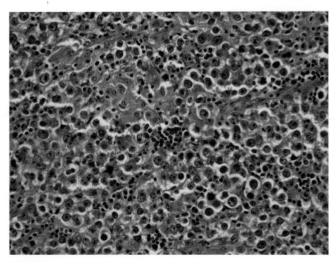

FIGURE 4

Dysgerminoma. An example of a more sheetlike architecture.

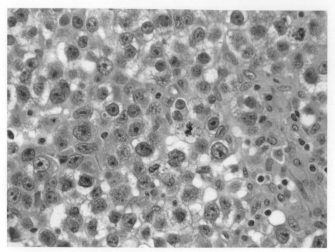

FIGURE 5

Dysgerminoma. At high power the cells have abundant clear to eosinophilic cytoplasm and round to oval nuclei. There are prominent violaceous nucleoli, and mitoses are common.

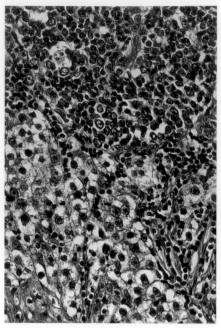

FIGURE 6

Dysgerminoma. Tumor-infiltrating lymphocytes are commonly seen.

YOLK SAC TUMOR

DEFINITION—A malignant germ cell tumor with endodermal sinus or vitelline differentiation.

CLINICAL FEATURES

EPIDEMIOLOGY

- The majority of patients are in their teens or twenties, although cases commonly occur in the first and fourth decades of life as well. The mean age is 19 years.
- Yolk sac tumors are the second most common malignant germ cell tumor (dysgerminoma is the most common) but are relatively rare overall.

PRESENTATION

- Most patients present with abdominal pain and enlargement.
- If measured before surgery, alpha fetoprotein (AFP) levels are usually elevated.
- Imaging studies often reveal a unilateral, large, and solid to partially cystic mass.

PROGNOSIS AND TREATMENT

- The overall prognosis is good, with around 80% of all cases cured after surgery (unilateral salpingo-oophorectomy) and modern chemotherapy regimens (cisplatinum, etoposide, bleomycin).
- Pure hepatoid or glandular variants have been reported to be slightly less responsive to chemotherapy and thus have a more guarded prognosis.
- AFP levels are monitored after surgery to detect metastasis or recurrence.

PATHOLOGY

HISTOLOGY

- The most common pattern is the microcystic pattern admixed with the endodermal sinus pattern, although any pattern may be seen in a tumor.

- Intensely eosinophilic hyaline droplets may be seen in any of the aforementioned patterns.
- Numerous histologic patterns of yolk sac tumor have been identified:
  - Microcystic/macrocystic: A lacelike network of small to large cystic spaces that tends to form a honeycomb-like pattern. The cysts are lined by flattened cells with hyperchromatic and pleomorphic nuclei.
  - Myxomatous: Abundant myxoid matrix with scattered cells forming strands and occasional glandlike structures.
  - Solid: Sheetlike arrangement of cells with clear cytoplasm and large nuclei. Occasional microcyst formation may be present but is typically focal.
  - Endodermal sinus: This pattern contains the classic Schiller-Duval body, which is composed of a vascular structure lined by a layer of cuboidal to columnar epithelial-like cells. The presence of these structures is diagnostic of yolk sac tumor; however, they may not be seen in every case.
  - Polyvesicular: Vesicle or cysticlike spaces that are lined by flattened cells. The vesicles may align and form a soap bubble–like pattern with intervening constrictions.
  - Alveolar-glandular: Glandlike or alveoli-like spaces lined by flat, cuboidal or columnar cells set in a myxoid stroma.
  - Papillary: True papillary structures with fibrous cores that are lined by markedly pleomorphic cells.
  - Hepatoid: Nest and cords of large eosinophilic cells with granular cytoplasm and well-defined cellular borders. Collections of these cells bear a remarkable resemblance to liver parenchyma.
  - Glandular (intestinal): Primitive cells in a glandular or nested pattern that are separated by stroma. The glands may be sparse and seen in varying levels of differentiation. Occasionally the glands may be well differentiated and resemble endometrial or colonic glandular epithelium. Be aware that there are rare examples of hybrid endometrioid/clear-cell and yolk sac tumors, seen in older women.

IMMUNOPATHOLOGY (INCLUDING IMMUNOHISTOCHEMISTRY)

- Yolk sac tumors are often positive for AFP, alpha-1-antitrypsin, and keratins. The tumors are negative for CD30 and vascular markers, differentiating them from embryonal carcinomas and vascular tumors, respectively.

- Embryonal carcinoma—more pronounced nuclear atypia, syncytiotrophoblastic differentiation.
- Vascular tumors—positive for vascular markers.
- Retiform Sertoli-Leydig cell tumors—inhibin positive.
- Juvenile granulosa cell tumors—inhibin positive.
- Metastatic hepatocellular carcinoma (hepatoid variant)—consider if monomorphic and bilateral.

MAIN DIFFERENTIAL DIAGNOSIS

- Clear-cell carcinoma.
- Dysgerminoma.

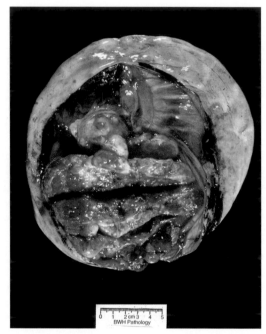

FIGURE 1
Yolk sac tumor with a solid and cystic cut surface.

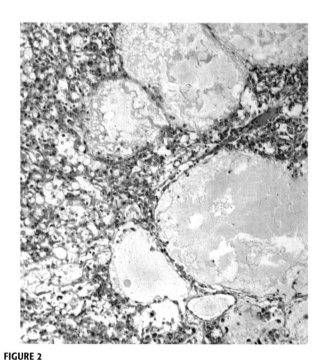

FIGURE 2
Yolk sac tumor. The polyvesicular pattern consisting of cystic spaces arranged in a soap bubble–like configuration.

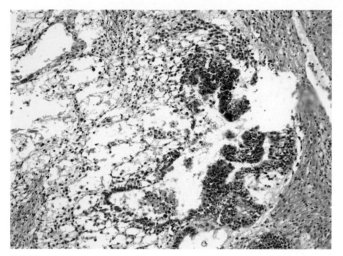

FIGURE 3

Yolk sac tumor. The microcystic pattern composed of a lacelike arrangement of primitive malignant cells.

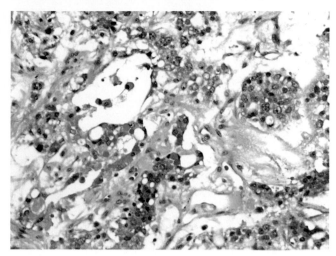

FIGURE 4

Yolk sac tumor. Numerous round, brightly eosinophilic hyaline bodies may be seen.

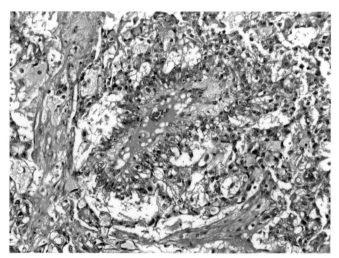

FIGURE 5

Yolk sac tumor. The endodermal sinus pattern composed of small to large Schiller-Duval bodies.

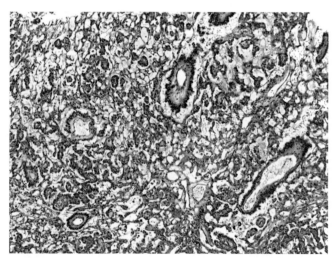

FIGURE 6

Yolk sac tumor. Numerous Schiller-Duval bodies can be seen.

EMBRYONAL CARCINOMA

DEFINITION—A malignant, primitive germ cell tumor of the ovary with embryonic differentiation.

CLINICAL FEATURES

EPIDEMIOLOGY

- Rare; represents less than 5% of all malignant ovarian germ cell tumors.
- Most cases arise in patients in their teens or twenties with a median age in the mid-teens.

PRESENTATION

- Rapidly growing ovarian mass.
- Most are stage I when diagnosed.
- Elevated serum levels of alpha fetoprotein (AFP) and, in many cases, human chorionic gonadotropin (HCG).

PROGNOSIS AND TREATMENT

- High relapse rate by surgery alone.
- Highly sensitive to chemotherapy (bleomycin, etoposide, and cisplatin).
- Cure rate exceeds 95% even with bulky metastatic disease.
- Prognostic data is limited because of small number of cases in the literature, but long-term remissions are seen with chemotherapy.

PATHOLOGY

HISTOLOGY

- Gross examination of the ovary will reveal a solid gray to tan with variable hemorrhage and necrosis.

- The low-power appearance is characterized by aggregates of primitive tumor cells that resemble malignant germ cells (dysgerminoma) but are arranged in glandlike structures, papillae with unpolarized cells and sheets.
- The tumor cells have large, variably shaped, vesicular nuclei with eosinophilic nucleoli, and very large nuclei may be seen as well as indistinct cell borders.
- There can be marked variability in nuclear size; giant cells or syncytiotrophoblastic cells may be seen, but cytotrophoblasts are absent except in true mixed germ cell tumors with choriocarcinoma.

IMMUNOPATHOLOGY (INCLUDING IMMUNOHISTOCHEMISTRY)

- Positive for SOX2, NANOG, OCT-3/4, and CAM5.2.
- Negative for D2-40.

MAIN DIFFERENTIAL DIAGNOSIS

- Yolk sac carcinoma—less atypia; growth patterns will distinguish from embryonal carcinoma.
- Clear-cell carcinoma or poorly differentiated carcinoma—older age in general and negative for SOX2, NANOG, and OCT-3/4.

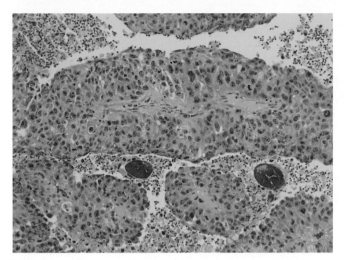

FIGURE 1

Embryonal carcinoma of the ovary. Note the papillary architecture and mildly polarized epithelioid cells with nuclear pleomorphism and nucleoli.

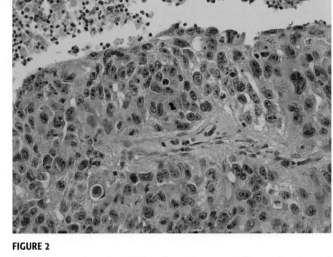

FIGURE 2

At higher power the cells exhibit nuclear enlargement with prominent nuclei. Note the more irregular nuclear spacing, a feature contrasting with conventional dysgerminoma.

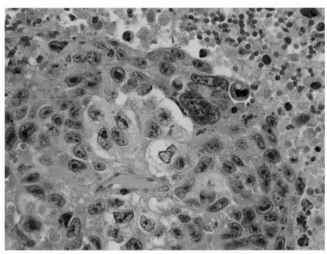

FIGURE 3

Very large nuclei can be seen in these tumors.

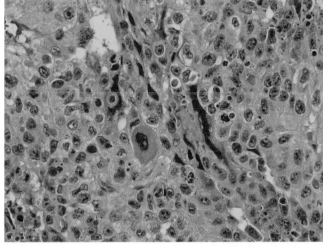

FIGURE 4

Syncytial giant cells *(center)* in an embryonal carcinoma can be associated with an elevated level of HCG.

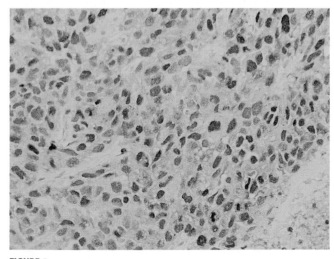

FIGURE 5

Staining for SOX2 highlights tumor cell nuclei.

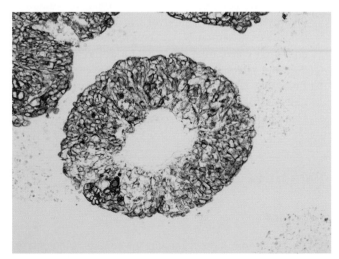

FIGURE 6

Strong staining for CAM5.2 will distinguish this tumor from a pleomorphic dysgerminoma.

IMMATURE TERATOMA

DEFINITION—A malignant germ cell tumor recapitulating fetal somatic differentiation.

CLINICAL FEATURES

EPIDEMIOLOGY

- Rare, comprising less than 1% of all germ cell tumors but third most common malignant germ cell tumor in young women.
- Mean age of 19 years; 75% are under age 35.

PRESENTATION

- Pelvic mass.
- Always unilateral, although some (about 15%) will have a contralateral mature cystic teratoma.

PROGNOSIS AND TREATMENT

There are five categories of management.

- Stage I grade I immature teratomas require no more therapy (95% cure rate).
- Stage I grade II or III teratomas will require chemotherapy (bleomycin, ~75% cure rate). There is no evidence that contralateral oophorectomy or radiation therapy will improve survival.
- Gliomatosis peritonei is a concurrent or subsequent condition where glial tissue is of a different origin and does not affect outcome.
- Enlarging teratoma syndrome is an expanding terminally differentiated teratoma post chemotherapy. Curable with complete excision.

PATHOLOGY

HISTOLOGY

- These tumors have a mixture of somatic elements in various stages of immaturity.

- Rarely, tumors may have only mild immaturity, and such neoplasms behave in a benign fashion.
- Grading is based principally on the amount of immature neuroepithelium, either as tubules or other primitive neuroectodermal differentiation.
  - Grade I—immature neural tissue is seen in less than a single 40× field per slide.
  - Grade II—immature neural tissue exceeds grade I but not more than three 40× fields per slide.
  - Grade III—primitive neural tissue exceeds three 40× fields per slide.
- One pitfall is overinterpreting germinal matrix or cerebellum as immature neuroepithelium.

IMMUNOPATHOLOGY (INCLUDING IMMUNOHISTOCHEMISTRY)

- Noncontributory.

MAIN DIFFERENTIAL DIAGNOSIS

- Primitive neuroblastic tumors (PNET) in mature teratomas—these tumors are monomorphic and lack other immature elements.
- Germinal matrix differentiation in mature cystic teratomas.
- Rarely mature solid teratomas will be encountered and must be sampled carefully to exclude immature elements.

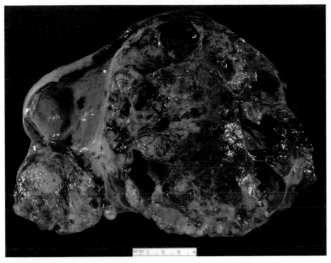

FIGURE 1

Immature teratoma. The tumor is a large encapsulated mass containing tissues of different consistency, some of which resemble cartilage.

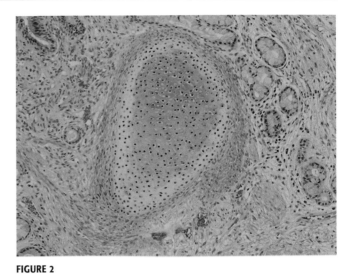

FIGURE 2

Immature cartilage in an immature teratoma. This is not used for the purposes of grading.

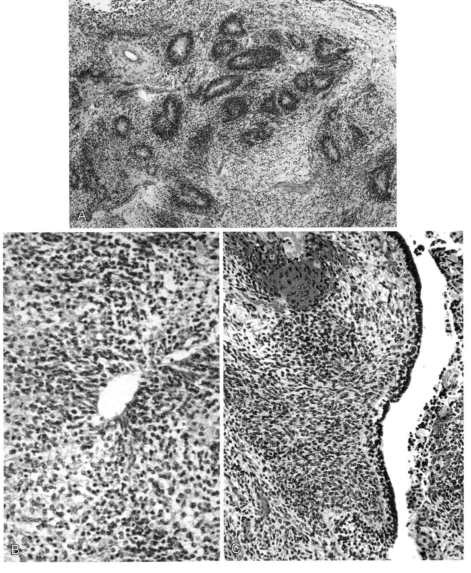

FIGURE 3

Grading of immature teratoma is based on the quantity of immature neuroepithelium, present as organized tubules **(A)** or disorganized primitive neuroecto-dermal cells **(B)**. Immature mesenchyme **(C)** for comparison.

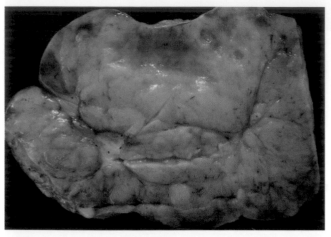

FIGURE 1

Mixed embryonal carcinoma and dysgerminoma. This tumor is predominantly dysgerminoma, and hence there is relatively little necrosis or hemorrhage.

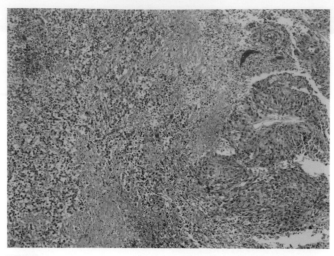

FIGURE 2

Embryonal carcinoma on the right versus dysgerminoma on the left.

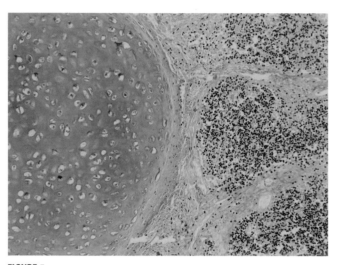

FIGURE 3

Mixed teratoma and yolk sac tumor. This focus contains immature cartilage and poorly preserved stroma.

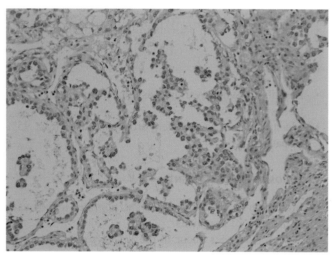

FIGURE 4

Mixed teratoma and yolk sac tumor. This focus contains yolk sac carcinoma.

THECOMA-FIBROMA

DEFINITION—A benign ovarian stromal tumor composed of cells resembling ovarian stroma with variable theca cell differentiation.

CLINICAL FEATURES

EPIDEMIOLOGY

- Fibromas are common, typically solitary, and found most commonly after menopause.
- Pure thecomas are rare and account for less than 1% of all ovarian tumors.
- Multiple fibromas can be encountered in Gorlin's syndrome, specifically in younger women.

PRESENTATION

- Unilateral ovarian mass (less than 5% are bilateral).
- Postmenopausal women; about a decade older than women with fibromas.
- Mean age is 59 years.
- Fibromas usually are not associated with endocrine manifestations but hyperestrinism is present in about half of patients with thecomas and usually present as abnormal uterine bleeding.
- Thecomas are associated with endometrial hyperplasia or low-grade endometrioid carcinomas.
- Luteinized thecomas present with androgenic manifestations in 10% of patients.
- Luteinized thecomas are rarely associated with sclerosing peritonitis.

PROGNOSIS AND TREATMENT

- Excellent; these are benign tumors.
- Excision is curative.

PATHOLOGY

HISTOLOGY

- *Thecoma:*
  - Grossly, thecomas are solid, smooth-surfaced masses with tan to yellow cut surfaces.
  - At low power thecomas are composed of nodules, sheets, and fascicles of plump spindled cells.
  - The tumor cells are fusiform, with vesicular oval nuclei, delicate nuclear membranes, and moderate to abundant amounts of palely eosinophilic cytoplasm.
  - Cytologic atypia is minimal, if present at all.
  - The stroma is composed of brightly eosinophilic collagen, and calcifications can be seen.
- *Luteinized thecoma:*
  - This type of thecoma is notable for the presence of either single luteinized cells or small clusters of luteinized cells.
  - The luteinized cells are small and round, with abundant clear cytoplasm.
- *Fibroma and Fibroma-thecoma:*
  - There is a significant degree of morphologic overlap between fibromas and thecomas; if there is a significant component of both, then the tumor should be termed "fibroma-thecoma" (the term thecoma should be reserved for tumors composed purely of thecoma cells).

IMMUNOPATHOLOGY AND SPECIAL STAINS (INCLUDING IMMUNOHISTOCHEMISTRY)

- Positive for inhibin (diffuse) and CD10.
- Negative for keratin.
- Reticulin demonstrates positivity around each individual cell.

MAIN DIFFERENTIAL DIAGNOSIS

- Adult-type granulosa cell tumor—spindled variants will exhibit nested cell groups by reticulin staining.

- Fibrosarcoma—a rare tumor with atypia and high mitotic index.
- Smooth muscle tumor—look for classic smooth muscle fascicles.
- Sclerosing stromal tumor—these tumors exhibit a classic regional pattern of fibrosis.

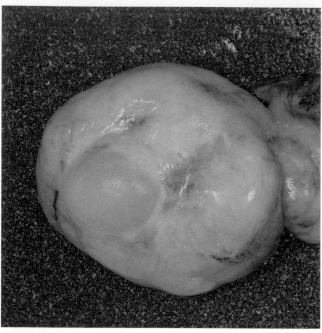

FIGURE 1

Thecoma gross image. Note the solid, vaguely nodular cut surface.

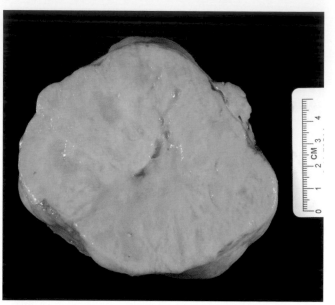

FIGURE 3

Luteinized thecoma. Note the yellow appearance in this gross image.

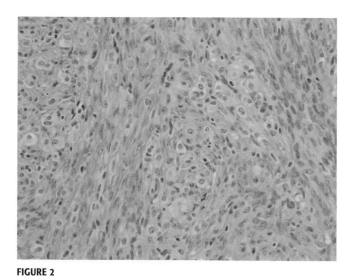

FIGURE 2

Thecoma-fibroma. Note the monotonous, somewhat fascicular population of bland cells. The nuclei are round to oval and have moderate amounts of cytoplasm.

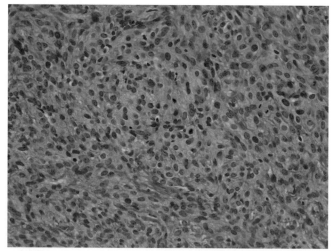

FIGURE 4

Luteinized thecoma. Note the plump-appearing cells with a vague spindled appearance.

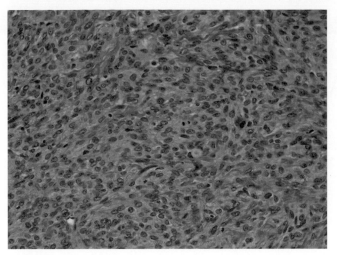

FIGURE 5

Luteinized thecoma. Note the plump-appearing cells with a vague spindled appearance.

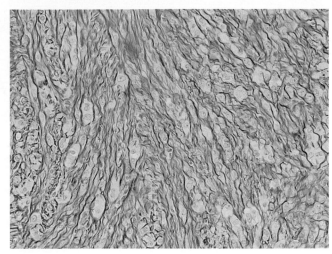

FIGURE 6

Thecoma-fibroma. A reticulin stain highlights individual cells. This is important for distinguishing this entity from a spindled granulosa cell tumor.

FIBROMA WITH MINOR SEX CORD ELEMENTS

DEFINITION—A benign ovarian fibroma with nests or cords of sex cord elements.

CLINICAL FEATURES

EPIDEMIOLOGY

- Rare.

PRESENTATION

- Incidental.
- Presentation is the same as that for typical fibroma.

PROGNOSIS AND TREATMENT

- Excellent; these are benign tumors.
- Excision is curative.

PATHOLOGY

HISTOLOGY

- At low power the majority of the tumor is identical to typical fibroma.
- The spindle cells are arranged in a storiform pattern with variable amounts of eosinophilic stroma.

- Scattered about the typical fibroma (accounting for less than 10% of the total tumor volume) are small tubules and/or cords of sex cord elements.
- The sex cord elements are composed of relatively large, epithelioid cells with abundant clear cytoplasm.

IMMUNOPATHOLOGY (INCLUDING IMMUNOHISTOCHEMISTRY)

- Positive (sex cord elements) for inhibin.
- Negative (sex cord elements) for keratin and EMA.

MAIN DIFFERENTIAL DIAGNOSIS

- Granulosa cell tumor—these typically appear as cellular fibromas or fibro-thecomas with nested spindled areas as opposed to discrete sex cord elements. A recticulin stain will distinguish these areas of spindled granulosa cell tumor from the fibroma.
- Sertoli cell tumor—this tumor exhibits a broader distribution of tubules or blends a more poorly differentiated spindle cell component with the tubules (as in an intermediate-grade tumor). Leydig cells will also be seen in many instances.

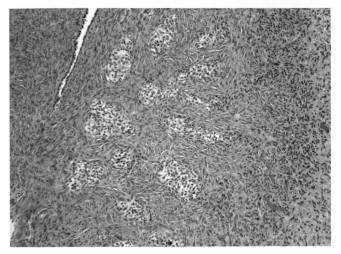

FIGURE 1

Fibroma with minor sex cord elements. At low power the background is that of a typical fibroma, but there is a second population of larger cells with abundant cytoplasm.

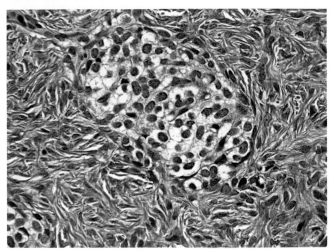

FIGURE 2

Fibroma with minor sex cord elements. At high power the sex cord elements are notable for their epithelioid appearance and nested growth pattern.

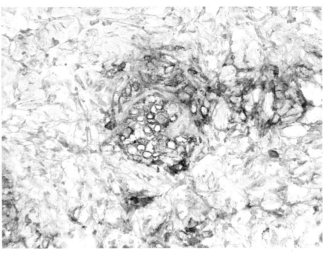

FIGURE 3

Fibroma with minor sex cord elements, inhibin stain. The sex cord elements are inhibin positive.

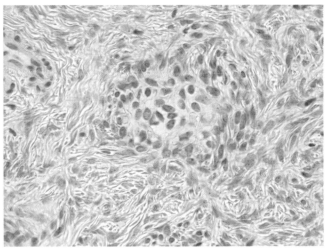

FIGURE 4

Fibroma with minor sex cord elements, keratin stain. The sex cord elements are keratin negative.

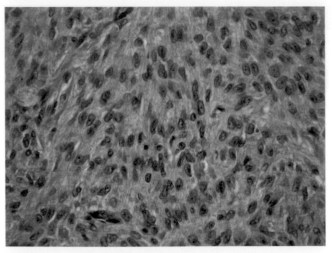

FIGURE 7
Adult-type GCT. Note the "coffee bean" nuclei.

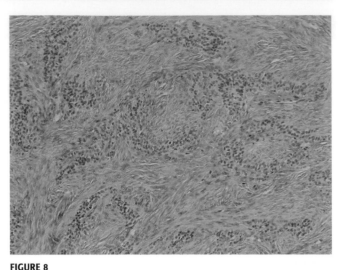

FIGURE 8
Adult-type GCT. The alternating tumor cell aggregates and fibrous stroma create a wavelet pattern (watered silk).

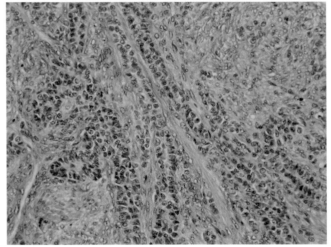

FIGURE 9
Adult-type GCT with a prominent trabecular pattern.

GRANULOSA CELL TUMOR VARIANTS

PITFALL

DEFINITION—Diagnostically challenging variant patterns include those with nuclear atypia, cystic architecture, thecoma-like, luteinized, and sertoliform.

CLINICAL FEATURES

EPIDEMIOLOGY

- Uncommon. The granulosa cell tumor (GCT) comprises less than 2% of ovarian tumors. Over 90% will be adult type (versus juvenile GCT).
- Perimenopausal or postmenopausal women.
- Mean age at presentation is in the mid-50s.

PRESENTATION

- Androgenic or estrogenic symptoms; anovulatory pattern endometrium on endometrial biopsy is typical.
- Unilateral ovarian mass (less than 10% are bilateral).

PROGNOSIS AND TREATMENT

- Most (more than 90%) of patients present with stage I disease, and the 10-year survival is at least 85%.
- Five-year survival for patients who present with more advanced disease (stage 2 and above) is less than 50%.
- Recurrence occurs within the first 5 years after diagnosis.

PATHOLOGY

HISTOLOGY

- Thecoma-like pattern is predominantly spindle cells. The important features of GCT are more rounded nuclei and focal loss of the spindle cell morphology. A reticu-

lin stain is key to identifying the nests of tumor granulosa cells.
- Cystic GCTs may mimic cystic follicles. The number of neoplastic granulosa cells in the cyst lining may vary, and multiple sections may be needed to reveal these cells.
- Nuclear atypia can be profound in both adult and juvenile GCTs. By itself it does not portend a worse outcome.
- The sertoliform variant may demonstrate ribbons or multiple acinar structures. The characteristic coffee bean nuclei and older age are helpful parameters for distinguishing this from a Sertoli-Leydig cell tumor.

IMMUNOPATHOLOGY (INCLUDING IMMUNOHISTOCHEMISTRY)

- Positive for calretinin, inhibin, and CD99.
- Negative for keratins (including CK7), EMA, and neuroendocrine markers.
- Reticulin staining will reveal nests of cells in the spindled variant.

MAIN DIFFERENTIAL DIAGNOSIS

- Spindle cell pattern—fibroma-thecoma, leiomyoma, and leiomyosarcoma.
- Cystic pattern: large follicle cyst.
- GCT with atypical nuclei—mesenchymal tumors and carcinosarcoma.
- Sertoliform—Sertoli cell tumor, trabecular carcinoid, and struma or strumal carcinoid.
- Luteinized—stromal luteoma and luteinized thecoma-fibroma.

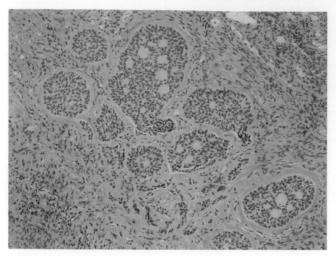

FIGURE 1

Microscopic GCT in the ovary.

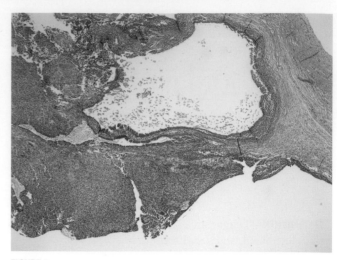

FIGURE 2

Cystic adult-type GCT.

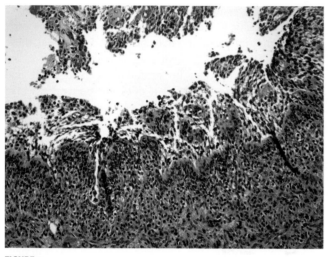

FIGURE 3

Cystic adult-type GCT. Note theca cells at the base of the granulosa cell–lined cyst.

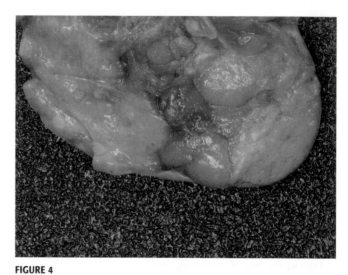

FIGURE 4

Luteinized adult-type GCT. Gross image. This luteinized example is solid and fleshy on cut section. Note the tan/white to yellow appearance.

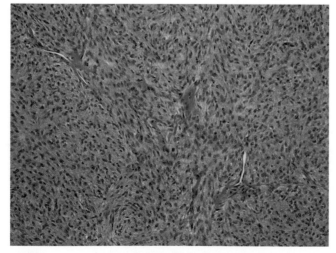

FIGURE 5

Luteinized GCT.

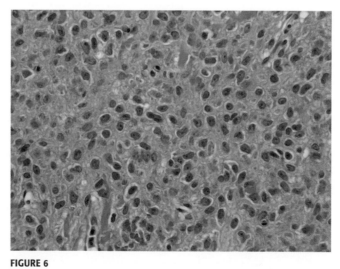

FIGURE 6

Luteinized GCT at higher power. Note the abundant cytoplasm and spaced nuclei.

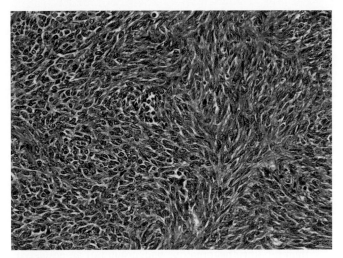

FIGURE 7

GCT with spindle features. The field at left has a faint nesting pattern in contrast to the more spindled appearance at upper right.

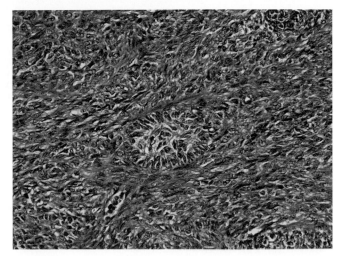

FIGURE 8

GCT with spindle features. Note the single sertoliform nest in the center.

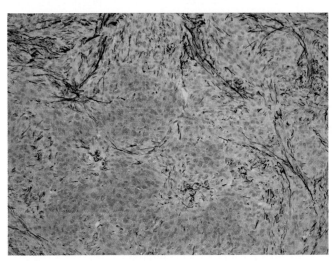

FIGURE 9

A reticulin stain highlights granulosa cell nests in a spindle cell GCT.

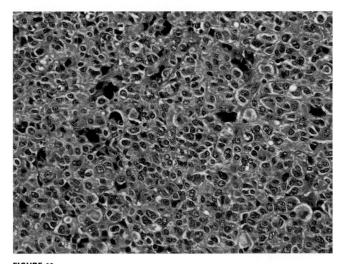

FIGURE 10

Adult-type GCT with marked atypia.

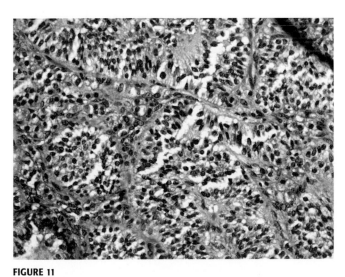

FIGURE 11

Adult-type GCT with tubules mimicking Sertoli cell tumor.

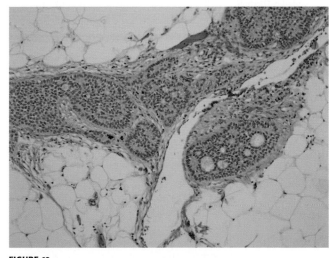

FIGURE 12

Metastatic GCT to the peritoneum.

JUVENILE GRANULOSA CELL TUMOR

PITFALL

DEFINITION—A sex cord–stromal tumor seen in the first decades of life that closely resembles the developing follicle.

CLINICAL FEATURES

EPIDEMIOLOGY

- Granulosa cell tumors (GCTs) comprise less than 2% of ovarian tumors.
- Juvenile GCTs comprise less than 10% of all GCTs.
- Accounts for only 10% of ovarian tumors in patients younger than age 20.
- Nearly all (more than 95%) occur before age 30, and 40% occur before age 10.

PRESENTATION

- Unilateral ovarian mass; less than 2% are bilateral.
- Isosexual pseudoprecocity is not uncommon in young patients, owing to estrogens produced by the tumor.
- In postpubertal patients, abdominal pain, swelling, and abnormal uterine bleeding are common presenting symptoms.

PROGNOSIS AND TREATMENT

- Prognosis and outcomes are closely linked to stage.
- More than 95% of patients present at stage Ia, and the 10-year survival approaches 90%.
- Surgical excision (unilateral salpingo-oophorectomy) is the treatment for early-stage tumors.
- Debulking and combination chemotherapy are reserved for advanced or metastatic disease.
- Less than 10% of patients experience disease recurrence.

PATHOLOGY

HISTOLOGY

- In contrast to the varied patterns of adult-type GCT, the juvenile-type GCT is characterized by a nodular and diffuse pattern of tumor cell growth.

- The cells are set in a myxoid or edematous matrix rather than the fibrothecomatous background of an adult-type GCT; in some cases, the background may be extensively hyalinized.
- Call-Exner bodies are rarely seen, but follicle-like spaces of various size and shape are prominently scattered throughout the tumor.
- The cells lining the cystic follicle-like spaces can exhibit a hobnail appearance.
- The tumor cells themselves are large and hyperchromatic, without prominent nuclear grooves.
- Cytologic atypia can be prominent, and atypical mitoses may be seen.
- The cytoplasm is relatively abundant and may be palely eosinophilic to vacuolated.
- Spindled theca cells can be seen surrounding tumor cell nodules or admixed with the granulosa cells.
- Foci of adult-type GCT are not uncommon.

IMMUNOPATHOLOGY (INCLUDING IMMUNOHISTOCHEMISTRY)

- Positive for inhibin and calretinin.
- Variably positive for WT1, EMA, keratin, S100, and SMA.

MAIN DIFFERENTIAL DIAGNOSIS

- Germ cell tumor—inhibin negative.
- Small cell carcinoma may be difficult given the presence of pseudofollicles; inhibin negative.
- Epithelial malignancy—rare cases of solid or undifferentiated epithelial growth; inhibin or calretinin negative.
- Adult-type GCT.

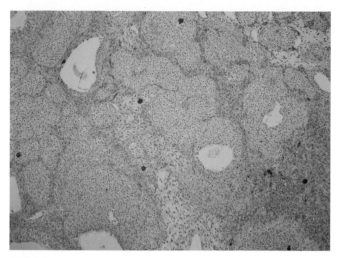

FIGURE 1

Juvenile-type GCT. The tumor is growing in a nodular pattern. Note the multiple follicle-like spaces.

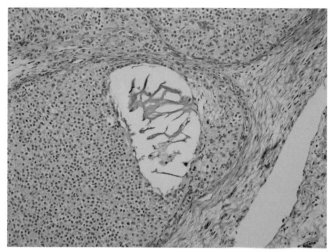

FIGURE 2

Juvenile-type GCT. Note the relatively abundant pale eosinophilic cytoplasm and the follicle-like spaces. Call-Exner bodies are absent.

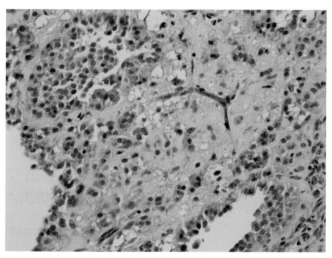

FIGURE 3

Juvenile-type GCT. At high power the myxoid background is apparent. Note the lack of nuclear grooves.

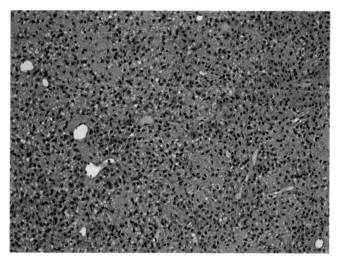

FIGURE 4

Juvenile-type GCT. In this image the background is alternately myxoid and hyalinized. The tumor cells are only mildly pleomorphic.

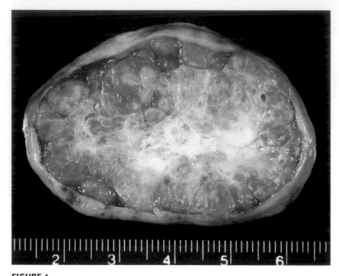

FIGURE 1

Sertoli-Leydig cell tumor (SLCT) with a characteristic golden brown appearance.

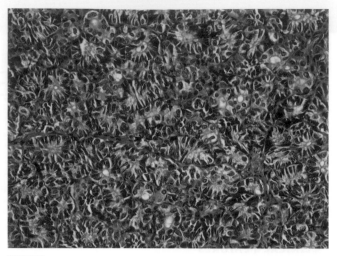

FIGURE 2

Well-differentiated SLCT with uniform tubules and interspersed Leydig cells.

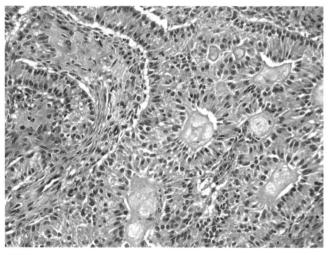

FIGURE 3

Well-differentiated SLCT with tall columnar cells lining tubules.

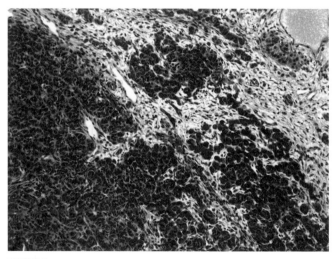

FIGURE 4

Intermediate SLCT with cordlike Sertoli cells in an edematous stroma.

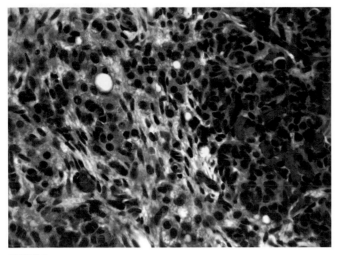

FIGURE 5
Intermediate SLCT with admixture of Sertoli cells and Leydig cells.

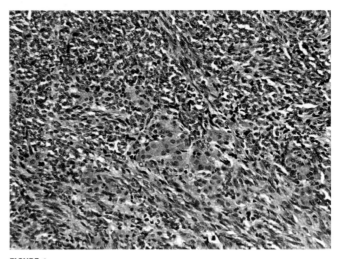

FIGURE 6
Poorly differentiated SLCT.

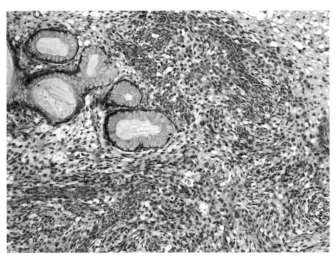

FIGURE 7
SLCT with heterologous elements.

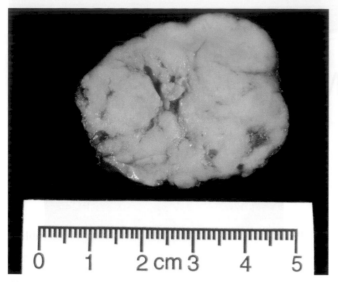

FIGURE 1

Sclerosing stromal tumor. The tumor shows a white to yellow appearance.

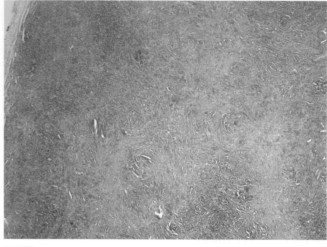

FIGURE 2

Sclerosing stromal tumor. Note the alternating cellular and more sparsely cellular collagenized zones.

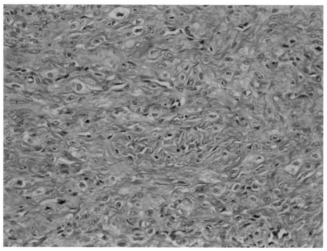

FIGURE 3

Sclerosing stromal tumor. Higher magnification depicts an area with prominent spindled fibroblasts and collagen deposition.

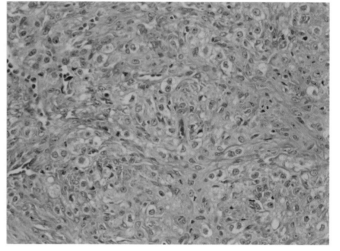

FIGURE 4

Sclerosing stromal tumor. In this area there are conspicuous luteinized cells within the collagen.

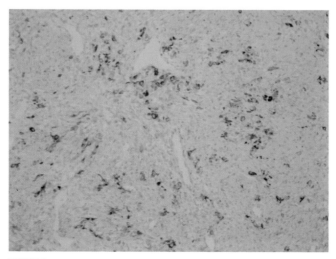

FIGURE 5

Sclerosing stromal tumor. The luteinized cells are strongly inhibin positive.

SMALL CELL CARCINOMA OF HYPERCALCEMIC TYPE

DEFINITION—A malignant rhabdoid tumor associated with hypercalcemia and mutations and inactivation in the SMARCA4 gene.

CLINICAL FEATURES

EPIDEMIOLOGY

- Presents between childhood and menopause, predominating in the late teens and early twenties.
- Rarely familial, but kindreds with mutations in the SMARCA4 gene have recently been described.

PRESENTATION

- Unilateral.
- Elevated calcium level in nearly two thirds.
- Extraovarian spread in half.
- Solid, lobulated, and cream colored with necrosis and hemorrhage.

PROGNOSIS AND TREATMENT

- These tumors have a high mortality. One third of stage Ia cases survived in one study.
- Most with higher stage will not survive, although occasional extended survivors have been reported with combination radiotherapy and chemotherapy with platinum-based agents and etoposide.

PATHOLOGY

HISTOLOGY

- Diffusely distributed, closely packed round tumor cells with a high nuclear-to-cytoplasmic (N/C) ratio and a high mitotic rate.

- Follicle-like structures, islets of cells, and cords or trabeculae.
- Variable cytoplasmic differentiation with large vesicular nuclei and prominent nucleoli. This can produce appearances of both small and large cell variants, particularly after chemotherapy.
- Occasionally other elements including mucin-producing epithelium.

IMMUNOPATHOLOGY (INCLUDING IMMUNOHISTOCHEMISTRY)

- Stains for WT1, p53, CD10, and EMA are usually positive.
- Neuroendocrine markers are typically negative.
- Staining for SMARCA4 should be negative due to loss of gene function.

MAIN DIFFERENTIAL DIAGNOSIS

- Sex cord–stromal neoplasms—inhibin positive.
- Primitive neuroectodermal tumor—EMA negative.
- Rhabdomyosarcoma—desmin positive.
- Intraabdominal desmoplastic small round cell tumor.
- Neuroblastoma—EMA negative.
- Metastatic pulmonary small cell carcinoma—chromogranin positive and TTF-1 positive.
- Small cell carcinoma of the ovary (neuroendocrine type)—chromogranin positive and will often exhibit other epithelial components.

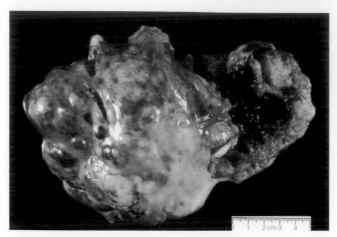

FIGURE 1

Small cell carcinoma, hypercalcemic type. Note the lobulated appearance, punctuated by hemorrhage and necrosis.

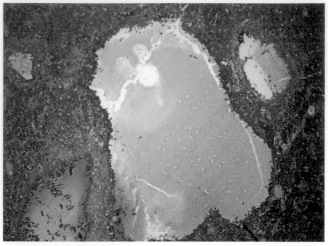

FIGURE 2

Small cell carcinoma, hypercalcemic type. At low magnification note the largely featureless landscape of blue cells punctuated by follicle-like spaces.

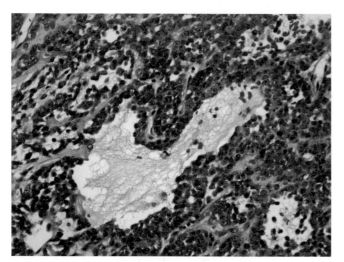

FIGURE 3

Small cell carcinoma, hypercalcemic type. At higher magnification another cystic space surrounded by small cells with a high N/C ratio.

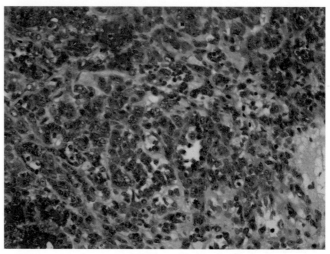

FIGURE 4

Small cell carcinoma, hypercalcemic type. Tumor cells are partially aligned in cordlike arrangements.

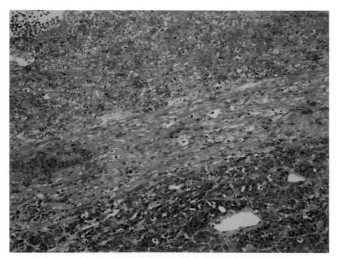

FIGURE 5

Small cell carcinoma, hypercalcemic type. An interface between viable tumor and necrosis with hemorrhage.

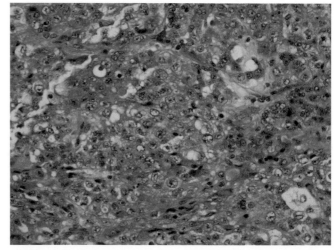

FIGURE 6

Small cell carcinoma, hypercalcemic type. Foci like this are seen in many tumors, with more abundant cytoplasm (large cell type), vesicular nuclei, and prominent nucleoli.

SMALL CELL CARCINOMA OF PULMONARY (NEUROENDOCRINE) TYPE

DEFINITION—A malignant small cell ovarian tumor with features of pulmonary neuroendocrine carcinomas.

CLINICAL FEATURES

EPIDEMIOLOGY

- Mean age of 48 years, which is over 20 years older than the small cell carcinoma of hypercalcemic type (SCCHT).
- *Not* associated with mutations in the SMARCA4 gene.

PRESENTATION

- Unilateral.
- Abdominal pain, nausea, and pelvic mass.
- Average duration of symptoms of 4 months (vs. 1 month for SCCHT).
- Solid tumor with necrosis and hemorrhage.
- Over half are stage 2 or greater when diagnosed.
- Elevated Ca125 in over 80%.

PROGNOSIS AND TREATMENT

- These tumors have a high mortality similar to SCCHT.
- Ten-year survival of 20%.
- Management is based primarily on chemotherapy (e.g., platinum, taxol, etoposide).

PATHOLOGY

HISTOLOGY

- Closely packed round tumor cells with a high nuclear-to-cytoplasmic (N/C) ratio and a high mitotic rate.

- Nuclear molding.
- Geographic necrosis.

IMMUNOPATHOLOGY (INCLUDING IMMUNOHISTOCHEMISTRY)

- Stains for chromogranin and synaptophysin are usually positive.
- Stains for vimentin and WT1 should be negative.
- Staining for SMARCA4 gene should be positive due to preservation of gene function.

MAIN DIFFERENTIAL DIAGNOSIS

- Sex cord–stromal neoplasms—inhibin positive.
- Primitive neuroectodermal tumor—EMA negative.
- Rhabdomyosarcoma—desmin positive.
- Intraabdominal desmoplastic small round cell tumor—desmin positive (dotlike pattern), WT1 positive, and EWS-WT1 gene fusion.
- Neuroblastoma—EMA negative.
- Metastatic pulmonary small cell carcinoma—chromogranin positive and TTF-1 positive.

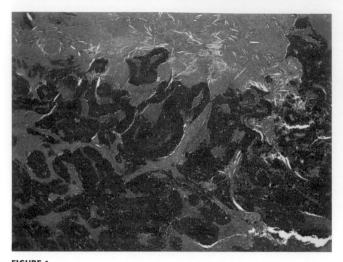

FIGURE 1

Small cell carcinoma, pulmonary type. At low magnification a featureless landscape of blue cells with necrosis.

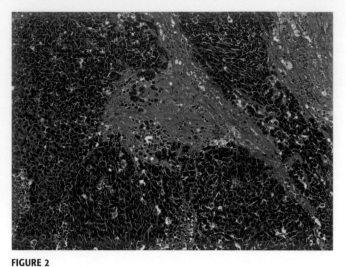

FIGURE 2

Small cell carcinoma, pulmonary type. At higher magnification, discohesive sheets of small tumor cells with necrosis.

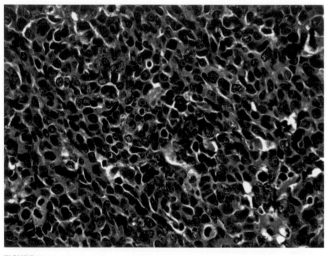

FIGURE 3

Small cell carcinoma, pulmonary type. At high magnification a nonuniform population of cells with dense nuclear chromatin and a high N/C ratio.

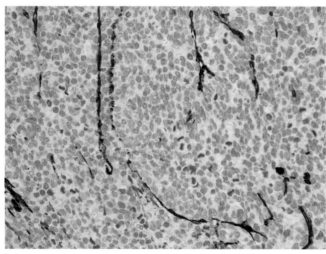

FIGURE 4

Small cell carcinoma, pulmonary type. A negative WT1 stain.

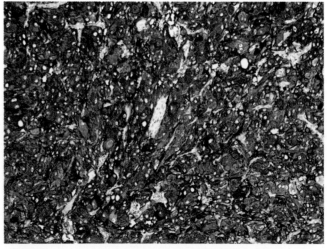

FIGURE 5

Small cell carcinoma, pulmonary type. Strong positivity for synaptophysin.

SEX CORD TUMOR WITH ANNULAR TUBULES

DEFINITION—A sex cord stromal tumor with annular tubules and features of both granulosa and Sertoli cell tumors.

CLINICAL FEATURES

EPIDEMIOLOGY

- These are rare tumors, comprising about 6% of sex cord stromal tumors and less than 1% of ovarian tumors.
- One third of cases are associated with Peutz-Jeghers syndrome.

PRESENTATION

- Typically (if not invariably) unilateral, larger, cystic, and solid in nonsyndromic cases, with a median age of presentation in the third decade.
- Typically bilateral, smaller, multinodular, and calcified when associated with Peutz-Jeghers syndrome, with a median age in the fourth decade.
- Can present with sexual precocity and abnormal bleeding.

PROGNOSIS AND TREATMENT

- Typically behave benign with excellent prognosis in cases associated with Peutz-Jeghers syndrome.
- Nonsyndromic tumors are considered low-grade malignancies similar to granulosa cell tumors. Approximately 10% behave in a malignant fashion.
- Spread is typically via retroperitoneal lymph nodes; hence nodal dissection is often performed.
- Recurrences treated by combination of chemotherapy and radiation.

- Recurrences can be followed by extended periods of remission.

PATHOLOGY

HISTOLOGY

- Multiple cystic and/or solid areas.
- Cysts or solid areas are punctuated by small annular tubules suspended in a matrix, surrounding eosinophilic hyaline bodies containing basement membrane material as seen on electron microscopy.
- Endometrium can exhibit hyperestrogenic features; in some cases even decidual change is seen with sexual precocity implying progesterone production as well.

IMMUNOPATHOLOGY (INCLUDING IMMUNOHISTOCHEMISTRY)

- Positive for inhibin.

MAIN DIFFERENTIAL DIAGNOSIS

- Either Sertoli or granulosa cell tumors may share features with sex cord tumor with annular tubules (SCTAT), but the latter has the classic repetitive tubules.

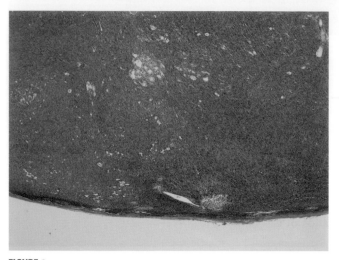

FIGURE 1

Gastrointestinal stromal tumor (GIST) involving the ovary and replacing the parenchyma.

FIGURE 2

At higher power the spindle cell population is arranged in rather compact but less sharply defined fascicles.

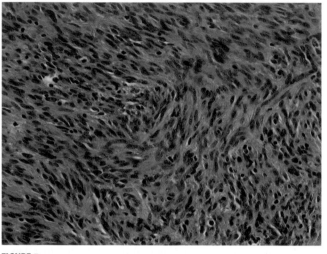

FIGURE 3

Fascicle formation in a GIST. Nuclei are elongated and show some palisading albeit less orderly than in a schwannoma.

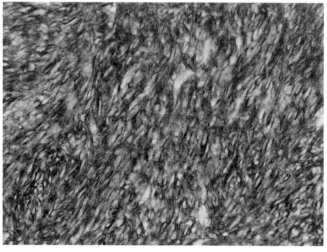

FIGURE 4

Staining for c-KIT is positive.

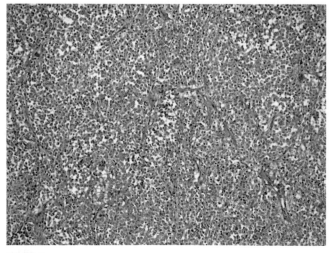

FIGURE 5

An epithelioid pattern in this GIST.

PRIMITIVE NEUROECTODERMAL TUMOR

DEFINITION—A rare, poorly differentiated embryonal neuroectodermal tumor sometimes associated with a teratoma that mimics the central type of primitive neuroectodermal tumor (PNET).

CLINICAL FEATURES

EPIDEMIOLOGY

- Extremely rare in the ovary.
- Belongs in the Ewing's family of tumors
- Ovarian tumors arise from neural tissue and are analogous to the "central" PNETs as opposed to the peripheral PNETs that contain a unique t(11:22)(q24;q12) translocation specific for the PNET/Ewing's sarcoma family.

PRESENTATION

- In the ovary the tumor may be found incidentally or within an enlarging teratoma.

PROGNOSIS AND TREATMENT

- In small series the prognosis was a function of stage, with over 80% surviving if the tumor was limited to the ovary. Stage III and IV tumors have a poor prognosis irrespective of radiation and chemotherapy.

PATHOLOGY

HISTOLOGY

- Monomorphic population arranged in sheets or nests with rosette-like structures in a fibrillar background (small, blue, round cell tumor).

- Often but not always associated with the primitive neuroepithelium of an existing immature teratoma.

IMMUNOPATHOLOGY (INCLUDING IMMUNOHISTOCHEMISTRY) AND OTHER STUDIES

- Strong CD99 staining characteristic of a central PNET.
- EWS/FLI-I chimeric RNA detected by reverse transcription polymerase chain reaction (RTPCR).

MAIN DIFFERENTIAL DIAGNOSIS

- In the ovary the main exclusion is an immature teratoma, which closely resembles embryonic neural tissue, whereas the PNET shows more anaplastic neural differentiation.

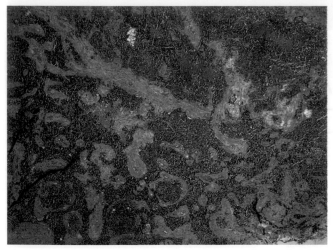

FIGURE 1

Desmoplastic small round cell tumor (DSRCT). A geographic arrangement of dense populations of oval cells in a desmoplastic stroma. Note the patchy necrosis.

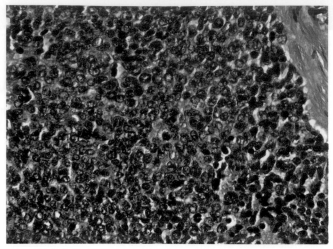

FIGURE 2

At high magnification the tumor cell displays a high N/C ratio, with crowding and nuclear overlap.

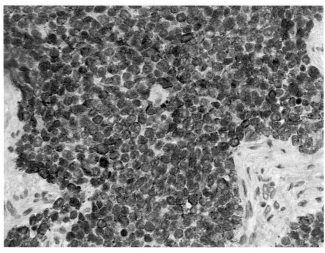

FIGURE 3

Cytokeratin staining in a DSRCT.

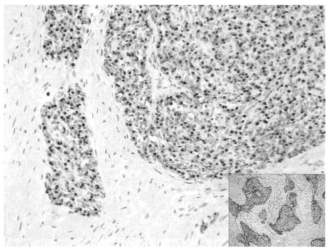

FIGURE 4

Dotlike desmin staining in this DSRCT (hematoxylin and eosin [H&E] in inset).

BENIGN CYSTIC MESOTHELIOMA

DEFINITION—A rare benign disease consisting of multiloculated mesothelial-lined cysts in the peritoneum. Also termed "multiloculated peritoneal cyst."

CLINICAL FEATURES

EPIDEMIOLOGY

- Rare.
- Reproductive-age women.
- History of a prior abdominal procedure or surgery is often noted.
- Controversy as to whether this is a neoplasm or reactive process.

PRESENTATION

- Most patients present with abdominal pain.
- Imaging studies show a peritoneal mass.
- Intraoperatively the multicystic mass is found attached to the peritoneum and/or abdominal and pelvic organs.

PROGNOSIS AND TREATMENT

- Excellent; this is a benign condition.
- Occasional recurrences.

PATHOLOGY

HISTOLOGY

- The gross appearance is that of a multicystic mass, with variably sized cysts.
- The cysts are filled by serous fluid.
- At low power the cysts have thin fibrous walls and are lined by a single layer of bland cuboidal cells.
- The lining cells are typically cuboidal to flattened, but occasionally hobnailing is apparent.
- Cilia are not present on the lining cells.
- Nuclear atypia can be seen, but mitoses are rarely identified.
- Solid growth of the mesothelial lining cells and/or invasion into adjacent stroma is not present.

IMMUNOPATHOLOGY (INCLUDING IMMUNOHISTOCHEMISTRY)

- Positive for calretinin, WT1, and cytokeratin.

MAIN DIFFERENTIAL DIAGNOSIS

- Benign serous cyst—this will be lined by a ciliated epithelium.
- Malignant mesothelioma—greater proliferation of mesothelial cells with tubulopapillary architecture (see Papillary mesothelioma).
- Cystic adhesions—these typically have much more delicate fibrous septa, often lined by flattened, rather cuboidal mesothelial cells.

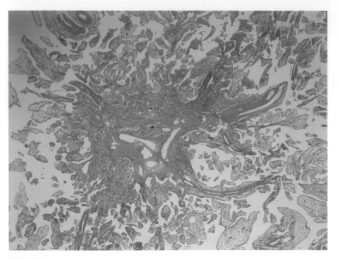

FIGURE 1

Well-differentiated papillary mesothelioma. This low-power microphotograph depicts the delicate papillae with mild stromal edema.

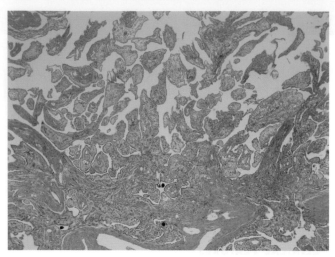

FIGURE 2

Well-differentiated papillary mesothelioma. Note the combination of papillary architecture and focal interdigitation with the underlying stroma *(bottom center)*.

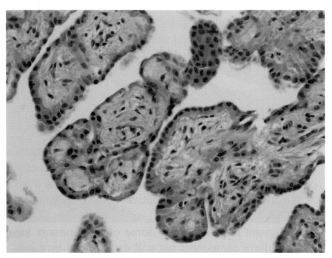

FIGURE 3

Well-differentiated papillary mesothelioma. Higher magnification showing a single layer of cuboidal lining cells without atypia.

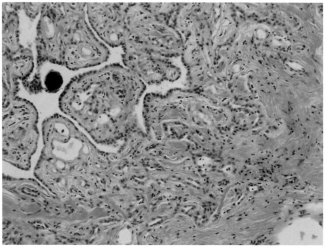

FIGURE 4

Interdigitation of small mesothelial cell-lined acini with stroma. This should not be confused with invasion (see Malignant Mesothelioma).

PAPILLARY MESOTHELIAL HYPERPLASIA

DEFINITION—A benign, reactive condition consisting of hyperplastic mesothelial cells seen in association with acute and chronic irritation of the peritoneal surface.

CLINICAL FEATURES

EPIDEMIOLOGY

- Papillary mesothelial hyperplasia is often found in cases of pelvic inflammatory disease, tubo-ovarian abscess, and upper genital tract tumors.
- Occasional cases may be associated with cardiac, renal, and hepatic insufficiency as well.

PRESENTATION

- Commonly found incidentally at the time of surgery or pelvic washings.
- Patients should not present with an abdominal mass or symptoms.

PROGNOSIS AND TREATMENT

- The prognosis is dependent on the inciting event; however, as this is a reactive process, no treatment is warranted.

PATHOLOGY

HISTOLOGY

- Mesothelial hyperplasia may present with a number of histologic patterns including solid, papillary, and tubulopapillary.

- The cells comprising the lesion are small with ample, eosinophilic cytoplasm; round nuclei; and variable (one to three) numbers of small, pinpoint nucleoli.
- Adjacent cells may display a cleft or "window" between them as a result of microvilli (seen ultrastructurally).
- Reactive mesothelial cells may be enlarged with more prominent nuclei and nucleoli.
- Mitotic figures are typically easily identifiable, and no necrosis should be present.

IMMUNOPATHOLOGY (INCLUDING IMMUNOHISTOCHEMISTRY)

- Several reports state that EMA is negative in reactive, hyperplastic mesothelial conditions and positive in malignant mesothelial conditions; however, this is controversial.
- Mesothelial cells, both benign and malignant, are positive for keratins, calretinin, WT1, h-caldesmon, and D2-40.

MAIN DIFFERENTIAL DIAGNOSIS

- Malignant mesothelial processes—these will demonstrate invasion and atypia.
- Implants of serous borderline tumor or low-grade serous carcinoma—distinction may be difficult in small foci, in which case special stains will usually discriminate mesothelial from epithelial (PAX8-positive and calretinin-negative) cells. However, we have seen cases that straddle this divide, with both calretinin and PAX8 staining.

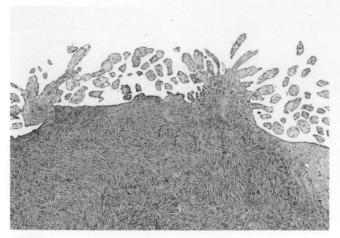

FIGURE 1

Papillary mesothelial hyperplasia. Papillary projections lined by mesothelial cells.

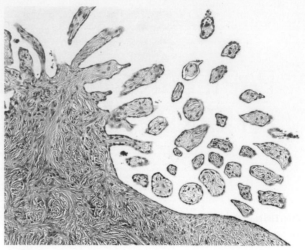

FIGURE 2

Papillary mesothelial hyperplasia. The lining cells are flattened; however, occasional cells with ample, eosinophilic cytoplasm can be seen in the upper right aspect.

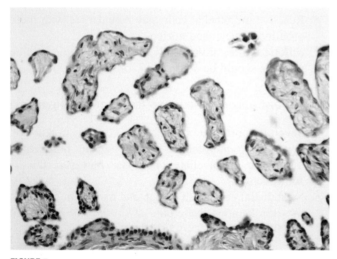

FIGURE 3

Papillary mesothelial hyperplasia. Indistinct cells with eosinophilic cytoplasm lining papillary structures.

MALIGNANT MESOTHELIOMA

DEFINITION—Malignancy comprised of mesothelial cells.

CLINICAL FEATURES

EPIDEMIOLOGY

- Malignant mesothelioma is an uncommon neoplasm that most often is found involving the pleura.
- Cases have been described within the abdomen; however, the majority of these cases have been described in men.
- The majority of cases occur later in life, between the sixth and ninth decades.
- Asbestos exposure is a risk factor for the development of mesothelioma, although some reports suggest that the association may not be as strong as in the pleural cavity.

PRESENTATION

- Patients present with ascites, abdominal swelling, and pain.
- Large lesions may present with mass effect or vague gastrointestinal symptoms.

PROGNOSIS AND TREATMENT

- The prognosis in malignant mesothelioma is poor.
- Numerous clinical and morphologic features such as age, extent of disease, completeness of resection, nuclear atypia, and mitotic rate have all been associated with outcome.
- Therapy consists of aggressive debulking with interoperative and perioperative intraperitoneal chemotherapy; however, with these treatment modalities the prognosis is still grim.

PATHOLOGY

HISTOLOGY

- Mesothelioma may have a strikingly heterogeneous growth pattern.

- The majority of tumors present with eosinophilic cells with an epithelioid cytology. Described patterns have included solid, papillary, tubular, and mixtures of all three.
- Tumors may appear well differentiated or very poorly differentiated, and frequently a sarcomatoid pattern may be focally present.
- The tumor cells are frequently round with moderate amounts of eosinophilic cytoplasm.
- The nuclei contain coarse, clumped chromatin and prominent nucleoli.
- Mitoses (including atypical forms), necrosis, and psammoma bodies are commonly identified.
- The tumor can be seen invading surrounding structures.

IMMUNOPATHOLOGY (INCLUDING IMMUNOHISTOCHEMISTRY)

- Mesothelial cells, both benign and malignant, are positive for keratins (CK5\6), calretinin, WT1, h-caldesmon, and D2-40 and should be negative for Ber-EP4, MOC31, and B72.3.

MAIN DIFFERENTIAL DIAGNOSIS

- Papillary serous carcinoma—both tumors can have a similar distribution. In virtually all cases this tumor will be PAX8 positive and calretinin negative or heterogeneous. Rarely tumors will be encountered that have both müllerian and mesothelial differentiation.
- Papillary mesothelioma—this is a well-differentiated variant without invasion.
- Unspecified high-grade sarcoma or carcinoma—some tumors will be difficult to classify and will necessitate immunostains to resolve or narrow the diagnosis.

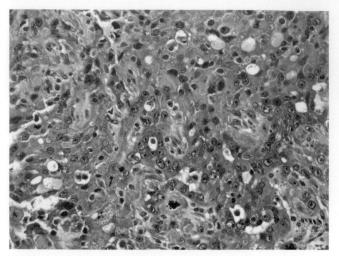

FIGURE 1

Malignant mesothelioma. Epithelioid malignant mesothelioma with marked atypia and prominent atypical mitotic figures.

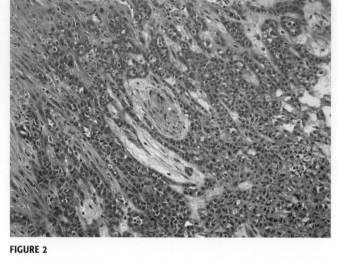

FIGURE 2

Malignant mesothelioma. Malignant cells arranged in a cordlike growth pattern. Note how the cells in this example are relatively monomorphic.

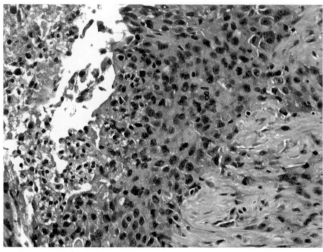

FIGURE 3

Malignant mesothelioma. Epithelioid malignant mesothelioma with large eosinophilic cells.

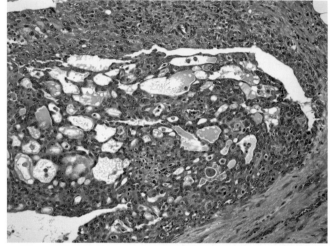

FIGURE 4

Malignant mesothelioma. Epithelioid malignant mesothelioma with pseudo-glandular spaces.

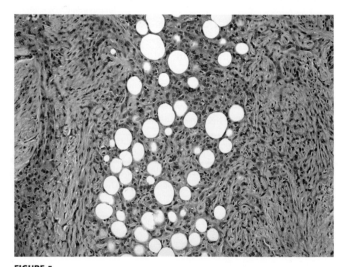

FIGURE 5

Malignant mesothelioma. Invasion of adipose tissue by malignant mesothelial cells.

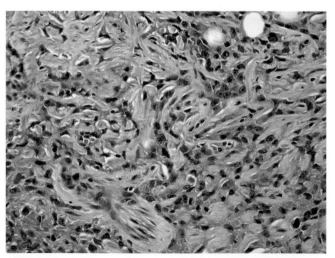

FIGURE 6

Malignant mesothelioma. Spindled (or sarcomatoid) growth in a malignant mesothelioma.

Gestational

GESTATIONAL SAC

DEFINITION—The membranous sac that envelops the developing embryo.

CLINICAL FEATURES

EPIDEMIOLOGY

- The gestational sac can be identified in the majority of samples from previable pregnancies.
- The gestational sac confirms an intrauterine pregnancy, even in cases in which embryonic tissue cannot be identified.

PRESENTATION

- In spontaneous abortions patients present with signs and symptoms of pregnancy loss, including cramping, vaginal bleeding, and passage of products of conception.
- In a missed abortion the patient has not yet passed the products of conception.
- The gestational sac can often be identified by the clinician at the time of dilation and curettage (D&C).

PROGNOSIS AND TREATMENT

- In a spontaneous or missed abortion, D&C is performed to ensure complete removal of the products of conception.
- If the ultrasound confirms no remaining products, treatment is not required.

PATHOLOGY

HISTOLOGY

- The gestational sac consists of a single scantly cellular layer of stroma lined by trophoblasts.
- A large cavitation is often present.
- The cavitation occasionally resembles the central cavitations seen in a molar pregnancy; however, all other features of a molar gestation are absent.
- An empty gestational sac should be suspected whenever a single, large, villouslike structure is identified.

IMMUNOPATHOLOGY (INCLUDING IMMUNOHISTOCHEMISTRY)

- Noncontributory.

MAIN DIFFERENTIAL DIAGNOSIS

- May be confused with a hydropic villous with a cistern, and hence misinterpreted as a molar pregnancy.

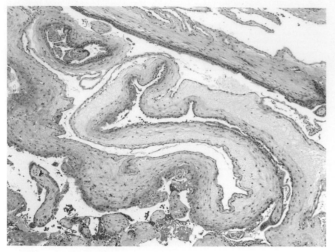

FIGURE 1

Gestational sac. Low power showing a minimally cellular stroma lined by a single layer of trophoblasts.

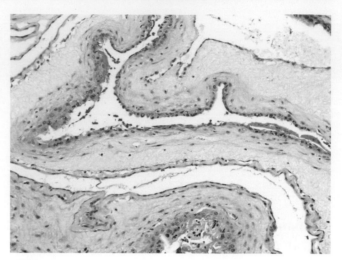

FIGURE 2

Gestational sac. The thin delicate lining is the amnion, and the shaggier side lined by large trophoblasts is the chorion.

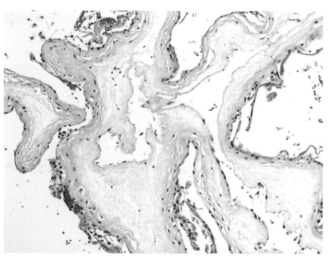

FIGURE 3

Gestational sac. A large central cavitation is present, but other features of a molar pregnancy are absent.

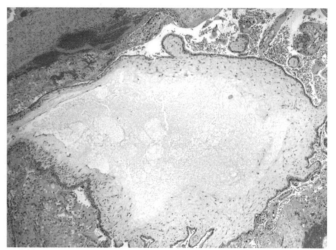

FIGURE 4

An empty gestational sac, resembling a hydropic villous.

FRESH IMPLANTATION SITE

PITFALL

DEFINITION—The area adjacent to the gestational sac where intermediate trophoblasts and fibrinoid can be found permeating the decidua.

CLINICAL FEATURES

EPIDEMIOLOGY

- Normal structure.

PRESENTATION

- Implantation site (IS) is frequently identified on the maternal surface of the placenta.
- In previable pregnancies it can be identified admixed with other products of conception.
- Identification of fresh IS can confirm an intrauterine pregnancy.

PROGNOSIS AND TREATMENT

- In a spontaneous or missed abortion, dilation and curettage may be undertaken to ensure complete removal of the products of conception.
- If the ultrasound confirms no residual products of conception, treatment is not required.

PATHOLOGY

HISTOLOGY

- IS is identified at scanning magnification by its brightly eosinophilic hue when compared with the background.

- The brightly eosinophilic material is known as Nitabuch's fibrin.
- Extravillous trophoblasts are identified migrating through the fibrinoid substance (Nitabuch's fibrin).
- The extravillous trophoblasts are dark and smudgy, with irregularly shaped nuclei and cytoplasm.
- There should not be significant trophoblastic atypia or mitotic activity in a normal IS.
- Mitoses are not identified.

IMMUNOPATHOLOGY (INCLUDING IMMUNOHISTOCHEMISTRY)

- Noncontributory.

MAIN DIFFERENTIAL DIAGNOSIS

- Decidua—decidual cells may at times appear atypical, usually as a function of degeneration, and may mimic implantation. A keratin stain will make this distinction, particularly if when excluding ectopic pregnancy.
- Molar IS—the extravillous trophoblasts are "more atypical" than usual, with larger and more hyperchromatic nuclei.
- Placental site nodule or older IS—these are composed of epithelioid extravillous trophoblasts arranged in a more homogeneous aggregate intertwined with fibrin-like material.

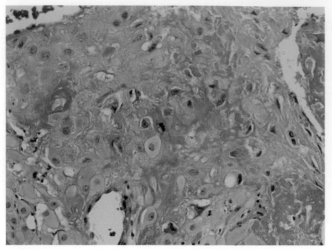

FIGURE 1

Fresh IS. Brightly eosinophilic fibrinoid material stands out from the background of decidualized endometrium. Dark, smudgy trophoblasts are scattered throughout Nitabuch's fibrin.

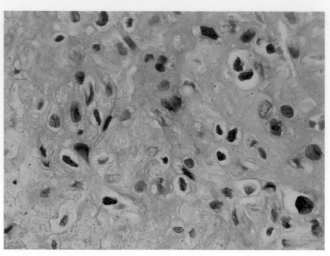

FIGURE 2

Fresh IS. The trophoblasts are irregularly shaped but not atypical. The chromatin is uniform and smudgy. The trophoblasts have abundant cytoplasm with indistinct cell borders. Mitoses are not present.

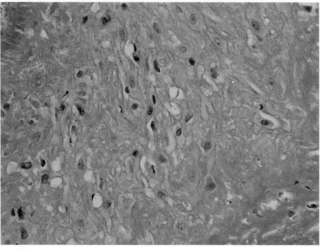

FIGURE 3

Fresh IS. In some areas the trophoblasts appear slightly spindled and also have prominent cell membranes in this focus.

IMPLANTATION SITE NODULE

DEFINITION—A collection of extravillous trophoblasts within hyalinized stroma, indicative of a previous pregnancy.

CLINICAL FEATURES

EPIDEMIOLOGY

- Implantation site nodules are common and typically have the same immunophenotype as epithelioid trophoblasts seen in the membranes, maternal surface, and intervillous fibrin.
- Can be identified in endometrial samples months to years following intrauterine pregnancies.

PRESENTATION

- The vast majority are identified incidentally upon endometrial sampling (or hysterectomy) for other indications.

PROGNOSIS AND TREATMENT

- Implantation site nodules are benign and incidental.
- No further treatment is warranted.

PATHOLOGY

HISTOLOGY

- Implantation site nodules are characterized by a collection of extravillous epithelioid trophoblasts set within hyalinized stroma.

- Fibrin is indicative of a recent implantation site and is by definition absent in placental site nodule (PSN).
- The trophoblasts show degenerative nuclear features.
- Nuclear atypia and mitotic activity are absent.

IMMUNOPATHOLOGY (INCLUDING IMMUNOHISTOCHEMISTRY)

- Ki-67 immunostaining may be helpful in determining the level of proliferative activity.
- Immunostains are noncontributory in the vast majority of cases. However, the cells should be immunopositive for inhibin and p63. Mel-cam staining will highlight only a subset of these cells in contrast to early implantation site.

MAIN DIFFERENTIAL DIAGNOSIS

- Implantation site, recent. This is early implantation site, not epithelioid trophoblast. Look for Nitabuch's fibrin.
- Exaggerated implantation site. This is an exaggeration of the early implantation site trophoblast and is not arranged in nodules. There will often be some Nitabuch's fibrin present.
- Epithelioid trophoblastic tumor, especially in small samples. Look for cellular atypia, increased proliferative (greater than 10% Ki-67 positive nuclei) activity.

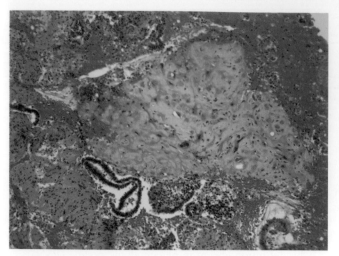

FIGURE 1

Implantation site nodule. At medium magnification a discrete fragment of hyalinized tissue is seen with a few hyperchromatic nuclei.

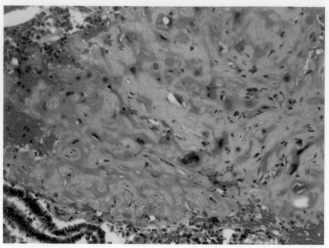

FIGURE 2

Implantation site nodule. At higher magnification a few hyperchromatic trophoblasts are seen in the hyalinized matrix. This matrix is composed of fibrinoid material elaborated by the extravillous trophoblast. A similar scenario plays out near the chorionic plate, within intervillous fibrin, and near the maternal surface of the placenta.

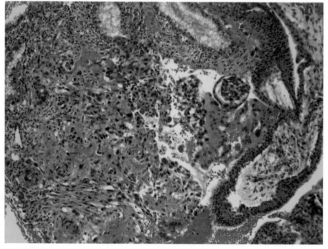

FIGURE 3

Implantation site in an early gestation. The origin of these cells is distinct from the implantation site nodule as they emanate from the trophoblastic columns during early gestation and invade the decidua and inner myometrium.

SPONTANEOUS ABORTION

DEFINITION—Unavoidable loss of viability in the first 12 weeks.

CLINICAL FEATURES

EPIDEMIOLOGY

- Approximately one third of clinically known pregnancies terminate in the first 12 weeks.
- Forty to fifty percent have a chromosomal anomaly.
- Twenty percent have trisomy aneuploidies, and 6% are triploid.
- The risk of a chromosomal abnormality increases with multiple losses.

PRESENTATION

- Typically detected on ultrasound as the absence of a fetus or abnormal fetal growth.
- Vaginal bleeding.

PATHOLOGY

HISTOLOGY

- Several important patterns should be appreciated that may cause confusion.
- Early previllous trophoblast may be confused with trophoblastic neoplasia.
- Villous enlargement and hydrops are common in early gestational loss. A key feature is the gradual differences in villous size that is typical of nonmolar pregnancies.
- Extravillous trophoblast may be exuberant; a key feature of benign trophoblastic changes is an eccentric orientation in the villi.
- Dysmorphic villi, scattered enlarged villi, and trophoblastic inclusions are features seen in aneuploidy gestations.
- Conspicuous cisterns in villi (a mimic is gestational sac) combined with prominent disparity in villous size are a feature of partial hydatidiform mole.

IMMUNOPATHOLOGY (INCLUDING IMMUNOHISTOCHEMISTRY)

- Noncontributory with the exception of p57kip2, which will exclude about 99% of early complete moles by its expression in cytotrophoblast and stromal cells.

MAIN DIFFERENTIAL DIAGNOSIS

- Choriocarcinoma—marked trophoblastic atypias.
- Placental site trophoblastic tumor (PSTT)—implantation site trophoblast atypias with clear-cut myometrial invasion.
- Early complete mole—diffuse mild villous enlargement, basophilic villous stroma, apoptosis, mild or moderate thickening of the villous trophoblast, and dysmorphic villi with knucklelike projections.
- "Partial mole" conspicuously enlarged villi, cisterns, some villous irregularity, and/or increased trophoblast.

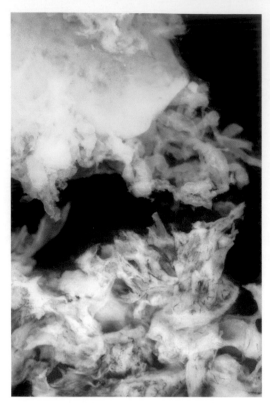

FIGURE 1

Dissecting microscopic image of early chorionic villi *(upper)*. Note the absence of vessels in contrast to the endometrial tissue *(lower)*.

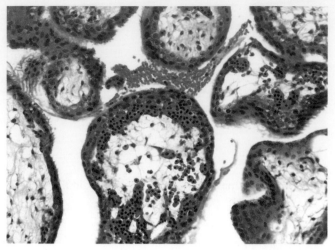

FIGURE 2

Immature chorionic villi at 6 weeks. Note the prominent nucleated red blood cells.

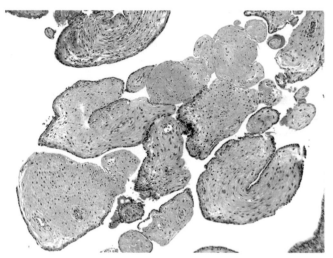

FIGURE 3

Villous sclerosis associated with embryonic death.

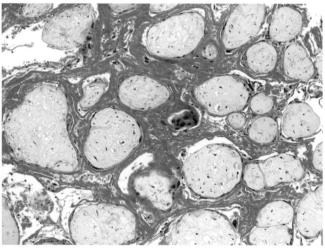

FIGURE 4

Villous edema with perivillous fibrin, commonly seen in early gestations.

ECTOPIC PREGNANCY

DEFINITION—Implantation of the embryo that occurs outside the uterine cavity or in an abnormal location within the uterus.

CLINICAL FEATURES

EPIDEMIOLOGY

- Ectopic pregnancies account for around 2% of all documented pregnancies in the United States.
- Ectopic pregnancy is associated with prior manipulation of the fallopian tube, infertility, and prior ectopic pregnancies. Ninety-five percent occur in the tube, 2.5% in the cornu, and the rest in the ovary.
- Inflammatory conditions, including pelvic inflammatory disease, affecting the fallopian tube are a major risk factor.

PRESENTATION

- Patients classically present with pelvic or abdominal pain and vaginal bleeding.
- Sexual and reproductive history, beta-HCG levels, and transvaginal ultrasound are helpful.
- If a gestational sac is not identified, endometrial sampling may be undertaken to rule out ectopic pregnancy.

PROGNOSIS AND TREATMENT

- If identified early and treated appropriately, ectopic gestations have a low, though significant, risk of maternal morbidity and mortality.
- Maternal morbidity and mortality are due to rupture and intraabdominal hemorrhage.

- If an intrauterine pregnancy cannot be identified, several treatment options exist including watchful waiting and medical management (methotrexate).
- Surgical exploration may be indicated in medically unstable patients.

PATHOLOGY

HISTOLOGY

- Endometrial samples from suspected ectopic pregnancies should be entirely submitted and carefully examined for evidence of uterine implantation.
- Structures that indicate the presence of a uterine pregnancy include embryonic tissue, placental villi, gestational sac, and fresh implantation site.
- Hormonally related endometrial changes, including Arias-Stella effect, are not sufficient to diagnose an intrauterine pregnancy and are often present in the setting of an ectopic pregnancy.

IMMUNOPATHOLOGY (INCLUDING IMMUNOHISTOCHEMISTRY)

- Noncontributory.

MAIN DIFFERENTIAL DIAGNOSIS

- Previous pregnancy (implantation site nodule).
- Shed tissue from an ectopic pregnancy (scant villi).
- Molar pregnancy.
- Contamination (i.e., "floaters") from another case.

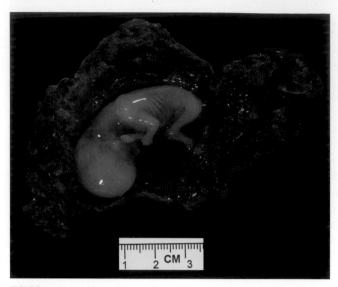

FIGURE 1

Tubal ectopic pregnancy. Gross example of an ectopic pregnancy discovered at a late stage in the fallopian tube.

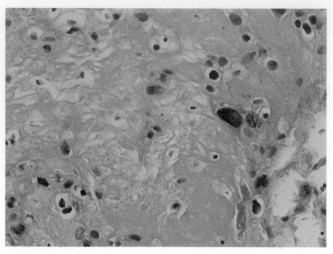

FIGURE 2

Example of fresh implantation site in an endometrial biopsy. This is indicative of an intrauterine pregnancy. However, be aware that a paired intrauterine and extrauterine gestation will occur in approximately one in 10,000 pregnancies.

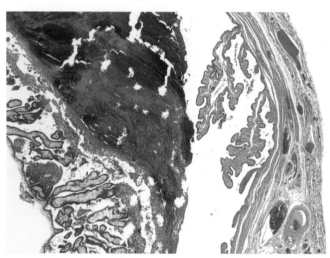

FIGURE 3

Ectopic pregnancy. Fallopian tube *(fimbria on right)* with immature placenta and implantation site with underlying hemorrhage.

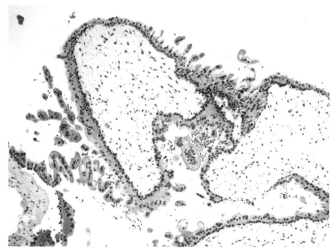

FIGURE 4

An ectopic molar pregnancy. This must always be excluded as it may often recur if unnoticed. High vascularity and elevated beta-HCG levels are common features but half are not suspected on ultrasound.

COMPLETE HYDATIDIFORM MOLE

PITFALL

DEFINITION—An abnormal gestation in which all of the genetic material is paternally derived.

CLINICAL FEATURES

EPIDEMIOLOGY

- Molar pregnancies have a biphasic age distribution, with increased incidence at the reproductive extremes: before age 20 and after age 40.
- Increased incidence has also been noted in women of Asian descent.
- Other risk factors include low socioeconomic status, prior molar pregnancies, and nulliparity.

PRESENTATION

- In classic complete hydatidiform mole (CHM) patients present with vaginal bleeding, vomiting, thyrotoxicosis, and markedly elevated levels of beta-human chorionic gonadotropin (HCG).
- Ultrasonographic evaluation shows a "snowstorm" or "Swiss cheese" appearance, which corresponds to the swollen, hydropic villi (hydatidiform, meaning grapelike).
- Early CHMs typically do not exhibit the classic signs and may be detected clinically as a missed abortion.
- In early CHM, beta-HCG levels are only mildly elevated.
- The diagnosis of an early CHM may not be apparent until histologic examination of the products of conception.

PROGNOSIS AND TREATMENT

- CHM carries a risk of developing a postmolar tumor.
- Initial treatment is usually evacuation of the uterus by suction dilation and evacuation (D&E), but hysterectomy may be employed in patients who have completed childbearing.
- Following D&E or hysterectomy, patients are followed with weekly serum beta-HCG determinations until they are normal for 4 consecutive weeks, then monthly for an additional 5 months.
- Approximately 15% to 20% of patients with CHM go on to develop persistent gestational trophoblastic disease (GTD), including 2% to 3% who develop choriocarcinoma.
- There are no histologic features that can predict which patients will develop progressive disease.
- Factors that are associated with an increased risk of recurrence include patient age, length of time to diagnosis, uterine size, and beta-HCG levels.
- Almost 100% of patients should be cured if followed appropriately.

PATHOLOGY

HISTOLOGY

CLASSIC (LATE) CHM:
- Late CHMs, those identified after 12 weeks, are characterized by a uniform population of large, hydropic villi with frequent central cavitations (cisterns).
- Trophoblastic hyperplasia is concentric, has a lacy appearance, and is conspicuous.
- Concentric trophoblast hyperplasia is often described as having a Medusa head–like configuration.
- Mild to moderate trophoblastic atypia is present but not necessarily conspicuous.
- Embryonic tissue, including nucleated fetal red blood cells, is absent.
- Atypical implantation site is often seen; however, this feature is also present in partial molar pregnancies.

EARLY CHM:
- Early CHMs, those presenting at 8 to 12 weeks gestation, are often grossly indistinguishable from a missed abortion.
- Villous morphology is the most helpful feature.

741

PARTIAL HYDATIDIFORM MOLE

DEFINITION—Gestational trophoblastic disease in which the conceptus contains a triploid (3n) amount of genetic material (typically 1n maternal and 2n paternal).

CLINICAL FEATURES

EPIDEMIOLOGY

- Partial moles are 10 times more common than complete moles.
- The risk factors for partial molar pregnancy are the same as for complete molar pregnancy and include age greater than 40 and less than 20, Asian descent, low socioeconomic status, prior molar pregnancies, and nulliparity.

PRESENTATION

- The majority present as a missed abortion with vaginal bleeding and a small uterus.
- Beta-human chorionic gonadotropin (HCG) levels are only mildly elevated.
- Partial mole is not suspected clinically in most cases.

PROGNOSIS AND TREATMENT

- Partial hydatidiform moles are associated with low risk of developing postmolar persistent disease (less than 15%) and choriocarcinoma (less than 1%).
- Therapy consists of complete removal (suction curettage) of the products of conception.
- Serial beta-HCG levels are checked weekly until normal values are attained.
- Follow-up beta-HCG levels are then followed monthly for 6 months.
- In addition, patients complete a 6-month course of contraceptive therapy.

PATHOLOGY

HISTOLOGY

- Partial moles consist of a biphasic population of small, fibrotic, normal villi and larger hydropic villi.

- The hydropic villi may display cistern formation and may have focal trophoblastic proliferation.
- The larger, dysmorphic villi will frequently have a scalloped contour resembling knuckles or fingers and toes.
- Trophoblastic "inclusions" are present within the villous stroma.
- These "inclusions" represent tangential sectioning of the irregular villous surface.
- Villous blood vessels, fetal nucleated red blood cells, membranes, and fetal parts may be identified and are a helpful finding in distinguishing from an early complete mole.
- Implantation site atypia may be present but is much less common that in complete moles.
- If fetal tissues are identified, they may contain malformations.
- The most common finding in association with partial moles is syndactyly (fusion) of the third and fourth or second and third fingers.

IMMUNOPATHOLOGY (INCLUDING IMMUNOHISTOCHEMISTRY)

- The villous mesenchymal cells and cytotrophoblasts are positive for p57.

MAIN DIFFERENTIAL DIAGNOSIS

- Early complete mole. Look for dysmorphic villi, basophilic stroma, loss of p57kip2 staining in stromal cells, and cytotrophoblast.
- Hydropic abortus. The distinction from partial mole is not always possible but uniform swelling of villi and graduated variations in villous size with absence of cisterns is helpful.
- Nonmolar aneuploidy. Typically differences in villous size are not marked and cisterns are absent.
- Mesenchymal dysplasia. Seen as asymmetric enlargement of stem villi. Cisterns are absent as is trophoblastic proliferation.

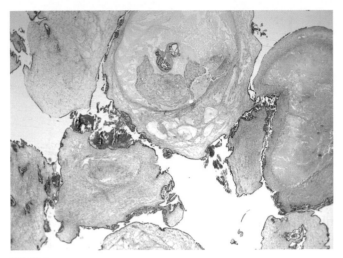

FIGURE 1

Partial hydatidiform mole. Low-power image showing a dual population of large edematous villi and smaller, more fibrotic-appearing villi.

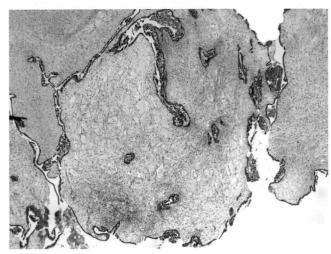

FIGURE 2

Partial hydatidiform mole. Large edematous villi with several so-called trophoblastic "inclusions." The villous contours are irregular. Concentric trophoblastic hyperplasia is not present.

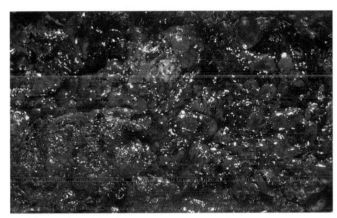

FIGURE 3

Immature placenta with focal villous hydrops suggesting partial mole.

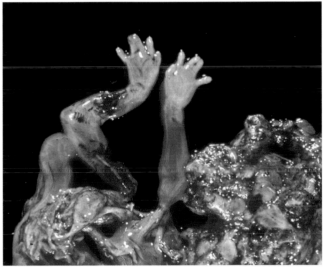

FIGURE 4

Characteristic 3-4 syndactyly in a triploid fetus associated with a partial mole.

CHORIOCARCINOMA

DEFINITION—A trophoblastic malignancy composed of syncytiotrophoblasts and cytotrophoblasts, intermediate trophoblasts of both.

CLINICAL FEATURES

EPIDEMIOLOGY

- At least half of choriocarcinomas follow a molar pregnancy, but only 2% to 3% of complete moles are followed by a diagnosis of choriocarcinoma.
- The remainder of choriocarcinomas follow a spontaneous abortion (25%), a normal gestation (20%), or an ectopic pregnancy (2.5%).
- Rare cases occurring more than a decade after the last gestation have been described.

PRESENTATION

- Choriocarcinoma is typically detected several months after pregnancy.
- Elevated serum beta-human chorionic gonadotropin (HCG).
- Patients present with abnormal uterine bleeding, which is due to endomyometrial invasion by choriocarcinoma.
- A metastatic lesion involving (in decreasing order of frequency) the lungs, brain, or liver is a not uncommon presentation.
- Because most patients are treated with chemotherapy based on their beta-HCG levels and imaging studies, the histologic diagnosis is not made in many patients (i.e., invasive mole vs. choriocarcinoma).

PROGNOSIS AND TREATMENT

- Cases that are detected early and treated with appropriate chemotherapy have better outcomes than patients who present later in the course of their disease.
- Advanced disease may be fatal despite aggressive surgical and medical therapy.
- Choriocarcinoma occurring after a diagnosis of complete hydatidiform mole is thought to have a better prognosis, although this is likely due to close clinical follow-up of these patients.
- Even with appropriate therapy, choriocarcinoma is fatal in about 10% of cases.

PATHOLOGY

HISTOLOGY

- Choriocarcinoma presents as a hemorrhagic, well-circumscribed nodule within the endomyometrium.
- Microscopic sections are characterized by a biphasic tumor composed of multinucleated syncytiotrophoblasts and either cytotrophoblasts or intermediate trophoblasts.
- Marked cytologic and nuclear atypia are common.
- In some cases only rare syncytiotrophoblasts can be identified.
- A background of abundant hemorrhage and necrosis is typical.
- In some cases only rare syncytiotrophoblasts can be identified.
- Placental villi should not be present.

IMMUNOPATHOLOGY (INCLUDING IMMUNOHISTOCHEMISTRY)

- Both syncytiotrophoblasts and intermediate trophoblasts are for HCG and for hPL.
- Syncytiotrophoblasts are strongly positive for HCG whereas intermediate trophoblasts are only weakly positive.
- All of the trophoblastic tumor cells should stain strongly and diffusely for cytokeratin.
- Inhibin is negative.

MAIN DIFFERENTIAL DIAGNOSIS

- Residual benign trophoblasts from an early gestation.
- Persistent molar tissue—this will be seen as atypical implantation site. Presence of villi effectively excludes choriocarcinoma. Necrosis should be minimal.
- Invasive mole—defined as villi in the myometrium excluding choriocarcinoma.

- Placental site trophoblastic tumor—lacks the biphasic trophoblast of choriocarcinoma and the high serum b-HCG levels.
- Undifferentiated carcinoma, particularly in metastatic lesions—typically seen in older age groups. Serum HCG is low.

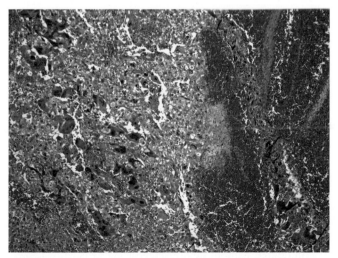

FIGURE 1

Gross appearance of choriocarcinoma, consisting of a hemorrhagic mass involving the endomyometrium.

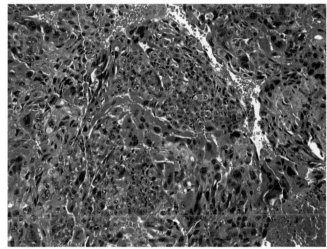

FIGURE 3

Choriocarcinoma. A biphasic carcinoma with characteristic wrapping by the syncytiotrophoblasts. Marked cytologic atypia is present in both populations of trophoblasts.

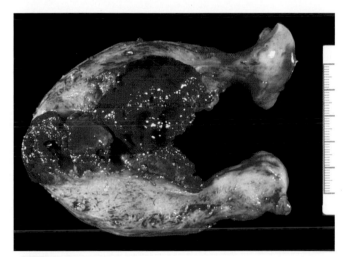

FIGURE 2

Choriocarcinoma. Low-power image shows a hemorrhagic and necrotic background. A clearly biphasic tumor is present.

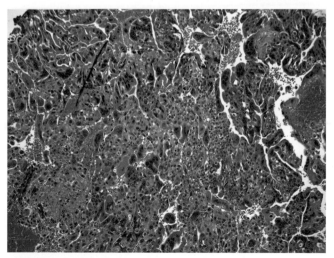

FIGURE 4

Choriocarcinoma. A biphasic carcinoma composed of an admixture of trophoblasts. Biphasic atypia is apparent.

INTRAPLACENTAL CHORIOCARCINOMA

PITFALL

DEFINITION—Choriocarcinoma occurring concurrently with a normal pregnancy.

CLINICAL FEATURES

EPIDEMIOLOGY

- Intraplacental choriocarcinoma is exceedingly rare.

PRESENTATION

- Intraplacental choriocarcinoma is occasionally diagnosed before delivery when symptomatic metastasis occurs.
- In rare cases the disease is diagnosed when the infant presents in early life with metastatic disease.
- Disease is most often detected at the time of placental examination.

PROGNOSIS AND TREATMENT

- Patients with disease that is detected early and treated with appropriate chemotherapy have a better outcome than patients who present later in the course of their disease.
- Beta-human chorionic gonadotropin (HCG) can be followed in both the mother and the newborn to monitor for metastatic disease, which can be fatal.
- Systemic chemotherapy is the most common treatment modality.
- Hysterectomy is performed in some cases.

PATHOLOGY

HISTOLOGY

- Grossly, intraplacental choriocarcinoma mimics placental infarction and appears as either single or multiple scattered tan nodules.

- Microscopic examination demonstrates a solid nodule composed of an admixture of atypical cytotrophoblastic and syncytiotrophoblastic cells.
- The tumor cells are present in the intervillous spaces and are histologically similar to choriocarcinoma seen in other settings.
- Both components are markedly atypical.

IMMUNOPATHOLOGY (INCLUDING IMMUNOHISTOCHEMISTRY)

- Cytokeratins are diffusely positive in the tumor cells.
- Syncytiotrophoblasts are strongly positive for HCG and weakly positive for human placental lactogen (hPL).
- Intermediate trophoblasts are weakly positive for both HCG and hPL.

MAIN DIFFERENTIAL DIAGNOSIS

- Complete hydatidiform mole—this is not a problem in the mature placenta. It can be a difficult distinction in a postmolar curetting without villi.
- Intraplacental trophoblastic proliferation with admixed fibrin—these occasionally occur, but the trophoblasts are extravillous in nature.
- Chorangioma-associated trophoblastic proliferation—this can be striking at times, and there have been rare reports of so-called "chorangiocarcinoma." However, the trophoblastic proliferation in chorangiomas is typically adherent to the exterior of the tumor and is modest in degree without hemorrhage or necrosis.

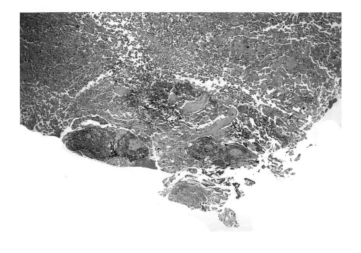

FIGURE 1

Intraplacental choriocarcinoma. Low-power image depicts a discrete proliferation of atypical epithelioid cells present in the intervillous spaces.

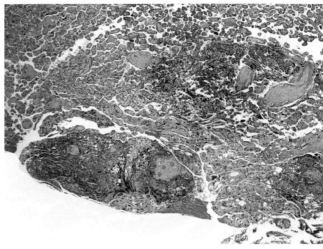

FIGURE 2

Intraplacental choriocarcinoma. Low-power image depicts a discrete proliferation of atypical epithelioid cells present in the intervillous spaces.

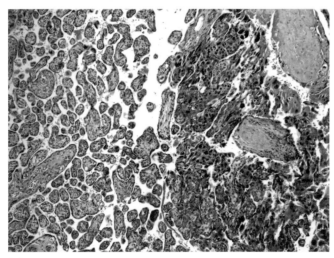

FIGURE 3

Intraplacental choriocarcinoma. Note the juxtaposed normal placental parenchyma and the highly atypical trophoblastic epithelium of the intraplacental
choriocarcinoma. The neoplastic epithelium is associated with sclerotic villous
remnants.

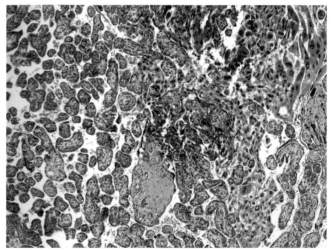

FIGURE 4

Intraplacental choriocarcinoma. Another field illustrating the marked disparity
in trophoblastic density between tumor *(center)* and surrounding villi.

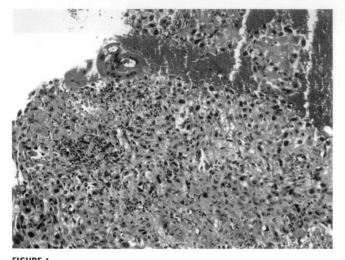

FIGURE 1

Molar IS. Brightly eosinophilic fibrinoid material is infiltrated by a population of atypical cells with dark, irregularly shaped nuclei. Compare to nonmolar IS.

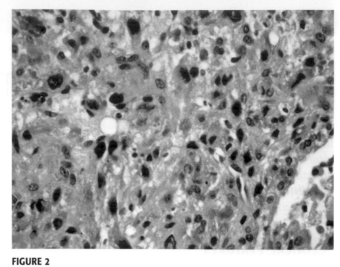

FIGURE 2

Molar IS. At higher magnification note that virtually all of the extravillous trophoblasts are hyperchromatic.

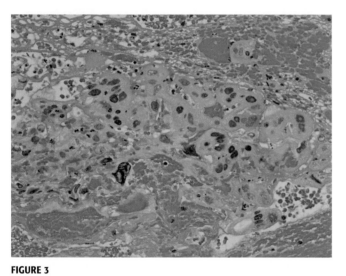

FIGURE 3

Molar IS. The trophoblasts are well spaced in the fibrinoid matrix but note the considerable variations in nuclear size and staining.

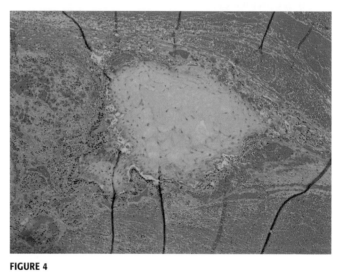

FIGURE 4

A rare degenerating molar villous was associated with the molar IS shown in Figure 3.

EPITHELIOID TROPHOBLASTIC TUMOR

DEFINITION—A subset of extravillous trophoblastic tumor that is thought to arise from an extravillous (transitional) trophoblast that forms a transition from villous cytotrophoblast to mature extravillous trophoblast. These cells are found in the chorionic membrane, maternal surface of the placenta, and where intervillous fibrin is deposited.

CLINICAL FEATURES

EPIDEMIOLOGY

- Rare.
- Occurs in reproductive-age women.
- Epithelioid trophoblastic tumors (ETTs) are an unusual type of extravillous trophoblastic tumor.
- Both ETTs and placental site trophoblastic tumors (PSTTs) are almost always seen following a term delivery.

PRESENTATION

- Patients present with irregular vaginal bleeding.
- The preceding pregnancy may have been months or years earlier.
- The beta-human chorionic gonadotropin (HCG) level is only mildly increased.
- The clinical impression may be that of a missed abortion.
- Uterine enlargement or an intrauterine mass may be identified. Occasional cases are found outside the uterus, presumably from residual trophoblasts exposed to the peritoneal cavity following cesarean section.
- Patients may have metastatic disease at the time of diagnosis.

PROGNOSIS AND TREATMENT

- The prognosis is variable.
- Features associated with adverse clinical outcome include increased mitotic rate (>5 mitosis per 10 hpf) and presentation more than 2 to 4 years after previous pregnancy.
- The majority of patients undergo hysterectomy.
- Adjuvant chemotherapy may be appropriate in some cases.

PATHOLOGY

HISTOLOGY

- Grossly, ETT appears as a solitary, circumscribed, solid and cystic hemorrhagic mass that invades into the myometrium or cervical stroma.
- Microscopically ETT is composed of medium-sized, relatively monomorphic epithelioid cells with prominent cell borders that resemble intermediate trophoblasts.
- The cells have abundant eosinophilic cytoplasm and are arranged in nests and cords which coalesce to form large expansile sheets and nodules of tumor.
- Occasional large or markedly atypical cells can be seen, but overall, ETT has a bland uniform appearance.
- A prominent hyalinized eosinophilic extracellular material is present and often associated with necrotic debris.
- In some cases ETT grows along the surface of the endometrium and cervix and can resemble an in situ cervical squamous lesion.

IMMUNOPATHOLOGY (INCLUDING IMMUNOHISTOCHEMISTRY)

- Negative for human placental lactogen (hPL), and only focally positive for MelCAM.
- Positive for p63, inhibin, and cytokeratins (AE1/AE3).
- Ki-67 labeling indexes of less than 10% are consistent with an placental site nodule.

CHORANGIOMA

DEFINITION—Benign expansile nodule of capillaries and stromal cells.

CLINICAL FEATURES

EPIDEMIOLOGY

- Uncommon; this finding is seen in less than 0.5% of placentas.
- Associated with twin gestations and preeclampsia.

PRESENTATION

- Term placenta.
- Incidental firm, tan nodule located at the disk edge or in the subchorion.

PROGNOSIS AND TREATMENT

- Varies with size; small lesions are nearly always incidental.
- Intermediate-sized lesions are associated with intrauterine growth restriction and may be noted on ultrasound examination.
- Large lesions (>9 cm) can cause arteriovenous shunting and subsequent polyhydramnios, hydrops, and even fetal death.
- Platelet sequestration within the chorangioma can rarely lead to disseminated intravascular coagulation in the fetus.

PATHOLOGY

HISTOLOGY

- A circumscribed nodule of small capillary channels is apparent at low power.
- Within the nodule there are varying amounts of bland stromal cells and collagen separating vascular spaces.
- In localized chorangiosis the changes are isolated to a single-stem villous, with all of the smaller villi containing excess numbers of capillary channels.
- An area of distended villous capillary channels should not be mistaken for chorangiosis.

IMMUNOPATHOLOGY (INCLUDING IMMUNOHISTOCHEMISTRY)

- Noncontributory.

MAIN DIFFERENTIAL DIAGNOSIS

- Intraplacental choriocarcinoma—the extravillous trophoblast at the periphery of a chorangioma will sometimes display some atypias that might be mistaken for a trophoblastic neoplasm. There have been rare reports of "chorangiocarcinomas" that might be an extreme example. However, the vast majority of trophoblastic proliferations on the perimeter of a chorangioma are benign.
- Diffuse chorangiosis—this will usually not be a problem, inasmuch as the process is not as discrete as a chorangioma.

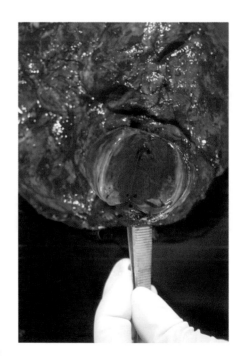

FIGURE 1

Chorangioma, shown here in the parenchyma as a discrete circumscribed red nodule with a pale rim.

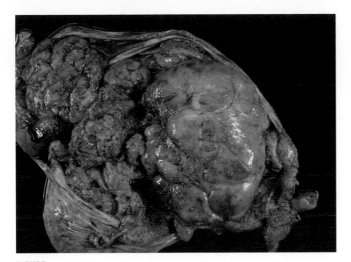

FIGURE 2

A very large chorangioma on the right side of the placental disk.

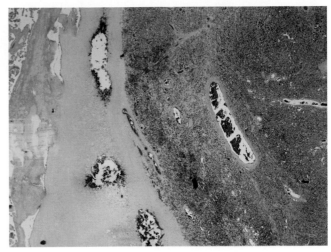

FIGURE 3

Chorangioma. Low-power image showing a circumscribed nodule within the placental parenchyma.

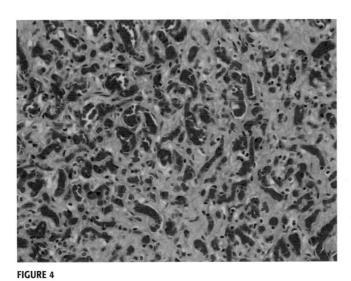

FIGURE 4

A proliferation of small, capillary-sized channels lined with a single layer of bland endothelial cells. The stroma is composed of dense eosinophilic material and scattered bland stromal cells.

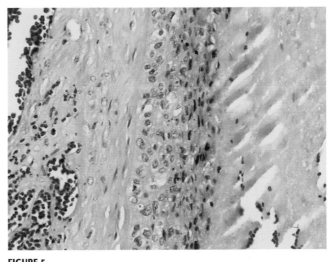

FIGURE 5

Extravillous trophoblast on the perimeter of the chorangioma might show some nuclear atypia.

KNOTS IN THE UMBILICAL CORD

DEFINITION—True knots in the umbilical cord.

CLINICAL FEATURES

EPIDEMIOLOGY

- Uncommon, occurring in 1% to 2% of pregnancies.
- Nuchal cord (around neck) is more common, in up to 25% of pregnancies.
- Constricting knots rarer, approximately 1:2000 pregnancies.
- Associated with large babies, long umbilical cords.

PRESENTATION

- Most often an incidental finding when not constricting.
- Reduced fetal movement if constriction and hypoxia occur.

- Rarely a primary cause of fetal death.
- May be detected by ultrasound (e.g., hanging noose sign, four-leaf clover).

PROGNOSIS AND TREATMENT

- Outcome is typically uneventful, but risk of death is up to 10-fold greater than with unknotted cords.

MAIN DIFFERENTIAL DIAGNOSIS

- "False knots" in the cord are common, the consequence of vascular ectasia from varices.

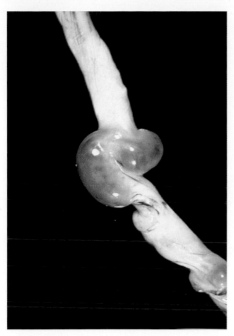

FIGURE 1
False knot created by a common vascular ectasia.

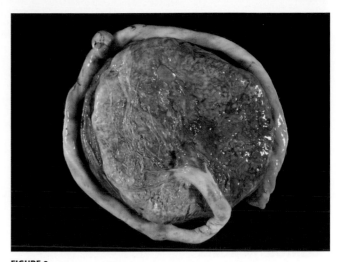

FIGURE 2
True knot in a case of fetal hypoxic demise.

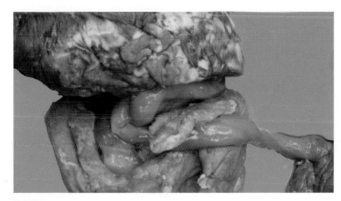

FIGURE 3
Constricting nuchal cord resulting in fetal death.

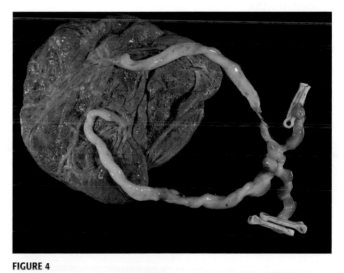

FIGURE 4
A dramatic case of cord entanglement of twin placentas. Both twins survived.

SINGLE UMBILICAL ARTERY (SUA)

DEFINITION—Umbilical cord with two vessels; one umbilical artery and one vein.

CLINICAL FEATURES

EPIDEMIOLOGY

- Common; noted in 1% to 3% of all gestations.
- More frequent in spontaneous abortions.
- More frequent in white women than black or Asian women.

PRESENTATION

- Commonly found with other anomalies.
- Sixteen percent of live-born infants with *isolated* SUA have a renal malformation, half of which are minor.

PROGNOSIS AND TREATMENT

- Excellent if not associated with other fetal anomalies.

PATHOLOGY

HISTOLOGY

- Umbilical cord contains two vessels: one artery and one vein.
- The usual embryonic remnants can still be present in the cord.

IMMUNOPATHOLOGY (INCLUDING IMMUNOHISTOCHEMISTRY)

- Noncontributory.

MAIN DIFFERENTIAL DIAGNOSIS

- Incomplete sectioning of cord can give the illusion of a single umbilical artery. It is important to ensure that the entire segment is represented in the section.

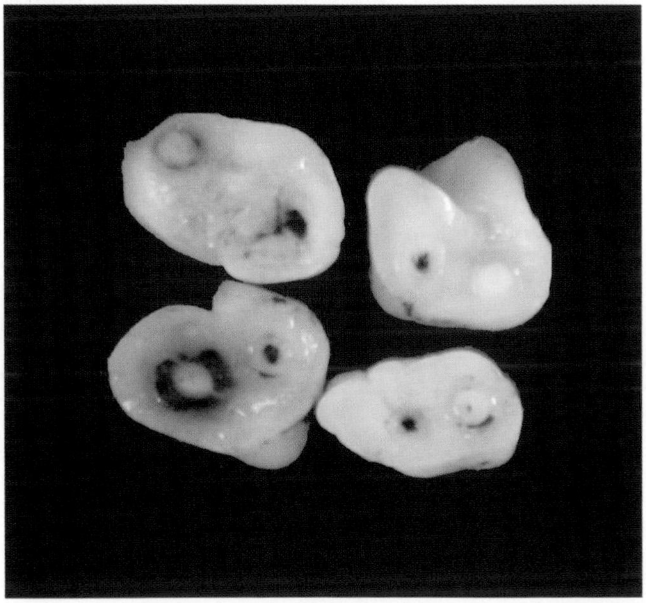

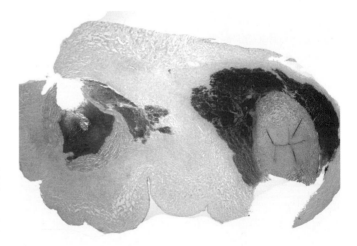

FIGURE 2

Single umbilical artery. Microscopic section shows a single umbilical artery *(right)* accompanied by the usual single umbilical vein *(left)*.

FIGURE 1

Two-vessel cord seen on cross section of several segments.

HYPERCOILED AND HYPOCOILED UMBILICAL CORD

■ **Kathleen Sirois, BA**

DEFINITION

- Hypercoiled cord: Defined as an umbilical coiling index ([UCI] measured as 1/average distance between coils in cm) of greater than 0.3.
- Hypocoiled cord: Defined as a UCI of less than 0.1.

CLINICAL FEATURES

EPIDEMIOLOGY

- Coiling of the cord is considered a function of the nature of the surrounding Wharton's jelly, genetic factors, and fetal movement.

PROGNOSIS

- Hypocoiled cords have been associated with growth retardation, fetal distress, and even Trisomy 21. Cords with a UCI (measured as 1/average distance between coils in cm) of under 0.1.
- Hypercoiled cords have a wide range of frequencies, ranging from 1% to 18%. Believed by some to result from deep placenta implantation into the decidua.

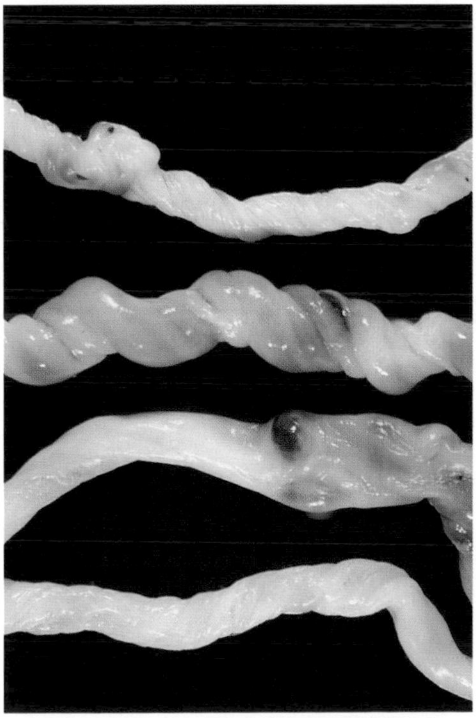

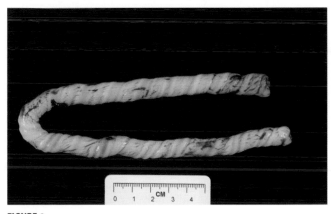

FIGURE 2

Hypercoiled umbilical cord.

FIGURE 1

Examples of cord twist. The UCI is defined as 1 divided by the distance between coils in centimeters. On average there should be about one coil per 5 cm.

VARIATIONS ON CORD INSERTION (MARGINAL, MEMBRANOUS, FURCATE)

■ **Kathleen Sirois, BA**

DEFINITION—Marginal cord insertion is defined as insertion within 2 cm of the periphery of the disk. With a membranous (velamentous) cord insertion, the cord vessels insert into the placental disk within the membranes, in the absence of Wharton's jelly. Furcate cord insertion appears as a forklike division of the cord prior to insertion into the placental disk.

CLINICAL FEATURES

EPIDEMIOLOGY AND PATHOGENESIS

- Marginal cord insertion occurs in less than 10% of single pregnancies but is more common in twin pregnancies, seen in up to one fourth. It is not significantly associated with any growth restriction or preterm delivery.
- Membranous (velamentous) cord insertion may occur as a function of asymmetric placental growth and involution during pregnancy, with the cord migrating from the center to the periphery. One percent of singleton gestations but 15% of monochorionic twin gestations.
- Furcate cord insertion.

PATHOLOGY

- In marginal cord insertion the cord emerges within 2 cm of the edge of the placenta.

- In membranous (velamentous) cord insertion vessels branch out into the membranes above the disk.
- Furcate cord insertion.

PROGNOSIS

- Membranous (velamentous) cord insertions have been associated with a wide range of complications including fetal growth restriction, death (this can occur with vasa previa, when the vessels are compressed by the fetus during delivery), low Apgar scores, and fetal distress; however, the risk in singleton pregnancies is considered very low. In contrast, it is associated with growth restriction of the affected fetus in monochorionic pregnancies. When detected on ultrasound, the pregnancy will be monitored more closely.
- In marginal cord insertion the cord emerges within 2 cm of the edge of the placenta.
- Furcate cord insertion.

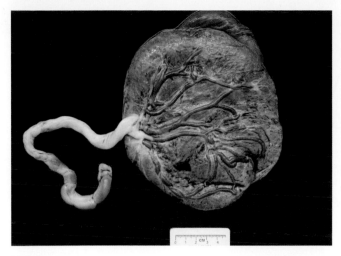

FIGURE 1

Marginal cord insertion. The cord emerges within 2 cm of the periphery of the disk.

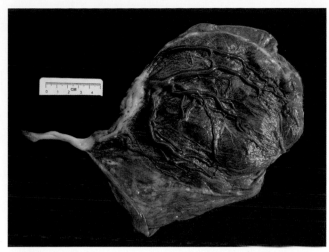

FIGURE 2

Membranous cord insertion. The cord enters the membrane prior to insertion into the disk.

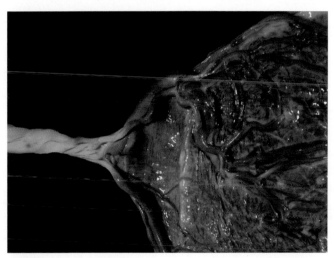

FIGURE 3

Membranous cord insertion. Note the branched cord vessels coursing through the membranes.

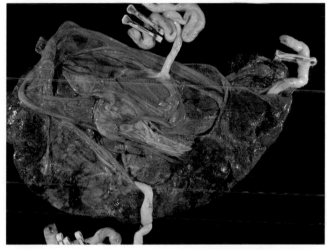

FIGURE 4

Another example of membranous cord insertion in this twin placenta.

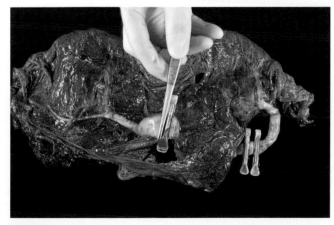

FIGURE 5

Furcate placenta. The cord bifurcates above the insertion with loss of Wharton's jelly.

CIRCUMMARGINATE AND CIRCUMVALLATE PLACENTAS

■ **Kathleen Sirois, BA**

DEFINITION—Variations in membranous insertions on the placental disk.

CLINICAL FEATURES

EPIDEMIOLOGY

- Circummarginate membranes are not strongly associated with any abnormality other than possibly fetal malformations in one study.
- Circumvallate membranes have a wide range of frequencies, ranging from 1% to 18%. Believed by some to result from deep placenta implantation into the decidua. Associated with abruption.

PRESENTATION

- Circummarginate membranes: Rather than joining the disk at the margin, the membranes arise concentrically directly from the fetal surface inside the margin. The zone between the membrane edge and the periphery of the placenta is yellow in appearance.

- Circumvallate membranes: The membranes join the placenta at the margin, but a concentric, redundant, duplicated rim of membrane, like the whitewall of a tire, covers the periphery of the disk.

PROGNOSIS AND TREATMENT

- None.

PATHOLOGY

- Histologic examination of the placenta with circumvallate membranes should include careful exam of the membrane role and maternal surface for hemosiderin-laden macrophages, which could signify prior retroplacental bleeding.

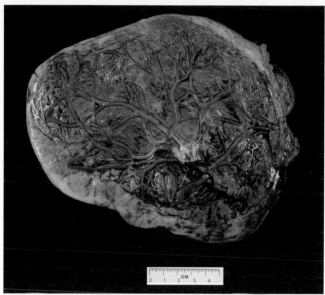

FIGURE 1

Circummarginate membranes. Note the insertion of the membranes is at the periphery of the disk.

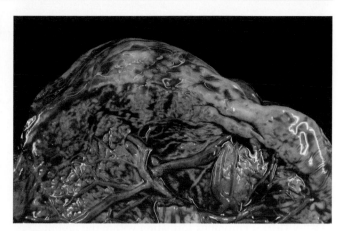

FIGURE 2

Circummarginate membranes.

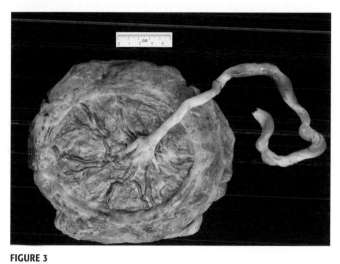

FIGURE 3

Circumvallate membranes. Note the duplicated membrane centrally, which is sharply demarcated.

FETAL VASCULAR THROMBOSIS

DEFINITION—Thrombus formation within the umbilical cord, within its tributaries on the placental surface, or within stem villi.

CLINICAL FEATURES

EPIDEMIOLOGY

- Common; seen in 3% to 10% of placentas.
- Increased incidence with maternal diabetes.

PRESENTATION

- Very large or multifocal (40% to 60% of placental mass) thromboses can cause sudden intrauterine fetal demise.
- Small or localized fetal vascular thrombosis (FVT) is generally an incidental finding.
- If FVT occurs early in gestation or in a somatic vessel, the infant can present with cerebral infarcts or limb reductions.

PROGNOSIS AND TREATMENT

- Usually incidental.
- Rarely the presence of FVT can identify newborns with inherited coagulopathies or those at risk of somatic thrombi.
- Rarely associated with childhood stroke.

PATHOLOGY

HISTOLOGY

- Microscopic examination shows wedge-shaped zones of infarction, with the base oriented toward the fetal surface, following the distribution of the thrombosed stem villous.
- An inflammatory infiltrate is absent.
- Downstream terminal villi exhibit ischemic change, with endothelial disruption, stromal karyorrhexis, and red blood cell extravasation.
- If the thrombus is remote, the terminal villi are collagenized and sclerotic (ghost villi).
- Thrombi are similar to those seen at other sites with attachment to the vessel wall, endothelial disruption, and expansion of the vessel lumen by a multilayered clot.
- Older thrombi show organization, with fibrosis and recanalization of the vessel lumen.
- Early fetal vascular thromboses can be confirmed by the presence of red cell extravasation into the vessel wall.

IMMUNOPATHOLOGY (INCLUDING IMMUNOHISTOCHEMISTRY)

- Noncontributory.

MAIN DIFFERENTIAL DIAGNOSIS

- Placental infarcts of maternal origin may interrupt fetal blood supply to nearby villi, producing villous sclerosis.
- Chronic villitis, when moderate or severe, can lead to vascular obliteration. In some instances the villitis may not be conspicuous.

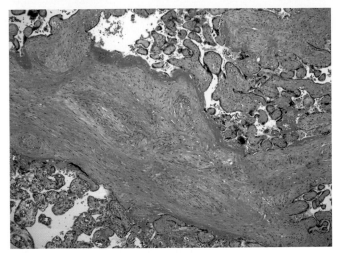

FIGURE 1

FVT. Thrombosed and nearly obliterated fetal vessels *(center)* are associated with sclerotic, avascular villi in the upper right. The avascular villi lack stromal inflammation or other features to suggest a chronic villitis.

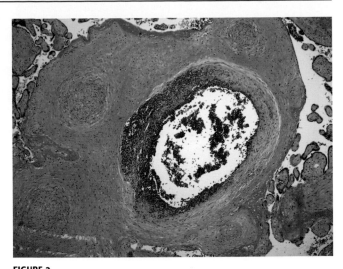

FIGURE 2

FVT. Fetal vessel with early thrombosis. Note the disruption of the vessel wall.

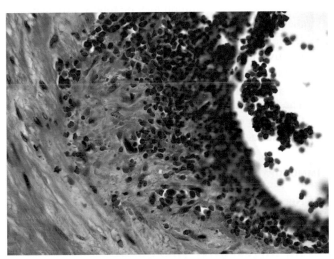

FIGURE 3

FVT. Higher power of an early vascular lesion shows extravasation of red blood cells into the vessel wall. Inflammation is absent.

MATERNAL FLOOR INFARCT/MASSIVE PERIVILLOUS FIBRIN DEPOSITION

DEFINITION—Diffuse or multifocal fibrin deposition that fills and obliterates the intervillous space along a significant portion of the chorionic plate.

CLINICAL FEATURES

EPIDEMIOLOGY

- Uncommon (less than 1% of placentas).
- Occasionally associated with abnormal maternal clotting (APhA, ATIII deficiency).

PRESENTATION

- Sudden intrauterine fetal demise in the third trimester.
- Can present with recurrent spontaneous abortions.

PROGNOSIS AND TREATMENT

- Tends to recur in subsequent pregnancies.
- If fibrin deposition involves at least 40% to 50% of the parenchyma, it is uniformly fatal.
- Maternal floor infarction is also associated with intrauterine growth restriction.

PATHOLOGY

HISTOLOGY

- Amorphous eosinophilic material (fibrin) surrounds individual villi or groups of villi.

- Mononuclear intermediate trophoblasts persist.
- Surrounded villi or groups of villi are widely separated from one another.
- The findings occupy a "significant" portion of the placenta.

IMMUNOPATHOLOGY (INCLUDING IMMUNOHISTOCHEMISTRY)

- Noncontributory.

MAIN DIFFERENTIAL DIAGNOSIS

- Sampling from the placental margin only—this region typically exhibits abundant intervillous fibrin, but the remainder of the placenta should be unaffected.
- Placental infarct—early infarcts might not have collapse of villous structures, but the trophoblasts have the telltale dusky appearance of early degeneration. In contrast, although focal villous infarction often is present in maternal floor infarct, the majority of the syncytiotrophoblasts are still viable. Cytotrophoblasts will often abandon the villi to differentiate into vacuolated (p63 positive) and mature extravillous trophoblast.

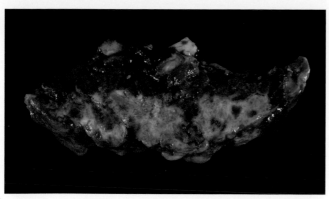

FIGURE 1

Massive perivillous fibrin. Gross example showing a diffuse process along the entirety of the maternal surface of the placenta, as seen on cut section.

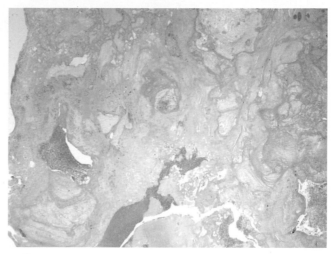

FIGURE 2

Massive perivillous fibrin. Widely separated groups of villi are apparent. There is abundant fibrin deposition along the maternal surface of the placenta. Note on the left clusters of extravillous trophoblast that have migrated from the villi into the fibrin. On the right there are a number of vague villous outlines signifying villous infarction. The key feature is the separation of villi, viable or dead, by abundant fibrin.

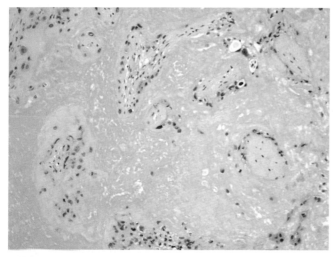

FIGURE 3

Massive perivillous fibrin. At high power the villi are viable. There is dense pink fibrin deposition completely surrounding the villi.

CHORIOAMNIONITIS

DEFINITION—Ascending infection of the amniotic fluid leading to a fetal and maternal inflammatory response.

CLINICAL FEATURES

EPIDEMIOLOGY

- Acute chorioamnionitis (ACA) is detected in approximately 25% of preterm deliveries, and gestational age of babies born with ACA is significantly younger than those born without ACA.
- Chorioamnionitis is a common end outcome of several infectious agents.
- May occur at any stage during pregnancy.
- Common cause of second-trimester inevitable abortion.
- Risk increased with cervical dilatation, premature rupture of membranes, or foreign bodies.

PRESENTATION

- Preterm premature rupture of membranes, resulting in preterm labor.
- Signs and symptoms of infection including fever and malaise.
- Uterine pain and tenderness may be present.

PROGNOSIS AND TREATMENT

- The prognosis is variable and highly dependent on the infectious agent, gestational age, duration, and severity of infection.
- Delivery is the most common method of treatment, with intensive unit care for the infant.
- The principal adverse neonatal outcomes are death, sepsis, pneumonia or bronchopulmonary dysplasia, intraventricular hemorrhage, and ultimately cerebral palsy. To what degree these complications are directly related to the ACA versus premature delivery is unclear. Some have linked ACA to a higher frequency of preterm neonatal morbidity, and increasing severity of histologic chorioamnionitis has been associated with intraventricular neonatal hemorrhage. ACA has also been linked to a *lower risk* of respiratory distress syndrome (RDS) and neonatal death in premature infants.
- Corticosteroids or antibiotics are often used to counteract the inflammatory effects on the fetus, although controlled trials evaluating their effectiveness are needed.

PATHOLOGY

HISTOLOGY

- The placenta displays opaque membranes and fetal surfaces in severe cases.
- A characteristic odor may be present in some specific infections, such as *Listeria*, *Fusobacterium*, or *Bacteroides*.
- Histologically the distinct fetal and maternal responses can be distinguished.
- The fetal neutrophilic response is seen in the umbilical cord and chorionic plate vessels.
- Nonspecific indicators of fetal distress, such as nucleated red blood cells, can also be seen.
- The maternal response consists of acute inflammation in the membranes, chorionic plate, and subchorion.
- Neutrophils present within the chorion and subchorion are not diagnostic of infection and should not be diagnosed as chorioamnionitis.
- Attempts have been made to categorize the extent of the inflammatory infiltrate (grade and stage) based on the distribution and extent of inflammation; however, these schemes do not correlate well with outcome.
- In general, a maternal response indicates an early infection, and the addition of an identifiable fetal response suggests a more chronic infection.
- Nonspecific, postmortem maternal inflammation may be seen that can mimic ascending infection; the presence of a fetal inflammatory response is helpful in ruling in infection in these cases.
- Amniotic fluid infection results in the presence of neutrophils within the alveolar spaces and gastrointestinal tract lumens, which can be a useful clue in cases of prolonged intrauterine fetal demise.

- In prolonged intrauterine demise of noninfectious causes, neutrophils should not be present within the alveolar spaces or along the gastrointestinal tract.
- Careful examination of the surface of the cord is important inasmuch as microabscesses on the surface could signify *Candida* infection and should prompt special stains to exclude this possibility.

IMMUNOPATHOLOGY (INCLUDING IMMUNOHISTOCHEMISTRY)

- Noncontributory.

MAIN DIFFERENTIAL DIAGNOSIS

- Specific infections such as viral, fungal, or bacterial infections, including *Listeria* or beta-streptococcus, spread hematogenously and will also be associated with an acute intervillositis.
- Subchorionitis or other maternal-derived inflammatory responses may be found following intrauterine fetal death and prolonged rupture of membranes prior to delivery. This is not related to fetal death and is considered an incidental finding.

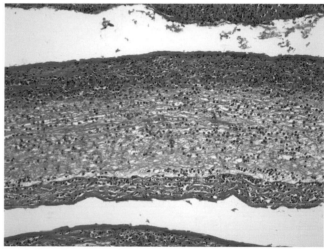

FIGURE 3

ACA. Necrotizing ACA with necrosis of the amnion and abundant neutrophils.

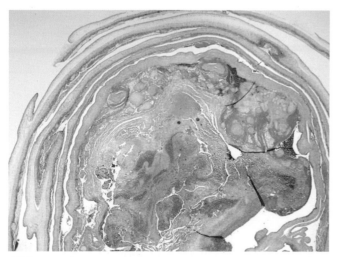

FIGURE 1

ACA. Gross image of a placenta with nearly completely opaque, white to greenish membranes.

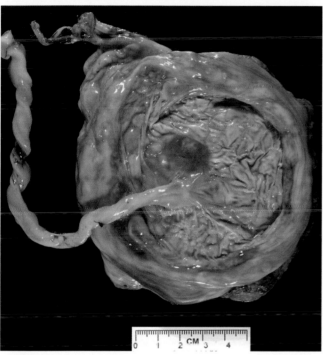

FIGURE 2

ACA. Low-power microscopic image of the membrane roll showing a dense inflammatory infiltrate of the chorion *(center)*. High-power examination *(not shown)* also revealed neutrophils in the amnion.

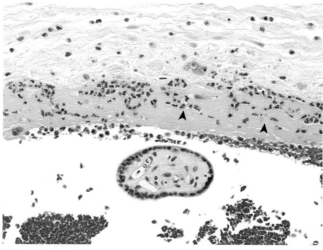

FIGURE 4

Subchorionitis, reflecting (by itself) early or mild infection. The maternal space is below with a single villous in this field. The subamnionic mesenchyme is above. The neutrophils in the chorionic plate are highlighted by the arrows.

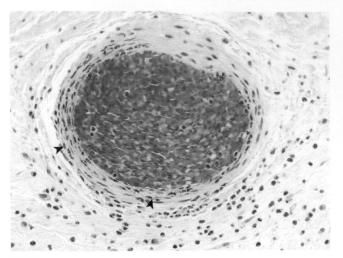

FIGURE 5

Chorionic plate vascular inflammation, a fetal neutrophilic response seen in vessels in the chorionic plate *(arrows)*.

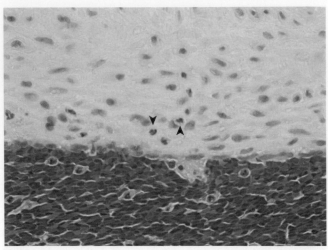

FIGURE 6

Umbilical cord vascular inflammation. This can be mimicked by early autolysis in the cord vessel subendothelial mesenchymal cells in second-trimester deliveries, which can mimic neutrophils. In this case the neutrophils in the vessel wall are easily seen *(arrows)*.

TABLE 1

Stages of Acute Amniotic Fluid Infection

Stage	Maternal	Fetal
I	Acute chorionitis, subchorionitis	Umbilical phlebitis
II	ACA	Umbilical arteritis, perivasculitis
III	Necrotizing chorioamnionitis	Concentric perivasculitis

TABLE 2

Template for Amniotic Fluid Infection

Inflammation characteristic of amniotic fluid infection

Maternal inflammatory response (choose all that apply below)
- ACA
- Acute subchorionitis, consistent with an early or mild amniotic
- Fluid infection
- Acute deciduitis

Fetal inflammatory response (choose all that apply below)
- Umbilical cord vasculitis
- Chorionic plate vasculitis
- Fungal funisitis

Inflammatory abruption (specify: marginal, retroplacental, subchorionic, intervillous) bleeding

Note: Amniotic fluid infection associated with extreme preterm delivery in midgestation raises concern for cervical incompetence. Clinical correlation may be helpful in this regard.

GESTATIONAL *CANDIDA* INFECTION

DEFINITION—Infection by any species of *Candida* during the gestational period.

CLINICAL FEATURES

EPIDEMIOLOGY

- Vaginal infection by *Candida* is common and is thought to occur in up to 25% of all pregnancies.
- Ascending infection of the placenta and/or fetus is rarer and occurs in less than 1% of all candidal infections during pregnancy.
- Risk factors for candidal chorioamnionitis include concurrent vaginal infection, cervical cerclage, and intrauterine device usage.

PRESENTATION

- Chorioamnionitis.
- Preterm delivery.
- Intrauterine fetal demise.

PROGNOSIS AND TREATMENT

- The prognosis is variable and dependent on the extent of the infection and the corresponding inflammatory response.

PATHOLOGY

HISTOLOGY

- *Candida* infection should be suspected grossly when small 1 to 2 mm white to yellow plaques or nodules are present on the umbilical cord or fetal surfaces of the placenta.
- A wedge-shaped abscess with yeast forms is characteristic microscopically.
- Accompanying chorioamnionitis should be identified.
- Severe cases may result in funisitis (inflammation of the umbilical cord) with or without necrosis.

IMMUNOPATHOLOGY (INCLUDING IMMUNOHISTOCHEMISTRY)

- Special stains for fungus (periodic acid–Schiff [PAS] with diastase and Grocott's methenamine silver [GMS]) may be helpful in identifying the fungal organisms.

MAIN DIFFERENTIAL DIAGNOSIS

- Chorioamnionitis of different infectious etiologies.

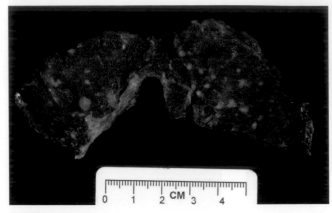

FIGURE 1

Listeria placentitis. Gross appearance. Small white patches are the gross correlate of the characteristic intervillous microabscesses.

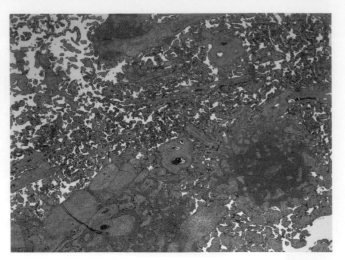

FIGURE 2

Listeria placentitis. Low power shows multifocal patchy intervillous inflammation forming microabscesses.

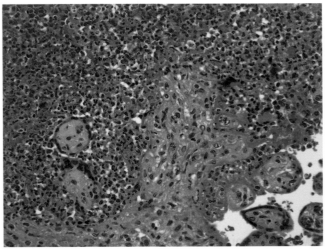

FIGURE 3

Listeria placentitis. The microabscesses are composed of neutrophils and are primarily intervillous. Note the noninflamed villi on the right. Organisms can be demonstrated with a gram stain in these areas.

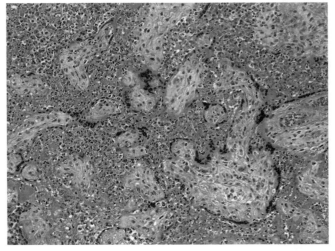

FIGURE 4

Listeria placentitis. Note that while the intervillous space is full of inflammation, the villi themselves appear uninvolved.

CHRONIC VILLITIS

DEFINITION—Maternal chronic inflammatory cells within terminal villi, not attributable to any known infection.

CLINICAL FEATURES

EPIDEMIOLOGY

- Present in 5% to 10% of examined placentas.
- More often seen in women with autoimmune disorders such as systemic lupus erythematosus.
- Thought by some to be an autoimmune phenomenon, and some authors consider it a maternal-placental graft rejection.
- Others suspect that chronic villitis (CV) represents a response to an as-of-yet unidentified organism.

PRESENTATION

- Presentation varies greatly with severity.
- Often noted as an incidental finding at the time of placental examination.
- Is associated with both intrauterine growth restriction and (rarely) fetal death.

PROGNOSIS AND TREATMENT

- Recurs with subsequent pregnancies in about 20% of cases, and recurrence is often more severe.
- Other than supportive care, no useful treatment protocol currently exists.

PATHOLOGY

HISTOLOGY

- The low-power clue to identification is that villi appear hypercellular.
- At higher power, aggregates of villi with stromal fibrosis, vascular obliteration, and chronic inflammatory cells are present.

- In some foci, lymphocytes and mononuclear histiocytes may be present (spill out) in the intervillous spaces.
- Not all villi are affected, and normal and inflamed villi are often intermixed.
- Viral inclusions are not present.
- Plasma cells should not be present in idiopathic CV; they are most commonly seen in infection, particularly cytomegalovirus (CMV).

IMMUNOPATHOLOGY (INCLUDING IMMUNOHISTOCHEMISTRY)

- Special stains for infectious organisms are negative.
- Immunostains for viruses such as CMV are negative.

MAIN DIFFERENTIAL DIAGNOSIS

- Viral infection, especially CMV—viral inclusions should be present. Villous necrosis and calcifications may also be seen.
- *Toxoplasma gondii* infection.
- Fetal vascular thrombosis—this is in the differential when there is extensive villous sclerosis, which can be caused by both an obliterative villitis and fetal vascular thrombosis. The latter is more likely if there is evidence of proximal vascular occlusion with recanalization, villous karyorrhexis, and absence of CV.

DIAGNOSTIC TERMINOLOGY

- If localized: Chronic nonspecific villitis.
- If involving multiple fields: Extensive CV.

A comment that extensive CV may recur and be associated with potential growth restriction or adverse fetal outcome may be included as appropriate.

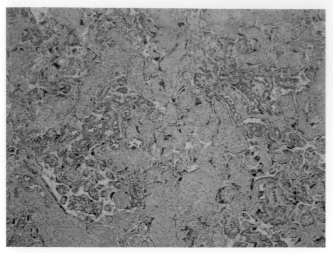

FIGURE 1

CV. Low-power image. An admixture of large, hypercellular villi and small normocellular villi.

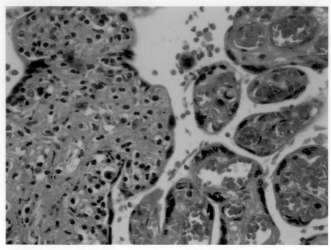

FIGURE 2

CV. High power contrasting normal villi on the right, with CV on the left. The villous on the left is infiltrated by lymphocytes, lacks normal vasculature, and had stromal fibrosis.

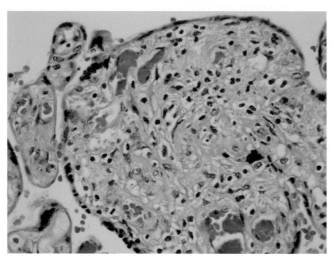

FIGURE 3

CV. A villous with numerous stromal lymphocytes and stromal fibrosis.

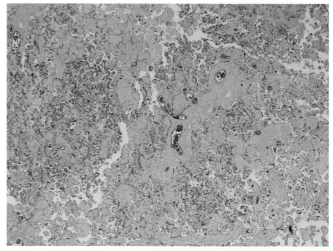

FIGURE 4

Severe CV. Note the widespread inflammation and villous obliteration, most prominent in the upper left of the image.

CHRONIC HISTIOCYTIC INTERVILLOSITIS

DEFINITION—Infiltration of the intervillous space by a monomorphic population of histiocytes.

CLINICAL FEATURES

EPIDEMIOLOGY

- Uncommon.
- Histiocytic intervillositis is associated with spontaneous abortion and recurrent pregnancy loss.
- Rare cases of maternal malaria or recurrent sepsis have been documented.

PRESENTATION

- Chronic histiocytic intervillositis may present as spontaneous abortion in the first or second trimester.
- In the third trimester it is associated with intrauterine growth restriction and stillbirth.
- Some patients present with a history of multiple early pregnancy losses.

PROGNOSIS AND TREATMENT

- The prognosis in diagnosed cases is poor.
- Some studies indicate that three out of four cases result in fetal demise.
- The only known treatment option is aggressive immunosuppressive therapy.

PATHOLOGY

HISTOLOGY

- The intervillous space is diffusely infiltrated by histiocytic cells admixed with lymphocytes.
- Intervillous fibrin deposition is also usually seen, although it is not present in all cases.
- By definition, classic chronic villitis is absent.

IMMUNOPATHOLOGY (INCLUDING IMMUNOHISTOCHEMISTRY)

- The histiocytic cells are strongly and diffusely positive for CD68.
- Special stains for infectious organisms are negative.

MAIN DIFFERENTIAL DIAGNOSIS

- Chronic villitis—here the inflammatory cells are mainly confined to the villi. Some intervillositis may be present, but it is mostly lymphocytic.
- Acute and chronic intervillositis—if neutrophils are abundant, B-strep or *Listeria* must be considered.

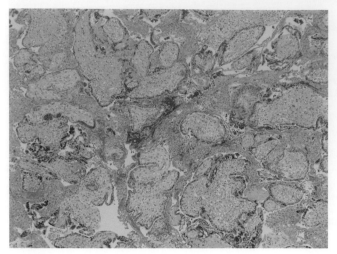

FIGURE 1

Chronic histiocytic intervillositis. Low power shows a diffuse intervillous process composed of a mixture of chronic inflammatory cells, histiocytes, and fibrin deposition.

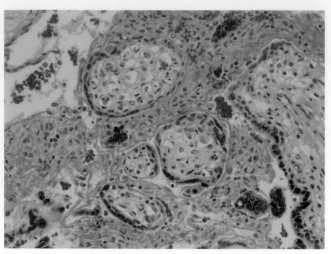

FIGURE 2

Chronic histiocytic intervillositis. High power shows that the infiltrate is composed predominantly of large histiocytic cells with abundant eosinophilic cytoplasm. Occasionally lymphocytes are present.

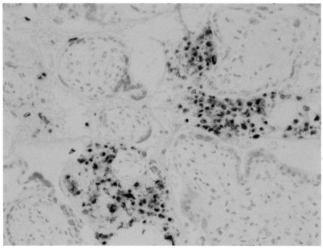

FIGURE 3

Chronic histiocytic intervillositis. An immunostain for CD68 is strongly and diffusely positive in the intervillous histiocytic infiltrate.

CONGENITAL SYPHILIS

DEFINITION—Infection resulting from the spirochete *Treponema pallidum*.

CLINICAL FEATURES

EPIDEMIOLOGY

- The frequency of congenital syphilis in developed countries is much lower; however, a recent rise in the incidence has been noted. It is rarely encountered in our practice.

PRESENTATION

- Congenital syphilis causes premature delivery and stillbirth.
- Screening tests are used to detect the majority of cases; however, mothers with no prenatal care may present at the time of delivery.

PROGNOSIS AND TREATMENT

- Congenital syphilis carries a high rate of neonatal morbidity in the form of premature birth and neurologic deficits and mortality.
- Aggressive antibiotic therapy may lessen the chance of neonatal infection to an incidence of around 14%.

PATHOLOGY

HISTOLOGY

- Examination of the placenta characteristically consists of villous changes including enlarged, hypercellular villi; acute and/or chronic villitis; and fetal vascular changes that include "onion skinning" of the vessel wall and vascular obliteration.
- Necrotizing funisitis may be present.

IMMUNOPATHOLOGY (INCLUDING IMMUNOHISTOCHEMISTRY)

- Silver staining may reveal treponemal organisms.
- Detection of treponemal DNA by polymerase chain reaction (PCR) is the most sensitive method for diagnosis.

MAIN DIFFERENTIAL DIAGNOSIS

- Acute and chronic villitis, unspecified.

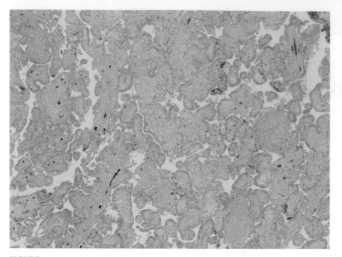

FIGURE 2

Placenta from a GM1 gangliosidosis. Note the slight villous enlargement with pallor, due to the abundant histiocytes.

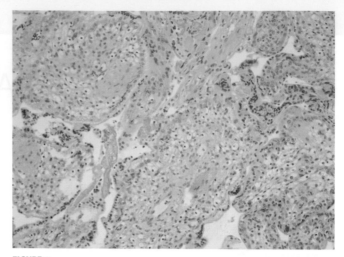

FIGURE 3

At higher magnification the villi are seen to contain numerous mononuclear cells.

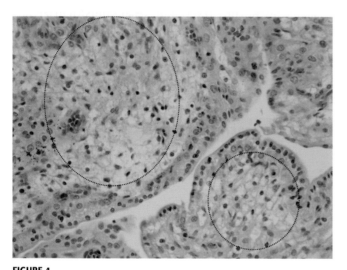

FIGURE 4

At higher magnification the numerous macrophages with small nuclei are evident *(see circles)*.

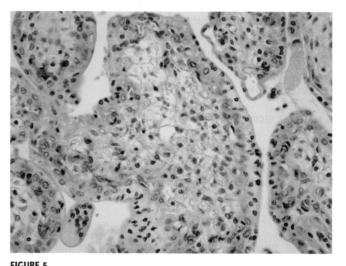

FIGURE 5

Alcian blue stain highlights the lysosomal contents as a faint blue.

INFLAMMATORY ABRUPTION

DEFINITION—Early separation of the placental disk from the underlying maternal surface.

CLINICAL FEATURES

EPIDEMIOLOGY

- Placental abruption is a relatively common event, with an overall incidence of 1%.
- Numerous predisposing factors are thought to lead to abruption but the focus recently has been on chronic inflammatory changes such as infarcts, decidual necrosis, and inflammation in the membranes and cord vessels. Bleeding early in pregnancy is also a risk factor.

PRESENTATION

- Patients present with uterine bleeding and preterm labor.
- Abruption at the time of delivery may not be detected until the time of placental examination.

PROGNOSIS AND TREATMENT

- Small foci of retroplacental hemorrhage are often seen and are generally insignificant; this should not be confused with significant placental abruption.
- Abruption carries a significant risk of morbidity and mortality for both mother and infant.
- The extent of abruption directly impacts the chances of fetal demise.
- Any infarction in a preterm placenta is abnormal and should be carefully investigated.
- Small infarcts in term placentas are usually insignificant, but large (>3 cm) or multifocal infarcts are abnormal and associated with worse perinatal outcomes.
- Maternal morbidity can result from blood loss, disseminated intravascular coagulation, and/or renal failure.

PATHOLOGY

HISTOLOGY

- Grossly, chronic abruption is suspected by the presence of a retroplacental hematoma.
- Peripartum hemorrhage is common and seen in nearly all placentas and should be distinguished from a potentially significant finding.
- If the clot is easily removed, then it is recent and likely related to the birth process.
- Clots of true chronic placental abruption will be adherent and often contain lines of Zahn on cut section.
- Another clue is the appearance of the underlying maternal surface; if the surface appears normal when the clot is removed, it is unlikely to be significant. If the clot creates a large defect or depression in the parenchyma, it may be a significant finding.
- A significant hematoma will block blood flow to the villous tree and causes a "halo" of ischemic placental infarction and villous collapse.
- Villous collapse is identified histologically by the loss of the intervillous space and confirmed by identifying the surrounding adherent hematoma.
- Acute abruptions are characterized by dissection of blood into the basal intervillous space; the time elapsed is generally not sufficient to form a true clot, and this diagnosis requires correlation with the clinical findings and impression at the time of delivery.
- Dissection of blood into the placental parenchyma may be seen as intravillous hemorrhage, although this is not always identified in cases of acute abruption.
- In some cases sudden acute abruption may produce a "ball-and-socket" appearance with a necrotic hemorrhagic core surrounded by infarcted placental parenchyma.

- Overall the histologic findings in both chronic and acute placental abruptions are nonspecific and should be correlated with the gross impression and clinical scenario.

IMMUNOPATHOLOGY (INCLUDING IMMUNOHISTOCHEMISTRY)

- Noncontributory.

MAIN DIFFERENTIAL DIAGNOSIS

- Adherent blood clot (gross) is not uncommon at delivery. Conversely an abruption might not be appreciated

if it dissects out from beneath the disk. A history of copious amounts of blood discharged at delivery or large blood clots found at cesarean section is supportive.

- Hypertensive infarct (ball-in-socket infarct) is a form of abruption where a spiral artery ruptures and produces a basal thrombus that is usually just within the parenchyma of the placenta. Unlike inflammatory abruption, which typically is diffuse and associated with chorioamnionitis, a hypertensive infarct is sharply circumscribed and associated with maternal hypertension or preeclampsia.

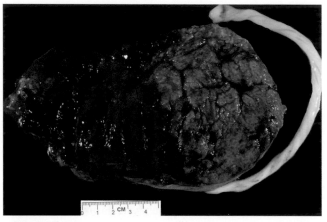

FIGURE 1

Placental abruption. Gross image of a placenta with a large (>3 cm) adherent hematoma with intraparenchymal dissection of blood.

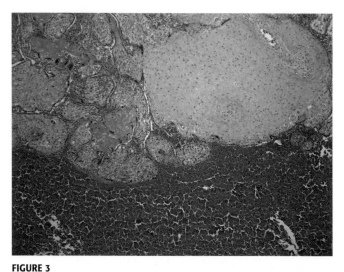

FIGURE 3

Inflammatory abruption. An acute abruption where the clot has not yet organized. There is minimal intraparenchymal dissection in this image.

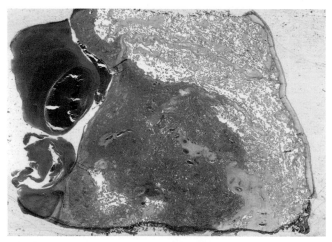

FIGURE 2

Inflammatory abruption. Note the large thrombus on the maternal surface on the left and the conspicuous zone of subjacent ischemia in the overlying placental tissue *(center)*, consisting of infarct and/or intravillous hemorrhage.

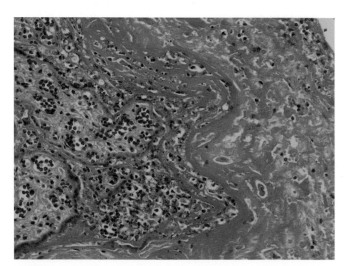

FIGURE 4

Higher magnification shows numerous neutrophils. This case was associated with a preexisting acute chorioamnionitis.

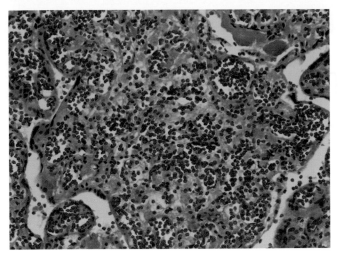

FIGURE 5

Intravillous hemorrhage in adjacent villi strongly suggests abruption; however, it can be reproduced by therapeutic terminations.

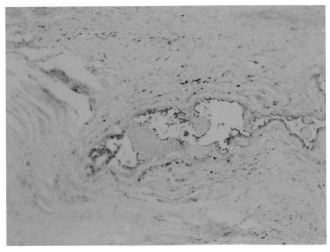

FIGURE 6

Hemosiderin on the maternal surface highlighted by an iron stain. This indicates a prior or chronic abruption and is not uncommonly found near acute retroplacental bleeding, given prior abruptions predispose the placenta to repeated bleeding.

FETAL LEUKEMIA

DEFINITION—A primary white blood cell malignancy arising in the fetus.

CLINICAL FEATURES

EPIDEMIOLOGY

- Fetal leukemia is exceedingly rare and has an incidence of approximately four to five per million live births.
- Fetal leukemia is the leading cause of neoplastic death in the neonate.
- All, or nearly all, infant leukemias are thought to originate in utero.

PRESENTATION

- Polyhydramnios, hydrops, and hepatosplenomegaly can be seen on ultrasound.
- At birth the infant can exhibit hydrops fetalis (nonimmune) or may appear normal.
- In some forms of leukemia the infant has numerous skin nodules (blueberry muffin baby).
- Hydrops may be seen in all fetal malignancies, as well as other conditions, and is not specific.
- Prenatal umbilical cord sampling can reveal malignant cells in the fetal blood.

PROGNOSIS AND TREATMENT

- Fetal leukemia carries a very poor prognosis.
- Clinical remission, even with treatment, is rare.

PATHOLOGY

HISTOLOGY

- If involved by the fetal leukemias, the placenta often exhibits placentomegaly.

- Microscopic evaluation reveals malignant leukocytes present in, and distending, the fetal vessels.
- Expansion or spillage of leukemic cells into the villous stroma is not prominent.

IMMUNOPATHOLOGY (INCLUDING IMMUNOHISTOCHEMISTRY)

- Immunohistochemical markers and flow cytometry are used to determine the lineage of the malignancy.
- The cytogenetic aberrations seen in these malignancies are unique and distinct from those present in other childhood and adult leukemias.
- Selection and application of these tests are outside of the scope of this chapter.

MAIN DIFFERENTIAL DIAGNOSIS

- Reactive fetal leukoerythroblastosis.
- Transient abnormal myelopoiesis, seen in 10% of newborns with Down syndrome.
- Exclusion of these entities requires a detailed hematological workup.

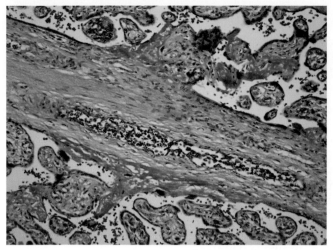

FIGURE 1

Fetal leukemia. In an infant with known leukemia, placental evaluation reveals foci of dark atypical cells in an otherwise normal appearing placenta.

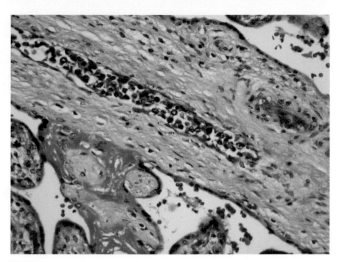

FIGURE 2

Fetal leukemia. At higher power the cells are highly atypical and morphologically consistent with blast forms.

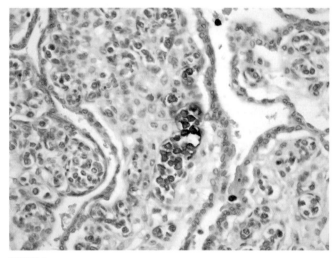

FIGURE 3

Fetal leukemia. A myeloperoxidase stain (MPO) highlights leukocytes within a fetal vessel.

PLACENTA CRETA

DEFINITION—Abnormal adherence of the placenta to the uterine wall.

CLINICAL FEATURES

EPIDEMIOLOGY

- Placenta creta occurs in 1 in 2500 pregnancies.
- Historically all subtypes of placenta cretas were rare.
- More than 80% of cases occur in patients with a prior cesarean section (C-section), and the rise in incidence is presumed to be due to the increased rate of C-section.
- Other risk factors include fibroids, Asherman's syndrome, previous uterine surgery (including curettage), high parity, and abnormal implantation.

PRESENTATION

- Most patients present during labor with difficulty delivering the placenta or increased uterine bleeding following delivery.
- Mild cases of placenta accreta may be asymptomatic.
- In severe cases of placenta increta or percreta, patients may present with abdominal pain due to impending uterine rupture.
- The diagnosis can be suspected on ultrasound.

PROGNOSIS AND TREATMENT

- Prognosis is dependent on the extent and depth of the creta.
- Manual removal of the placenta is sufficient in half of cases.
- Sutures or artery ligation to stop bleeding may be required in about a fifth of cases.

- Uncontrollable bleeding in any form of creta may require hysterectomy.
- Placenta percreta may require hysterectomy.

PATHOLOGY

HISTOLOGY

- Grossly, the placenta is often fragmented or grossly incomplete.
- In cases of hysterectomy the placenta is directly applied to the myometrium without intervening decidua (accreta), invades into the myometrial wall (increta), or rarely invades through the full thickness of the myometrial wall (percreta).
- Microscopic examination will reveal the presence of placental villi in direct contact with the myometrium, without intervening decidua.
- Implantation site fibrin with accompanying trophoblasts is present and should not be considered decidua.

IMMUNOPATHOLOGY (INCLUDING IMMUNOHISTOCHEMISTRY)

- Noncontributory.

MAIN DIFFERENTIAL DIAGNOSIS

- Abnormal or exaggerated implantation site.

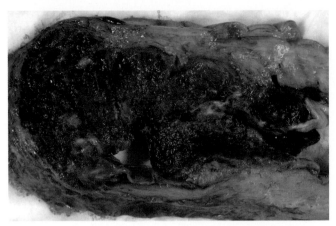

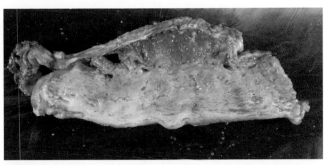

FIGURE 1

Placenta creta. Gross image of a gravid hysterectomy for placenta percreta. The placental parenchyma invades through the full thickness of the myometrial wall to involve the uterine serosa *(upper left)*.

FIGURE 2

Placenta creta. Cross section from a gravid hysterectomy. The placenta is adherent directly to the myometrium, without intervening decidua.

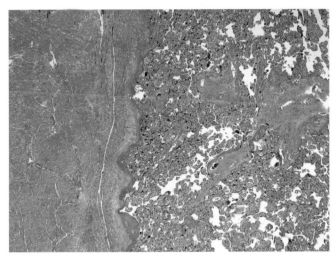

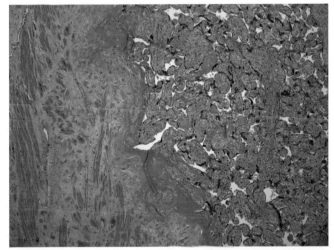

FIGURE 3

Placenta creta. Low-power image of placenta accreta. The placenta is directly adherent to the smooth muscle of the uterine wall. Decidua is absent.

FIGURE 4

Placenta creta. Placental villi are directly adherent to the myometrium but do not invade into the myometrial wall. Trophoblasts set in brightly eosinophilic fibrin are present (implantation site), but decidua is absent.

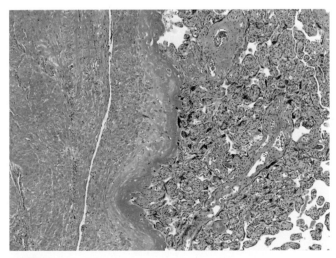

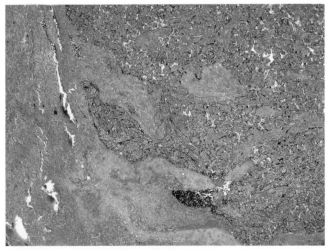

FIGURE 5

Placenta creta. Only implantation site separates placental villi from the smooth muscle of the uterine wall, consistent with a diagnosis of placenta accreta.

FIGURE 6

Placenta creta. Low-power image showing placental villi invading into the myometrial wall, diagnostic of placenta increta.

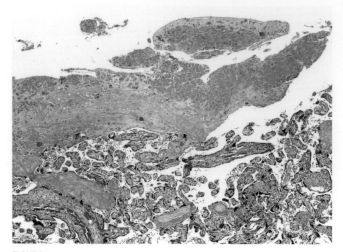

FIGURE 7

Muscle fibers adherent to the basal plate (maternal surface of the placenta, *upper right*), suggestive of placenta accreta.

PLACENTA PREVIA

DEFINITION—Placental implantation within the lower uterine segment, overlying the cervical os.

CLINICAL FEATURES

EPIDEMIOLOGY

- Placenta previa is a common finding in early pregnancy.
- The majority of cases spontaneously resolve during gestation.
- Less than 1% of cases persist until delivery.

PRESENTATION

- Most cases are identified through ultrasonographic examination during routine prenatal care visits.
- Occasionally cases may present with vaginal bleeding.
- If abruption occurs, vaginal bleeding can be severe and life threatening for the mother and infant.
- Previa may be complete (complete cervical occlusion) or partial (incomplete cervical occlusion).

PROGNOSIS AND TREATMENT

- Prognosis for the fetus is guarded as there is a significant risk of fetal hemorrhage due to vasa previa (rupture) if the previa does not resolve.
- Early in the pregnancy, distal vaginal examination is deferred.
- In the third trimester the onset of labor may be stalled until fetal lung maturity is reached (around 36 weeks) to allow for a planned cesarean section (C-section).

PATHOLOGY

HISTOLOGY

- If hysterectomy is performed, the placenta can be seen overlying the cervical os.
- Any other gross findings in placenta previa may be suggestive but are nonspecific.
- If only the placenta is received, many cases have an eccentrically placed cord, and/or the site of membrane rupture is close to the placental disk.

- Thinning of the placental disk or disruption of the maternal surface may be appreciated.
- Cases of previa also appear entirely normal, with no significant gross findings.
- There are no specific histologic findings.

IMMUNOPATHOLOGY (INCLUDING IMMUNOHISTOCHEMISTRY)

- Noncontributory.

MAIN DIFFERENTIAL DIAGNOSIS

- Placental or membrane disruption due to C-section (gross differential).
- Placental abruption (if hemorrhage occurs).

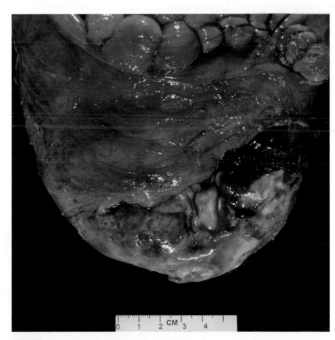

FIGURE 1

Placenta previa. Gross image showing the placenta extending over and out through the cervical os *(below)*. Sutures from the C-section are present above.

TOXOPLASMOSIS

DEFINITION—A parasitic infection often contracted by handling cat litter, which can result in significant fetal morbidity if primary maternal infection occurs in the first trimester.

CLINICAL FEATURES

EPIDEMIOLOGY

- Affects approximately 3500 newborns each year in the United States.
- Primary maternal infection results in fetal transmission in 25% of cases.
- Particularly common in France.

PRESENTATION

- Primary maternal infection is usually asymptomatic.
- Ultrasound may reveal intracranial calcifications or growth restriction in the fetus.
- Large, pale placenta.

PROGNOSIS AND TREATMENT

- Approximately 10% of infections result in fetal death; most newborns with acute congenital toxoplasmosis will die.
- Encephalitis is the most severe manifestation of congenital infection; chorioretinitis and hydrops may also develop.
- Approximately 70% of congenital infections are subclinical at birth, with ocular problems (for example) developing later in life.

PATHOLOGY

HISTOLOGY

- Histology is variable; in two thirds of cases placentas are normal appearing, even with severe fetal disease.
- Chronic villitis, sometimes with granulomatous features, can be seen.
- Organisms are rarely found; when present, the 200 μm encysted organisms are most easily identified in the umbilical cord, chorionic plate, or amniotic membranes.
- Organisms are PAS positive.

IMMUNOPATHOLOGY (INCLUDING IMMUNOHISTOCHEMISTRY)

- Fluorescent antibody tests are available; however, they are not as reliable as polymerase chain reaction (PCR).

MAIN DIFFERENTIAL DIAGNOSIS

- Other toxoplasmosis, other agents, rubella, cytomegalovirus, and herpes simplex (TORCH) infections.

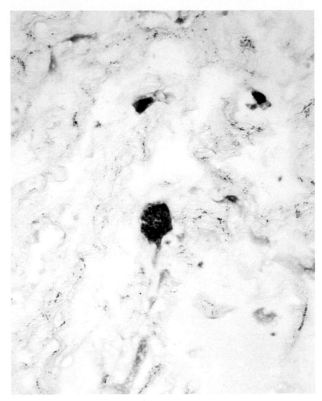

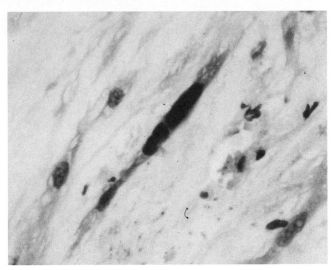

FIGURE 2
Toxoplasmosis.

FIGURE 1
Toxoplasmosis. Encysted organisms are seen in Wharton's jelly.

TOXEMIA

DEFINITION—A hypertensive disorder that arises during pregnancy; there are five types.

CLINICAL FEATURES

EPIDEMIOLOGY

- Hypertensive disorders that fall under the umbrella of "toxemia of pregnancy" are common occurrences.
- Their presentations are varied and described in the following section.

PRESENTATION

- Preeclampsia: Hypertension after 20 weeks gestation with accompanying proteinuria (>300 mg/24 hours or 1+ urine protein on dipstick). Patients usually present after 32 weeks gestation, unless associated with gestational trophoblastic disease, in which case they will present earlier. Preeclampsia may present with headache, visual problems, abdominal pain, elevated serum creatinine, oliguria, elevated liver enzymes, thrombocytopenia, fetal growth restriction, and pulmonary edema. This is the most common presentation of toxemia.
- Eclampsia: Patients display the symptoms of preeclampsia but have the additional finding of seizure.
- Gestational hypertension: Blood pressure greater than 140/90 mm Hg occurring for the first time during the pregnancy. Should resolve within 12 weeks after delivery.
- Chronic hypertension: Hypertension that is present before pregnancy, lasts longer than 12 weeks after pregnancy, or is present before 20 weeks in the absence of gestational trophoblastic disease.
- Superimposed preeclampsia on chronic hypertension: Proteinuria (>300 mg/24 hours) in the presence of chronic hypertension or the elevation of proteinuria, blood pressure, or thrombocytopenia in the presence of chronic hypertension and existing proteinuria.

PROGNOSIS AND TREATMENT

- The prognosis for the various types is highly variable depending on the type and severity of the toxemia.
- Mild cases of preeclampsia may resolve weeks after delivery, while severe cases of eclampsia may result in coma or maternal death.
- Delivery is the definitive treatment; however, mild cases may be treated with bed rest, dietary restriction, and medication.

PATHOLOGY

HISTOLOGY

- In any type of toxemia the most common finding is a small placenta (less than 10th percentile for gestational age).
- Vascular changes and accompanying placental infarcts are also commonly seen.
- The vascular changes consist of maternal vessels that retain their smooth muscle walls, which is known as incomplete transformation of the spiral arterioles, or decidual arteriopathy.
- In more severe forms the decidual arteriopathy exhibits fibrinoid necrosis of the vessel wall with or without acute atherosis.
- These vascular changes are best seen in the membrane roll where it is clear which vessels are maternal in origin.
- Reactive changes within the placenta indicative of fetal stress are usually present.
- Increased syncytial knotting of the terminal villi, terminal villous hypoplasia, increased fetal nucleated red blood cells, and release of meconium with meconium staining of the membranes and chorionic plate are all signs of fetal distress.

IMMUNOPATHOLOGY (INCLUDING IMMUNOHISTOCHEMISTRY)

- Noncontributory.

MAIN DIFFERENTIAL DIAGNOSIS

- Infection with fetal and maternal vasculitis.
- Other causes of fetal hypoxia.

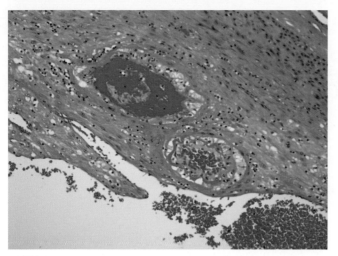

FIGURE 1

Toxemia of pregnancy. Low power of the membrane roll showing abnormal maternal vessels.

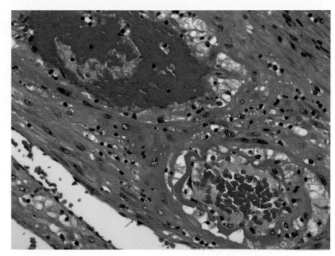

FIGURE 2

Toxemia of pregnancy. At high power the abnormal maternal vessels are characterized by a persistent smooth muscle wall and brightly eosinophilic fibrinoid change of the vessel wall. Acute atherosis is present.

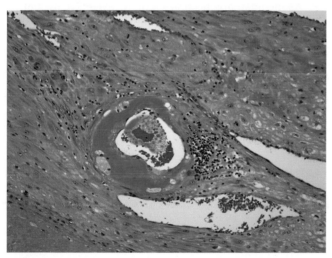

FIGURE 3

Toxemia of pregnancy. Maternal vessel showing acute fibrinoid necrosis, characterized by brightly eosinophilic change with occasional macrophages.

PLACENTAL INFARCTION

DEFINITION—Infarction of the fetal villi due to lack of intervillous perfusion.

CLINICAL FEATURES

EPIDEMIOLOGY

- Localized infarction within term placentas is very common.
- Abnormal infarction occurs in the setting of the intervillous hemorrhage of abruption, thrombosis, or vasoconstriction of the maternal spiral arteries.

PRESENTATION

- Small infarcts are asymptomatic and incidental.
- Peripheral infarcts are seen in a large proportion of term placentas.
- Large infarcts (>3 cm) are associated with fetal hypoxia, morbidity, and mortality.
- Placental infarction in the first two trimesters is always abnormal.

PROGNOSIS AND TREATMENT

- Prognosis and treatment are dependent on the extent and severity of infarction, as well as the antecedent cause.
- The vast majority of infarctions are found in the periphery of term placentas and import no risk to the infant.

PATHOLOGY

HISTOLOGY

- Grossly, a placental infarct is identified by a focus of villous pallor.

- Remote infarcts may be firm, fibrotic, and very pale.
- Early placental infarction is characterized by coalescence of the terminal villi with preservation of the trophoblasts.
- The coalescence is due to loss of the intervillous space.
- Over time, trophoblastic death leads to loss of nuclear detail and villous "ghosts" will remain.
- As the infarction becomes remote, extensive hyalinization may occur.
- In abruption-related infarction, intervillous hemorrhage will often be surrounded by a rim of placental infarction (i.e., the ball-and-socket infarct).

IMMUNOPATHOLOGY (INCLUDING IMMUNOHISTOCHEMISTRY)

- Noncontributory.

MAIN DIFFERENTIAL DIAGNOSIS

- Intervillous fibrin—may be impossible to distinguish from an aged infarct.
- Intervillous thrombus—may mimic an acute infarct.
- Intraplacental choriocarcinoma—reason enough to *sample all suspected intravillous thrombi.*

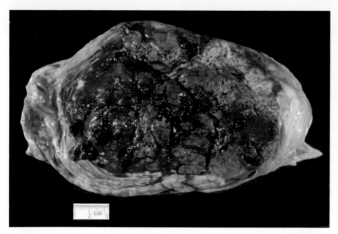

FIGURE 1

Placental infarction. The gross photo of the maternal surface reveals a markedly abnormal placental parenchyma. The discolored areas in the center correspond to recent infarcts; the pale granular areas at the upper right correspond to older infarcts.

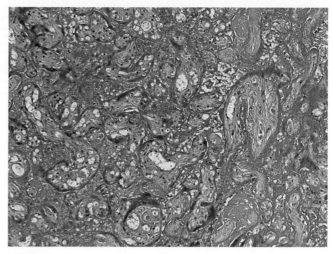

FIGURE 2

Placental infarction. A relatively recent infarct with degenerated trophoblast and collapse of the villous space.

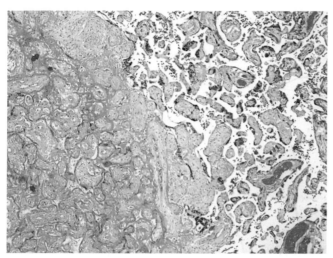

FIGURE 3

Placental infarction. A slightly older infarct on the left with juxtaposed uninfarcted but ischemic parenchyma on the right, with increased syncytial knots.

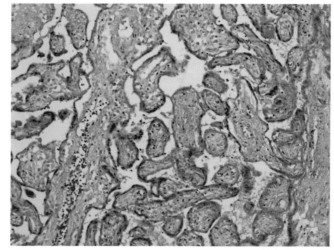

FIGURE 4

Placental infarction. This is a rather recent example, and note that the intervillous space is still preserved.

MECONIUM STAINING

DEFINITION—Discoloration of the placenta and membranes due to staining with meconium.

CLINICAL FEATURES

EPIDEMIOLOGY

- Meconium release is a relatively common event in term deliveries.
- Much debate exists about the pathologic nature of meconium and whether it represents a normal occurrence or is always pathologic.
- Meconium release is strongly associated with fetal stress near the time of delivery.

PRESENTATION

- Meconium staining is obvious at birth as a green to brown discoloration of the placenta and fetal membranes.
- Severe or remote cases may result in discoloration of the umbilical cord.

PROGNOSIS AND TREATMENT

- Meconium passage has variable effects on the newborn ranging from none to severe meconium aspiration.
- The prognosis depends on the amount of meconium passage, length of time of exposure, and the predisposing stressor leading to meconium release.
- Supportive care in symptomatic cases is the only realistic treatment option.

PATHOLOGY

HISTOLOGY

- Meconium staining is best appreciated within the membranes as a globular green to brown to orange pigment that is within macrophages.
- The amniotic surface often shows reactive changes of the amniocytes and occasionally shows necrosis.
- In severe or longstanding cases the pigment can even be identified within the umbilical cord, with associated inflammation, and rarely vascular necrosis.
- There may be a neutrophilic fetal inflammatory response that is out of proportion to the maternal inflammatory response.

IMMUNOPATHOLOGY (INCLUDING IMMUNOHISTOCHEMISTRY)

- Noncontributory.

MAIN DIFFERENTIAL DIAGNOSIS

- Hemosiderin.
- Deposition of another type of pigment.
- Inflammation due to infection.

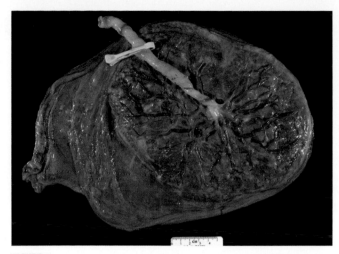

FIGURE 1

Meconium. Gross image of a meconium-stained placenta. There is greenish discoloration of the membranes and the fetal surface. The maternal surface *(not pictured)* will have normal coloration.

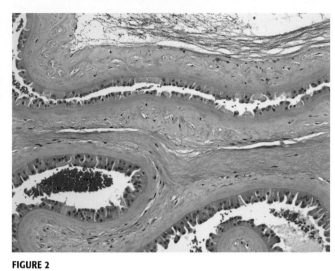

FIGURE 2

Meconium. At low power, meconium is not usually visible. Reactive amniocytes are identified by their prominence, with hobnailing and enlarged nuclei.

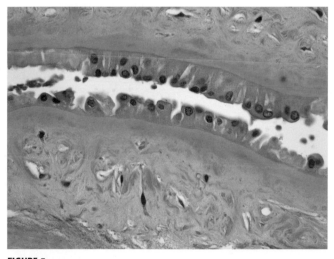

FIGURE 3

Meconium. At high power, greenish-brown pigment is seen engulfed by macrophages in the subchorionic tissue.

DISTAL VILLOUS PATHOLOGY

DEFINITION—Abnormalities in distal villous maturation that occur late in pregnancy and are emblematic of underperfusion, including increased syncytial knots, distal villous hypoplasia (DVH), aggregated terminal villi, and chorangiosis.

CLINICAL FEATURES

EPIDEMIOLOGY

- Seen as abnormal development of the distal villous tree as a consequence of multiple factors, including diabetes, smoking, anemia, pregnancy at high altitudes, and a number of genetic and epigenetic factors.
- Distal villous pathology (DVP) is associated with underperfusion and placental ischemia, specifically reversed end-diastolic flow.
- Linked to intrauterine growth restriction, intrauterine fetal death, and adverse neonatal neurological outcome.

PRESENTATION

- Should be typically looked for in small-for-dates placentas or fetuses, intrauterine fetal death (IUFD), or retrospectively in the case of adverse neurologic outcome.
- In many instances these changes may be encountered in normal placentas.

PROGNOSIS AND TREATMENT

- Management is directed toward monitoring the neonate. In cases of IUFD these changes in a placenta may help determine cause of death.

PATHOLOGY

HISTOLOGY

- DVH: The hallmark of DVH is small often widely spaced terminal villi with prominent syncytial knots.
- Terminal agglutination of villi.
- Increased syncytial knots.

- Chorangiosis: This has been associated with gestational diabetes, smoking, and pregnancy at high altitudes. It has been defined as at least 10 foci in the placenta containing at least 10 villi with 10 or more vessels seen at medium power (Altschuler criteria).

IMMUNOPATHOLOGY (INCLUDING IMMUNOHISTOCHEMISTRY)

- Noncontributory.

MAIN DIFFERENTIAL DIAGNOSIS

- Normal villous maturation late in pregnancy will feature syncytial knots; however, the terminal villi are not small.

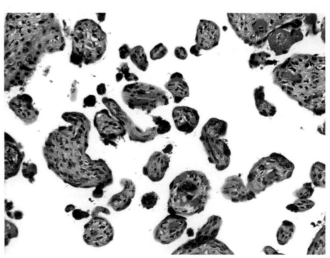

FIGURE 1

Increased syncytial knots. This is a generic correlate of placental ischemia that signifies "hypermaturity" and thus is evaluated in the context of the gestational age. It is characterized by groups of prominent syncytiotrophoblasts along stem and terminal villi.

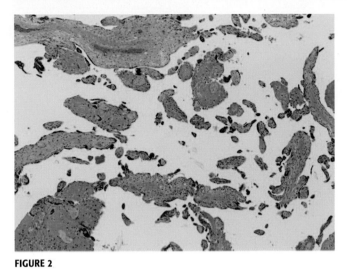

FIGURE 2

DVH. In this field there is a sudden transition from stem to small terminal villi, creating open space.

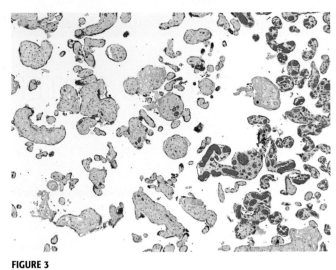

FIGURE 3

DVH at higher magnification showing the sharp contrast between very small terminal villi and stem villi.

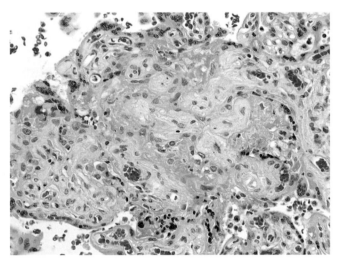

FIGURE 4

Aggregated terminal villi in which villi appear congealed in fibrin.

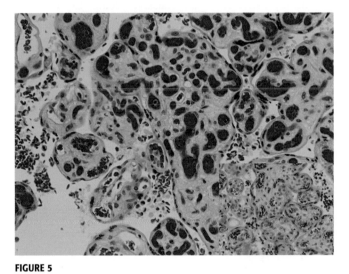

FIGURE 5

Chorangiosis. Here several villi contain at least 10 vessels each. Compare with normal villi (inset, lower right).

FETAL TO MATERNAL HEMORRHAGE

DEFINITION—Bleeding under low pressure into the placental parenchyma of fetal origin.

CLINICAL FEATURES

EPIDEMIOLOGY

- Cause is unknown.
- Rarely severe, with massive fetal to maternal hemorrhage.

PRESENTATION

- Small fetal to maternal hemorrhages are found incidentally in the placenta as intervillous thrombi (IVTs).
- Massive hemorrhage may not be detected and may be appreciated only as a pale placenta due to exsanguination and dispersal of the fetal blood into the maternal circulation.

PROGNOSIS AND TREATMENT

- There is no treatment.

PATHOLOGY

HISTOLOGY

- Grossly, small IVTs present as irregular laminated thrombi with minimal compression of the surrounding parenchyma.

- Focal adjacent infarcts or ischemic parenchymal changes might be appreciated.
- Massive fetal to maternal hemorrhage may be unappreciated with the exception of a pale placenta. In such cases a Kleihauer-Betke test for fetal erythrocytes in the maternal circulation will determine the extent of hemorrhage.

IMMUNOPATHOLOGY (INCLUDING IMMUNOHISTOCHEMISTRY)

- Noncontributory normally, although fetal to maternal hemorrhage has been documented by appropriate immunohistochemistry.

MAIN DIFFERENTIAL DIAGNOSIS

- Intervillous fibrin: may be impossible to distinguish from an old IVT.
- Intraplacental choriocarcinoma: reason enough to *sample all suspected IVTs*.

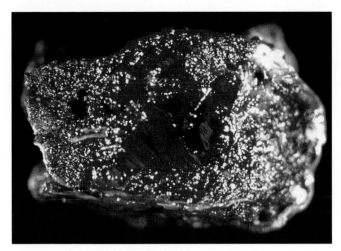

FIGURE 1

Cross section of placental disk with fresh IVT *(center)*.

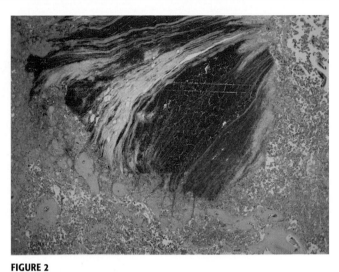

FIGURE 2

IVT. Note the layering of fibrin and blood characteristic of a thrombus. The interface of thrombus and parenchyma is not sharply circumscribed unlike a ball-in-socket infarct. However, the interface at the lower left displays some parenchymal changes in keeping with ischemia.

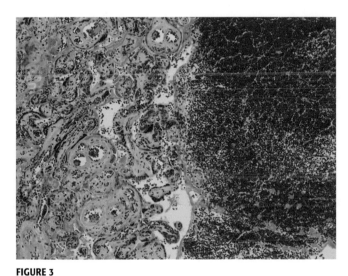

FIGURE 3

IVT. The interface with normal parenchyma displays a few ischemic villi with early trophoblastic degeneration.

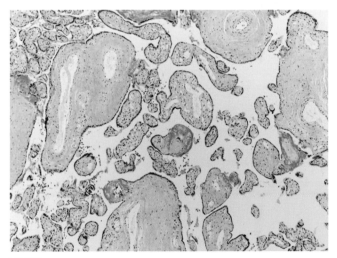

FIGURE 4

Markedly hypovolemic fetal vessels from a massive fetal to maternal hemorrhage, associated with a pale placenta. This underscores a specific cause of late intrauterine fetal death that will not provide evidence of intraplacental hemorrhage, yet like cord accident, must always be kept in the differential diagnosis until ruled out by appropriate tests.

COMMON PITFALLS IN DIAGNOSTIC GYNECOLOGIC AND OBSTETRIC PATHOLOGY

Topic	Mistaken for	Comments
Candidiasis	A premalignant lesion (vulvar intraepithelial neoplasia [VIN])	Chronically rubbed skin can produce a striking acanthosis. A yeast infection must always be kept in mind if there is minimal atypia or *any* epithelial neutrophils.
Syphilis	Inflammatory dermatosis	This is still a rare disease in vulvar pathology. However, any dense lymphoplasmacytic infiltrate, including those accompanied by acanthosis or which are arranged around vessels, should be investigated.
Psoriasis	VIN1	We have seen these occasionally misdiagnosed as VIN1.
Chronic erosive herpes	Noninfectious inflammatory conditions	Epithelial hyperplasia rather than erosion may be seen. The viral inclusions may not be obvious.
Sclerotic hidradenoma	Invasive adenocarcinoma	The degree of sclerosis can be striking with epithelial entrapment. Adenocarcinoma can be excluded with a p63 stain, which will highlight the basal cells.
Basal cell carcinoma	Adenoid basal carcinoma	These can be misclassified as adenoid cystic carcinomas. Basal-squamous lesions may be difficult to classify as well.
Pseudobowenoid papulosis	HIVIL or bowenoid papulosis	The abundant pseudomitoses seen with apoptosis can be confusing. At the same time similar changes can be seen in high-grade VIN, so caution is needed in both directions.
VIN with superimposed lichen simplex chronicus	Differentiated VIN or lichen simplex chronicus	Presumably if a VIN is rubbed or scratched, a prominent superimposed lichen simplex chronicus can occur. This may either make the lesion less conspicuous or prompt a diagnosis of differentiated VIN. Classic VIN can be confirmed with a p16 immunostain.
Pagetoid VIN	Glandular or urothelial lesion	A p16 stain may be helpful to support VIN; CK7/CK20/CDX2 can be used to investigate for spread from a gastrointestinal (GI) or urothelial primary.
VIN with columnar differentiation	Paget's disease	CK7 and GATA3 positivity is seen in Paget's disease cells (normal epithelium is CK5/6 positive).
Epstein-Barr virus (EBV)–like atypia	Classic VIN or atypia not otherwise specified (NOS)	A history of immunosuppression may be helpful.
Giant condyloma (GC)	Verrucous or papillary squamous carcinoma	GC can occur on the vulva, vagina, and cervix. Care should be exercised in making the diagnosis of a "verrucous" carcinoma in a young woman with an exophytic well-differentiated squamous lesion in this region. Most will be large condylomas.
Pseudoepitheliomatous hyperplasia (PEH)	Squamous cell carcinoma	The key is lack of atypia and the characteristic interlacing strands of epithelium. Also watch out for a granular cell tumor, syphilis, and the like, and be aware that some carcinomas can mimic PEH.
Keratoacanthoma	Underdiagnosis or overdiagnosis of squamous carcinoma	Remains a controversial diagnosis.
Aggressive angiomyxoma	Usually overdiagnosed	Look for the deep location and characteristic vascular pattern. Clinically it may be difficult to completely resect, and it may be locally invasive.

Continued

Topic	Mistaken for	Comments
Synovial sarcoma of vulva	Müllerian or vulvar adenocarcinoma or carcinosarcoma	The epithelium, if prominent, can be disarmingly benign appearing, and the stroma may not be markedly atypical, mimicking endometrial stroma. Müllerian markers (PAX8) will be absent; the presence of TLE1 would support synovial sarcoma.
Prepubertal fibroma	Angiomyxoma	Ill-defined, asymmetric, prominent collagen deposition.
Hymenal ring	Condyloma	A common pitfall. These are small filiform polyps without atypia.
Melanoma	Undifferentiated carcinoma or sarcoma	Vaginal melanoma may not have pigment and may not initially be clinically recognized. Always consider melanoma when confronted with a poorly differentiated spindle or epithelioid lesion in the vagina.
Spindle cell epithelioma	Sarcoma	The epithelial component is often quite subtle, but the spindle cells are bland appearing and well circumscribed. Cytokeratin stains will be focally positive.
Pseudocrypt pattern of invasive squamous carcinoma	High-grade squamous intraepithelial lesion (HSIL) with crypt involvement	Stromal reaction, loss of cell polarity, and central necrosis typify pseudocrypt involvement by carcinoma.
Lymphoepithelial-like carcinoma	Lymphoma, undifferentiated carcinoma	The squamous nests may be subtle but are strongly p63 positive.
Superficial adenocarcinoma in situ (AIS)	Tubal metaplasia, nonspecific changes	Mitoses and atypia may be inconspicuous or absent; look for discrete appearance, apoptosis, and luminal eosinophilia. p16 stain is very helpful.
Endocervicosis	Adenocarcinoma/ adenosarcoma	More typically the problem is not whether the lesion is malignant but why it is in the odd location. Best explanation is misplaced endocervix from a prior cesarean section (C-section).
Extensive cervical AIS	Invasive adenocarcinoma	Controversial and cutoffs are difficult to define; however, approach any extensive AIS with caution.
Signet-ring cell carcinoma of the cervix	Metastatic breast or GI carcinoma	This is a diagnosis of exclusion, but look for evidence of a precursor (AIS) lesion. Immunostains can be helpful.
Adenoid basal carcinoma	Squamous cell carcinoma	Look for the uniform nests, lack of desmoplasia, and the tell-tale rim of basal-type cells around the squamous nests.
Prostatic metaplasia	Adenoid basal carcinoma, squamous intraepithelial lesion	Look for the signature finding of small acini suspended in the squamotransitional nests.
Microglandular hyperplasia (MGH) of the endocervix	Adenocarcinoma	This can occur with solid growth, lacking significant acinar architecture. p16 will be patchy in MGH versus diffuse in carcinoma.
Mesonephric carcinoma	Sarcoma, conventional adenocarcinoma	The spindled variety tends to be remarkably uniform; glandular elements can resemble endometrial or sex cord differentiation and are typically closer to the surface, with the blander mesonephric histology at the periphery. The presence of GATA3 is supportive of mesonephric origin.
Minimal deviation adenocarcinoma (MDA)	Endocervical hyperplasia	Can be mistaken for each other. Irregular glands and intraglandular papillae with mitoses and atypia are key for MDA or its precursor. Remember both MDA and sex cord tumor with annular tubules (SCTATs) are associated with Peutz-Jeghers syndrome.
Adenosarcoma of the cervix, atypical polyp, adenomyoma	All three can be confused with each other	Beware that all three of these entities can have overlapping morphologic features. Smooth muscle fascicles are seen in adenomyoma.
Stromal breakdown	Adenocarcinoma and vice versa	The key is separating congealed aggregates of stroma from clusters of tumor cells. Rimming of stromal aggregates by reactive epithelium can help identify breakdown.
Yolk sac tumor of the vagina	Müllerian adenocarcinoma	A primitive-appearing vaginal carcinoma in a young woman raises this possibility.
Pyometra	Malignant and vice versa	May need to resample to confirm or exclude malignancy.
Exfoliation artifact	Adenocarcinoma or endometrial intraepithelial neoplasia (EIN)	Note that the adjacent stroma will usually demonstrate preservation artifacts and hemorrhage. Transition from normal to "abnormal" may be gradual and superficial.
Atypical polypoid adenomyoma (APA)	Myoinvasive carcinoma and vice versa	A compact investing smooth muscle component typifies APA.
Squamous cell carcinoma of endometrium	Benign squamous epithelium or metaplasia	The neoplastic squamous epithelium may be papillary and can be remarkably bland-appearing in endometrial primaries.

Topic	Mistaken for	Comments
Microacinar endometrioid carcinoma	Microglandular changes in the cervix	Collagen stroma separates acini more typical in benign MGH; slightly more amphophilic glands and a "soft" appearance to the glands in carcinoma.
Involvement of adenomyosis by adenocarcinoma	Myoinvasive adenocarcinoma	This cuts both ways. Extensive "vertical" growth or myxoid stromal reaction may indicate myoinvasion. Most important if present deeper than 50% of the myometrial thickness.
Intraperitoneal keratin granulomas	Metastatic carcinoma	Glandular epithelium is absent.
Histiocytes	Neoplastic cells	Histiocytes can form sheets with mitotic activity; lack of cell polarity, nuclear folds/grooves, and indistinct edges.
Ischemic atypia	Clear-cell or serous carcinoma	Seen most commonly in necrotic polyps; typically there is stromal hyaline change in a zonal configuration reflecting partial ischemic degenerative changes.
Adenocarcinoma with spindle features	Carcinosarcoma	Juxtaposed well-differentiated adenocarcinoma and plump spindled cells (keratin positive).
PEComa	Epithelioid smooth muscle tumor	Inherent overlap between the two tumor types. Prominent capillary vascular network and clear or eosinophilic cytoplasm in PEComa, including endometrial stromal sarcoma (ESS)–like invasion. HMB45 stain is helpful but will not always discriminate the two.
Myxoid low-grade ESS	Adenomyosis or adenomyomatosis, leiomyoma	Exceedingly bland with numerous normal-appearing vessels, but the growth pattern is distinctly ESS like.
Pregnancy- and inflammatory-related tubal atypia	Tubal intraepithelial or invasive carcinoma	Look for cilia, normal/wild-type p53 expression pattern, and low nuclear-to-cytoplasmic (N/C) ratio in Arias-Stella–like atypias.
Secretory cell outgrowths (benign epithelial hyperplasia)	Endometrioid/tubal neoplasia	These foci closely resemble endometrioid epithelium and have an increased proliferative index but are self-limited with normal p53 expression.
Tangentially sectioned follicle	Stromal tumor	Typically small and concentric with indistinct interface with the ovarian stroma; mitoses are common.
Clear-cell (CCC) and yolk sac tumors (YST)	Either and occasionally both in one tumor	Classic Schiller-Duval bodies and SALL4 favor YST; HNF1b, PAX8, CK7 present in CCC. Consider YST in middle-aged women if the immunophenotype does not fit for CCC, as a pure YST might respond dramatically to appropriate chemotherapy.
Spindled granulosa cell tumor	Fibrothecoma and rarely a smooth muscle tumor	Carefully evaluate highly cellular "thecomas," particularly with foci of nested epithelioid areas, high mitotic index. Pericellular reticulin preservation is common in fibrothecomas.
Follicle cyst	Cystic granulosa cell tumor	Look for monotonous growth pattern of granulosa cells, Call-Exner bodies, and nuclear grooves in the cystic germ cell tumor (GCT).
Juvenile granulosa cell tumor	Small cell carcinoma, hypercalcemic type	Granulosa cell tumors can exhibit considerable nuclear atypia. WT1 positive in small cell carcinoma.
Retiform Sertoli-Leydig cell tumor (RSLCT)	Borderline serous tumor	Young patients, retiform pattern in a portion of the lesion, heterologous elements, strong inhibin staining typify RSLCT.
Heterologous elements in sex cord tumors	Metastatic carcinoma, sex cord differentiation, sarcomas	Hepatic differentiation can mimic breast carcinoma; the latter is positive for GATA3.
Benign germinal matrix in teratomas	Immature teratoma	Be aware of normal cerebellar differentiation. Immature neuroepithelium typically contains abundant mitoses and apoptosis.
Extravillous trophoblast	Choriocarcinoma	No necrosis or marked trophoblastic atypia. Be familiar with previllous trophoblast.
Degenerating decidual cells	Can mimic mature extravillous trophoblast and vice versa	Cytokeratin stains.
Focal mature villi or an old implantation site in first-trimester curetting	Intrauterine pregnancy	Mature villi, old implantation site, and even recent implantation site (via contamination) can mimic a current intrauterine pregnancy.
Localized endometrial proliferation of pregnancy	EIN or adenocarcinoma	Found typically in a "products of conception" specimen.
Early complete mole	Hydropic abortus	Watch out for stromal basophilia and karyorrhexis, mild concentric thickening of the trophoblastic rim.
Intraplacental choriocarcinoma	Infarct	Sample all infarcts for histologic exam!

Continued

Topic	Mistaken for	Comments
Placental site trophoblastic tumor (PSTT)	Exaggerated implantation site	MelCAM/MIB1 staining should highlight over 15% of cells in PSTT. Look for sheets of tumor cells between smooth muscle fascicles.
Epithelioid leiomyoma	Epithelioid trophoblastic tumor in a small sample	Desmin positive. Cytokeratins may stain both tumors.
Mesenchymal dysplasia	Partial mole	Abnormally large stem villi. Lack of cistern formation in mesenchymal dysplasia.
Histiocytic intervillositis	Unremarkable abortus	The histiocytes can be present but unappreciated in early second-trimester pregnancy. This can recur and be associated with repeated pregnancy loss.
Listeria	Conventional intervillositis	Acute intervillositis; order appropriate stains for microorganisms.
Fetal thrombotic vasculopathy (FTV)	Chronic villitis, fetal death	Chronic villitis can be inconspicuous in villitis-mediated villous sclerosis; remote fetal death will cause widespread villous changes mimicking FTV.
Maternal-fetal hemorrhage	No abnormality	Look for pale placenta, bloodless villi, and normoblastemia. Order a Kleihauer-Betke test.
Candida chorioamnionitis	Conventional chorioamnionitis	Can be lethal if undetected. Search for neutrophils on the surface of the cord.

INDEX

Page numbers followed by "f" indicate figures and "t" indicate tables.

A

Ablation artifact, 368, 369f
Abortion, spontaneous, 737
Acanthosis, in eczematous dermatitis, 3, 4f
AIS. *see* Adenocarcinoma in situ (AIS).
Actinomycosis, pseudoactinomycotic radiant
  granules versus, 355
Acute herpes simplex virus infection, 40, 41f
Acute salpingitis, versus follicular salpingitis,
  517
Adenocarcinoma
  with apocrine features, 75f, 78f
  breakdown mimicking neoplasia versus,
    341
  clear cell, 221, 222f
  endometrioid, 223, 224f-225f
  of fallopian tube, 549-550, 550f
  high-grade, squamous and morular
    metaplasia versus, 385
  of lower uterine segment, 400, 401f
  mixed-pattern, 426, 427f
  radiation atypia versus, 286
  with spindle cell features, 445, 445f-446f
  vaginal adenosis versus, 204
  well-differentiated, atypical polypoid
    adenomyoma versus, 374
Adenocarcinoma in situ (AIS)
  cervical, endometriosis versus, 280
  conventional, 274f-275f
    clinical features of, 273
    differential diagnosis of, 274
    pathology of, 273-274
  extensive, versus invasion, 292, 293f-294f
    clinical features of, 292
    differential diagnosis of, 292
    pathology of, 292
  intestinal variant of, 278, 279f
  radiation atypia versus, 286
  reactive atypia in endocervix versus, 284
  stratified, 276, 277f
  superficial (early), 270, 271f-272f
    clinical features of, 270
    differential diagnosis of, 270
    pathology of, 270
Adenofibroma, 527, 527f-528f
  endometrioid, 620, 621f
  of ovary, 578f
Adenoid basal carcinoma, 308, 309f
  cervical
    conventional squamous cell carcinoma
      versus, 263
    pseudocrypt involvement by squamous
      cell carcinoma versus, 266

Adenoid cystic carcinoma, 74, 74f-75f, 77f
  adenoid basal carcinoma versus, 308
  clinical features of, 74
  differential diagnosis of, 74
  pathology of, 74
Adenoma, Bartholin's, 70, 72, 73f
  clinical features of, 72
  differential diagnosis of, 72
  hyperplasia of Bartholin's gland versus, 70
  pathology of, 72
Adenoma malignum, myoinvasion and, 406,
    409f
Adenomatoid tumor, 472, 473f-474f
  clinical features of, 472
  differential diagnosis of, 472
  pathology of, 472
Adenomyoma
  atypical endocervical polyp versus, 324
  versus atypical endometrial polyp, 469
  cervical adenosarcoma versus, 331
  of cervix, 326, 327f
Adenomyomatous polyp, 351, 352f
Adenomyosis-like pattern, of myoinvasion,
    406, 408f-409f
Adenosarcoma
  cervical adenomyoma versus, 326
  cervical schwannoma versus, 333
  of cervix, 331, 332f
  of endometrium, 466-467, 467f-468f
    clinical features of, 466
    differential diagnosis of, 467
    pathology of, 466-467
  of ovary, 594, 595f-596f
    carcinosarcoma versus, 592
    clinical features of, 594
    differential diagnosis of, 594
    pathology of, 594
Adenosis, vaginal, 204, 205f
Adenosquamous carcinoma, 144, 145f
Adherent blood clot
  versus hypertensive bleeding infarct, 798
  versus inflammatory abruption, 796
Adrenal rest, 511, 512f
Amniotic bands, 776, 777f
Amniotic fluid infection, 780
  stages of, 782t
  template for, 782t
Anal carcinoma, 195, 196f
Anal condyloma, 190, 191f-192f
  clinical features of, 190
  differential diagnosis of, 190
  pathology of, 190
Anal intraepithelial neoplasia II and III, 193,
    194f

Anal Paget's disease, 197, 198f-199f
  clinical features of, 197
  differential diagnosis of, 197
  pathology of, 197
Angiofibroma, cellular, 168, 169f
Angiokeratoma, 183, 184f
Angiomatosis, bacillary, 52, 53f
Angiomyofibroblastoma, 163, 164f
Angiomyxoma, 165, 165f
  superficial, 166, 167f
Anovulatory endometrium, with persistent
    follicle, 343, 344f
Antivirals, for HSV infection, 40
APA. *see* Atypical polypoid adenomyoma
    (APA).
Arias-Stella effect
  clear cell adenocarcinoma versus, 221
  clear-cell carcinoma versus, 434
  endometrial intraepithelial carcinoma versus,
    418
  high-grade intraepithelial neoplasia versus,
    542, 544f
  ischemic atypias of endometrium versus, 419
  low-grade serous tubal intraepithelial
    neoplasia versus, 536
  radiation atypia versus, 286
  reactive atypia versus
    in endocervix, 284
    in endometrium, 421
  tubal, 524, 525f-526f
    clinical features of, 524
    differential diagnosis of, 524
    pathology of, 524
Atrophy
  high-grade vaginal intraepithelial neoplasia
    III versus, 216
  including squamous intraepithelial lesion in
    atrophy, 249, 250f-251f
    clinical features of, 249
    differential diagnosis of, 249
    pathology of, 249
Atypia
  epidermodysplasia verruciformis-like, 106,
    107f
  metaplastic, minor p16-positive, 252,
    253f-254f
  moderate, and STIN, 536
Atypical polyp
  endocervical, 324, 325f
  endometrial, 469, 470f-471f
Atypical polypoid adenomyoma (APA), 374,
    375f
  adenomyomatous polyp versus, 351
  versus atypical endometrial polyp, 469

Atypical polypoid adenomyoma (APA)
  (Continued)
  clinical features of, 374
  differential diagnosis of, 374
  pathology of, 374
Atypical proliferations, 414, 415f-416f
Atypical verruciform hyperplasia. *see* Vulvar
  acanthosis with altered differentiation.

B

Bacillary angiomatosis, 52, 53f
Bacterial vaginosis, 36, 37f
Ball-in-socket infarct. *see* Hypertensive infarct.
Bartholin's adenoma, 70, 72, 73f
  clinical features of, 72
  differential diagnosis of, 72
  hyperplasia of Bartholin's gland versus,
    70
  pathology of, 72
Bartholin's duct cyst, 57, 58f
  Bartholin's adenoma versus, 72
  clinical features of, 57, 58f
  main differential diagnosis of, 57
  pathology of, 57
Bartholin's gland
  carcinoma of, 76
  hyperplasia of, 70, 71f
Basal atypia, 110
Basal cell carcinoma, 141, 142f-143f
  adenoid variant, 75f, 77f
  clinical features of, 141
  differential diagnosis of, 141
  pathology of, 141
Basaloid carcinoma, 75f, 78f
  cervical, conventional squamous cell
    carcinoma versus, 263
  occasional primitive, papillary squamous
    carcinoma versus, 219
  squamous, 142f
Benign adnexal tumors, versus mucous cyst of
  vagina, 59
Benign epithelial hyperplasia, 529, 530f-531f
  clinical features of, 529
  differential diagnosis of, 529
  high-grade serous tubal intraepithelial
    neoplasia versus, 542
  low-grade serous tubal intraepithelial
    neoplasia versus, 536
  pathology of, 529
Benign hyperplasia, 345, 346f
  anovulatory endometrium with persistent
    follicle versus, 343
  clinical features of, 345
  differential diagnosis of, 345
  endometrial intraepithelial neoplasia versus,
    371
  pathology of, 345
Benign or proliferative struma
  malignant struma versus, 653
  reactive changes in, 655f
Benign papillary hyperplasia, in struma,
  654f
Benign serous tumors, 579f
Biliary carcinoma, metastatic, 641f-642f
Biphasic carcinoma, 397
Borderline Brenner tumor
  benign Brenner tumor versus, 629
  malignant Brenner tumor versus, 631

Borderline clear-cell adenofibroma, 638, 639f
  in a case of mixed clear-cell carcinoma and
    YSC of ovary, 637f
  clinical features of, 638
  differential diagnosis of, 638
  pathology of, 638
"Borderline endometrioid tumor", 622
Borderline mucinous tumors, mucinous
  carcinoma versus, 607
Borderline serous tumors
  müllerian mucinous and seromucinous
    tumors of ovary versus, 626
  versus papillary mesothelioma, 723
  serous cystadenomas and cystadenofibromas
    versus, 577
Bowenoid dysplasia, 100, 100f-101f
  associated with HPV 16, 101f
  seborrheic keratosis versus, 88
BRCA1 mutations, and low-grade serous tubal
  intraepithelial neoplasia, 535
BRCA2 mutations, and low-grade serous tubal
  intraepithelial neoplasia, 535
Breast carcinoma, metastatic, 641f-642f
  signet-ring cell cervical adenocarcinoma
    versus, 305
Breast tissue, ectopic, 61, 62f
Brenner tumor
  benign, 629, 630f
  malignant, 631, 632f
  proliferative, low-grade endometrioid
    adenocarcinoma with squamotransitional
    or spindle features versus, 590
Broad front pattern, of myoinvasion, 406
Bullous pemphigoid, 18, 19f

C

Calretinin, cortical inclusion cysts stained with,
  581f
Cancer, risk for, and risk reducing salpingo-
  oophorectomy, 545
Candida infection
  gestational, 783, 784f
  with LSC, 6f
Candidiasis, vulvovaginal, 34, 35f
Carcinoid, benign Brenner tumor versus, 629
Carcinoma
  versus adenocarcinoma with spindle cell
    features, 445
  adenoid cystic, 74, 74f-75f, 77f
  with adenomyosis, 406, 407f
  adenosquamous, 144, 145f
  adnexal or apocrine, 74
  anal, 195, 196f
  Bartholin's gland, 76
  basal cell, 75f, 77f, 141
  basaloid, 75f, 78f
    squamous, 142f
  cloacogenic, 151, 152f
  versus endometrial histiocytes, 412
  endometrioid or clear-cell, 437, 438f-439f
  Merkel cell, 149, 150f
  papillary squamous, 219, 220f
  undifferentiated
    of endometrium, 432, 433f
    versus uterine serous carcinoma, 424
  verrucous, 135f
  well-differentiated, telescoping artifacts
    mimicking neoplasia versus, 347

Carcinosarcoma, 440, 441f-444f, 592, 593f
  adenoid basal carcinoma versus, 308
  adenosarcoma versus
    of endometrium, 467
    of ovary, 594
  clinical features of, 440, 592
  differential diagnosis of, 440, 592
  low-grade endometrial stromal sarcoma
    versus, 456
  mixed-pattern adenocarcinoma versus,
    426
  pathology of, 440, 592
  retiform SLCT versus, 696
  synovial sarcoma of vulva versus, 179
  Wilms' tumor versus, 447
CD10, myoinvasion and, 406
Cellular angiofibroma, 168, 169f
  clinical features of, 168
  differential diagnosis of, 168
  pathology of, 168
  prepubertal vulvar fibroma versus, 187
Cellular leiomyoma, 477, 478f
  clinical features of, 477
  differential diagnosis of, 477
  pathology of, 477
  versus renal cell carcinoma syndrome, 497
  stromomyoma versus, 451
Cerebellar differentiation, in mature cystic
  teratoma, 646, 647f
Cervical cancer, lower uterine segment
  adenocarcinoma versus, 400
Cervical cone biopsy, for conventional
  adenocarcinoma in situ, 273
Cervical endometriosis, 280, 281f
Cervical intraepithelial neoplasia 1, 237-238,
  238f-239f
Cervical intraepithelial neoplasia II, 240-241,
  241f-242f
Cervical intraepithelial neoplasia III, 240-241,
  241f-242f
Cervical neuroendocrine carcinoma, versus
  neuroendocrine carcinoma, 430
Cervical schwannoma, 333, 334f
Cervix
  adenosarcoma of, 331, 332f
  mesonephric remnants in, 310, 311f
  microglandular hyperplasia of, 328,
    329f-330f
  pregnancy-related changes in, 282, 283f
  in situ and invasive adenocarcinoma of, with
    gastric differentiation, 300-301, 301f
  squamous cell carcinoma of, endometrial
    squamous carcinoma versus, 389
Chancroid, 46, 47f
Chemotherapy, for undifferentiated uterine
  sarcoma, 464
Chorangioma, 764, 764f-765f
Chorangioma-associated trophoblastic
  proliferation, versus intraplacental
  choriocarcinoma, 754
Choriosis, 817f
  diffuse, versus chorangioma, 764
Chorioamnionitis, 780-781
  acute, 781f
  clinical features of, 780
  differential diagnosis of, 781
  from gestational *Candida* infection, 784f
  pathology of, 780-781

Choriocarcinoma, 752-753, 753f
  clinical features of, 752
  differential diagnosis of, 753
  intraplacental, 754, 755f-756f
    versus choriangioma, 764
    clinical features of, 754
    differential diagnosis of, 754
    pathology of, 754
  molar implantation site versus, 759
  pathology of, 752
  placental site trophoblastic tumor versus, 758
  spontaneous abortion versus, 737
Chorionic plate vascular inflammation, 782f
Chorionic villi, early, 738f
Chronic erosive herpes simplex, 42, 43f
Chronic erosive lichen planus, 14
Chronic salpingitis, versus pseudoxanthomatous salpingiosis, 513
Circummarginate placenta, 772, 773f
Circumvallate placenta, 772, 773f
Clear-cell adenocarcinoma, 221, 222f
  clinical features of, 221
  differential diagnosis of, 221
  microglandular cervical hyperplasia versus, 328
  pathology of, 221
  pregnancy-related changes in cervix versus, 282
Clear-cell adenofibroma, borderline clear-cell adenofibroma versus, 638
Clear-cell carcinoma, 434, 435f-436f, 633, 634f-635f
  of cervix, 298, 299f
  clinical features of, 434, 633
  differential diagnosis of, 633
  embryonal carcinoma versus, 670
  versus endometrioid or clear-cell carcinoma, 437
  exfoliation artifact versus, 364
  versus ischemic atypias of endometrium, 419
  pathology of, 434, 633
  radiation atypia versus, 286
  reactive atypia in endometrium versus, 421
  uterine serous carcinoma versus, 424
Cloacogenic carcinoma, 151, 152f
  clinical features of, 151
  differential diagnosis of, 151
  glandular, 196f
  pathology of, 151
Clomiphene, for polycystic ovarian syndrome, 566
Clonal evolution, mixed pattern endometrium versus, 349
"Clue cells", 36, 37f
  multiple, 37f
Colon cancer, metastatic, 642f
Colonic carcinoma, metastatic, 553f, 641f
Complete mole
  early, versus spontaneous abortion, 737
  hydatidiform, 741-742, 742f-743f
    clinical features of, 741
    differential diagnosis of, 742
    early, 741-742, 742f-743f
      versus intraplacental choriocarcinoma, 754
    late, 741
    pathology of, 741-742

Condyloma, 79, 81f
  anal, 190, 191f-192f
  clinical features of, 79
  containing koilocytotic atypia, 81f
  differential diagnosis of, 79
  flat, 92, 93f
  hymenal ring versus, 208
  immature, 245, 246f
  multiple, 80f
  nonkoilocytotic variant of, 81f
  pathology of, 79
  versus seborrheic keratosis, 88
Condyloma acuminatum, 80f-81f
  immature condyloma versus, 245
Condyloma lata, 44
Cone biopsy, for intestinal variant of adenocarcinoma in situ, 278
Cord insertion, variations on, 770
  furcate. see Furcate cord insertion
  marginal. see Marginal cord insertion
  membranous. see Membranous cord insertion
Corpus luteum
  cortical inclusion cysts associated with, 581f
  of pregnancy, 561f-562f
    decidualized endometrioma versus, 575
    histology of, 561
Cortical inclusion cysts (CICs), 580, 581f
  clinical features of, 580
  differential diagnosis of, 580
  extensive, serous cystadenomas and cystadenofibromas versus, 577
  pathology of, 580
Cortical invasion, by low-grade serous carcinoma, 603f
Cortical stromal hyperplasia, 569-570, 570f
Crohn's disease
  versus granulomatous salpingitis, 520
  of vulva, 30, 31f
Crystalloids of Reinke, 700f
Curettings, microglandular endometrial adenocarcinoma in, 393, 394f-395f
Cystadenofibromas, 577
  clinical features of, 577
  differential diagnosis of, 577
  paratubal, 578f
  pathology of, 577
  serous, 579f
Cystic adhesions, versus benign cystic mesothelioma, 721
Cysts
  Bartholin's duct, 57, 58f
  benign serous, versus benign cystic mesothelioma, 721
  cortical inclusion, 580, 581f
  epidermal inclusion
    versus Bartholin's duct cyst, 57
    versus mucous cyst of vagina, 59
  Gartner's duct, versus mucous cyst of vagina, 59
  mucous. see Mucous cyst
  multiloculated simple/mesothelial, borderline clear-cell adenofibroma versus, 638
  paratubal, serous cystadenomas and cystadenofibromas versus, 577
  Skene's duct
    versus Bartholin's duct cyst, 57
    versus mucous cyst of vagina, 59
  solitary luteinized follicle, 564, 565f

Cytomegalovirus (CMV) infection, versus chronic villitis, 787

D

Darier's disease, 24, 25f
  clinical features of, 24
  differential diagnosis of, 24
  versus epidermolytic hyperkeratosis, 26
  pathology of, 24
Decidua, versus fresh implantation site, 733
Decidualized endometrioma, 575, 576f
Dedifferentiated liposarcoma, 177
Deep aggressive angiomyxoma, prepubertal vulvar fibroma versus, 187
Degenerative repair, 378, 379f
Dermatitis
  eczematous, 3, 4f
  seborrheic, 9, 10f
Dermatofibroma, 170, 171f
Dermatofibrosarcoma protuberans, 172, 173f
Desmoplastic noninvasive implants, 605, 606f
Desmoplastic small round cell tumor, 719, 720f
Diffuse laminar glandular hyperplasia, 317
Dilation and curettage (D&C), 731
Disseminated intraperitoneal leiomyomatosis, 493, 494f
Distal villous pathology (DVP), 816, 816f-817f
Divergent differentiation, and low-grade endometrial stromal carcinoma, 455-456
DNA poxvirus, 38
Donovan bodies, 48, 49f
DVP. see Distal villous pathology (DVP).
Dysgerminoma, 664-665, 665f-666f
  clinical features of, 664
  differential diagnosis of, 665
  versus mixed germ cell tumor, 675
  pathology of, 664
Dyskeratoma, warty, 84, 85f
Dyskeratotic cells, 24
Dysplasia
  bowenoid, 100, 100f-101f
  mesenchymal, 750, 751f
Dysplastic nevus, 159, 160f

E

Early complete hydatidiform mole, 741-742, 742f-743f
Eclampsia, toxemia and, 810
Ectopic breast tissue, 61, 62f
  clinical features of, 61
  differential diagnosis of, 61
  with fibroadenoma, 64f
  pathology of, 61
Ectopic pregnancy, 739, 740f
  clinical features of, 739
  differential diagnosis of, 739
  fetiform teratoma versus, 648
  pathology of, 739
  tubal, 740f
Eczematous dermatitis, 3, 4f
  clinical features of, 3
  differential diagnosis of, 3
  versus lichen simplex chronicus and prurigo nodularis, 5
  pathology of, 3
EIN. see Endometrial intraepithelial neoplasia (EIN).

Embryonal carcinoma, 670, 671f
  clinical features of, 670
  differential diagnosis of, 670
  versus dysgerminoma, 676f
  pathology of, 670
Embryonal rhabdomyosarcoma, 230, 231f
Empiric therapy, for neuroendocrine carcinoma, 430
Endocervical adenocarcinoma
  adenoma malignum variant of
    cervical adenomyoma versus, 326
    cervical schwannoma versus, 333
  early invasive
    conventional adenocarcinoma in situ versus, 274
    extensive adenocarcinoma in situ versus invasion and, 292
  glandular hyperplasia versus, 317
  infiltrative, 295-296, 296f-297f
  microglandular cervical hyperplasia versus, 328
  superficial, 290, 291f
Endocervical adenocarcinoma in situ, pregnancy-related changes in cervix versus, 282
Endocervical adenosarcoma, low-grade, atypical endocervical polyp versus, 324
Endocervical glandular neoplasia, endometrial involvement by, 376-377, 377f
Endocervical hyperplasia
  benign, in situ and invasive adenocarcinoma of cervix with gastric differentiation versus, 301
  glandular, 317, 318f
Endocervical microglandular change, microglandular endometrial adenocarcinoma in curettings versus, 393
Endocervical polyp
  atypical, 324, 325f
  benign atypical, cervical adenosarcoma versus, 331
  cervical schwannoma versus, 333
Endocervix
  reactive atypias in, 284, 285f
  superficial adenocarcinoma of. see Endocervical adenocarcinoma, superficial
Endometrial adenocarcinoma
  endometrioid, metastatic low-grade, cervical endometriosis versus, 280
  in Lynch syndrome, 403, 404f
  microglandular, in curettings, 393, 394f-395f
  microglandular cervical hyperplasia versus, 328
  myoinvasion in, 406, 407f-409f
  small endometrioid carcinoma in, 551f
  squamous and morular metaplasia versus, 385
  with squamous differentiation, ichthyosis uteri versus, 387
Endometrial adenosarcoma, low-grade, versus atypical endometrial polyp, 469
Endometrial carcinoma
  conventional, with squamous differentiation, endometrial squamous carcinoma versus, 389
  metastatic, cervical mesonephric remnants versus, 310

Endometrial histiocytes, foamy stromal macrophages and, 412, 413f
Endometrial intraepithelial neoplasia (EIN), 370-371, 371f-373f
  anovulatory endometrium with persistent follicle versus, 343
  atypical polypoid adenomyoma versus, 374
  benign hyperplasia versus, 345
  clinical features of, 370
  degenerative repair versus, 378
  differential diagnosis of, 371
  pathology of, 370-371
  telescoping artifacts mimicking neoplasia versus, 347
Endometrial neoplasia, proliferative repair versus, 380
Endometrial polyps
  adenomyomatous polyp versus, 351
  anovulatory endometrium with persistent follicle versus, 343
  atypical endometrial polyp versus, 469
  benign hyperplasia versus, 345
  chronic endometritis versus, 354
  endometrial intraepithelial neoplasia versus, 371
  necrotic, ablation artifact and, 368
  prolapsed, atypical endocervical polyp versus, 324
  submucosal leiomyoma versus, 361
Endometrial stromal nodule, 449, 450f
  clinical features of, 449
  differential diagnosis of, 449
  versus low-grade endometrial stromal sarcoma, 456
  pathology of, 449
Endometrial stromal sarcoma (ESS)
  adenosarcoma of the endometrium versus, 467
  endometrial stromatosis versus, 453, 454f
  low-grade. see Low-grade endometrial stromal sarcoma
  myxoid variant, intravenous leiomyomatosis versus, 489
  stromomyoma versus, 451
  uterine tumor resembling sex cord stromal tumor versus, 459
Endometrial stromal tumor, submucosal leiomyoma versus, 361
Endometrial stromatosis, 453, 454f
Endometrioid adenocarcinoma, 223, 224f-225f, 396-397, 398f-399f
  clinical features of, 223, 396
  differential diagnosis of, 223, 397
  endometrial intraepithelial neoplasia versus, 371
  grade 3, versus neuroendocrine carcinoma, 430
  low-grade, endometrial involvement by endocervical glandular neoplasia versus, 377
  metastatic, mesonephric carcinoma versus, 312
  p53-positive, 428, 429f
  pathology of, 223, 396-397
  with secretory differentiation
    clear cell adenocarcinoma versus, 221
    clear-cell carcinoma versus, 434
  with spindle cell component, synovial sarcoma of vulva versus, 179

Endometrioid adenofibroma, 620, 621f
Endometrioid atypia, involving plica, 551f
Endometrioid carcinoma
  grade II, versus mixed-pattern adenocarcinoma, 426
  low-grade, proliferative (borderline) endometrioid adenofibroma versus, 623
  metastatic to cervix, 321, 322f-323f
    clinical features of, 321
    differential diagnosis of, 321
    pathology of, 321
  with transitional or spindle cell differentiation, malignant Brenner tumor versus, 631
  uterine serous carcinoma versus, 424
Endometrioid endometrial cancer (EEC)
  diagnosis of, 397
  morphologic patterns in, 396-397
  traditional low-grade, 396
Endometrioid glands, divergent differentiation in, 455-456
Endometrioid or clear-cell carcinoma, 437, 438f-439f
Endometrioma
  with atypia, 573, 574f
  decidualized, 575, 576f
  with mucinous metaplasia, 571, 572f
Endometriosis
  adenosarcoma arising in, cervical adenosarcoma versus, 331
  with atypia, proliferative (borderline) endometrioid adenofibroma versus, 623
  cervical, 280, 281f
  polypoid, 206, 207f
  vaginal adenosis versus, 204
Endometritis, chronic, 353-354, 354f
Endometrium
  ischemic atypias of, 419
  mixed pattern, 349, 350f
  reactive atypia in, 421
  undifferentiated carcinoma of, 432, 433f
Endosalpingeal implants, from remote tumors, 552, 553f
Endosalpingiosis, 582, 583f
  clinical features of, 582
  differential diagnosis of, 582
  invasive implants versus, 605
  pathology of, 582
Enlarging teratoma syndrome, 672
Epidermal inclusion cyst
  versus Bartholin's duct cyst, 57
  versus mucous cyst of vagina, 59
Epidermodysplasia verruciformis-like atypia, 106, 107f
Epidermolytic hyperkeratosis, 26, 27f
Epithelial tumors
  metastatic carcinoid versus, 659
  with yolk sac carcinoma, versus mixed germ cell tumor, 675
Epithelioid leiomyosarcoma, 503, 504f
  clinical features of, 503
  differential diagnosis of, 503
  versus epithelioid trophoblastic tumor, 762
  pathology of, 503
Epithelioid placental site nodule, versus epithelioid trophoblastic tumor, 762

Epithelioid trophoblastic tumor, 761-762, 762f-763f
  clinical features of, 761
  differential diagnosis of, 762
  pathology of, 761
Epithelioma, spindle cell, 228, 229f
Erythema
  of labia minora and majora, 35f
  occasional, 32
ESS. see Endometrial stromal sarcoma (ESS).
Exfoliation artifact, 364, 365f
  clinical features of, 364
  differential diagnosis of, 364
  endometrial intraepithelial carcinoma versus, 418
  pathology of, 364
Exophytic low-grade squamous intraepithelial lesion, 235, 236f
External genitalia, giant condyloma of, 134, 135f-136f

F

Fallopian tube
  adenocarcinoma of, 549-550, 550f
  adenofibroma and, 527
  Arias-Stella effect of, 524, 525f
  versus papillary hyperplasia, 539
  prolapsed, 200, 201f
    vaginal adenosis versus, 204
  sectioning of, versus salpingitis isthmica nodosum, 519
  torsion of, 522, 523f
"False knot," in cord, versus umbilical cord knots, 766, 767f
Fasciitis, necrotizing, 54, 54f
Female adnexal tumor of wolffian origin (FATWO), 554, 555f
  adenocarcinoma of fallopian tube versus, 550
  clinical features of, 554
  differential diagnosis of, 554
  pathology of, 554
Fetal leukemia, 802, 803f
Fetal to maternal hemorrhage, 818, 819f
Fetal vascular thrombosis, 774, 775f
  versus chronic villitis, 787
  clinical features of, 774
  differential diagnosis of, 774
  pathology of, 774
Fetiform teratoma, 648, 649f
Fetus in fetu, fetiform teratoma versus, 648
Fibrin, implantation site and, 735
Fibroadenoma, 63, 64f
Fibroepithelial papilloma, 79
Fibroepithelial stromal polyp, 86, 87f
  anal condyloma versus, 190
  clinical features of, 86
  condyloma versus, 79
  differential diagnosis of, 86
  hymenal ring versus, 208
  pathology of, 86
  prepubertal vulvar fibroma versus, 187
Fibroma
  with minor sex cord elements, 680, 681f
  versus sclerosing stromal tumor, 705
Fibroma-thecoma
  cortical stromal hyperplasia and hyperthecosis versus, 570
  sclerosing stromal tumor versus, 705

Fibromyxoid sarcoma, low-grade, 174, 175f
Fibrothecoma
  versus gastrointestinal stromal tumor, 715
  histology of, 677
Fibrous histiocytoma. see Dermatofibroma.
"Fish net pattern", 20
Flat condyloma, 92, 93f, 237-238, 238f-239f
  clinical features of, 92, 237
  differential diagnosis of, 238
    and pitfalls, 92
  pathology of, 92, 237-238
Florid benign microglandular change, signet-ring cell cervical adenocarcinoma versus, 305
Florid endocervical adenocarcinoma in situ, villoglandular adenocarcinoma of cervix versus, 288
Focal atypia, in struma ovarii, 652f
Follicle, with granulosa cells, 685f
Follicular dysfunction, mixed pattern endometrium versus, 349
Follicular salpingitis, 517, 518f
  clinical features, 517
  differential diagnosis, 517
  histology, 517
  versus salpingitis isthmica nodosum, 519
FOXJ1, cortical inclusion cysts stained with, 581f
Fresh implantation site, 733, 734f
Furcate cord insertion, 770, 771f

G

Gartner's duct cyst, versus mucous cyst of vagina, 59
Gastric carcinoma, metastatic, 641f
  signet-ring cell cervical adenocarcinoma versus, 305
Gastrointestinal stromal tumor, 715, 716f
Genital-type nevus, 157, 158f
Germ cell tumor, mixed, 675, 676f
Germinal matrix differentiation, in mature cystic teratoma, 646, 647f
Gestational Candida infection, 783, 784f
Gestational sac, 731, 732f
Giant condyloma, 243, 244f
  of external genitalia, 134, 135f-136f
Glial polyp, of cervix, 335, 336f
Gliomatosis peritonei, 672
Granular cell tumor, 185, 186f
Granulation tissue, 202, 203f
  clinical features of, 202
  differential diagnosis of, 202
  pathology of, 202
  prolapsed fallopian tube versus, 200
Granuloma, intraperitoneal keratin, 410, 411f
Granuloma inguinale, 48, 48f-49f
Granulomatous endometritis, tubercular endometritis versus, 359
Granulomatous salpingitis, 520, 521f
  clinical features, 520
  differential diagnosis, 520
  pathology, 520
  versus xanthogranulomatous salpingitis, 515
Granulosa cell tumor(s), 684, 685f
  adult-type, 685f-686f, 689f
  benign Brenner tumor versus, 629

Granulosa cell tumor(s) (Continued)
  clinical features of, 684, 687
  cystic adult-type, 685f, 688f
  differential diagnosis of, 684, 687
  epidemiology of, 684, 687
  histology of, 684, 687
  immunopathology of, 684, 687
  juvenile. see Juvenile granulosa cell tumor
  luteinized, 688f
    adult-type, 688f
  metastatic, 689f
  in ovary, 688f
  pathology of, 684, 687
  presentation of, 684, 687
  prognosis and treatment of, 684, 687
  versus sex cord tumor with annular tubules, 711
  with spindle features, 689f
  variants of, 687
"Gumma," of tertiary syphilis, 44
Guttate psoriasis, 7

H

Haemophilus ducreyi, 46
Hailey-Hailey disease, 22, 23f
  clinical features of, 22
  differential diagnosis of, 22
  versus epidermolytic hyperkeratosis, 26
  pathology of, 22
Hemangioma, angiokeratoma versus, 183
Hemorrhage, fetal to maternal, 818, 819f
Hemorrhoids, anal condyloma versus, 190
Herpes simplex virus infection
  acute, 40, 41f
  chronic erosive, 42, 43f
Herpes zoster (shingles), 55
Herpetic ulcers, 41f
Hidradenitis suppurativa, 28, 29f
Hidradenoma, 65, 67f
  clinical features of, 65
  differential diagnosis of, 65
  fibroadenoma versus, 63
  pathology of, 65
Hidradenoma papilliferum (HP), 66f-67f
  apocrine differentiation in, 66f
  sclerotic, 67f
High-grade endometrial stromal sarcoma, 461, 462f-463f
High-grade müllerian carcinomas
  endometrioid differentiation in, 550f
  transitional pattern in, 551f
High-grade serous carcinoma
  classic type, 586, 587f
  exophytic, 550f
  serous borderline tumor versus, 597
  with set patterns, 588, 589f
High-grade serous tubal intraepithelial neoplasia, 541-542, 542f-544f
  clinical features of, 541
  differential diagnosis, 542
  pathology, 541-542
High-grade squamous intraepithelial lesion (HSIL)
  anal condyloma versus, 190
  cervical intraepithelial neoplasia II and III, 240-241, 241f-242f
  metaplastic, stratified adenocarcinoma in situ versus, 276

High-grade squamous intraepithelial lesion (HSIL) *(Continued)*
papillary, 132f
pseudocrypt involvement by squamous cell carcinoma versus, 266
High-grade stromal sarcoma, versus undifferentiated uterine sarcoma, 464
High-grade tubal intraepithelial neoplasms, versus low-grade serous tubal intraepithelial neoplasia, 536, 536f
High-grade vaginal intraepithelial neoplasia III, 215-216, 216f
Higher-grade carcinoma with transitional differentiation, low-grade endometrioid adenocarcinoma with squamotransitional or spindle features versus, 590
Hilar cell tumor, 698, 699f-700f
Hilar cells, versus adrenal rest, 511
Hilus cell hyperplasia, cortical stromal hyperplasia and hyperthecosis versus, 570
Histiocytes, endometrial, 412, 413f
Histiocytic intervillositis, chronic, 789, 790f
Hormonal effect, mixed pattern endometrium versus, 349
Hormone replacement therapy, submucosal leiomyoma and, 361
HSIL. *see* High-grade squamous intraepithelial lesion (HSIL).
Hydatidiform mole
complete, 741-742, 742f-743f
invasive, 745, 746f-747f
partial, 748, 749f
Hydropic leiomyoma, 479, 480f
clinical features of, 479
differential diagnosis of, 479
versus leiomyomatosis, 485
pathology of, 479
Hydrosalpinx, serous cystadenomas and cystadenofibromas versus, 577
Hymenal ring, 208, 209f
Hypercoiled umbilical cord, 769, 769f
Hypergranulosis, 4f
Hyperkeratosis, 4f
epidermolytic, 26, 27f
Hyperplasia
of Bartholin's gland, 70, 71f
benign, 345, 346f
epithelial, 529, 530f-531f
papillary, in struma, 654f
cortical stromal, 569-570, 570f
diffuse laminar glandular, 317
lobular glandular, 317
microglandular. *see* Microglandular hyperplasia
papillary, 539, 540f
pseudoepitheliomatous, 137, 138f
theca-lutein, of pregnancy, 561, 562f
Hyperreactio luteinalis, 561, 563f
Hypertension, chronic, toxemia and, 810
Hypertensive infarct
bleeding, 798, 799f
versus inflammatory abruption, 796
Hyperthecosis, 569-570, 570f
Hypocoiled umbilical cord, 769
Hypoplasia, distal villous, 817f

Hysterectomy, for intestinal variant of adenocarcinoma in situ, 278

I

Ichthyosis uteri, 387, 388f
Immature condyloma, 245, 246f
Immature neuroepithelium, mature cystic teratoma versus, 646, 647f
Immature teratoma, versus primitive neuroectodermal tumor, 717
Immunostaining, for clear-cell carcinoma, 434
Implantation site nodule, 735, 736f
clinical features of, 735
differential diagnosis of, 735
versus molar implantation site, 759
pathology of, 735
Infarction, placental, 812, 813f
Infection
amniotic fluid, 780
Candida
gestational, 783, 784f
with LSC, 6f
congenital parvovirus, 800, 801f
cytomegalovirus, versus chronic villitis, 787
herpes simplex virus
acute, 40, 41f
chronic erosive, 42, 43f
Toxoplasma gondii, versus chronic villitis, 787
yeast, versus lichen simplex chronicus and prurigo nodularis, 5
Infiltrating glands pattern, of myoinvasion, 406
Infiltrative endocervical adenocarcinoma, 295-296, 296f-297f
clinical features of, 295
differential diagnosis of, 296
pathology of, 295-296
Inflammatory abruption, 795-796, 796f-797f
Insular carcinoid tumor, low-grade endometrioid adenocarcinoma versus, 617
Intervillositis, acute and chronic, versus chronic histiocytic intervillositis, 789
Intervillous fibrin, versus placental infarction, 812
Intervillous thrombi, 818, 819f
versus placental infarction, 812
Intestinal mucinous carcinoma, immunopathology of, 607
Intraabdominal desmoplastic small round cell tumor
versus small cell carcinoma of pulmonary (neuroendocrine) type, 709
versus solitary fibrous tumor, 713
Intraepithelial carcinoma, mucinous borderline tumor with, 615, 616f
Intraepithelial neoplasia II and III, anal, 193, 194f
Intraperitoneal keratin granuloma, 410, 411f
Intraplacental choriocarcinoma, 754, 755f-756f
versus chorangioma, 764
clinical features of, 754
differential diagnosis of, 754
pathology of, 754
versus placental infarction, 812
Intraplacental trophoblastic proliferation, with admixed fibrin, versus intraplacental choriocarcinoma, 754

Intravillous thrombus, versus hypertensive bleeding infarct, 798
Invasive hydatidiform mole, 745, 746f-747f
clinical features of, 745
differential diagnosis of, 745
pathology of, 745
Invasive implants, 605, 606f
Ischemic atypia
of endometrium, 419, 420f
versus reactive atypia in endometrium, 421

J

Juvenile granulosa cell tumor, 690, 691f-692f
clinical features of, 690
differential diagnosis of, 690
pathology of, 690

K

Keratinizing squamous cell carcinoma, versus epithelioid trophoblastic tumor, 762
Keratoacanthoma, 139, 140f
clinical features of, 139
versus condyloma, 79
differential diagnosis of, 139
pathology of, 139
versus vulvar squamous carcinoma, 123
Keratosis, inverted, 127f
Ki-67 immunostaining, 735
Klebsiella granulomatis, 48
Knots, in umbilical cord, 766, 767f

L

Large-cell keratinizing squamous cell carcinoma, cervical, 262-263, 263f
Large-cell nonkeratinizing squamous cell carcinoma, cervical, 262, 264f
Leiomyoma
versus adenofibroma, 527
atypical, 483, 484f
intravascular, 487, 488f
intravenous, versus intravenous leiomyomatosis, 489
versus low-grade endometrial stromal sarcoma, 456
mitotically active, 481, 482f
Leiomyomatosis, 485, 486f
clinical features of, 485
differential diagnosis of, 485
disseminated intraperitoneal, 493, 494f
disseminated peritoneal, versus morcellation-related dissemination of smooth muscle neoplasia, 491
hereditary, and renal cell carcinoma syndrome, 497, 497f-498f
intravenous, 489, 490f
pathology of, 485
Leiomyosarcoma, 499, 500f
versus cellular leiomyoma, 477
clinical features of, 499
differential diagnosis of, 499
epithelioid, versus epithelioid trophoblastic tumor, 762
gastrointestinal stromal tumor versus, 715
high-grade endometrial stromal sarcoma versus, 461
leiomyomatosis versus, 485

Leiomyosarcoma *(Continued)*
  low-grade endometrial stromal sarcoma
    versus, 456
  myxoid, 501, 502f
  pathology of, 499
  renal cell carcinoma syndrome versus, 497
  undifferentiated carcinoma of endometrium
    versus, 432
  undifferentiated uterine sarcoma versus, 464
Lentiginous nevus, lentigo versus, 155
Lentigo, 155, 156f
Leukemia, fetal, 802, 803f
Leydig cell (hilar) tumor, 698, 699f-700f
LGFMS. *see* Low-grade fibromyxoid sarcoma
  (LGFMS).
Li-Fraumeni syndrome, versus p53 signatures,
  532, 534f
Lichen planus, 14, 15f
Lichen sclerosus, 12f-13f
  early, 11, 12f
    clinical features of, 11
    differential diagnosis of, 11
    pathology of, 11
  with superimposed lichen simplex chronicus,
    13f
Lichen simplex chronicus, 5, 6f
  classic vulvar intraepithelial neoplasia with,
    98, 99f
  clinical features of, 5
  differential diagnosis of, 5
  pathology of, 5
  verruciform, 114, 114f-115f
Lipoleiomyoma, 475, 476f
  versus adenomatoid tumor, 472, 474f
  clinical features of, 475
  differential diagnosis of, 475
  pathology of, 475
Lipoma, 176, 176f
  clinical features of, 176
  differential diagnosis of, 176
  versus lipoleiomyoma, 475
  pathology of, 176
Liposarcoma, 177, 178f
Listeria placentitis, 785, 786f
Lobular glandular hyperplasia, 317
Localized intraepithelial endometrioid
  carcinomas, versus benign epithelial
  hyperplasia, 529
Loop electrosurgical excision procedure
  (LEEP), for intestinal variant of
  adenocarcinoma in situ, 278
Low-grade endometrial stromal sarcoma,
  455-456, 456f-458f, 459
  versus cellular leiomyoma, 477
  clinical features of, 455
  differential diagnosis of, 456
  versus high-grade endometrial stromal
    sarcoma, 461
  pathology of, 455-456
  versus undifferentiated uterine sarcoma, 464
Low-grade endometrioid adenocarcinoma, 617,
  618f-619f
  clinical features of, 617
  differential diagnosis of, 617
  pathology of, 617
  with squamotransitional or spindle features,
    590, 591f

Low-grade fibromyxoid sarcoma (LGFMS),
  174, 175f
Low-grade serous carcinoma
  implants of, versus papillary mesothelial
    hyperplasia, 725
  invasive, of ovary, 602, 603f-604f
  versus papillary mesothelioma, 723
Low-grade serous tubal intraepithelial
  neoplasia, 535-536, 536f-538f
  clinical features, 535
  differential diagnosis, 536
  with moderate atypia, 536
  pathology, 535-536
Low-grade serous tumors, versus retiform
  SLCT, 696
Low-grade squamous intraepithelial lesion
  (LSIL)
  exophytic, 235, 236f
  flat condyloma/cervical intraepithelial
    neoplasia 1, 237-238, 238f-239f
  giant condyloma, 243, 244f
  immature condyloma, 245, 246f
  stratified adenocarcinoma in situ versus, 276
Low-grade vaginal intraepithelial lesion,
  210-211, 211f
Lower-grade tubal intraepithelial neoplasms,
  versus high-grade serous tubal
  intraepithelial neoplasia, 542
Lower uterine segment (LUS), adenocarcinoma
  of, 400, 401f
LSIL. *see* Low-grade squamous intraepithelial
  lesion (LSIL).
Lung carcinoma, metastatic to ovary, 643f
Luteal phase defect, mixed pattern
  endometrium versus, 349
Luteinized thecoma, histology of, 677,
  678f-679f
Luteoma
  pregnancy, 703, 704f
  stromal, 701, 702f
Lymphoepithelial-like squamous carcinoma,
  268, 269f
Lymphoma
  in cervix, lymphoepithelial-like squamous
    carcinoma versus, 268
  versus neuroendocrine carcinoma, 430
  reproductive tract, 507
  versus undifferentiated carcinoma of
    endometrium, 432
Lynch syndrome, endometrial adenocarcinoma
  in, 403, 404f
  clinical features of, 403
  screening of, 403
Lysosomal storage disorder, 793, 793f-794f

M
Macrophages
  versus adrenal rest, 511
  foamy, 412, 413f
Malakoplakia, 584, 585f
Malignancy, excluding, versus torsion of tube
  and ovary, 522
Malignant mesothelial processes, versus
  papillary mesothelial hyperplasia, 725
Malignant mesothelioma, 727, 728f
  versus benign cystic mesothelioma, 721
  clinical features of, 727

Malignant mesothelioma *(Continued)*
  differential diagnosis of, 727
  versus papillary mesothelioma, 723
  pathology of, 727
Malignant nodules, 610
Malignant struma, 653, 654f
Marginal cord insertion, 770, 771f
Marked chronic inflammation, versus
  reproductive tract lymphoma, 507
Massive perivillous fibrin deposition, 778, 779f
Maternal floor infarct, 778
Mature cystic teratoma, normal neural
  differentiation, 646
MAV. *see* Multinucleated atypia of the vulva
  (MAV).
Meconium staining, 814, 815f
Melanoma, 161, 162f, 226, 227f
  anal Paget's disease versus, 197
  clinical features of, 161, 226
  conventional squamous cell carcinoma
    versus, 263
  differential diagnosis of, 161, 226
  pathology of, 161, 226
Membranous cord insertion, 770, 771f
Menopausal endometrium, submucosal
  leiomyoma and, 361
Merkel cell carcinoma, 149, 150f
Mesenchymal dysplasia, 750, 751f
Mesonephric carcinoma, 312, 313f-314f
  cervical mesonephric remnants and, 310
  clinical features of, 312
  differential diagnosis of, 312
  pathology of, 312
  versus uterine tumor resembling sex cord
    stromal tumor, 459
  versus Wilms' tumor, 447
Mesonephric "hyperplasia," cervical
  mesonephric remnants and, 310
Mesonephric remnants, in cervix, 310, 311f
Mesothelial cells, invasive implants versus, 605
Mesothelial hyperplasia, versus papillary
  mesothelioma, 723
Mesothelioma
  benign cystic, 721, 722f
  serous borderline tumor versus, 597
Metaplasia
  squamous and morular, 384-385, 385f-386f
    clinical features of, 384
    differential diagnosis of, 385
    pathology of, 384
  tubal and eosinophilic (oxyphilic), 391,
    391f-392f
    clinical features of, 391
    differential diagnosis of, 391
    pathology of, 391
Metaplastic atypia, with columnar
  differentiation, stratified adenocarcinoma
  in situ versus, 276
Metastatic carcinoid, 659, 660f
  clinical features of, 659
  differential diagnosis of, 659
  insular, 660f-661f
  pathology of, 659
Metastatic carcinoma
  colonic
    low-grade endometrioid adenocarcinoma
      versus, 617

Vulva *(Continued)*
  metastatic carcinoma of, 153, 154f
  Paget's disease of, 146, 147f-148f
  polynucleated atypia of, 108
  synovial sarcoma of, 179, 180f
Vulvar acanthosis with altered differentiation
    (VAAD), 116, 117f
  clinical features of, 116
  versus condyloma, 79
  differential diagnosis and pitfalls of, 116
  pathology of, 116
Vulvar fibroma, prepubertal, 187, 188f-189f
Vulvar intraepithelial neoplasia (VIN)
  classic, 94, 95f-97f, 100, 143f
    clinical features of, 94
    versus condyloma, 79
    differential diagnosis and pitfalls of, 94
    with lichen simplex chronicus, 98, 99f
    or differential, versus lichen simplex
        chronicus and prurigo nodularis, 5
    pathology of, 94
  with columnar differentiation, 104, 105f
  containing diffuse nuclear atypia, 91f
  differentiated, 110, 111f-113f
  with multinucleation, 109f
  pagetoid, 102, 103f
  versus seborrheic keratosis, 88
  tangential sectioning of, versus vulvar
      squamous carcinoma, 123

Vulvar Paget's disease, anal Paget's disease
    versus, 197
Vulvar psoriasis, 8f
Vulvar squamous carcinoma, 123f
  basaloid and warty patterns, 122-123
  keratinizing pattern, 124-125, 125f-127f
    clinical features of, 124
    differential diagnosis of, 125
    pathology of, 124
Vulvodynia, 32, 33f
Vulvovaginal candidiasis, 34, 35f

W

Warty dyskeratoma, 84, 85f
Well-differentiated serous carcinomas, serous
    borderline tumor versus, 597
White sponge nevus, hymenal ring versus, 208
Wilms' tumor
  of endometrium, 447, 448f
  extra renal, synovial sarcoma of vulva
      versus, 179

X

Xanthogranulomatous salpingitis, 515, 516f
  clinical features of, 515
  differential diagnosis of, 515
  pathology of, 515
  versus pseudoxanthomatous salpingiosis,
      513

Xanthoma, verruciform, 82, 83f
  clinical features of, 82
  differential diagnosis and pitfalls of, 82
  pathology of, 82
  versus vulvar acanthosis with altered
      differentiation, 116
Xanthomatous pseudotumor, decidualized
    endometrioma versus, 575

Y

Yeast infections, versus lichen simplex
    chronicus and prurigo nodularis, 5
Yolk sac carcinoma, 667-668, 668f-669f
  clinical features of, 667
  differential diagnosis of, 668
  embryonal carcinoma versus, 670
  with endometrioid differentiation, ovarian
      adenocarcinoma with yolk sac
      differentiation versus, 636
  mixed teratoma and, versus mixed germ cell
      tumor, 676f
  pathology of, 667-668

Z

Zoon's vulvitis, 16, 17f

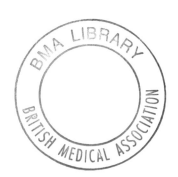